THE GROWTH OF GASTROENTEROLOGIC KNOWLEDGE DURING THE TWENTIETH CENTURY

THE GROWTH OF GASTROENTEROLOGIC KNOWLEDGE DURING THE TWENTIETH CENTURY

Joseph B. Kirsner, M.D., Ph.D., M.A.C.P., D.Sc. (Hon.)

The Louis Block Distinguished Service Professor of Medicine and Attending Physician
Bernard Mitchell Hospital, University of Chicago

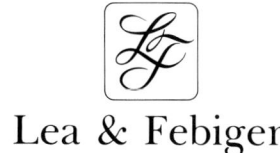

Lea & Febiger

PHILADELPHIA · BALTIMORE · HONG KONG
LONDON · MUNICH · SYDNEY · TOKYO

A WAVERLY COMPANY
1994

Lea & Febiger
Box 3024
200 Chester Field Parkway
Malvern, Pennsylvania 19355-9725
U.S.A.
(215) 251-2230

Executive Editor—Michael Brown
Development Editor—Frances M. Klass
Manuscript Editor—Jessica Howie Martin
Production Manager—Samuel A. Rondinelli

Library of Congress Cataloging-in-Publication Data

The growth of gastroenterologic knowledge during the twentieth century
  / edited by Joseph B. Kirsner.
        p.   cm.
    Includes bibliographical references and index.
    ISBN 0-8121-1592-9
    1. Gastroenterology—History—20th century. I. Kirsner, Joseph
B., 1909–   .
    [DNLM: 1. Gastroenterology—history. 2. Digestive System. WI
11.1 G884 1994]
    RC801.G76   1994
    616.3′3′00904—dc20
    DNLM/DLC
    for Library of Congress   93-35579
                                                                 CIP

NOTE: Although the author(s) and the publisher have taken reasonable steps to ensure the accuracy of the drug information included in this text before publication, drug information may change without notice and readers are advised to consult the manufacturer's packaging inserts before prescribing medications.

Reprints of chapters may be purchased from Lea & Febiger in quantities of 100 or more. Contact Sally Grande in the Sales Department.

PRINTED IN THE UNITED STATES OF AMERICA

Print number: 5 4 3 2 1

About the Author

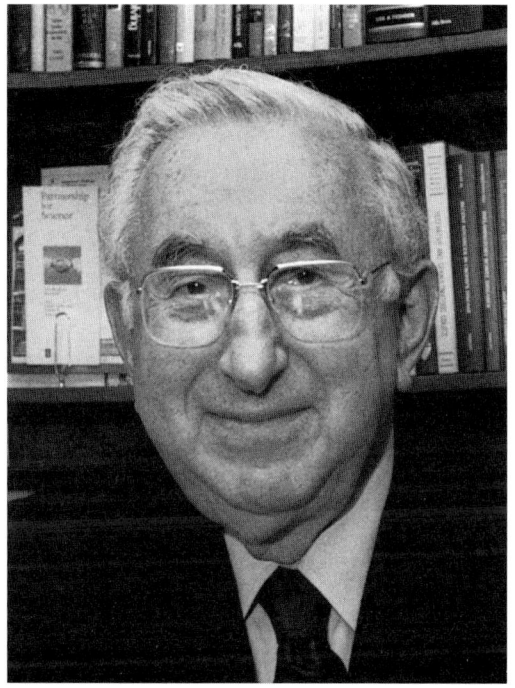

Joseph B. Kirsner's medical career began in 1933, when he obtained his medical degree from Tufts University School of Medicine in Boston and continued with an internship and residency in Chicago. He began his nearly 60-year association with the University of Chicago in 1935.

Dr. Kirsner participated in the founding of many gastroenterologic societies and has served as president of the American Gastroenterological Association, among others. He also has been a member of the editorial boards of major medical journals, including Gastroenterology and Annals of Internal Medicine.

During his long career, Dr. Kirsner has received many awards, including the Friedenwald Medal presented by the American Gastroenterological Association, the John Phillips Memorial Award of the American College of Physicians, the Rudolph Schindler Award from the American Society for Gastrointestinal Endoscopy, the Gold Key Award in 1979 and the 1989 Alumni Award from the University of Chicago Alumni Association, and the Distinguished Service Award from the National Foundation for Ileitis and Colitis.

In 1986 the Joseph B. Kirsner Center for the Study of Digestive Diseases was dedicated at the University of Chicago. The Kirsner Center houses the entire Gastroenterology Section and includes a GI procedure unit, research laboratories, and office space.

Dr. Kirsner has published 12 textbooks relating to gastroenterology. At this time, he is working on the Fourth Edition of *Inflammatory Bowel Disease.* He continues to present named lectures throughout the world and maintains his interest in research, writing, and treating patients as a full-time member of the Department of Medicine of the University of Chicago.

Dedication

This book is respectfully dedicated to all who support the spirit of inquiry and the essentiality of clinical and basic research toward the better understanding and management of gastrointestinal disease.

Preface

> "The past is not dead history, it is living material out of which man. . . . builds for the future."
>
> René Dubos (1901–1982)

Awareness of the digestive system dates back to the dawn of civilization, when man, influenced by the feeding habits of animals in the surrounding environment, experimented with foods, edible and inedible. This perception reached unusual levels in ancient Egypt (4500–2500 BC), where the royal court included "the Physician of the Belly of the Pharaoh" and the "Guardian of the Anus," who was responsible for the administration of clysters (enemas) and purges. At a time when religion and medicine were one discipline and knowledge of disease did not exist, all symptoms were shrouded in mystical and supernatural beliefs involving actions of evil spirits. The clinical observations of Hippocrates (460–370 BC) introduced some rationale into the care of the sick, but medicine was dominated and retarded for centuries by strange concepts of illness, in particular the humoral (blood, phlegm, yellow bile, black bile) theory, originating with Empedocles (5th century) and expanded by Hippocrates, Aristotle, and Galen. This concept reappeared 2000 years later, during the latter part of the 18th century, as the fallacy of William Cullen of Edinburgh and his pupil, Benjamin Rush of America, who attributed all illness to increased tension within the nervous and vascular systems that could be relieved only by bloodletting or purging. These misconceptions persisted despite early descriptions of individual diseases (pneumonia, tetanus) by Aretaeus the Cappadocian (2nd and 3rd centuries); the differentiation of smallpox and measles by Rhazes of Persia (9th century); recognition of the natural history of individual diseases by Thomas Sydenham (1624–1689); the perceptive clinical-pathologic correlations of G. B. Morgagni (1761); M. F. X. Bichat's Anatomie Générale, which oriented disease to distinct and differing bodily tissues rather than to the indefinable "humors;" W. W. Gerhard's differentiation of typhoid fever and typhus (1837); and Rudolf Virchow's establishment of cellular pathology (1858). Virchow's insight, in particular, was decisive: "There are no general diseases . . . From now on we shall recognize only diseases of organized cells."

Interest in the digestive system increased with identification of the digestive organs, the writings of Galen, and especially the anatomic discoveries of Andres Vesalius (1514–1564) in the 16th and 17th centuries. Also identified were the intestinal lacteals (Aselli, 1622); thoracic duct (Pecquet, 1651); submaxillary gland (Wharton, 1656); parotid duct (N. Stensen, 1662); lymphoid follicles of the intestine (J. Peyer, 1677); intestinal glands (Brunner, 1686; Lieberkuhn, 1745), and pancreatic ducts (Wirsung, 1642; Santorini, 1775).

For centuries, speculation on digestion had focused upon control by an internal "spirit" and upon mechanisms of mechanical grinding or trituration, putrefaction, maceration, chemical fermentation, and chemical solution, until the issue was resolved by the studies of R. de Reameur (1752), L. Spallanzani (1760), and J. Hunter (1786), W. Prout's confirmation of the secretion of hydrochloric acid by the stomach (1824), and the observations of William Beaumont on Alexis St. Martin (1825–1834).

Although Regner de Graaf (1641–1679) had constructed pancreatic and biliary fistulas in the dog in the 17th century, not until Claude Bernard's (1813–1878) classic studies of the role of the pancreas in digestion and the metabolic activities of the liver during the mid-nineteenth century was significant attention directed to the physiology of the gastrointestinal tract. However, another 50 years were to pass before active physiologic research on the digestive system resumed during the early part of the 20th century, led by I. P. Pavlov of Russia and J. C. Dalton, W. B. Cannon, S. J. Meltzer, W. C. Alvarez, A. J. Carlson, J. Earl Thomas, S. A. Komarov, Frank Mann, A. C. Ivy, Charles F. Code, Morton Grossman, and Horace W. Davenport of the United States, among many others.

The development of laboratories for biochemistry (J. Von Liebig, 1824) and physiology (Purkinje, 1824) in Germany during the 19th century inaugurated the basic sciences and was followed by the identification of gastric pepsin (T. Schwann, 1835) and its purification (E. Brucke, 1861), and the isolation of the pancreatic enzyme trypsin (W. Kuhne, 1867). The discovery of secretin in 1902 by W. M. Bayliss and E. H. Starling of England, J. S. Edkin's identification of gastrin, and Bayliss's 1905 use of the term "hormone," originally invented by Hardy, established the discipline of gastrointestinal endocrinology.

For centuries, abdominal surgery had been an almost impossible, extremely dangerous, and torturous procedure until it was dramatically improved during the latter part of the nineteenth century by the recognition of bacteria as the cause of disease 200 years after their initial visualization by A. Leeuwenhoeck (1671), the discovery of antisepsis by Joseph Lister in 1867, and the identification of the anesthetics nitrous oxide (Humphrey Davy, 1798) and ether (J. C. Warren and W. Morton, 1846).

Influenced by the careful methodic clinical studies of French physicians including R. Laennec and P. Louis during the first half of the nineteenth century, clinical medicine in America under the leadership of Drs. Joseph Parrish, James Jackson, Jr., Alfred Stille, Thomas D. Mutter, and Austin Flint, Sr. advanced gradually from the superficial to the more complete examination of the patient and from clinical assumptions to organized clinical studies, typified by Reginald Fitz's classic descriptions of acute appendicitis and acute pancreatitis.

Diagnostic approach to the hitherto inaccessible gastrointestinal tract improved rapidly with the discovery of the x-ray by W. C. Roentgen in 1895, the semiflexible gastroscope by Rudolf Schindler (1932), and Basil Hirschowitz's development of the flexible fiberoptic endoscope. The interdependence of knowledge and technology in the progress of gastroenterology is beautifully illustrated in the development of flexible fiberoptic endoscopes, a sequence of events beginning in 1879 with the observation of the British physicist, John Tyndall, that light follows the path of a flowing stream of water. Subsequent progress in the physics of optics and optical fibers and technologic improvements produced the fiberoptic gastroscope, sigmoidoscope, colonoscope, enteroscope, and fiberoptic instruments for viewing other bodily cavities.

The growth of specialization in medicine and in gastroenterology during the latter part of the nineteenth and early part of the twentieth centuries coincided with a series of important concurrent developments: an enlarging body of knowledge; new, increasingly complex diagnostic techniques (gastric analysis, x-ray); the addition of specialized subjects to the medical curriculum (chemistry, pathology); the increasing influence of hospitals; and growing public awareness of the potential benefits of medical and surgical progress. Gastroenterology as a distinct clinical specialty began in 1885 when Ismar Boas of Germany established the first clinic devoted exclusively to digestive problems. In the United States, specialization in gastroenterology advanced with Max Einhorn, J. C. Hemmeter, J. Friedenwald, C. G. Stockton, D. Riesman, and B. W. Sippy. Worldwide, early gastroenterologists included A. Kussmaul and C. Ewald of Germany, A. F. Hurst and J. Ryle of England, G. Banti and C. Fregoni of Italy, N. Svartz and B. Ihre of Sweden, R. Gutmann and F. Moutier of France, and T. Billroth of Vienna. Prominent American gastroenterologic surgeons included S. D. Gross, W. S. Halsted,

N. Senn, C. Fenger, J. B. Murphy, and W. J. Mayo. Although de facto specialization had existed in the United States since the beginning of the 20th century, gastroenterology was not certified as a specialty of internal medicine in the United States until 1940, and most academic departments of gastroenterology in this country were not established until the 1950s and 1960s. The American Gastroenterological Association, beginning in 1897 and continuing into the 20th century, and later the American College of Gastroenterology, the American Society for Gastrointestinal Endoscopy, the American Association for the Study of Liver Disease, the American College of Surgeons, and other surgical organizations, improved standards of training and practice, expanded educational programs, and supported research through fellowship and training grants. Generally, however, fundamental research in gastroenterology during the early part of the 20th century lagged behind that in other medical specialties.

All branches of medicine, including gastroenterology, and the biomedical sciences benefited from the increased governmental and private support of research after World War II during the 1950s and 1960s. The National Institutes of Health and The General Medicine Study Section of the National Institute of Arthritis, Metabolic and Digestive Diseases, including such authorities as F. Ingelfinger, J. B. Kirsner, J. Ruffin, and S. Wolf, in particular, played a major role in the rapid expansion of gastroenterologic research and the increased number of academic gastroenterologic divisions.

This brief overview of some of the notable events in the origins of gastroenterology provides a rich background for the still more remarkable achievements of the past half century, when much of the fundamental knowledge of gastroenterology has been acquired. During this period, the crude methodology of the past was replaced by sophisticated techniques from biochemistry, cellular biology, radioimmunoassay, and molecular medicine. Gastroenterology advanced from the examination of organs and tissues to the study of individual cells, and increasingly perceptive clinicians adopted more critical attitudes toward the acquisition of clinical data.

In retrospect, the growth of gastroenterologic knowledge spanned four periods in history:

a. Antiquity through the 16th century—Initial awareness of the digestive system.
b. 17th century to mid-19th century—Early clinical and physiologic observations, recognition of individual disease.
c. Latter 19th century to mid-20th century—Discovery of bacterial causes of disease, antisepsis, and anesthesia improving surgery; discovery of x-ray and endoscopy facilitating diagnosis; specialization in medicine and gastroenterology.
d. Mid-20th century to present—The greatest growth of fundamental knowledge of the digestive system in history; paralleling extraordinary advances in the biomedical and basic sciences (the major focus of this book).

Gastroenterology today is a broadly oriented multidisciplinary and interdisciplinary composite of many clinical areas and organizations focused on individual organs, diagnostic and therapeutic endoscopy, and radiologic imaging and many scientific disciplines including biochemistry, pathology, physiology, cell biology, neuroendocrinology, immunology, molecular biology, and genetics. Research questions have changed from the amount of hydrochloric acid secreted by the stomach to the molecular basis of gastric acid secretion, from the balloon measurement of peristaltic contractions to studies of the sensory, motor, and interneurons of the enteric nervous system, "from the epidemiology of gallstones to the sequence of physicochemical events in the formation of gallstones," from catarrhal jaundice to the molecular biology of the viruses of hepatitis, and from the "psychogenic" cause of ulcerative colitis to the molecular events modifying gastrointestinal cellular defenses.

How did all this come about? Who made the insightful observations, what were the "revolutionary" ideas? Who provided unifying themes? What were the critical events in this brief span of 50 years? And what were the contributions of the biomedical sciences and of technology to the advance of gastroenterology?

All things considered and recalling such individual accomplishments as Bernard's discovery of the metabolic activities of the liver, Roentgen's discovery of the x-ray, and Cannon's application of the x-ray to investigate gastrointestinal physiology, W. I. Beveridge's comment (The Art of Scientific Discovery, W. W. Norton, New York 1927) is most appropriate: "Elaborate apparatus plays an important part in the science of today but I sometimes wonder if we are not inclined to forget that the most important instrument in research must always be the mind of man."

In *The Growth of Gastroenterologic Knowledge During the Twentieth Century*, 31 leading gastroenterologic authorities in the United States have answered these and related questions in a comprehensive and scholarly account of the scientific maturation of one of medicine's most important disciplines, and provide a revealing insight into the origin and development of today's concepts of the human digestive system.

Chicago   Joseph B. Kirsner, M.D., Ph.D.

Acknowledgments

I am pleased to recognize the interest of Carroll Cann and Executive Editor Michael Brown of Lea & Febiger in this project and to Developmental Editor Frances Klass, Manuscript Editor Jessica Howie Martin, and Production Manager Samuel Rondinelli for their expertise in facilitating the excellent technical quality of the publication.

I am especially pleased to acknowledge the invaluable editorial assistance of my Administrative Assistant, Arlene Willett; and the assistance of my secretary, Donna Rogers, and the librarians of the John Crerar and Joseph Regenstein libraries of the University of Chicago.

I am most grateful to the Gastro-Intestinal Research Foundation of Chicago, whose generous support made this project possible.

Contributors

James L. Achord, M.D.
Professor and Director
Division of Digestive Diseases
University of Mississippi School of Medicine
The University of Mississippi Medical Center
Jackson, Mississippi

M. Mazen Anbari, M.D., J.D.
Resident
Mallinckrodt Institute of Radiology
St. Louis, Missouri

Ulrich Beuers, M.D.
Postdoctoral Associate
Yale University School of Medicine
New Haven, Connecticut

Henry J. Binder, M.D.
Professor of Medicine
Department of Internal Medicine
Section of Digestive Diseases
Yale University
New Haven, Connecticut

H. Worth Boyce, Jr., M.D., F.A.C.P.,
  M.A.C.G.
Professor of Medicine
Director, Center for Swallowing Disorders
Hugh F. Culverhouse Chair for Esophageal
  Disorders
University of South Florida College of
  Medicine
Tampa, Florida

James L. Boyer, M.D.
Professor of Medicine
Chief, Division of Digestive Diseases
Director, Liver Center
Department of Internal Medicine
Yale University School of Medicine
New Haven, Connecticut

Michael Camilleri, M.D.
Professor of Medicine
Consultant in Gastroenterology and Physiology
Gastroenterology Research Unit
Mayo Clinic
Rochester, Minnesota

Donald O. Castell, M.D.
Kimbel Professor and Chairman
Department of Medicine
The Graduate Hospital
Philadelphia, Pennsylvania

James Christenson, M.D.
Professor, Internal Medicine
Gastrointestinal Motility
University of Iowa College of Medicine
University Hospitals and Clinics
Iowa City, Iowa

Horace W. Davenport, Ph.D., D.Sc.
William Beaumont Professor of Physiology
  Emeritus
University of Michigan
Ann Arbor, Michigan

Jules L. Dienstag, M.D.
Associate Professor of Medicine
Harvard Medical School
Associate Physician
Massachusetts General Hospital
Boston, Massachusetts

Eugene F. DiMagno, M.D.
Professor of Medicine
Mayo School of Medicine
GI Diagnostic Unit
Mayo Clinic
Rochester, Minnesota

Robert M. Donaldson, Jr., M.D.
David Paige Smith Professor of Medicine
Yale University School of Medicine
New Haven, Connecticut

Douglas A. Drossman, M.D.
Professor of Medicine and Psychiatry
Division of Digestive Diseases
University of North Carolina at Chapel Hill
Chapel Hill, North Carolina

Norton J. Greenberger, M.D.
Professor and Chairman
Department of Internal Medicine
University of Kansas Medical Center
Kansas City, Kansas

William S. Haubrich, M.D.
Clinical Professor of Medicine
University of California at San Diego
La Jolla, California

Basil Hirschowitz, M.D.
Professor of Medicine
Division of Gastroenterology
University of Alabama at Birmingham
Birmingham, Alabama

Eugene D. Jacobson, M.D.
Professor of Medicine and Physiology
University of Colorado School of Medicine
Denver, Colorado

Joseph B. Kirsner, M.D., Ph.D., M.A.C.P.,
    D.Sc.
Louis Block Distinguished Service Professor
    of Medicine
The University of Chicago Medical Center
Chicago, Illinois

Nicholas F. LaRusso, M.D.
Professor and Chairman
Division of Gastroenterology
Center for Basic Research in Digestive
    Diseases
Rochester, Minnesota

Igor Laufer, M.D.
Professor of Radiology
Chief, GI Radiology
University of Pennsylvania
Hospital of the University of Pennsylvania
Department of Radiology
Philadelphia, Pennsylvania

Michael D. Levitt, M.D.
Associate Chief of Staff for Research
Professor of Medicine
Veterans Affairs Medical Center
University of Minnesota
Minneapolis, Minnesota

Charles S. Lieber, M.D.
Professor of Medicine and Pathology
Mt. Sinai School of Medicine
Director, Alcohol Research and Treatment
    Center
Bronx VA Medical Center and Mt. Sinai
    School of Medicine
Bronx, New York

Jay W. Marks, M.D.
Associate Professor of Medicine
Associate Director, Division of
    Gastroenterology
Department of Medicine
Cedars-Sinai Medical Center
Los Angeles, California

Loren K. Murphy, M.A.
Basic Science Program Liaison
Cedars-Sinai Medical Center
Inflammatory Bowel Disease Center
Los Angeles, California

John O. Phillips, Ph.D., M.D.
Clinical Investigator Fellow
Chairman, Division of Gastroenterology
Director, Center for Basic Research in
    Digestive Diseases
Mayo Clinic
Rochester, Minnesota

Sidney F. Phillips, M.D.
Professor of Medicine
Gastroenterology Research Unit
Mayo Clinic
Rochester, Minnesota

Ian R. Sanderson, M.D.
Assistant Professor of Pediatrics
Harvard Medical School
Mucosal Immunology Laboratory
Combined Program in Pediatric
    Gastroenterology and Nutrition
Massachusetts General Hospital
Boston, Massachusetts

Leslie J. Schoenfield, M.D., Ph.D.
Director, Gastroenterology
Professor of Medicine
UCLA Cedars-Sinai Medical Center
Los Angeles, California

Marvin M. Schuster, M.D.
Professor of Medicine and Psychiatry
The Johns Hopkins School of Medicine
Director, Division of Digestive Diseases
Francis Scott Key Medical Center
Baltimore, Maryland

Michael D. Sitrin, M.D.
Professor of Medicine and the Committee on
    Human Nutrition and Nutritional Biology
University of Chicago
Pritzker School of Medicine
Chicago, Illinois

Thomas E. Starzl, M.D.
Professor of Surgery
Director, Transplantation Institute
The Falk Clinic
Pittsburgh, Pennsylvania

Stephan R. Targan, M.D.
Professor of Medicine
UCLA School of Medicine
Director, Cedars-Mt. Sinai Medical Centers
Inflammatory Bowel Disease Center
Feintech Family Chair in Inflammatory Bowel
    Diseases
Los Angeles, California

Andrea Todisco, M.D.
Instructor of Internal Medicine
Department of Internal Medicine
University of Michigan Medical Center
Ann Arbor, Michigan

W. Allan Walker, M.D.
Conrad Taft Professor of Nutrition and
    Pediatrics
Harvard Medical School
Mucosal Immunology Laboratory
Combined Program in Pediatric
    Gastroenterology and Nutrition
Massachusetts General Hospital and the
    Children's Hospital
Boston, Massachusetts

Wilfred M. Weinstein, M.D.
Professor of Medicine
Division of Gastroenterology
UCLA Center for Health Sciences
Los Angeles, California

Russell H. Wiesner, M.D.
Professor of Medicine
Mayo Clinic
Rochester, Minnesota

Sidney J. Winawer, M.D.
Professor of Medicine
Chief, Gastroenterology and Nutrition Service
Member and Head, Laboratory for
    Gastrointestinal Cancer Research
Head, World Health Organization
Collaborating Center for the Prevention of
    Colorectal Cancer
Memorial Sloan-Kettering Cancer Center
New York, New York

Jackie D. Wood, Ph.D.
Professor and Chairman
Department of Physiology
College of Medicine
The Ohio State University
Columbus, Ohio

Tadataka Yamada, M.D.
Professor of Medicine
Chief, Gastroenterology Section
University of Michigan
Ann Arbor, Michigan

Contents

Esophagus

1

Esophageal Motility and Benign Disorders

DONALD O. CASTELL

During this century, great strides have been made in our understanding of both normal and abnormal esophageal function. In the early 1900s, Cannon described esophageal peristalsis and lower esophageal sphincter (LES) dynamics from fluoroscopic studies. Subsequently, greater understanding has evolved of many details of esophageal motility, including the defects occurring in diseases such as achalasia, spastic disorders, and gastroesophageal reflux.

NORMAL FUNCTION OF THE ESOPHAGUS AND ITS SPHINCTERS

Esophageal Peristalsis

In the early years of this century, the two methods used to study esophageal motility and the effect of pharmacologic agents were radiographic techniques and intraesophageal balloons to obtain kymographic records. As a result of Cannon's pioneering studies, the potential value of contrast radiography to observe the movement of ingested material down the esophagus became well established. Differences in the movement of barium through the esophagus were noted with changes in body position and with varying consistency of the liquid material. The importance of the squirt of pharyngeal pressure to drive the bolus initially into the esophagus was shown to be greater with a thinner barium mixture and with the subject in the upright position, utilizing the effect of gravity. The final importance of the peristaltic wave was best identified with the subject in the horizontal position. The significance of a lumen-obliterating contraction to move the tail of the bolus throughout the esophagus also was recognized. Because of the radiation exposure, radiographic methods were limited to brief periods of observation. Balloon kymography was developed as a method for the in vivo recording of esophageal contractions. This technique offered the advantage of prolonged periods of observation and the ability to be adapted to the continuous recording of intraluminal pressures. The disadvantage of this technique is the requirement that the balloon be inflated within the esophagus to allow the recording of changes in volume during muscular contractions. The distended balloon created a local stimulus for pressure activity and produced an artifact of almost continuous contractile activity. These limitations led to the development of intraluminal manometry through the work of Quigley and associates (1), followed by a series of experiments from the laboratories of both Code and Ingelfinger beginning at about the midpoint of this century. These early studies, using small, water-filled, open-tipped catheters and external transducers, established many of the characteristics of the intraluminal pressure wave in response to deglutition. Sequential contractions measured by the placement of intraluminal pressure sensors at different levels within the esophagus established the nature of the primary peristaltic response induced by swallowing. These studies determined that the average velocity of this primary peristaltic wave varied from 2 to 3 cm per second but grossly underestimated the amplitude of the contraction because of the limitation of the recording accuracy of noninfused catheters. Kramer and Ingelfinger used a small intraesophageal balloon to produce secondary peristaltic contractions in the human esophagus (2).

Quantitation of contractile pressures within the human esophagus was achieved as a result of experiments performed in the laboratory of Harris. Using small syringes injecting cumulative microliter quantities of fluid, Harris et al. developed a technique of constant slow infusion within intraluminal catheters which allowed a more accurate quantitation of intraluminal squeezing pressures within the esophagus than had been provided by fluid-filled noninfused catheters (3). These studies initially were performed measuring human anal sphincter pressure and subsequently applied to LES pressures and peristaltic contractions. Studies performed in the laboratories of both Castell and Dodds comparing peristaltic pressures measured by small intraluminal transducers with those recorded by catheters with slow infusion rates demonstrated that the latter underestimated peristaltic pressures. These investigators established that normal contraction pressures in the human esophagus in response to a 5 mL water bolus averaged between 80 and 100 mm Hg and that accurate recording of these pressures required more rapid perfusion rates into intraluminal catheters (4). These studies helped to establish reliable techniques for the recording of esophageal peristaltic pressures; either a low compliance pneumohydraulic pressure system or small intraluminal strain gauge transducers provide accurate recording of the transient pressure increases produced by the peristaltic wave. These techniques have continued to be used over the past 20 years.

Early radiographic studies of the human esophagus had identified the phenomenon of "deglutitive inhibition," defined as an absence of peristalsis during a series of repetitive swallows, followed by a large clearing contraction with the termination of swallows. This event has been confirmed through the use of intraluminal manometry, with the physiologic mechanism being studied in greater detail. By changing the timing between subsequent swallows in a series,

Meyer and Castell demonstrated that both neural inhibition and smooth muscle refractoriness combined to produce this phenomenon (5). These same investigators also evaluated the events occurring within the human esophagus during the production of pain by rapid ingestion of cold liquid, previously ascribed to induced "esophageal spasm." In a series of studies using both intraluminal manometry and radiography, a total absence of contractile activity was shown to occur within the esophagus when pain followed repeated ingestion of cold material (6).

The simultaneous radiographic and manometric studies performed in the laboratories of Dodds during the past decade have clarified the role of squeezing pressures within the esophagus during bolus transport in both normal subjects and patients (7). These studies have demonstrated that a lumen-obliterating peristaltic contraction is essential for the orderly transport of swallowed barium. Contractions that do not obliterate the lumen radiographically, such as tertiary contractions seen on barium x-ray examinations, often do not result in an identifiable pressure response on the manometric recording. A contractile pressure exceeding 40 to 45 mm Hg is required to obliterate the lumen and transport the bolus. In addition, these studies have determined that the tail of the barium bolus is best identified manometrically by the onset or upstroke of the peristaltic wave, rather than the peak of the contraction.

Lower Esophageal Sphincter (LES) Function

At the beginning of this century, Cannon identified the presence of a physiologic sphincter at the esophagogastric junction that would open to permit passage of a swallowed bolus, yet maintain sufficient closure to prevent reflux of gastric contents. An enormous number of studies on the regulation of the LES have been performed during this century. The early manometric studies from the laboratories of both Code and Ingelfinger confirmed the presence of a high-pressure zone in this region which relaxed with deglutition (2). The magnitude of the resting tone, however, was underestimated by these noninfused catheters as demonstrated by the subsequent studies by Pope and Harris, using continuous slow infusion to accurately record resting LES tone (3). The physiologic mechanisms responsible for the constant resting tone of the LES have been studied in great detail. Animal experiments have indicated that resting LES pressure is not neurally dependent because it persists despite proximal vagotomy or the injection of the generalized neurotoxin tetrodotoxin. Studies by Fox and Daniel initially demonstrated that LES tone was primarily myogenic and largely dependent on calcium ions (8). These observations have subsequently been supported by other in vivo experiments in both animals and humans which showed decreases in LES pressure following administration of calcium channel antagonists (9). On the other hand, the relaxation of the LES in response to swallowing is primarily dependent on neural mechanisms. Animal experiments have indicated that stimulation of the vagus nerve leads to relaxation of this sphincter and that this response can be completely blocked by tetrodotoxin. Search for the specific neurotransmitter responsible for LES relaxation has been arduous. The classical adrenergic and cholinergic neurotransmitters have been shown in these experiments to have no important effect on LES relaxation. Early speculation suggested that this nonadrenergic, noncholinergic (NANC) neurotransmitter might be ATP or another "purinergic" agent. Rattan and Goyal published a series of experiments during the past decade indicating that vasoactive intestinal polypeptide (VIP) was the most likely candidate for the elusive transmitter of sphincter relaxation (10). More recent evidence indicates that this relaxation depends on the generation of nitric oxide, possibly cofunctioning in concert with VIP (11).

A report from the laboratory of Harris in 1970 demonstrated that dramatic increases in resting LES pressure occurred after injection of pentagastrin (12). This was the first indication that gastrointestinal peptides might play a role in the regulation of LES pressure, and it stimulated a series of investigations on possible hormonal regulation of the LES. Subsequent studies have shown that secretin, cholecystokinin, glucagon, and VIP, all decrease LES pressure, whereas motilin, substance P, and pancreatic polypeptide (in addition to gastrin) increase pressure. At present, the unresolved question relative to these observations is whether any of these peptides plays an important physiologic role in control of LES pressure because these studies utilized intravenous injections that would better qualify as "pharmacologic" effects. It has been shown, however, that various types of meals affect LES pressure, raising the question whether release of peptides after food ingestion might be responsible for some of these effects. The dramatic decreases in LES pressure seen after ingestion of high-fat meals provides evidence for a possible role of cholecystokinin as a regulator of LES pressure and has provided important insight into a possible explanation for the high prevalence of gastroesophageal reflux disease (GERD) in Western civilization.

An important new concept regarding the effectiveness of the LES as a barrier against reflux of gastric contents has evolved from the studies in the laboratory of Dodds during the past decade. Using the technique of prolonged recordings of LES pressures via a 6 cm Dent sleeve, it has been shown that frequent spontaneous relaxations of the LES occur throughout the day in both normal subjects and patients with GERD. These transient LES relaxations (TLESR) are normally of short duration, with the resultant acid reflux being cleared quickly by secondary peristalsis. TLESRs also are an important component of the normal mechanism of belching. Patients with GERD were shown to have a greater frequency of TLESRs than normal subjects, leading to greater acid exposure in the distal esophagus (13). A major conclusion from these observations has been to confirm the primary importance of LES pressure as the anti-reflux barrier. Reflux, measured by an intraesophageal pH electrode, was demonstrated in both the normal subjects and the GERD patients *only* when LES pressure was low relative to gastric pressure in one of three scenarios: chronically weak LES tone, borderline LES pressure exceeded by increased intra-abdominal pressure, or TLESRs.

Hiatus Hernia Controversy

Since the studies of Cannon at the beginning of this century, the relative importance of a diaphragmatic contribution to the tonus of the LES has been explored. As a corollary, the importance of a sliding hiatus hernia in the production of GERD has been a controversy that has raged throughout the last half of this century. The absolute importance of a proximally displaced EG junction in the etiology of reflux was the conventional wisdom before the studies from the laboratory of Harris which indicated that chronic heartburn depended primarily on low resting LES pressure rather than on the presence or absence of a hiatus hernia (14). This observation appeared to explain the observation by Palmer, a prominent "esophagologist" during the middle years of this century, that some patients with severe GERD did not have the expected hiatus hernia (15). Investigations by Mittal have reinforced the contribution provided by the muscles of the right crus of the diaphragm in the cyclic changes in resting LES pressure produced by respiration (16). These studies have clearly demonstrated that the tonic component of the LES pressure is dependent on myogenic tension of the circular smooth muscle of the sphincter itself, whereas the cyclic respiratory variations are produced by diaphragmatic contraction. There is good evidence to indicate that the antireflux competence of the sphincteric high pressure zone depends on both of these pressure components. The most recent evidence in support of the concept that a hiatus hernia is not essential to the development of reflux esophagitis comes from the report by Hirschowitz of his experience with 663 patients with upper GI symptomatology evaluated over 15 years (17). In this report, it was noted that the endoscopic presence of esophagitis was not directly associated with the finding of a hiatus hernia. Esophagitis also was not associated with gastric hypersecretion in these patients.

ESOPHAGEAL MOTILITY DISORDERS

Achalasia

Idiopathic dilation of the human esophagus was well known before the 20th century. Sir Thomas Willis is reported to have successfully dilated the distal esophagus of one such patient with a whalebone in 1674. At the beginning of this century, the term "simple ectasia" was used to describe this entity. Because of the absence of identifiable stricture and the spastic appearance at the cardia noted on early barium studies, the term "cardiospasm" became popular. With the development of esophageal manometry, the abnormal relaxation of the LES in this disease was identified in the laboratory of Code in 1957 (18). As a result, the term achalasia (Greek: without relaxation) has become the accepted name. Subsequent manometric studies confirmed the typical absence of peristalsis in the distal esophageal body in this disease. Although the specific etiology of achalasia has not been clarified, studies in the 1960s by Cassella and colleagues demonstrated the denervation of the distal esophagus, including a decrease in the number of enteric ganglia in the myenteric plexus and also possible lesions in the vagus nerves (19). Hyper-responsiveness of the esophagus to Mecholyl was described by Kramer and Ingelfinger in 1951 (20). This clinical demonstration of "denervation supersensitivity" confirmed the prior pathologic findings. During the past decade, additional support for denervation in this disease has come from a variety of sources, including the finding of a paradoxic increase in LES pressure after administration of cholecystokinin, a paradoxic increase in tone of circular muscle strips from the LES of achalasia patients during in vitro electrical stimulation, and decrease in VIP concentrations in LES circular smooth muscle from achalasia patients.

The manometric criteria for the diagnosis of achalasia have evolved with the improving technology throughout this century. The earlier concept of a nonrelaxing LES reported with fluid-filled, noninfused catheters has been replaced with the more appropriate perspective of incomplete relaxation identified with infused catheters or solid state transducers. The absence of distal esophageal peristalsis has been a consistent finding over the years, perceived as the manometric expression of denervation. The description by Vantrappen et al. of the apparent return of peristalsis on manometric studies after successful pneumatic dilatation in selected patients has raised interesting speculation regarding pathophysiology in achalasia (21). Perhaps, the loss of peristalsis is not a primary event, but rather secondary to the distal obstruction produced by the dysfunctional LES. This question is fueled by other reports of occasional return in peristalsis following a myotomy or even with successful treatment with nifedipine.

A potential relation between achalasia and squamous carcinoma of the esophagus was described before the 20th century. During this century, numerous case reports and occasional reviews have confirmed this relationship. The concept has remained controversial, however, with other reports failing to identify a definite cancer risk in achalasia patients. In a study from Yale University, Chuong et al. reported finding no cases of carcinoma in 91 patients with achalasia followed for over 6.5 years (22). A report from the Netherlands (Meijssen et al.) contradicts this observation, reporting an increased incidence of esophageal squamous cell carcinoma in 195 patients with achalasia successfully treated with pneumatic dilatation and followed for 15 years. It has not become common practice to perform routine surveillance endoscopy on patients successfully treated for achalasia, although these authors suggest that this should be seriously considered (23). The relationship between achalasia and cancer is confounded by the observation, first reported in 1968, that adenocarcinoma at the esophagogastric junction can produce a syndrome mimicking achalasia, so-called "secondary achalasia" (24). Subsequent reports have documented other malignant and nonmalignant conditions occasionally producing secondary achalasia. Although this is not highly likely, these observations have led to the current practice of requiring a careful view of the esophagogastric junction with the retroflexed endoscope in the stomach before definitive therapy for apparent idiopathic achalasia.

The treatment of achalasia has evolved dramatically during this century and no longer includes the whalebone of Willis. In 1913, Heller performed the first bilateral longitudinal myotomy in a patient with achalasia (25). Over the ensuing years, the most widely performed surgical repair of this entity has become the modified Heller myotomy, a single anterior incision. Beginning in the 1950s, the nonsurgical approach of forceful dilatation began to evolve, leading to the technique of pneumatic dilatation, which is currently considered by many authorities to be the preferred initial treatment for idiopathic achalasia. All techniques of forceful dilatation have been shown to carry a small risk of perforation. Surgical myotomy appears to have the potential for greater success, but to carry a greater risk of subsequent gastroesophageal reflux. In 1989, the only prospective randomized comparison of pneumatic dilatation and modified Heller myotomy was reported (26). The 81 patients in the study were followed for a median of 60 months, and the results confirmed observations perceived from the uncontrolled prior reports: overall success better with surgery than dilatation (95% versus 54%) and greater reflux after surgery (28% versus 8%). More recently, a prospective comparison of pneumatic dilatation and sublingual nifedipine in 30 patients with a mild to moderate degree of achalasia has reported equal results for either therapy with a mean follow up of 21 months (27).

Spastic Disorders of the Esophagus

Before this century, dating to the Crimean and Civil Wars, reports of young men with unexplained chest pain began to appear. In 1892, Sir William Osler reported on this syndrome in both men and women in civilian life and suggested "esophageal spasm" as a possible cause (28). Throughout this century, numerous observations have been made that esophageal spasm or related spastic disorders may be an important component of the unexplained chest pain syndrome, particularly when associated with other esophageal symptoms. The earliest manometric studies of diffuse esophageal spasm were reported from the laboratory of Code in 1958 (29). Numerous subsequent studies refined the manometric features in these patients, with the one constant finding being the presence of increased numbers of simultaneous contractions following swallows. When compared with results obtained using modern manometric techniques in normal individuals, excessive numbers of simultaneous contractions are best defined as occurring with at least 20% of wet swallows (30). Additional studies from the Mayo Clinic in 1962 reported a variety of abnormal esophageal motility patterns in patients being evaluated for unexplained chest pain (31). These manometric findings included the then newly described hypertensive lower esophageal sphincter and other forms of dysmotility and noted that typical diffuse spasm was not a common pattern in these patients. With the development of improved manometric technology, it was observed that the most common manometric change in patients with unexplained chest pain was the presence of high amplitude peristaltic contractions, the so-called "nutcracker esophagus" (32). With due respect to Dr. Osler, actual manometric documentation of esophageal spasm in patients with unexplained chest pain is unusual, documented in only 4% of 916 patients with chest pain studied in our laboratory (33). As we move toward the close of this century, the newly evolving technique of prolonged ambulatory pressure monitoring should provide some additional clarity to intermittent spastic disorders of the esophagus and their possible relationship to chest pain episodes.

Gastroesophageal Reflux

The modern concept of reflux esophagitis appears to have emerged from the publication by Winkelstein in 1935 which included the following statement (34):

> "One cannot avoid the suspicion that the disease in these five cases is possibly a peptic esophagitis; i.e., an esophagitis resulting from the irritant action on the mucosa of free hydrochloric acid and pepsin."

Although Winkelstein introduced the concept that esophagitis was caused by the digestive action of gastric juice on the esophageal mucosa, it was not until 1946 that Allison introduced the concept of chronic reflux of gastric contents and the term "reflux esophagitis" (35). Over the 20 years after the work of Allison and others, most investigators believed that GE reflux was mainly related to anatomic mechanical factors, particularly the presence of a hiatus hernia. However, reports began to appear in the literature, like that of Palmer (14), that many patients with hernias had neither reflux symptoms nor esophagitis, and that

other patients had esophagitis in the absence of a hiatus hernia. As discussed previously, the late 1960s and the 1970s could be considered the era of the LES because the importance of the sphincter as a primary mechanism against reflux became more firmly established.

The term GERD for gastroesophageal reflux disease has evolved to encompass the multiplicity of clinical manifestations seen in these patients. As early as 1968, Cherry and Margulies suggested that laryngeal abnormalities might be secondary to GE reflux (36), and in 1962 Kennedy implicated reflux in the production of pulmonary symptoms (37). Confirmation of these "extra esophageal" manifestations of GERD has recently become available through the development of prolonged ambulatory intraesophageal pH monitoring. With this technology, Sontag et al. demonstrated abnormal reflux in 82% of asthmatics (38), and studies from our laboratory documented abnormal reflux in 78% of patients with pharyngeal lesions and hoarseness (39). The development of the ability to monitor intraesophageal pH throughout a 24-hour period, resulting from the pioneering studies by Johnson and DeMeester in the 1970s (40), has provided some of the most profound advances in our understanding of mechanisms and therapy of reflux during this century. Most recently, ambulatory pH monitoring has revealed that reflux, rather than the esophageal spasm of Osler, may represent the most important esophageal abnormality producing recurring unexplained chest pain (41).

The many advances in knowledge of pathophysiology of GERD have led to greatly improved therapeutic strategies for this entity. Many of the conservative approaches, including dietary restrictions and elevation of the head of the bed, are supported by physiologic studies performed during the past 20 years. These conservative approaches form the base on which other therapies are developed and are now generally referred to as Phase I therapy of GERD (42). Since the development of H_2 receptor antagonists (H_2RAs) in the 1970s, numerous controlled trials have indicated that acid suppression with these agents will result in greater healing of esophagitis than previously achieved. Optimal acid suppression therapy is now achievable with omeprazole, an agent that inhibits the enzymatic release of acid into the lumen, the "proton pump." The past few years have seen numerous reports of even greater healing rates of esophagitis with this agent (approximately 80%) as opposed to those with H_2RAs (approximately 40%). The development of drugs that effectively increase LES pressure and improve gastric emptying (promotility agents) also represent advances in the treatment of GERD over the past 20 years. Following the initial report that cholinergic stimulation with bethanechol would improve GERD symptoms compared to placebo (43), other promotility drugs such as metoclopramide and cisapride have been shown to have a positive therapeutic effect in patients with GERD. Most of these studies indicate a positive degree of symptom control. Occasional reports have shown healing rates comparable to those with H_2RAs with these promotility drugs, but none have achieved the effectiveness of omeprazole in the treatment of GERD.

Over the past 50 years, the surgical approach to GERD has changed dramatically. Poor results with the simple repair of a hiatus hernia (the Allison procedure) seem consistent with the recognition that the pathophysiology of GERD was much more complex than that produced simply by a hiatus hernia. A wrap of the gastric fundus around the distal esophagus, a Nissen or Belsey fundoplication, will usually effectively control reflux. It is yet to be determined, however, whether a surgical repair at the esophagogastric junction or long-term modern medical therapy is the preferred treatment of GERD. Two prospective comparisons of medical versus surgical therapy of GERD have been reported in this century. In 1975, Behar et al. reported that fundoplication was superior to Phase I medical therapy over a 3-year period in the treatment of GERD (44). In 1992, Spechler et al. reported that fundoplication was superior to a combination of H_2RA plus metoclopramide in the treatment of GERD over a 2-year follow-up (45). Although these studies make a strong argument in favor of surgery, they suffer from design difficulties in that new and more effective medical therapies have become available while the studies were being performed. The remarkable improvement in the control of GERD with omepra-zole promises results with long-term medical therapy that are far superior to those studied in these two prospective trials.

REFERENCES

1. Brody PA, Werle JM, Meschan I, Quigley JP: Intralumen pressures of the digestive tract especially the pyloric region. Am J Physiol *130*:791, 1940.
2. Kramer P, Ingelfinger FJ: Motility of the human esophagus in control subjects and in patients with esophageal disorders. Am J Med *7*:168, 1949.
3. Harris LD, Winans CS, Pope CE: Determination of yield pressures. Gastroenterology *50*:754, 1966.
4. Hollis JB, Castell DO: Amplitude of esophageal peristalsis as determined by rapid infusion. Gastroenterology *63*:417, 1972.
5. Meyer GM, Gerhardt DC, Castell DO: Human esophageal response to rapid swallowing: Muscle refractory period or neural inhibition. Am J Physiol *241*:G129, 1981.
6. Meyer GM, Castell DO: Human esophageal response during chest pain induced by swallowing cold liquids. JAMA *246*:2057, 1981.
7. Kahrilas PJ, Dodds WJ, Hogan WJ: The effect of peristaltic dysfunction on esophageal volume clearance. Gastroenterology *94*:73, 1988.
8. Fox JA, Daniel EE: Role of Ca^{++} in genesis of lower esophageal sphincter tone and other active contractions. Am J Physiol *237*:E163, 1979.
9. Blackwell JH, Holt S, Heading RC: Effect of nifedipine on oesophageal motility and gastric emptying. Gut *21*:50, 1981.
10. Goyal R, Rattan S: VIP as a possible neurotransmitter of non-cholinergic, non-adrenergic inhibitory neurons. Nature *288*:378, 1980.
11. Sanders KM, Ward SM: Nitric oxide as a mediator of non-adrenergic noncholinergic neurotransmission. Am J Physiol *262*:G379, 1992.
12. Castell DO, Harris LD: Hormonal control of gastroesophageal sphincter strength. N Engl J Med *282*:886, 1970.
13. Dodds WJ et al.: Mechanisms of gastroesophageal reflux in patients with reflux esophagitis. N Engl J Med *307*:1547, 1982.
14. Cohen S, Harris LD: Does hiatus hernia affect competence of the gastroesophageal sphincter? N Engl J Med *284*:1053, 1971.
15. Palmer ED: The hiatus hernia-esophagitis-esophageal stricture complex: Twenty-year prospective study. Am J Med *44*:566, 1968.

16. Mittal RK, Rochester DF, McCallum RW: Electrical and mechanical activity in the human lower esophageal sphincter during diaphragmatic contraction. J Clin Invest *81*: 1182, 1988.

17. Hirschowitz B: A critical analysis, with appropriate controls of gastric acid and pepsin secretion in clinical esophagitis. Gastroenterology *101*:1149, 1991.

18. Creamer B, Olsen AM, Code CF: The esophageal sphincters in achalasia of the cardia (cardiospasm). Gastroenterology *33*: 293, 1957.

19. Cassella RR et al.: Achalasia of the esophagus: Pathologic and etiologic considerations. Ann Surg *160*:474, 1964.

20. Kramer P, Ingelfinger FJ: Esophageal sensitivity to Mecholyl in cardiospasm. Gastroenterology *19*:242, 1951.

21. Vantrappen G et al.: Achalasia, diffuse esophageal spasm, and related motility disorders. Gastroenterology *76*:450, 1979.

22. Chuong JJ, DuBovik S, McCallum RW: Achalasia as a risk factor for esophageal carcinoma. Dig Dis Sci *29*:1105, 1984.

23. Meijssen MA et al.: Achalasia complicated by oesophageal squamous cell carcinoma. Gut *33*:133, 1992.

24. Kolodny M et al.: Esophageal achalasia probably due to gastric carcinoma. Ann Intern Med *69*:569, 1968.

25. Heller E: Extramukose kardioplastik beim chronischen kardiospasms mit dilatation oesophagus. Mitt Grenzgeb Med Chir *27*: 141, 1914.

26. Csendes A, Braghetto I, Henriquez A, Cortes C: Late results of a prospective randomized study comparing forceful dilatation and oesophagomyotomy in patients with achalasia. Gut *30*:299, 1989.

27. Coccia G, Bartoletti M, Michetti P, Dodero M: Prospective clinical and manometric study comparing pneumatic dilatation and sublingual nifedipine in the treatment of oesophageal achalasia. Gut *32*:604, 1991.

28. Osler W: Principles and Practice of Medicine. New York, D. Appleton and Company, 1892.

29. Creamer B, Donoghue FE, Code CF: Pattern of esophageal motility in diffuse esophageal spasm. Gastroenterology *34*:782, 1958.

30. Richter JE et al.: Esophageal manometry in 95 healthy adult volunteers. Dig Dis Sci *32*: 583, 1987.

31. Schmidt CD et al.: The value of the esophageal motility test in evaluation of thoracic pain problems. Dis Chest *41*:303, 1962.

32. Benjamin SB, Gerhardt DC, Castell DO: High amplitude peristaltic contractions associated with chest pain and/or dysphagia. Gastroenterology *77*:478, 1979.

33. Dalton CB et al.: Diffuse esophageal spasm. Dig Dis Sci *36*:1025, 1991.

34. Winkelstein A: Peptic esophagitis: A new clinical entity. JAMA *104*:906, 1935.

35. Allison PR: Peptic ulcer of the esophagus. J Thoracic Surg *15*:308, 1946.

36. Cherry J, Margulies SI: Contact ulcer of the larynx. Laryngoscope *78*:1937, 1968.

37. Kennedy JH: "Silent" gastroesophageal reflux: An important but little known cause of pulmonary complications. Dis Chest *42*:42, 1962.

38. Sontag SJ et al.: Most asthmatics have gastroesophageal reflux with or without bronchodilator therapy. Gastroenterology *99*: 613, 1990.

39. Wiener GJ et al.: Chronic hoarseness secondary to gastroesophageal reflux disease: Documentation with 24 hour ambulatory pH monitoring. Am J Gastroenterol *84*:1503, 1989.

40. Johnson LF, DeMeester TR: Twenty-four hour pH monitoring of the distal esophagus: A quantative measure of gastroesophageal reflux. Am J Gastroenterol *62*:325, 1974.

41. Hewson EG, Sinclair JW, Dalton CB, Castell DO: Twenty-four hour esophageal pH monitoring: The most useful test for evaluating noncardiac chest pain. Am J Med *90*: 576, 1991.

42. Kitchin LI, Castell DO: Rationale and efficacy of conservative therapy for gastroesophageal reflux disease. Arch Intern Med *151*:448, 1991.

43. Farrell FL, Roling GT, Castell DO: Cholinergic therapy of chronic heartburn. A controlled trial. Ann Intern Med *80*:573, 1974.

44. Behar J et al.: Medical and surgical management of reflux esophagitis. N Engl J Med *293*:263, 1975.

45. Spechler J et al.: Comparison of medical and surgical therapy for complicated gastroesophageal reflux disease in veterans. N Engl J Med *326*:786, 1992.

2

Esophageal Malignancies and Premalignant Conditions

H. WORTH BOYCE, JR.

Esophageal cancer has been recognized for centuries. Over 2000 years ago in China, it was referred to as Ye Ge, which may be interpreted literally as dysphagia and belching. There was a Chinese saying in those days that "those discovered to suffer from esophageal cancer in the autumn will not live through the next summer" (1). And so it remains today. Only primary hepatic and pancreatic malignancies have a shorter survival time.

Until the past two decades, the term esophageal cancer was synonymous with squamous-cell carcinoma because this lesion was known to comprise over 95% of esophageal malignancies. Consequently, most of the reports on epidemiology, etiology, diagnosis, and therapy for esophageal cancer published in the 20th century refer to the squamous-cell variety. However, as the 21st century approaches, this imbalance favoring squamous cancer over primary adenocarcinoma of the esophagus in the United States is changing drastically. Reports from several medical centers during the past decade reveal about a tenfold increase in adenocarcinoma of the esophagus (2,3). The dramatic increase is occurring primarily in white men in the 40- to 70-age range in association with a columnar-lined (Barrett) esophagus. In this review, the term esophageal cancer refers to the squamous-cell type and adenocarcinoma is used specifically for this type of malignancy arising in the esophagus, usually associated with a columnar-lined (Barrett) esophagus. Unfortunately, many surgical reports fail to discriminate between the two and to exclude adenocarcinoma of the gastric cardia when reporting responses to therapy and survival statistics.

Malignant neoplasms of the esophagus other than squamous-cell carcinoma and adenocarcinoma are rare and are not reviewed here.

CHALLENGES OF ESOPHAGEAL MALIGNANCIES

The dismal prognosis in patients diagnosed with esophageal cancer has been virtually unchanged during this century. The biologic fact that symptoms occur late in this disease has proven to be the one constant that has thwarted all known diagnostic and therapeutic efforts.

The primary symptom of esophageal obstruction is dysphagia. For dysphagia to occur, the potential esophageal lumen diameter, normally about 2.5 to 3.0 cm, must be narrowed by either a large intraluminal tumor mass or stenosis caused by circumferential intramural growth through about 270° of the wall circumference. The time required for a lesion to develop to this extent has been variously estimated to require up to several years. During this asymptomatic interval, the carcinoma easily spreads through the 3- to 4-mm thick esophageal wall and, in the absence of the protective effect of a serosal layer, readily invades the mediastinal tissues and vital contiguous or-

11

gans. Lymphatic invasion occurs during the asymptomatic phase, with spread to mediastinal nodes as well as through intramural lymphatic channels that drain in both cephalad and caudad directions along the esophagus.

The incurability of symptomatic esophageal cancer has been difficult for physicians and surgeons to accept, and as a consequence, increasingly more radical, high-risk therapeutic methods have been tried in an uncontrolled manner, with improved survival achieved in only highly selected cases. The treatment of esophageal cancer is replete with surgical, radiotherapy, and chemotherapy reports that are initially enthusiastic and then discarded. The lack of prospective, controlled studies of available treatments in carefully evaluated and staged patients has delayed progress toward a cure. Accurate conclusions can be made only if treatment groups are randomized between the best treatments currently available, i.e., surgery and radiation.

The purpose of this chapter is to review current knowledge of the epidemiology, known risk factors, pre-malignant lesions of the esophagus, early diagnosis, the staging of esophageal carcinoma, and present surgery, radiation therapy and chemotherapy with added consideration of necessary and promising areas of future investigation. Because 95% of patients with esophageal cancer die within 5 years of diagnosis, the best palliative measures must be available for sustaining life with as much quality as possible. These patients can be likened to the lotus eaters, about whom Homer wrote: "and the men waste day by day with withering undelight."

EPIDEMIOLOGY AND PREDISPOSING FACTORS

The incidence of squamous-cell cancer of the esophagus in China is estimated at 236 in 100,000 in the highest-incidence areas, and in all areas, the incidence has remained fairly constant since the report in 1924 by Davies (4). Reports from Northern Iran, especially along the Caspian littoral made by Elgood in 1951, show an even higher peak incidence at 515 in 100,000 population (5). A high frequency has been recognized there since the 12th century. A unique form of chronic esophagitis has been identified in Iran and China as a predisposing condition for esophageal cancer (6). Other high-incidence areas around the world include such widely separated regions as South Africa, England and Wales, Puerto Rico, South Carolina, Washington, D.C., France, and Japan.

Predisposing factors have included dietary deficiencies, dietary carcinogens, race, heredity, tobacco, alcohol and other chemical injury, stagnation of esophageal contents, and esophageal dysplasia following prolonged gastroesophageal acid reflux.

Geographic Considerations

Wide variations in incidence of esophageal cancer have been noted among people in adjacent geographic areas and in the same region among populations with different lifestyles and eating habits. Several authors have reported very low incidence in Mormons and Seventh-Day Adventists (7–9). One dramatic variation among the neighboring regions of Gurjev, Kazakhstan, and Georgia in the Ukraine, which are about 500 miles apart, is the drop in frequency by 70-fold for men and 230-fold for women (10). In 1967, Doll reported that the worldwide incidence ranged 500-fold, a range greater than for almost any other type of cancer (11). By comparison, lung cancer shows a 40-fold worldwide variation between highest and lowest incidences. Persons in lower socioeconomic classes appear at higher risk for developing esophageal cancer (12). Blacks in this country appear significantly more prone than whites to develop squamous-cell esophageal cancer by a factor of two to ten times (13). By comparison, adenocarcinoma of the esophagus (nearly always associated with a columnar-lined or Barrett esophagus) may be as much as 10-fold greater in white men (14).

Variations Between the Sexes

Several authors have reported an increasing incidence of squamous-cell cancer among men over the past two decades (15–17). In 1930, the incidence in the United States was 3 in 100,000 men; in 1985 it was 5 in 100,000. The frequency among white men and women has not changed appreciably, but there has been a 30% increase in the black population over the last 30 years (18). King and Locke have reported that persons who were born in China or Japan and moved to the United States have a two to three times higher incidence for esophageal cancer than those of the same racial background born in this country (19).

Tylosis

In 1958, Howel-Evans et al. showed an unequivocal association between the hereditary condition of tylosis palmaris et plantaris (hyperkeratosis of palms and soles) and squamous-cell cancer of the esophagus in two families in Liverpool, England (20). After 30 years of followup of these families, 95% of those with tylosis had developed esophageal cancer by age 65. None of the family members without tylosis had developed esophageal cancer. An abnormality in vitamin A metabolism has been proposed as the cause of this malignant potential (21).

Caustic Injury

The etiologic relationship between lye injury of the esophagus and subsequent development of squamous cell cancer was first reported by Catel in 1896. The mean age of lye ingestion was at 6.2 years and carcinoma developed after a mean interval of 41 years (22). The risk of esophageal cancer in these patients was estimated to exceed 1000 times.

Alcohol and Tobacco

Young and Russell, in 1926, implicated alcohol, tobacco, and occupation in the development of squamous cancer of the esophagus (23). Thirty-two years later, Steiner in a case-control study confirmed the association among alcohol, tobacco, and esophageal carcinoma (24). This association has been substantiated by others (25,26), and in 1961, Wynder and Bross defined a clear dose response for both alcohol and tobacco independently (27). They also noted that spirits carried a much higher risk than beer and wine. Tuyns, in 1977, reported a synergistic effect of beer plus wine. He reported that habitual alcohol consumption with infrequent use of tobacco represented a higher risk than frequent use of tobacco

and moderate alcohol consumption (1). In 1982, it was estimated that in Europe, North America, and the Caribbean, alcohol and tobacco use probably could account for 90% of patients with esophageal carcinoma, especially in men (28). However, their explanation does not account for the increases of esophageal cancer in women in the series of Wynder and Bross, who reported that 41% of the women were nonsmokers and 43% rarely or never drank (27).

Dietary Deficiencies

By the 1960s, investigators recognized that worldwide variations in squamous esophageal cancer were too great to be explained by alcohol and tobacco consumption alone. In 1965, Wynder and Klein reported that in animal experiments, vitamin A and riboflavin can inhibit tumor development and riboflavin deficiency is related to squamous metaplasia in esophageal epithelium in mice (29). This discovery led to an investigation of the dietary intake of high- and low-incidence areas for esophageal carcinoma. In 1971, it was reported that excessive alcohol intake can result in nutritional deficiencies, not only because of the poor eating habits that can accompany addiction, but also because alcohol itself interferes with absorption of nutrients (30). One year later, Kmet and Mahboubi showed a negative association with rainfall and a partial correlation with many variables dependent on rainfall, such as vegetation, soil types, and crop patterns (31). In 1975, in the highest-incidence areas around the Caspian Sea, the barren steppe grasslands provided virtually no vegetables or fruits. The native diet had very low levels of animal proteins, vitamin A, riboflavin, and vitamin C (32). A later report contributed the risk to low intake of fruits and vegetables. They also reported that people in rural areas of northern Iran have the lowest economic status and generally have poor dietary intake (33). Pottern et al., in 1985, found an increased number of patients with esophageal cancer among black men in Washington, D.C. The group was characterized by excessive smoking and drinking and decreased intake of red meat, chicken, eggs, fruits, and vegetables (34).

In 1978, Fong and Newberne reported

that zinc had an important role in maintaining the integrity of epithelial tissue, and animal experiments showed that zinc deficiencies can promote the induction of esophageal tumors (35). Two years earlier, it had been shown that a high intake of bread rich in fiber, such as that eaten in high-incidence areas of northern Iran, causes an increase in fecal excretion of zinc and other minerals (36). On the other hand, in a 1985 study in China, a treatment group received retinol, riboflavin, and zinc to evaluate the effect on premalignant mucosal changes. No significant difference was found in the frequency of histologically diagnosed precancerous lesions in the treatment and placebo groups (37).

Dietary Carcinogens

Carcinogenic elements in the diet have been implicated in the development of squamous esophageal cancer. In 1966, Burell et al. in Transkei suggested that molybdenum deficiency in the soil causes a buildup of nitrates in plants which could be converted to nitrosamines in the stomach (38). One year later, it was shown not only that nitrosamines were carcinogenic, but also that they caused esophageal tumors in experimental animals (39). In 1978, Kaplan and Tsuchitani reported that, in high-incidence areas of China, molybdenum added to the seeds before planting reduced considerably the nitrate content of grains and increased the vitamin C content of the vegetables (40). A tea consumed widely in northern Iran and vitamin C apparently inhibited the development of nitrosamines in the stomach (41,42). Several years later, low levels of nitrosamines were reported in homemade ciders and apple brandies from Normandy and Brittany in France (43) and in a variety of foods in both high- and low-incidence regions of Iran (44).

Other carcinogens have been found in high-incidence areas around the world and are thought to contribute to an increased risk of developing esophageal cancer. In 1969, the shikimic acid contained in bracken fern was found to cause tumor growth in cattle (45). Ten years later, in high-incidence regions of Japan, a study in humans showed a twofold greater risk associated with the consumption of bracken fern (46).

In 1981, two separate studies showed that "pickled" vegetables, common in high-incidence regions of China, were found to be mutagenic for bacteria and produced hyperkeratosis and dysplasia of the esophagus in rats (47,48,49).

Physical Trauma to Esophageal Epithelium

Watson, in 1933, was the first to suggest that repeated ingestion of hot food and drinks increases the risk of squamous-cell esophageal carcinoma (50). This concept has been reported numerous times (51–53). In 1971, a twofold increase in risk was reported if the patient had been a frequent consumer of chagayo (hot rice tea) (54). Several years later, a geographic association was found between consumption of chagayo and incidence of cancer of the esophagus (55). De Jong et al. in Singapore reported a 3- to 15-fold increase in cancer risk for patients who preferred hot beverages (56). However, a report in 1977 revealed that patients often believed their tea was very hot when it was only warm. Such an observation suggests that their digestive problems made them more aware of the temperature (57). This may indicate a bias in reporting by the patients. A 1987 report indicates that in southern Brazil the consumption of excessively hot "maté" (a hot herbal infusion) over 40 to 50 years is associated with a twofold increase in esophageal cancer risk (58).

Another type of physical trauma possibly increasing the risk of esophageal cancer is the consumption of abrasive particles. In 1969, in Transkei, silica particles derived from grinding stones used to prepare maize flour were suggested to have an irritant effect on the esophagus (59). Ten years later, in high-incidence regions of Iran, there was a high frequency of abrasive seeds in bread and wheat samples (60). O'Neill et al., in 1980, found that in some seeds there were finely pointed silica fibers that could stimulate cell growth if lodged in the esophagus (61). Two years later, they reported that, in northern China, silica fragments from millet bran were found lodged in the mucosa surrounding esophageal tumors (62).

Upper Aerodigestive Carcinoma

Squamous-cell carcinoma of the esophagus has a remarkably high associated rate

(10 to 16.4%) of similar carcinomas in the oropharynx and larynx (63). If patients with esophageal cancer lived longer, this association of neoplasms with similar biologic behavior would probably be much more apparent, and surveillance would be more productive. Use of surveillance endoscopy is reasonable for screening patients with cancer in either location, although no precise interval for such screening examination has been established.

Carcinoma in a Skin Tube Interposition Graft

Although attempts to restore continuity by skin tubes were made as early as 1871 by Billroth and others, the first successful skin tube replacement of the esophagus was in 1894 by Bircher. The first report of carcinoma developing in a skin tube was 60 years later in a tube that had been in place for 30 years (64). In 1991, Horvath et al. reviewed the literature and found 22 cases of cancer in a skin tube esophagus. They call attention to the problem because, even though skin tubes are no longer used to replace the esophagus, use of skin replacements in the mouth and pharynx has been increasing, and they fear that similar long-term complications may arise (65).

Achalasia

Fagge, in 1872, was the first to report a relationship between achalasia and esophageal squamous-cell carcinoma. Since his initial observation, several authors have reported an increased risk of esophageal cancer in patients with long-standing achalasia, with incidences ranging from 1.7 to 20% (66–68). There also has been at least one report of no cancers developing in a large group of achalasia patients (69), which has led some authors to question the association (69,70). In 1919, Guisez first suggested that stasis was important in the development of carcinoma associated with achalasia. Rake, 8 years later, proposed that chronic esophagitis from stagnation eventually led to malignant degeneration (66). This theory has been disputed by several authors on the grounds that most carcinomas arise in the middle third of the esophagus in achalasia patients, whereas, if Rake's hypothesis were true, it would be most often found in the lower third (71,72). An alternative hypothesis may explain the middle-third location. Because most patients with achalasia have the level of retained fluid lying in the middle third, retained fat or other potential carcinogens that float at the fluid-air interface could be the responsible agents. There also is some evidence that the risk of cancer is highest in patients who have failed treatment or have never been treated, which supports a possible role for the effects of prolonged stagnation.

Columnar-Lined Esophagus (CLE)

In 1950, Barrett reported peptic ulceration in a tubular segment of the esophagus lined by columnar epithelium that he incorrectly believed was the stomach attached to a congenitally short esophagus (73). Three years later, Allison and Johnstone correctly pointed out that the segment lined by columnar epithelium was anatomically located within the esophagus (74). Although the squamo-columnar mucosal junction was displaced proximally in the tubular esophagus, these authors recognized that the columnar epithelium extended proximally to the lower esophageal sphincter, that the muscular layer surrounding this segment was typically esophageal, and that esophageal glands were located beneath the columnar epithelium. They also correctly proposed that this condition was acquired as a consequence of gastroesophageal acid reflux and that it may be a precursor of esophageal adenocarcinoma.

The development of CLE has been reported in several conditions known to be associated with gastroesophageal reflux, including scleroderma, postmyotomy achalasia, and the acid hypersecretory state associated with a gastrinoma (75,76).

There is some evidence for an inheritable basis for the columnar-lined esophagus related to a predisposition of the esophagus to develop the disorder or the tendency to severe gastroesophageal reflux (77). Jochem et al. recently reported six cases of columnar-lined esophagus in one family. They believe that the predisposition was definitely inherited and noted that it was associated with an early age of onset (78).

The detection of a multiple aneuploid population of cells in patients with columnar-lined esophagus may be considered a high risk for adenocarcinoma (79). Several studies have reported no significant relationship among alcohol intake, smoking, and development of adenocarcinoma with CLE (80,81). Casson et al. state that, after identification of the gene mutations for CLE, adenocarcinoma, and squamous cell carcinoma, there appears to be no link. They suggested that the carcinoma is caused by unknown intermediate events and not a genetic predisposition for malignant progression of the metaplastic epithelium (82).

Correlation Between Columnar-Lined Esophagus and Adenocarcinoma

Between 1952 and 1971, 11 cases of adenocarcinoma were reported with CLE. Hawe et al. added five more cases in 1973 and emphasized CLE as a premalignant condition that was increasing in frequency (83). In 1975, Naef et al. reported that 8.5% of their 140 patients with CLE had developed adenocarcinoma (84). The histologic evolution of carcinoma in CLE was clarified in 1978 by the proposal of Haggitt et al. that this malignancy probably evolves through a sequence of dysplasia and carcinoma in situ that is detectable by endoscopic biopsy (85). There has been no evidence to date that, once CLE has developed, prevention of gastroesophageal reflux will lead to alteration of the metaplastic columnar epithelium or reduce the predisposition to dysplasia and carcinoma. Consequently, once CLE is known to be present, the patient should be under surveillance by endoscopy and biopsy.

The columnar-lined esophagus (CLE) is the most established indicator for risk of adenocarcinoma of the esophagus (Table 2–1). In a 1986 report from Wang et al. of 35 esophageal cancers, adenocarcinoma accounted for 34% of all cancers and 60% of those occurring in the lower third of the esophagus (86). All adenocarcinomas were in men and all but one were associated with CLE. Table 2-1 lists the various published estimates for frequency of adenocarcinoma, expressed as cases per patient-years of follow-up. Wide variations are apparent, but all agree that the risk is much higher than in persons without CLE.

Increasing Prevalence of Adenocarcinoma

Esophageal adenocarcinoma is increasing at an alarming rate. Between 1926 and 1976, several reports indicated that adenocarcinomas accounted for 1.7 to 7.3% of esophageal cancers (Table 2–2). A report from Boston University tumor registries in 1989 revealed that 31% of esophageal cancers were adenocarcinomas, with 84% located in the lower third of the esophagus (3). They compared this report with an 8% frequency for adenocarcinoma among esophageal malignancies

Table 2–1
Reported Incidence of Adenocarcinoma in Patients with Barrett's Esophagus*

Source, Year	Incidence/Patient-Years of Follow-up Study	No. of Times Greater Than the Incidence in General Population
Hameeteman et al., 1989	1/52	125
Van der Veen et al., 1989	1/170	30
Robertson et al., 1988	1/56	62
Cameron et al., 1985	1/441	30
Skinner, 1989	1/175	40
Spechler et al., 1984	1/48	Not given
Ovaska et al., 1989	1/55	90
Sampliner et al., 1985	1/56	Not given
Ollyo et al., 1989	1/253	Not given
Williamson et al., 1991[181]	1/99	74.8

* Modified from Williamson et al. 1991

Table 2–2
Frequency of True Adenoma of the Esophagus*

	Years	Total Esophageal Carcinomas	No. of True Adenocarcinomas (%)
Turnbull et al.[183]	1926–66	1859	45 (2.4)
Smithers et al.[184]	1936–51	314	23 (7.3)
Bosch et al.[185]	1950–74	350	13 (3.7)
Webb and Busuttil[182]	1962–76	115	2 (1.7)
Boston University[3]	1980–86	262	47 (17.9)
Blot et al.[2]	1976–87	9405	1598 (17)
Massachusetts[3]	1982–84	868	231 (27)
Connecticut[3]	1983–86	680	156 (22.9)
Wang et al.[86]	1975–82	35	12 (34)

* Modified with permission from Hesketh PJ, et al.: Increasing frequency of adenocarcinoma of the esophagus. Cancer *64*:526, 1989.

reported in the National Cancer Survey for the years 1969 to 1971.

The increasing evolution of adenocarcinoma was confirmed by the 1991 report of Blot et al. (2). They reported on a review of cases of esophageal carcinoma collected between 1976 and 1987 by the nine population-based cancer registries that constitute the National Cancer Institutes' surveillance, epidemiology, and end results program. This registry accounts for 10% of the U.S. population. In this review of 9405 cases of esophageal cancer, adenocarcinoma accounted for 17%. Rates for squamous-cell cancer remained relatively constant, but the average annual rates of increase of adenocarcinoma were 9.4% among white men, 9.8% for black men, and 4.5% among white women. Between 1984 and 1987, adenocarcinomas accounted for 34% of esophageal cancers in white men. The rate of increase of this cancer in the 1970s and 1980s was higher than for any other malignancy. From 1976 to 1987, the rates of squamous-cell carcinoma were relatively stable, but increased more than 100% for adenocarcinoma and actually exceeded rates of squamous-cell cancer among white men below age 55 (2).

GROWTH AND METASTASIS OF ESOPHAGEAL CANCER

Growth Rate of Esophageal Cancer

Information regarding the growth rate of esophageal cancer is available only from high-incidence areas. The best data thus far have been obtained by follow-up studies on patients with early esophageal squamous cell cancer who have either refused therapy or been lost to follow-up. There appears to be a significant window for curative treatment when screening programs are able to detect lesions still localized to the mucosa and before intramural and regional lymph node metastasis.

In general, the natural history of esophageal carcinoma extends from the date when dysphagia is first recorded to the date of death, which is usually only 9 months to 1 year later. Esophageal carcinoma therefore has been considered a rapidly growing cancer. No correlation has been found between age, cancer location, sex and degree of differentiation, and the growth rate of esophageal carcinoma. There was, however, some suggestion that the plaque-like type of early esophageal squamous carcinoma (EESC) progressed more rapidly than the congestive or erosive type. The percentage of plaque-like carcinomas that progressed to overt malignancy was 61%, the corresponding figures being only 33% and 34% for erosive types of EESC. In China, many cases of EESC were detected, and the natural history of EESC was found to differ from that of advanced esophageal cancer. Age distributions of most cases of EESC ranged from 40 to 59 years, with an average of 52.7 years. Most advanced carcinomas occurred in patients 50 to 59 years old, with an average of 58.7 years. These data suggest that a period of several years may be needed for EESC to develop into an advanced stage. In 1976, a study of 19 cases reported the average period of EESC to progress to an advanced stage was 32.5 months, with a further 10.5 months for progress to death. In this report of 90 cases of EESC, a natural history of 4 to 5 years appears more likely for a carcinoma in situ to progress to advanced cancer. Based on this EESC data, squamous cancer is therefore considered a slowly progressing cancer, which permits detection of this disease at an early stage, at least in high-incidence areas. This paper reports a 5-year survival rate of 62.5% even for untreated EESC (87).

Anatomy of the Esophagus and the Spread of Cancer

From an anatomic viewpoint, the esophagus provides a fertile field for the silent development and spread of intrinsic cancer, and at the same time poses a serious and sometimes insurmountable obstacle to adequate surgical management (88). Watson, in 1933, reported that the esophagus was unique in the digestive tract in that it does not have a serosal covering. He also noted that it is richly supplied by lymphatics in the submucosal and muscular coats that provide a submucous pathway for dissemination of cancer (50). However, in the early 1900s it was disputed whether the esophageal carcinoma metastasized early or distant from its origin (89). In 1923, a review of the literature found several authors who reported no evidence of early metastasis, but conversely, many other authors found a high percentage of cases that metastasized early (89).

It is now widely accepted that the esophageal cancer that invades through the epithelium spreads early and distantly because of the anatomic structure of the esophagus (90). It is surrounded throughout its length by important and vital organs, which may be invaded early in the course of this cancer (50). The intramural lymphatic vessels distribute neoplastic cells in a longitudinal direction, often to a considerable distance above and below the visible or palpable limits of the primary cancer (88). The disease spreads by direct extension via lymphatics and through the blood stream (50).

DIAGNOSIS OF ESOPHAGEAL CANCER

Clinical

The historical presentation of esophageal cancer has changed little, if at all, during this century. Still, most patients and some physicians remain unaware of the significance of the cardinal symptoms that time has not altered. A history of dysphagia, weight loss, ill-defined mid-chest discomfort, odynophagia, and unexplained hiccups, alone or in combination, should suggest the possibility of esophageal cancer. Solid-food dysphagia occurs relatively late but is typically progressive for 3 to 6 months before a patient first seeks medical attention. Some patients report the earliest symptom to be a vague sensation or discomfort noted when swallowing a solid food bolus. These warning symptoms must be investigated completely by barium radiography and endoscopy with biopsy and cytology for histologic confirmation.

Radiographic

Esophageal cancer was one of the first lesions evaluated by radiography in 1897 by Rumpel (91) using bismuth subnitrate as the contrast medium. Over the ensuing decades, barium use and better equipment established contrast radiography as the first indicated procedure to diagnose these malignancies. The technique of double contrast radiography has significantly improved the resolution that allows detection of very early mucosal abnormalities (92). Good radiographic contrast study is essential for complete assessment of the patient suspected of having an esophageal malignancy.

Endoscopy

Esophagoscopy was pioneered in this country by Dr. Chevalier Jackson, a bronchoesophagologist in Philadelphia during the early 1900s. He developed rigid instruments and techniques that permitted relatively safe examination and biopsy of esophageal cancer. The first rigid esophagoscope in wide use among gastroenterologists was introduced by Hufford in 1949. This instrument was approximately 53 cm long with a 10-mm channel through which a biopsy forceps could be passed under direct vision, using a four-power telescope that allowed good visualization of the lesion 53 cm away. The earlier rigid esophagoscopes and most of those still used by otolaryngologists today have no telescopic capability for good mucosal examination.

Although Rudolf Schindler introduced the first semiflexible gastroscope in this country in the 1930s, and Hirschowitz developed the first fiberoptic gastroscope in 1957, it was not until Lo Presti developed the forward-viewing flexible fiberoptic esophagoscope in 1964 that precise, close-up examination and biopsy of the esophagus were possible (93). The evolution of fiberoptic endoscopes to current videoendoscopes has permitted close observations of minute alterations in esophageal mucosa and superb documentation by color prints and videotape recording. Reliable visual detection and guided biopsy confirmation of esophageal malignancies, even in their earliest stages, is now possible, making fiberoptic endoscopy with biopsy the primary diagnostic method for esophageal cancer.

Biopsy and Brush Cytology

The diagnostic accuracy of forceps biopsy for carcinoma approaches 100% in most reports, if at least eight specimens are taken. Cytologic diagnosis also approaches 100% when specimens are taken properly, by brush, from the tumor surface under direct endoscopic visual control. The use of combined forceps biopsy and brush cytology virtually ensures accurate diagnosis.

Chromoendoscopy

Although publicized for many years, the technique of mucosal staining with various dyes, called chromoendoscopy, is beginning to gain favor as a method to enhance mucosal examination, especially to diagnose early carcinomas and to define the mucosal alterations associated with the columnar-lined esophagus.

In 1933, Schiller used Lugol's iodine solution for vital staining and diagnosis of cervical cancer (94). Thirty-three years later,

Voegeli used this color reaction resulting from the iodine staining the glycogen of the squamous cells a brownish-black color in his in vitro study of esophageal mucosa. In 1972, Endo et al. were the first to use Lugol's solution for staining during endoscopy of the esophagus (95). Further study by several investigators, primarily from Japan, has shown the value of iodine staining for diagnosis of early cancer. Sugimachi has reported that iodine staining during endoscopy with biopsy is the best surveillance method for early esophageal cancer (96,97). Areas that fail to stain may represent neoplasia, severe inflammation and erosion, or nonsquamous (columnar) tissue (95,96,98). Guided biopsy of unstained areas permits accurate histologic diagnosis. Toludine blue dye also is useful for guided biopsy diagnosis because it reveals subtle topographic variations in surface contour and stains the surface of intestinalized metaplastic epithelium in both esophagus and stomach (99,100).

SCREENING FOR ESOPHAGEAL CANCER

Squamous-Cell Cancer

Accurate screening for esophageal squamous-cell cancer is most likely to be achieved by endoscopy and accessory procedures, although proper time intervals for surveillance have not been established. However, it is logical to recommend that patients at highest risk (i.e., with prior upper aerodigestive tract cancer, tylosis, long-standing caustic injury) have an endoscopic surveillance at 1- to 2-year intervals. In such patients, the likelihood of finding early mucosal cancer is greatly enhanced by using chromoendoscopy techniques with iodine and/or toluidine blue.

For screening large numbers of patients in high-incidence areas, several ingenious procedures have been developed using a nylon mesh over a balloon or a small plastic sponge inside a gelatin capsule attached to a string. The balloon apparatus is passed into the stomach, inflated, and slowly retracted, collecting esophageal specimens by abrasion in its mesh. Similarly, the Nabeya capsule is swallowed, and the sponge inside expands after the capsule melts and is pulled through the esophagus, collecting cells in the interstices of the sponge (101).

Adenocarcinoma

Patients with CLE are known to develop a premalignant dysplasia in the metaplastic intestinalized epithelium, which is characteristic of this condition. A precise surveillance interval has not been established, but most authorities recommend surveillance endoscopy at 1- to 2-year intervals with four quadrant biopsies at 2-cm intervals throughout the columnar-lined segment (102). Severe or high-grade dysplasia documented by an expert pathologist is now considered an indication for esophagectomy (103). Frank early carcinoma is found in about 30% of such cases. Flow cytometry appears to offer another approach for identifying patients with CLE who are at high risk for developing adenocarcinoma for surveillance (104).

Tumor Markers

The use of tumor markers may be useful in the near future, not only for early detection of esophageal carcinomas, but also for monitoring and follow-up of various therapeutic procedures. Because no current methods are available to detect small masses and focal areas that commonly remain as residual tumors after surgery, these biomarkers may be unique in their application. Markers are produced during biosynthesis or degradation processes in malignant cells and are distinct in either qualitative or quantitative aspects from normal cell products. Relatively few markers are associated with oral and esophageal malignancies. The most promising of these are the differentiation markers, which include those for cytoskeletal proteins such as keratins, involucrin, and the associated particulate transglutaminase. These are of particular interest because of their specificity for epithelial neoplasms. Growth factors, isoantigens, and some specific hormone/enzyme markers also are under investigation and appear to have promise, but much work is still needed to develop these into reliable diagnostic techniques. It is speculated that, with modern techniques and multidisciplinary approaches, there soon may be specific and accurate biomarkers for the detection of early esophageal cancers (105). This capability for diagnosis of the earliest lesions will provide the best chance for cure of both major types of esophageal cancer.

STAGING OF ESOPHAGEAL CANCER

Computed Tomography

Computed tomography (CT) initially was considered highly accurate for staging esophageal cancer. However, with further experience and comparison with surgical pathology, it was recognized that intramural and transmural invasion (T stage) often is not accurately detected, leading to understaging in up to 40% of cases. The overall accuracy of CT in evaluating mediastinal nodes is only about 50%. In 1989, Halvorsen and Thompson provided an excellent update on the limited role of CT in staging esophageal neoplasms (106). They specifically warned of the frailties of CT for staging carcinoma of the distal esophagus and cardia. The major advantage for CT for esophageal cancer staging is the detection of gross invasion of adjacent organs and distant metastases.

Endoscopic Ultrasonography

The latest diagnostic technique involved with staging evaluation of esophageal cancer is endoscopic ultrasonography (EUS), introduced in the 1980s. Although not capable of a histologic diagnosis or detecting distant metastasis, it is capable of determining the longitudinal, circumferential, and transmural extent of esophageal malignancy. The primary benefit of EUS in esophageal cancer is for staging lesions under the TNM system. Relatively high-frequency ultrasound (7.5 or 12 mHz) is used to provide excellent resolution of the four layers of the esophageal wall and nearby structures. Therefore it has proven to be excellent and superior to CT for determining the T stage (depth of wall penetration) and the N stage (regional lymph node metastasis) with about 85% and 75% accuracy, respectively. In most cases, it is not capable of evaluating distant metastasis (M stage), which is best done by CT, conventional ultrasound, and other methods (107).

The initial clinical studies with EUS began about 1980. Instruments, techniques, and results have improved dramatically over the past decade. Numerous studies have reported the various clinical applications of EUS, but staging of carcinoma has proven to be the primary indication at this time. It is too early to assess whether EUS has an effect on outcome, especially relative to any improvement in survival or cure. However, it is now clear that selection of patients for available therapeutic options is enhanced by EUS (108,109). A major advantage of EUS is to identify patients in whom resection for cure or even palliation is not indicated. Much needless risk and suffering from unnecessary surgery is thereby prevented. Future clinical trials will use EUS to correctly stage patients into more homogenous groups for evaluation of various treatment regimens in stage-dependent protocols. Currently, both EUS and CT are necessary for optimal staging accuracy (110).

Transendoscopic ultrasound probes with very high resolution provided by a 20 mHz transducer are under investigation and may provide more precise definition and staging of the earliest mucosal malignancies.

TREATMENT OF ESOPHAGEAL CANCER

Surgery

No malignancy has stimulated more concerted efforts to cure with less success than cancer of the esophagus. This cancer was undoubtedly the basis for the surgical efforts to resect the esophagus begun by Billroth in dogs in 1870. Seven years later, Czerny, one of Billroth's students, performed the first successful resection of an esophageal carcinoma. Sadly, the major indicator of success, then and now, is that the patient survived the operation rather than being cured of the disease. That first operation was performed to remove a carcinoma of the cervical esophagus in a 51-year-old woman. She returned to work and lived for 1 year before dying of a recurrence (1). Esophagectomy for cancer was performed in a few patients over the next several years, with mortality rates near 100%.

As the 20th century dawned, the first intrathoracic resection of esophageal cancer was performed. In 1901, Dobromysslov resected a small cancer and restored continuity by an end-to-end anastomosis (1). In 1905, Beck demonstrated by animal experiment that the greater curvature of the stomach could be fashioned into a tube long enough to reach into the chest (111).

In 1907, Cesar Roux in Switzerland used an isolated jejunal loop with intact blood supply to join cervical esophagus and stomach and to bypass the intrathoracic esophagus.

Colon interposition was first tried in 1911 by Kelling (1). In 1913, Denk described a "pull-through" operation in cadavers done without opening the chest. Ochsner and De-Bakey reported that only 3 of 32 patients survived this operation up to 1941. They also reported that an operation devised by Torek in 1913, using a rubber tube to connect stomach and proximal esophagus, had an operative mortality of over 70% (112). In Hurt's review of esophageal cancer surgery, up until 1938, 30 successful resections (17 of the 30 in 1938) were reported by 13 different surgeons and only two patients had survived for 5 years (1). In 1948, Sweet reported an operative mortality of 16.5% for 181 esophageal resections, whereas up until 1938 191 resections had been reported in the literature, with mortality rates between 59 and 91%.

All imaginable approaches and anatomic variations to restore esophagogastric or esophagoenteric continuity were attempted between 1905 and 1938, with generally poor results and operative mortality rates in excess of 50%. Further improvement in the mortality rate for esophagectomy came after World War II, with better anesthesia, blood transfusion, improved pre- and postoperative care, and surgical technique. Even so, advanced disease at diagnosis, malnutrition, infections, technical failures such as anastomotic leaks, and inadequate supportive measures all combined to make esophagectomy a high-risk procedure.

In 1946, Ivor Lewis of London presented his experience with preliminary laparotomy to mobilize the stomach, followed by a right thoracotomy with esophageal resection and esophagogastric anastomosis. The earlier approach through the left chest had proved difficult because the aortic arch obstructed access to the middle and upper esophagus making anastomosis difficult. The relative success of the Ivor Lewis technique led to renewed surgical enthusiasm, and it continues to be the operation performed most often today. All techniques of esophageal resection with anastomosis have had to contend with anastomotic leaks as a significant complication. The use of resection with a high esophagogastric anastomosis in the lower cervical area has resulted in a reduced frequency of anastomotic leak.

Earlam and Cunha-Melo reviewed the results of surgery for esophageal cancer in 83,783 patients reported in the world literature before 1980 (113). Many surgeons and numerous variations in operative technique were used, with 5 year survival of about 6%. The operative mortality for this large series was about 30%, a result that led the surgeons to conclude that surgery for esophageal cancer carried the highest operative mortality of any elective surgical procedure performed at that time.

"New" operations continue to be reported, but few are new in the true sense. The trans-hiatal esophagectomy (without thoracotomy) technique recommended in recent years by Orringer (114) and others (115,116) was first proposed in 1913 by Denk as a "pull-through" operation he developed in cadavers. In 1933, Turner in England revived the Denk "blind" esophagectomy without thoracotomy because of the high morbidity and mortality of transthoracic resection. Orringer has reported an operative mortality of 6% with a 4-year survival of 17% (114). Interestingly, most esophageal surgeons continue to favor the classic Ivor Lewis resection technique by means of laparotomy and right thoracotomy because it allows better visualization and lymph node resection.

Reports during the past decade by expert surgeons are showing slight improvement in survival and operative mortality in highly selected patients (Table 2–3). More accurate staging, better patient selection, improved supportive care, including pre- and postoperative parenteral nutrition, collectively, are helping to reduce the operative mortality and improve prolonged survival. Lu et al. reported 1025 esophageal resections for cancer performed between 1953 and 1973 at Peking Medical College Hospital. Incidentally, only 5 of 1025 were adenocarcinomas. The best results appear from such experience, i.e., an operative mortality of 4.9% and a 5-year survival after resection of 20.9% (117). When survival by subgroups was evaluated separately, 32.7% of those with cancer of the lower third of the esophagus lived 5 years. Of those in this subgroup with negative lymph nodes, 64.2% survived for 5 years. Proper understanding of survival data for this disease requires a detailed understanding of how surgeons separate patients into highly selected subgroups. Unfortunately, the overall 5-year survival in most reports remains in the vicinity of 5 to 10%.

Rarely is surgical enthusiasm over the operative approach tempered by the decades-

Table 2–3
Surgical Survival for Resection of Carcinoma of the Esophagus*

Author(s)	Year	No. of Cases	Operative Mortality (%)	5-Year Survival (%)
Dark et al.	1981	449	7.6	18
Griffith and Davis	1980	211	11.4	15
Jackson et al.	1979	216	18.0	14
Lea	1987	205	10.0	15
McKeown	1979	392	12.2	—
Earlam and Cunha-Melo[124]	1980	83,783	29 ± 16	4 ± 3
Giuli & Gignoux	1980	2,400	30.0	14

* Modified with permission from Hurt RL: Management of Esophageal Carcinoma. London, New York, Springer-Verlag, 1989.

old fact that surgical treatment for most patients with esophageal cancer is fraught with high complication and mortality rates in most hands, and very low 5-year survival rates. In 1990, Kimose et al. found that in 657 patients treated over 25 years, operative mortality varied from 10 to 27% and the cumulative 5-year survival ranged from 0 to 26% (118). They recommend a more selective surgical approach because of the high morbidity and mortality and low 5-year survival rate.

An excellent overview of surgical experiences at a major medical center was reported by Katlic et al. in 1990 (119). Of 701 patients with squamous carcinoma, 411 were operated on and 261 of these were resected. The large discrepancy between those operated upon and those resected is noteworthy. These authors reported a dramatic reduction in postoperative death rate from 30.5% in the 1950s to 10.4% in the 1970s. Their best survival followed resection plus radiotherapy in 85 cases, with 35% alive at 2 years and 20% at 5 years. Note, however, that these figures are for 85 of 701 patients, or only 12% of all patients (119).

The grim results for surgery of esophageal cancer reviewed above are for patients who present with the usual symptomatic lesions and associated sequelae. Kato et al. reported experience with esophagectomy in 92 patients with early lesions, referred to as superficial esophageal carcinoma (SEC), with an operative mortality of 5.4%. In 24 patients, the cancer was limited to the mucosa, and in 68 to the submucosa. The 5-year survival rate for patients with SEC limited to the mucosa was 83.5%, and for those with cancer in the submucosa it was 54.9% (120).

Knowledge gained through extensive surgical experience with esophageal cancer over the past several decades finally appears to be tempering some surgical enthusiasm for continuing operative treatment for most lesions that are clearly incurable when first seen by a physician. History indicates that surgical therapy for cure should be used only for highly selected, accurately staged patients who are the best operative risks, with lesions that are resectable for possible cure. Palliative surgery for patients based on their ability to survive the operation for 30 days hence no longer seems justified.

From 1954 to 1988, 446 squamous cell carcinomas, 124 located in the distal esophagus, were coded in the tumor registry of the Southern California Permanente Medical Group (121). Radiation and surgery were equally efficacious for lesions located in the distal esophagus without evidence of distant metastases. There was no survival benefit in those operated on. These authors recommend nonsurgical palliative therapy, reserving surgery for special circumstances.

Radiation Therapy

A few patients with tumors at the "root of the neck" were treated by external radiation in the early years with temporary relief of symptoms (1). Early experiences with radiation therapy during the first two decades of this century were encouraging but disastrous for patients over the short term and for the therapists later because of excessive radiation exposure. In 1933, Cleminson and Monkhouse reported success with radiation in reducing tumor mass, but the side effects were often fatal (122).

As early as 1904, Einhorn and Exner began trials using radium placed in a bougie or in grooves in a vulcanite tube inserted into the esophagus (1,123). In 1921, Guisez used radium in a tube or bougie inserted into the esophagus and reported favorable palliative results, with relief in three patients for as long as 5, 10, and 11 years (124). In 1925, radium was inserted into the esophagus in silver containers that were attached to the teeth by a string. Others suggested use of a Souttar tube (prosthesis) with radium seed attached to the outside and lowered on a string into the esophagus (122). It would appear from the methods described that the radiation probably was often applied only to the upper end of the esophageal neoplasm and the normal esophagus proximal to the lesion. In 1937, Souttar reported on the techniques used to implant radium needles and seeds directly into the esophagus. Serious side effects included unequal delivery of radiation, strictures, and perforation.

While the poor results with intralumenal radium therapy were being recorded in the 1930s, new technology for radiation delivery was developed. Pearson reported that, between 1931 and 1947, radium internally by means of bougie and ortho voltage radiation gave only a 19% survival for one year, 5% for 3 years, and 2% for 5 years. The first encouraging results were observed from 1948 to 1955, when orthovoltage was reported by Pearson to provide survivals of 47% for 1 year and 29% for 5 years (125).

The modern era of radiation therapy for esophageal cancer was ushered in during the mid-1950s with introduction of linear accelerators that produced megavoltage and featured peak ionization occurrence at great depths below the skin surface (126). This development greatly reduced the earlier restrictions on radiation dosage based on skin tolerance. Pearson's work continued to be prominent in the field, and he reported exceptional results with megavoltage and radiotherapy between 1955 and 1964 (125), including survival rates of 44% for 1 year, 27% for 3 years, and 22% for 5 years. These results were indeed exciting and encouraging, but to date have not been duplicated by other radiation therapists.

Pearson strongly recommended that cancer in the proximal and middle thirds of the esophagus is best treated by radiation, and in the lower third by combined radiation and surgery (127). This policy has been followed in some institutions since his 1977 report, and continues to be as acceptable as any treatment at this time.

In 1980, Earlam and Cunha-Melo reviewed the worldwide results of radiation therapy in more than 8000 patients (128). By comparing a similar review in the same year of over 83,000 patients reported to have surgical resection, these authors concluded that radiation appeared to be the better treatment (113).

A major frustration among radiation therapists, clinicians who care for patients with esophageal cancer, and at least one surgeon, has been the fact that there has never been a properly conducted comparative study between surgery and radiation for esophageal cancer. Earlam, a British surgeon, organized a randomized study of radiotherapy versus surgery that began in 1988 (129). However, the study was discontinued after 18 months because the bias of participating surgeons toward surgery prevented them from following the protocol for randomization.

Earlam proceeded to study the results of radiation therapy alone in 22 patients staged

as having resectable lesions (130). In 1990, he reported a 46% survival for 1 year, 27% for 2 years, and 14% for 5 years. These results are equal to or better than those in most reports of surgical treatment, except in highly selected patients.

The strong bias toward surgery for esophageal cancer in the medical profession has prevented resolution of the therapeutic dilemma. Over 90% of symptomatic esophageal cancers have either metastasized or extended directly through the esophageal wall at the time of diagnosis. There probably is no single treatment capable of ensuring a significant cure rate. Success with present therapy depends primarily on diagnosis of lesions confined to a limited area of the esophageal wall. Recent reports on treatment of the earliest form of esophageal cancer suggest that such lesions, staged as T1 (limited to mucosa), can be cured by photodynamic laser therapy or endoscopic mucosectomy—procedures that may prove superior to surgery or radiation for early lesions. These nonsurgical approaches may prove as effective as surgery for cure after long-term follow-up data are available (110).

Combined Radiation and Chemotherapy with Surgery

During the past decade, several large studies using various combinations of radiation, chemotherapy, and hyperthermia were concluded. In the 1988 report by Sugimachi et al., hyperthermia combined with radiation and chemotherapy (HCR) was prescribed for patients with resectable and nonresectable squamous-cell carcinoma (96). Five-year survival rates for those with HCR and resection was 43.2%, whereas those who had only chemotherapy and radiation (CR) with resection had a 5-year survival of 14.7%. Two-year survival rates for those with unresectable carcinoma receiving HCR or CR alone were 15.5% and 1.2% respectively. The authors reported no serious side effects and suggest that hyperthermia shows promise of providing a significant improvement with low risk.

Radiation and Surgery

Since the 1930s, much experience with radiation and surgery has been reported, with variable results. A 1970 study from Japan reported a 25% 5-year survival. However, in 1976 Marks et al. reported only a 13.9% 5-year survival. When taking into account all the studies conducted using the best surgical candidates, Hurt reported few benefits from preoperative radiotherapy and even fewer benefits in patients receiving postoperative radiotherapy (1).

External Radiation Combined with Intracavitary Radiation (Brachytherapy)

Following the disastrous radiotherapeutic exploits in the early years by Einhorn and Exner in 1904, Guisez in 1921, and Souttar in 1937, using radium in one form or another, intraluminal radiation therapy fell into disrepute. However, after the development of nuclear reactors during World War II, several radioactive agents (^{60}Co needles, ^{182}Ta ins, ^{198}Au seeds, and ^{192}Ir seeds) became available in the 1950s. The availability of these radioisotopes and afterloading methods for safer use sparked interest in their potential application. With the advent of ^{60}CO teletherapy and linear accelerators, interest in brachytherapy appeared to wane until the early 1980s (90).

In 1989, Flores reported results in 171 patients treated with intracavitary radiation either before or after external beam radiation. The combination appeared safe and simple, with survival for 1 year of 33%, for 2 years of 26%, and for 3 years of 19% (131).

As of 1993, the new techniques of intraluminal radiation or brachytherapy, alone or in combination with other treatments, are being applied more widely, but data are too preliminary at this time.

Chemotherapy

The history of chemotherapy for esophageal carcinoma is one of toxicity, poor response rates, and no predictable or proven effect on survival or palliation. The concept of using chemical agents for treating diseases has been accepted for centuries. Quinine, an extract from the bark of the chinchona tree in Peru, was used to treat malaria in the 1600s. One of the earliest uses of chemical agents for malignant disease was potassium arsenite used for treating chronic leukemias by Lissauer and for lymphosarcoma by Billroth et al. in 1865. During the first half of the twentieth century, no chemotherapeutic agents with efficacy in esophageal cancer had been discovered (132).

In 1957, Heidelberger et al. synthesized 5-fluorouracil and its derivatives, but this agent, although widely used, never produced significant benefit for esophageal cancer (133). Rundles in 1962 reported the first "successful" treatment of esophageal carcinoma, with a 2-year survival in a patient treated with cyclophosphamide (134). A miraculous total remission and 5-year survival after cyclophosphamide therapy was reported by Dark in 1968 (135). This response is so rare that one should either immediately question the diagnosis or simply accept the response as a biologic curiosity.

Many chemotherapeutic agents have been used singly, in combination, or as adjunctive therapy to radiation and/or surgery over the past 3 decades with generally poor results for both the disease and the patients. Kelsen has conducted many studies on chemotherapy in esophageal cancer and has reviewed the extensive literature on the subject (136). He found that, even with the best of single agent trials, the response rate was no better than 20% with a duration of effect of only 2 to 5 months. Improved response rates (up to 80%) have been obtained by using combinations of drugs, but different reporting methods make interpretation of "response rates" and results unreliable. The duration of these partial responses is a maximum of 7 months and the overall survival remains poor (137).

The many reports for various combined therapies is a reflection of the frustration of esophageal cancer therapists. In a 1992 report, Herskovic et al. compared patients with squamous-cell cancer treated by chemotherapy and radiation with a group treated by radiation alone (138). Concurrent therapy with cisplatin and fluorouracil plus radiation was superior to radiation alone in survival (only 2.6 months longer median survival), at a cost of significantly more severe and life-threatening side effects. The effort to gain a few additional weeks of life at the expense of severe side effects seems unjustified.

Chemotherapy for esophageal cancer, both squamous-cell and adenocarcinoma, to date has been disappointing. In his detailed monograph, *Management of Esophageal*

Carcinoma, Hurt has indicated that there can be no justification for the general use of cytotoxic chemotherapy in this disease (1). Kelsen has further emphasized the importance of using chemotherapy only in patients in controlled clinical trials (136).

Laser Palliation

Even though the theory of the laser was conceived early in this century, it was not until 1960 that the first ruby laser was developed. Four years later, the laser was reported to be successful in destroying malignant tissue (139). By the early 1970s, the laser was being evaluated for its possible role in the treatment of acute and chronic gastrointestinal bleeding (140). In 1982, Fleischer et al. reported the first use of the endoscopic laser in the palliation of a malignant stricture of the esophagus (141). After a few preliminary studies, the laser was reportedly successful in the palliative relief of dysphagia, with few complications (141,142). Reports indicate that lumen patency can be restored in a majority of cases (142–144), but this does not necessarily improve swallowing or the patient's nutritional status (143,145). Generally, swallowing improvement can be obtained in 70 to 80% of patients with esophageal cancer using the Nd:YAG laser. The most serious complication is perforation of the esophagus, which occurs with an incidence of 0 to 9% (146). Laser therapy is associated with an increase in the 1-year survival rate (10 to 16%) and the median survival time (142,147). To date, no reason has been determined for these minimal improvements in survival.

Photodynamic Therapy (PDT)

In 1924, Policord reported that the presence of endogenous porphyrins causes some tumors to display a red-orange fluorescence when exposed to ultraviolet light. Subsequent studies in rats demonstrated that systemic injections of hematoporphyrin gave the characteristic red-orange fluorescence in tumors but not in normal tissue. It has been found subsequently that a hematoporphyrin derivative (HPD) produces a higher degree of fluorescence in neoplastic tissue (148). In 1968, a 75 to 85% correlation was shown between diagnosis by cancer fluorescence from intravenous HPD and positive biopsy for esophageal squamous cell and adenocarcinoma. The purpose of this original work was to use fluorescence as a diagnostic technique (149). Four years later, Diamond and Granelli reported that after injection of HPD into experimental tumors, destruction could be obtained by exposing the tumors to visible or near-ultraviolet light (150). However, Daugherty and his co-workers were the true pioneers of photodynamic therapy in the treatment of malignant tumors of humans, beginning in 1978 with the successful destruction of skin metastases from breast cancer and other solid tumors with light-activated HPD (151).

Daugherty later extracted an active mixture from HPD called dihematoporphyrin ether (DHE), which is given intravenously and disseminates throughout the body. It begins to clear rapidly from normal tissues, but malignant neoplasms retain large concentrations. The tumor then is exposed to light at a wavelength of 630 nm, which activates the dye and produces singlet oxygen radicals that cause death of tumor tissue (148). PDT has been used to palliate advanced esophageal carcinoma and to relieve dysphagia with few complications. The most common complication is sunburn because skin tissue is rendered hypersensitive to sunlight for several weeks (152,153). During this time, the patient must remain out of sunlight to avoid side effects. More recently, PDT has been used to treat early (superficial) esophageal cancer and is reported to give a high complete response rate with very few recurrences after long-term follow-up (146,154,155).

Ethanol-Induced Tumor Necrosis (ETN)

Endoscopic local injections of absolute alcohol (ethanol) into gastric carcinomas to induce necrosis was first reported in 1984 (156). Three years later, Payne-James et al. reported the use of ETN in the relief of dysphagia caused by malignant strictures of the esophagus (157). Two studies report that ETN gives good palliative relief of dysphagia with no major complications. It has been suggested that this may be the best new form of palliation for dysphagia from esophageal carcinoma (158). ETN therapy is inexpensive, safe and relatively pain-free.

Endoscopic Esophageal Mucosal Resection (EMRT)

In 1990, Endo and Inoue reported on the development of a new method of endoscopic esophageal mucosal resection using a transparent tube (159). They used the Olympus EMRT overtube and a forward-viewing fiberscope. A tumor up to 2 cm in diameter can be resected and the lesion electrically excised with the resulting ulcer healing within 1 month. Endo reports complete resection of early-stage esophageal cancer with few complications (160). This technique and PDT currently are indicated as curative therapy only for patients with cancer confined to the mucosa, who are not considered good surgical risks or who refuse surgery.

Bipolar Electrocoagulation

In 1985, Johnston et al. reported on the development and experimental testing of a large bipolar coagulation tumor probe (BICAP) for the palliative treatment of obstructing esophageal carcinomas. The tumor probe is provided in several diameters with an active electrode banded around the circumference of a spindle-shaped segment. The size probe that fits the structured segment snugly is positioned on withdrawal over a guide wire, and coagulating current is applied at successive 1-cm intervals. The next larger size is passed similarly until a suitable lumen diameter is reached (161). Initial reports indicated that the probe was a useful palliative device with promise (162–164). In a comparative study of the Nd-YAG laser and the BICAP tumor probe, it was recommended that the probe be used in place of the laser because of its similar palliative results and significantly lower cost (163). However, it was recognized that the probe should be used only in completely circumferential tumors because of possible coagulation of normal tissue on any uninvolved wall leading to perforation. A new model with a 180-degree electrode has been developed to reduce the risk of perforation, but this ablation method is not often used at this time.

Palliative Intubation

The ideal palliation for dysphagia caused by malignant esophageal obstruction should be effective, safe, generally available, and relatively inexpensive. Palliative intubation for prosthesis or stent offers treatment with these characteristics for most patients with malignant obstruction.

In 1885, Symonds performed the first successful permanent esophageal intubation using a gum elastic tube passed blindly on a special introducer and held in place by an attached string tied around the patient's ear. This prosthesis remained in place for 8 months until the patient's death (165). In 1924, Souttar introduced a coiled silver wire tube that was introduced blindly. Needless to say, this technique was ineffective (166). In 1952, Berman attempted use of a plastic tube to surgically replace a resected segment of the esophagus. The expected high morbidity and mortality condemned this procedure (167).

Esophageal prosthesis palliation became more popular in 1954 after Kropff placed a polyurethane tube through an esophageal tumor by means of a cervical esophagostomy (168). In 1956, Mousseau and Barbin used a neoplex tube inserted by way of mouth and positioned by pulling the tube through a small gastrostomy incision (169). Three years later, Celestin developed a latex tube specially adapted for peroral placement with surgical assistance, similar to the Mousseau-Barbin technique (170). This surgical method proved to have unacceptable morbidity and mortality.

Expanded use of the peroral prosthesis followed the report of O'Connor et al. in 1963, reviewing their experience in 378 patients using a homemade polyethylene prosthesis (171). Their method proved to be simple, safe, and effective for dysphagia relief in most patients. This homemade prosthesis was modified years later by Boyce and Palmer using a polyvinyl tube and different peroral introducer apparatus over a guide wire (172,173). The technique is simple and safe, and offers the major advantage of tailoring the prosthesis specifically for each patient. Tytgat et al. introduced several modifications of the homemade polyvinyl prosthesis and added a wire spiral for structural support in the prosthesis shaft (174). A relatively high rate of perforation initially detracted from this technique. A more careful preparation by gradual esophageal dilation has reduced the perforation rate to less than 5%.

The first commercially made peroral pulsion esophageal (silicone) prosthesis with its Nottingham Introducer (Key Med) became available in 1977 (175). This prosthesis is made in two diameters and four lengths. Although it is effective, the perforation rate with this system also varied between 5 and 10% which is too high for a palliative method (176). The Wilson-Cook silicone prothesis is similar in design to the original homemade prosthesis and has a metal spiral support in the shaft walls. The Dumon introducer used over a guide wire has proved safe and easy to use. An excellent review of esophageal intubation for palliation of malignant esophageal obstruction was provided by Earlam and Cunha-Melo in 1982 (177).

A special prosthesis (Wilson-Cook) with an inflatable balloon on its shaft is being used for palliating esophagopulmonary fistulas that complicate esophageal cancer (178). This prosthesis has proven helpful in selected patients for relieving the debilitating cough and pulmonary soilage that occurs with these fistulas.

A major development in the potential for endoluminal prostheses was the introduction of the first expandable intravascular metal stent in 1985. In 1990, Domschke et al. described a metal mesh esophageal stent and reported the problem of tumor growth through the mesh (179). Reports in 1991 and 1992 described further modifications in the mesh construction and with silicone coating to reduce tumor ingrowth (180–182). Initial reports on experience with the expanding metal stents indicate that future modifications of this technique will revolutionize and broaden the clinical application of prostheses for the palliation of malignant dysphagia.

CONCLUSIONS

The history of progress and acquisition of knowledge about esophageal malignancies and premalignant conditions has been hindered mostly by our inability to understand the biologic nature of these disorders. Squamous-cell cancer and adenocarcinoma of the esophagus begin insidiously, grow steadily, and metastasize transmurally and to regional nodes readily—all before the patient becomes aware of any disturbing symptoms. Diagnosis also is delayed because the patient, even with significant dysphagia, often fails to seek medical help for 3 to 6 months. Further delay in diagnosis occurs when the physician fails to recognize the significance of dysphagia and other symptoms with or without weight loss. However, in the vast majority of patients, the diagnosis is promptly suspected on the basis of the medical history, precisely localized by barium esophagram, and accurately confirmed by fiberoptic endoscopy with guided biopsy. Diagnosis is not usually the problem. Therapy is the major problem and the focus of effort during this century by surgeons, radiotherapists, chemotherapists, and gastroenterologists. The accurate diagnostic techniques developed by gastroenterologists, radiotherapists, and surgeons undoubtedly represent the most tangible achievements in managing esophageal cancer since 1900. Most of the positive knowledge gained relates to palliation rather than to cure.

Future research and clinical efforts must be directed toward screening and earlier cancer diagnosis before transmural invasion and distant metastasis if cure rates are to improve. Surgical resection or radiotherapy offer the only current hope for curing symptomatic malignancies in a few highly selected patients who can be identified properly with the most modern staging methods. Chemotherapy should be considered only for controlled research trials. Knowledge most needed for the future includes development of sensitive and specific screening methods; identification of the populations at highest risk; specific, safe and effective chemotherapy regimens; and most importantly, methods to reduce risk and to prevent malignant transformation of esophageal epithelial cells.

ACKNOWLEDGMENT

The author wishes to express sincere appreciation to Sean Dingle for his careful, detailed literature research and to Joanne Penders for her expert typing and secretarial assistance.

REFERENCES

1. Hurt RL: Management of Esophageal Carcinoma. London, New York, Springer-Verlag, 1989.
2. Blot WJ, Devesa SS, Kneller RW, Fraumeni JF: Rising incidence of adenocarcinoma of the esophagus and gastric cardia. JAMA 265:1287, 1991.
3. Hesketh PJ, Clapp RW, Doos WG, Spechler SJ: Increasing frequency of adenocarcinoma of the esophagus. Cancer 64: 526, 1989.
4. Davies S: Cancer in China. Br Med J i:131, 1924.
5. Elgood CA: A medical history of Persia. London, Cambridge University Press, 1951.
6. Thurnham DI, Munoz N, Wahrendorf J, Crespi M: Aetiology of esophageal cancer. Lancet i:1500, 1987.
7. Wynder EL, Lemon FR, Bross IJ: Cancer and coronary artery disease among Seventh Day Adventists. Cancer 5:1016, 1959.
8. Enstrom JE: Cancer mortality among Mormons in California during 1965–75. J Natl Cancer Inst 65:1073, 1980.
9. Lyon JL, Gardner JW, West DW: Cancer incidence in Mormons and non-Mormons in Utah during 1967–75. J Natl Cancer Inst 65:1055, 1980.
10. Doll R: The geographical distribution of cancer. Br J Cancer 23:1, 1969.
11. Doll R: Prevention of cancer: Pointers from epidemiology. London, Nuffield Provincial Hospitals Trust, 1967.
12. Graham S, Levin M, Lilienfeld M: The socio-economic distribution of cancer of various sites in Buffalo, New York 1948–52. Cancer 13:180, 1960.
13. Waterhouse J, Muir C, Shanmugaratnam K, Powell J: Cancer incidence in five continents, vol IV. IARC, Lyon (IARC Scientific Publication no. 42), 1982.
14. Crespi M et al.: Esophageal lesions in Northern Iran: A premalignant condition? Lancet ii:217, 1979.
15. Cutler SJ, Devesa SS: Trends in cancer incidence and mortality in the USA. In: Doll R, Vodpija I (eds). Host environment interactions in the etiology of cancer in man. IARC, Lyon (Scientific Publications, no. 7), 1973, pp. 15–34.
16. Audigier JC, Tuyns AJ, Lambert R: Epidemiology of esophageal cancer in France. Digestion 13:209, 1975.
17. Tuyns A, Masse LMF: Mortality from cancer of the esophagus in Brittany. Int J Epidemiol 2:242, 1973.
18. Silverberg E, Boring CC, Squires TS: Cancer statistics, 1990. CA—A Cancer Journal for Clinicians. 40:119, Jan. Feb. 1990.
19. King H, Locke FB: Cancer mortality risk among Japanese in the United States, J Natl Cancer Inst 65:1149, 1980.
20. Howel-Evans W, McCowwell R, Clarke CA, Sheppard PM: Carcinoma of the esophagus with keratosis. Palmaris et Plantaris (Tylosis). QJ Med 27:413, 1958.
21. O'Mahony MY et al.: Familial tylosis and carcinoma of the esophagus. J Roy Soc Med 77:514, 1984.
22. Appelqvist P, Salmo M: Lye corrosion carcinoma of the esophagus: A review of 63 cases. Cancer 45:2655, 1980.
23. Young M, Russell WT: An investigation into the statistics of cancer in different trades and professions. Her Majesty's Stationery Office, London, 1926.
24. Steiner P: Aetiology and histogenesis of carcinoma of oesophagus. Cancer 9:436, 1956.
25. Martinez I: Factors associated with cancer of the oesophagus, mouth and pharynx in Puerto Rico. J Natl Cancer Inst 42:1069, 1969.
26. Hakulinen JS, Lehtimaki L, Lehtonen M, Tappo L: Cancer morbidity among two male cohorts with increased alcohol consumption in Finland. J Natl Cancer Inst 52: 1711, 1974.
27. Wynder EL, Bross IJ: A study of etiological factors in cancer of the esophagus. Cancer 14:389, 1961.
28. Day NE, Muñoz N, Ghadirian P: Epidemiology of oesophageal cancer. A review. In Correa P, Haenszel W (eds): Epidemiology of Cancer of the Digestive Tract. Netherlands, Martinus Nijhoff, 1982.
29. Wynder EL, Klein UE: The possible role of riboflavin deficiency in epithelial neoplasia. I. Epithelial changes of mice in simple deficiency. Cancer 18:167, 1965.
30. Vitalle JJ, Coffey J: Alcohol and vitamin metabolism. In Kissin B, Begleiter H (eds): Biology of Alcoholism, vol 1. Biochemistry. New York, Plenum Press, pp 327–352, 1971.
31. Kmet J, Mahboubi E: Esophageal cancer in the Caspian littoral of Iran: Initial studies. Science 175:846, 1972.
32. Hormozdiari H, Day NE, Aramesh R, Mahboubi E: Dietary factors and oesophageal cancer in the Caspian littoral of Iran. Cancer Res 35:3493, 1975.
33. Cook-Mozaffari P: The epidemiology of cancer of the oesphagus. Nutr Cancer 1:51, 1979.
34. Pottern LM et al.: Esophageal cancer among black men in Washington DC: Alco-

hol, tobacco and other risk factors. J Natl Cancer Inst *67*:777, 1985.

35. Fong LYY, Newberne PM: Nitrosbenzylmethylamine zinc deficiency and oesophageal cancer. *In* Griciute L, Lyle R (eds): Environmental aspects of N-nitroso compounds. Lyon IARC Scientific Publications, No. 19 pp. 503–516, 1978.

36. Reinbold JG et al.: Decreased absorption of calcium, magnesium, zinc and phosphorous by humans due to increased fibre and phosphorus consumption as wheat bread. J Nutr *106*:493, 1976.

37. Muñoz N et al.: No effect of riboflavin, retinol and zinc on prevalence of precancerous lesions of oesophagus. Lancet *iii*:111, 1985.

38. Burrell RJW, Roach WA, Shadwell A: Esophageal cancer in the Bantu of Transkei associated with mineral deficiency in garden plants. J Natl Cancer Inst *36*:201, 1966.

39. Magee PN, Barnes JM: Carcinogenic nitroso compounds. Adv Cancer Res *10*:168, 1976.

40. Kaplan HS, Tsuchitani PJ (eds): Cancer in China. New York, Alan R Liss, 1978.

41. Bogovski P, Castegnaro M, Pegnatelli B, Walker EA: The inhibiting effect of tannins on the formation of nitrosamines. *In* Bogovski P, Preussmann R, Walker EA (eds): N-nitroso compounds. Analysis and formation. Lyon, IARC Scientific Publications No. 3, pp. 127–129, 1972.

42. Mirvish SS, Wallcave L, Eagen M, Shubik P: Ascorbate-nitrate reaction: Possible means of blocking the formation of carcinogenic N-nitroso compounds. Science *177*: 65, 1972.

43. IARC Annual Report. World Health Organization, Lyon, France, 1975.

44. IARC Annual Report. World Health Organization, Lyon, France, 1976.

45. Pamukbu AM, Price JM: Induction of intestinal and urinary bladder cancer in rats by feeding bracken fern *(Pteris acquilina)*. J Natl Cancer Inst *43*:275, 1969.

46. Hirayama T: Diet and cancer. Nutr Cancer *1*:67, 1979.

47. Li MH: Studies of potential carcinogens in the diet of individuals of high risk for oesophageal cancer. *In* Marks PA (ed): Cancer research in the PRC and USA. New York, Grune and Stratton, 1981.

48. Lu SH et al.: Mutagenicity of extracts of pickled vegetables collected in Linxian county, a high-incidence area for oesophageal cancer in northern China. J Natl Cancer Inst *66*:33, 1981.

49. Doll R: Oesophageal cancer: A preventable disease? In: International Seminar on the Epidemiology of Oesophageal Cancer (syl-

labus). Bangalore, Indian Cancer Society and UICC, 1971.

50. Watson WL: Carcinoma of the esophagus. Surg Gynec Obst *56*:884, 1933.

51. Cheng PCL: Carcinoma of the oesophagus. A statistical study of forty-three cases. Chin Med J *67*:662, 1949.

52. Burrell RJW: Oesophageal cancer in the Bantu. S Afr Med J *31*:401, 1957.

53. Sato T: An approach method for finding causative agents of human cancer of environmental origin through the analyses of the relation between the distribution of the agents and the incidence rates of the cancer. Bull Inst Public Health, Tokyo *12*:160, 1963.

54. Hirayama T: An epidemiology study of cancer of the oesophagus in Japan, with special reference to the combined effect of selected environmental factors. In: International Seminar on the Epidemiology of Oesophageal Cancer. Bangalore, Indian Cancer Society and UICC, 1971.

55. Segi M: Tea gruel as a possible factor for cancer of the oesophagus. Gan No Rinsho *66*:199, 1975.

56. De Jong UW et al.: Aetiological factors in oesophageal cancer in Singapore Chinese. Int J Cancer *13*:291, 1974.

57. Cook-Mozaffari PJ et al.: Oesophageal cancer studies in the Caspian littoral of Iran: Results of a case-control study. Br J Cancer *39*:293, 1979.

58. Victoria CG et al.: Hot beverages and oesophageal cancer in southern Brazil: A case control study. Int J Cancer *39*:710, 1987.

59. Rose EF: The interplay of factors determining a cancer pattern. Progr Exp Tumour Res *12*:95, 1969.

60. Jarret WFH et al.: High incidence of cattle cancer with a possible interaction between an environmental carcinogen and a papilloma virus. Nature *274*:215, 1978.

61. O'Neill CH et al.: A fine silica contaminant of flour in the high oesophageal cancer area of Iran. Int J Cancer *26*:617, 1980.

62. O'Neill CH et al.: Silica fragments from millet bran in mucosa surrounding oesophageal tumors in patients in northern China. Lancet *i*:1202, 1982.

63. Grossman TW et al.: Role of esphagoscopy in the evaluation of patients with head and neck carcinoma. Ann Otol Rhinol Laryngol *92*:369, 1983.

64. Nakayma N et al.: A report of three cases with carcinoma developing after ante thoracic reconstructive surgery of the esophagus (by skin graft). Surgery *69*:800, 1971.

65. Horvath OP, Bajusz H, Borbly L: Skin cancer: A late complication of skin tube esophagus. Br J Surg *78*:1467, 1991.

66. Just-Viera JO, Haight C: Achalasia and carcinoma of the esophagus. Surg Gynecol Obstet *128*:1081, 1969.

67. Barrett NR: Achalasia of the cardia: Reflections upon a clinical study of over 100 cases. Br Med J *i*:1135, 1964.

68. Maijssen MA et al.: Achalasia complicated by esophageal squamous cell carcinoma: A prospective study in 195 patients. Gut *33*: 155, 1992.

69. Chuong J, DuBovik S, McCallum RW: Achalasia as a risk factor for esophageal carcinoma: A reappraisal. Dig Dis Sci *29*: 1105, 1984.

70. Wychulis AR, Woolam GL, Anderesen HA, Ellis FH: Achalasia and carcinoma of the esophagus. JAMA *215*:1638, 1971.

71. Williams JL: Carcinoma of the oesophagus as a complication of achalasia of the cardia. Thorax *11*:268, 1956.

72. Joske RA, Benedict EB: The role of benign esophageal obstruction in the development of carcinoma of the esophagus. Gastroenterology *36*:749, 1959.

73. Barrett NR: Chronic peptic ulcers of the esophagus and esophagitis. Br J Surg *38*: 175, 1950.

74. Allison PR, Johnstone AS, Royce GB: The esophagus lined with gastric membrane. Thorax *8*:87, 1953.

75. McKinley M, Sherlock P: Barrett's esophagus with adenocarcinoma in scleroderma. Am J Gastroenterology *79*:438, 1984.

76. Hennessy TPJ, Cuschieri A, Bennett JR: Reflux Oesophagitis. Boston and London, Butterworths, 1989.

77. Everhart CW, Holtzapple PG, Humphries TJ: Barrett's esophagus: Inherited epithelium or inherited reflux? J Clin Gastroenterology *5*:357, 1983.

78. Jochem VJ, Fuerst PA, Fromkes JJ: Familial Barrett's esophagus associated with adenocarcinoma. Gastroenterology *102*:1400, 1992.

79. Rabinovitch PS et al.: Progresion to cancer in Barrett's esophagus is associated with genomic instability. Laboratory Investigation *60*:65, 1988.

80. Levi F et al.: The consumption of alcohol, tobacco and the risk of adenocarcinoma in Barrett's esophagus. Int J Cancer *45*:852, 1990.

81. Gray JR, Coldman AJ, MacDonald WC: Cigarette and alcohol use in patients with adenocarcinoma of the gastric cardia or lower esophagus. Cancer *69(a)*:2267, 1992.

82. Casson AG et al.: Gene mutations in Barrett's epithelium and esophageal cancer. Cancer Research *51*:4495, 1991.

83. Hawe A, Payne WS, Wieland LH: Adenocarcinoma in the columnar epithelial lined lower (Barrett's) esophagus. Thorax *28*: 511, 1973.

84. Naef AP, Savary M, Ozzello L: Columnar-lined lower esophagus: An acquired lesion with malignant predisposition: Report on 140 cases of Barrett's esophagus with 12 adenocarcinomas. J Thorac Cardiovasc Surg *70*:826, 1975.

85. Haggitt RC, Tryzelaar J, Ellis HF, Colcher H: Adenocarcinoma complicating columnar epithelium-lined (Barrett's) esophagus. Am J Clin Pathol *70*:1, 1978.

86. Wang HH, Antonioli DA, Goldman H: Comparative features of esophageal and gastric adenocarcinomas: Recent change in type and frequency. Hum Pathol *17*:482, 1986.

87. Guanrei Y, Sonliang Q, He H, Guizen F: Natural history of early esophageal squamous carcinoma and early adenocarcinoma of the gastric cardia in the People's Republic of China. Endoscopy *20*:95, 1988.

88. Watson WL, Goodner JT, Miller TP, Pack GT: Torek esophagectomy: the case against segmental resection for esophageal cancer. J Thorac Surg *32*:347, 1956.

89. Helsley GF: The metastasizing tendency of esophagus carcinoma. Ann Surg *77*:272, 1923.

90. Perez CA: Principles and Practices of Radiation Oncology. Philadelphia, JB Lippincott Company, 1987.

91. Rumpel T: Die klinische diagnose der spindel formigen speiserohrenez Weiterung. Munch Med Wschr *44*:420, 1897.

92. Skucas J: The routine double-contrast examination of the esophagus. Crit Rev Diag Imag *11*:121, 1978.

93. LoPresti PA, Cifarelli PS, Dixit N, Kasinathan M: Successful examination of the esophagus and stomach with a new fiberoptic instrument. Gastrointest Endosc *3*:103, 1971.

94. Schiller W: Early diagnosis of carcinoma of the cervix. Surg Gyn Obstet *56*:210, 1933.

95. Endo M et al.: Observations of esophageal lesions with the use of endoscopic dyes. Prog in Dig Endosc *1*:34, 1972.

96. Sugimachi K et al.: Lugol-combined endoscopic detection of minute malignant lesions of the thoracic esophagus. Ann Surg *208*:179, 1988.

97. Shiozaki H et al.: Endoscopic screening of early esophageal cancer with the Lugol dye method in patients with head and neck cancers. Cancer *66*:2068, 1990.

98. Brodmerkel GJ: Schiller's test: An aid in esophagoscopic diagnosis. Gastroenterology *60*:813, 1971.

99. Herlin P et al.: A study of the mechanism of toluidine blue dye test. Endoscopy *15*:4, 1983.

100. Chobanian SJ et al.: In vivo staining with toluidine blue as an adjunct to the endoscopic detection of Barrett's esophagus. Gastrointest Endosc *33*:99, 1987.

101. Nabeya K, Ri S, Miyajima H: Mass-screening using capsulated brushing cytology for esophageal cancer. *In* Kassi M (ed): Esophageal Cancer. Current Clinical Practice Series, No. 40. Tokyo, Excerpta Medica, 1961.

102. Reid BJ et al.: Endoscopic biopsies can detect high grade dysplasia or early adenocarcinoma and Barrett's esophagus without grossly recognizable neoplastic lesions. Gastroenterology *94*:81, 1988.

103. Hamilton SR, Smith RRL: The relationship between columnar epithelial dysplasia and invasive adenocarcinoma arising in Barrett's esophagus. Am J Clin Pathol *87*:301, 1987.

104. Reid BJ, Haggitt RC, Rubin CE, Rabinovitch PS: Barrett's esophagus: Correlation between flow cytometry and histology in detection of patients at risk for adenocarcinoma. Gastroenterology *93*:1, 1987.

105. Mufti SI, Zirvi KA, Garewal HS: Precancerous lesions and biologic markers in esophageal cancer. Cancer Detection and Prevention *15*:291, 1991.

106. Halvorsen RA Jr., Thompson WM: CT of esophageal neoplasms. Radiol Clin North Am *27*:667, 1989.

107. Botet JF et al.: Endoscopic ultrasonography in the preoperative staging of esophageal cancer: A comparative study with dynamic CT. Radiology *181*:419, 1991.

108. Tio TL, Tytgat GN: Endoscopic ultrasonography in the assessment of intra and transmural infiltration of tumors in the oesophagus, stomach and papilla of Vater and detection of extraesophageal lesions. Endoscopy *16*:203, 1984.

109. Tio TL, Coene PPLO, Luiken GJHM, Tytgat GNJ: Endosonography in the clinical staging of esophagogastric carcinoma. Gastrointestinal Endsocopy *36*:S2, 1990.

110. Lambert R: Endoscopic therapy of esophago-gastric tumors. Endoscopy *35*:531, 1992.

111. Beck C: Demonstration of specimens illustrating a method of formation of a pre-thoracic esophagus. IMJ *7*:463, 1905.

112. Oschner A, DeBakey M: Surgical aspects of a carcinoma of the esophagus. J Thorac Surg *10*:401, 1941.

113. Earlam R, Cunha-Melo JR: Esophageal squamous cell carcinoma: I. A critical review of surgery. Br J Surg *67*:381, 1980.

114. Orringer MB: Transhiatal esophagectomy without thoracotomy for carcinoma of the thoracic esophagus. Ann Surg *200*:282, 1984.

115. Kirk RM: Partial and complete sternotomy for blunt esophagectomy. Br J Surg *74*:685, 1987.

116. Ochsner A Jr.: Discussion of Orringer MB, Sloan H: Esophagectomy without thoracotomy. J Thorac Cardiovasc Surg *76*:643, 1978.

117. Lu YK, Li VM, Gu YZ: Cancer of esophagus and esophagogastric junction: Analysis of results of 1,025 resections after 5 to 20 years. Ann Thorac Surg *43*:176, 1987.

118. Kimose H et al.: Independent predictors of operative mortality and postoperative complications in surgically treated carcinomas of the esophagus and cardia—Is the aggressive surgical approach worthwhile? Acta Chir Scand *156*:373, 1990.

119. Katlic MR, Wilkins EW, Jr, Grillo HC: Three decades of treatment of esophageal squamous carcinoma at the Massachusetts General Hospital. J Thorac Cardiovasc Surg *99*:929, 1990.

120. Kato H et al.: Superficial esophageal carcinoma: Surgical treatment and results. Cancer *66*:2319, 1990.

121. Harvey JC et al.: Squamous carcinoma of the distal esophagus: A survival study. J Surg Oncol *46*:97, 1991.

122. Cleminson FJ, Monkhouse JP: Carcinoma of esophagus treated with radiation. Proc Roy Soc Med *27*:365, 1933.

123. Einhorn M: Observations on radium. Med Rec *66*:164, 1904.

124. Baum SM: Esophageal-gastric carcinoma successfully treated by protracted fractional x-ray. Radiology *27*:58, 1936.

125. Pearson JG. The radiotherapy of carcinoma of the esophagus and post cricoid region in southeast Scotland. Clin Radiol *17*:242, 1966.

126. Swann GW: Optimization of Human Cancer Radiotherapy. Berlin, New York, Springer-Verlag, 1981.

127. Pearson JG: The present status and future potential of radiotherapy in the management of esophageal cancer. Cancer *39*:882, 1977.

128. Earlam R, Cunha-Melo JR: Esophageal squamous carcinoma: A critical review of radiotherapy. Br J Surg *67*:457, 1980.

129. Earlam R: An MRC prospective randomized trial of radiotherapy versus surgery for operable squamous cell carcinoma of the esophagus. Ann Roy Coll Surg Eng *73*:8, 1991.

130. Earlam RJ, Johnson L: 101 esophageal can-

cers: A surgeon uses radiotherapy. Ann Roy Coll Surg Eng *72*:32, 1990.

131. Flores AD et al.: Cancer of the esophagus and cardia: Overview of radiotherapy. Can J Surg *32*:404, 1989.

132. Burchenal JH: The historical development of cancer chemotherapy. Semin Oncol *4*: 135, 1977.

133. Heidelberger C, Chanduri NK, Danneberg P: Fluorinated pyrimidines, a new class of tumor-inhibitory compounds. Nature *179*: 663, 1957.

134. Rundles, W: Definition of clinical problems. Cancer Chemotherapy Reports *2*:1, 1962.

135. Dark JF: Apparent cure of cancer with cyclophosphamide. Brit Med J *19*:161, 1968.

136. Kelsen D: Chemotherapy of esophageal cancer. Semin Oncol *11*:159, 1984.

137. Kelsen KP et al.: Cisplatin, vindesine and bleomycin combination chemotherapy of local-regional and advanced esophageal carcinoma. Am J Med *75*:639, 1983.

138. Herskovic A et al.: Combined chemotherapy and radiotherapy compared with radiotherapy alone in patients with cancer of the esophagus. N Engl J Med *326*:1593, 1992.

139. Minton JP, Ketchum AS: The laser, a unique oncolytic entity. Am J Surg *108*:845, 1964.

140. Buset M et al.: Nd-YAG Laser, A new palliative alternative in the management of esophageal cancer. Endoscopy *15*:353, 1983.

141. Fleischer D, Kessler F, Hay O: Endoscopic Nd:YAG laser therapy for carcinoma of the esophagus: A new palliative approach. Am J Surg *143*:280, 1982.

142. Spinelli P, Dal Fante M, Mancini A: Endoscopic palliation of malignancies of the upper gastrointestinal tract using Nd:YAG Laser: Results and survival in 308 treated patients. Lasers Surg Med *11*:550, 1991.

143. Mellow M, Pinkas H: Endoscopic laser therapy for malignancies affecting the esophagus and gastroesophageal junction. Arch Intern Med *145*:1443, 1985.

144. Buset M et al.: Palliative endoscopic management of obstructive esophagogastric cancer: laser or prosthesis. Gastrointest Endosc *33*:357, 1987.

145. Mellow M, Pinkas H: Endoscopic therapy for esophageal carcinoma with Nd:YAG laser: Prospective evaluation of efficacy, complications and survival. Gastrointest Endosc *30*:334, 1984.

146. Overholt BF: Laser and photodynamic therapy of esophageal cancer. Semin Surg Oncol *8*:191, 1992.

147. Siegal H et al.: The effect of endoscopic laser therapy on survival of patients with squamous cell carcinoma of the esophagus. J Clin Gastroenterology *13*:142, 1991.

148. McCaughan JS, Jr: Photodynamic therapy of skin and esophageal cancers. Cancer Invest *8*:407, 1990.

149. Gregorie Jr H et al.: Hematoporphyrin-derivative fluorescence in malignant neoplasms. Ann Surg *167*:820, 1968.

150. Diamond I, Granelli S: Photodynamic therapy for malignant tumors. Lancet *ii*:1175, 1972.

151. Daugherty TJ et al.: Photoradiation therapy for the treatment of malignant tumors. Cancer Research *38*:2628, 1978.

152. McCaughan Jr J et al.: Photodynamic therapy for esophageal tumors. Arch Surg *124*: 74, 1989.

153. Hayata Y et al.: Photodynamic therapy with hematoporphyrin derivative in cancer of the upper gastrointestinal tract. Semin Surg Oncol *1*:1, 1985.

154. Tian M, Qui S, Ji Q: Preliminary results of hematoporphyrin derivative-laser treatment for 13 cases of early esophageal carcinoma. Adv Exp Med Biol *193*:21, 1985.

155. Fujimaki M, Nakayama K: Endoscopic laser treatment of superficial esophageal cancer. Semin Surg Oncol *2*:248, 1986.

156. Maruyama M et al.: Endoscopic treatment of gastric carcinoma by local injection of pure ethanol. Proceedings of European Gastrointestinal Endoscopy Congress (Lisbon 1984): abstract 29.

157. Payne-James JJ, Spiller RC, Misiewicz JJ, Silk DBA: Use of ethanol-induced tumor necrosis to palliate dysphagia in patients with esphagogastric cancer. Gastrointest Endosc *36*:43, 1990.

158. Nwokolo C et al.: Palliation of malignant dysphagia by ethanol-induced tumor necrosis (ETN). International Congress on Cancer of the Esophagus (abstract), June 7–10, 1992.

159. Inoue H, Endo M: Endoscopic esophageal mucosal resection using a transparent tube. Surg Endosc *4*:198, 1990.

160. Endo M: Endoscopic resection of mucosal cancer of the esophagus. International Congress on Cancer of the Esophagus (*abstract*). June 7–10, 1992.

161. Johnston JH, Fleischer D, Petrini J, Nord HJ: Palliative bipolar electrocoagulation of obstructing esophageal cancer. Gastrointestinal Endoscopy *33*:349, 1987.

162. Fleischer D: A comparison of endoscopic laser therapy and BICAP tumor probe therapy for esophageal cancer. Am J Gastroenterol *82*:608, 1987.

163. Jensen DM et al.: Comparison of low power

YAG laser and BICAP tumor probe for palliation of esophageal cancer strictures. Gastroenterology 94:1263, 1988.

164. McIntyre AS et al.: Palliative therapy of malignant esophageal strictures with the bipolar tumor probe and prosthetic tube. Gastrointest Endosc 35:531, 1989.

165. Symonds CJ: A case of malignant stricture of the esophagus illustrating the use of the new form of esophageal catheter. Trans Chir Soc Lond 18:155, 1885.

166. Souttar HS: Method of intubating the esophagus for malignant stricture. Br Med J i:782, 1924.

167. Berman EF: A plastic prothesis for resected esophagus. Arch Surg 65:916, 1952.

168. Kropff G: Intubation oesophagienne par tube en matiere plastique suivie de radium therapie dans le traitment du cancer de l'oesophage. Mem Acad Chir (Paris) 80:628, 1954.

169. Mousseau M, Le Forestier J, Barbin J, Hardy M: The indications for permanent intubation in the palliative treatment of carcinoma of the esophagus. Arch Mal App Digest 45:208, 1956.

170. Celestin LR: Permanent intubation in inoperable cancer of the esophagus and cardia. A new tube. Ann R Coll Surg Eng 25:165, 1959.

171. O'Conner T, Watson R, Lepley D, Weisel W: Esophageal prosthesis for palliative intubation. Arch Surg 87:275, 1963.

172. Boyce HW Jr, Palmer ED: Techniques of Clinical Gastroenterology. Springfield, Illinois, Charles C Thomas, 1975.

173. Boyce HW Jr.: Palliation of advanced esophageal cancer. Semin Oncol 11:186, 1984.

174. Tytgat GN, den Hartog Jarger FCA, Bartelsman JFWM: Endoscopic prosthesis for advanced esophageal cancer. Endoscopy 18:32, 1986.

175. Atkinson M, Ferguson R: Fiberoptic endoscopic palliative intubation of inoperable oesophagogastric neoplasms. Br Med J i:266, 1977.

176. Atkinson M, Ferguson R, Ogilvie AL: Management of malignant dysphagia by intubation at endoscopy. JR Soc Med 72:894, 1979.

177. Earlam R, Cunha-Melo JR: Malignant esophageal strictures: A review of techniques for palliative intubation. Br J Surg 69:61, 1982.

178. Sargeant IR, Thorpe S, Bown SG: Cuffed esophageal prosthesis: A useful device in desperate situations in esophageal malignancy. Gastrointest Endosc 38:669, 1992.

179. Domschke W, Foerster EC, Matek W, Rodl W: Self-expanding mesh stent for esophageal cancer stenosis. Endoscopy 22:134, 1990.

180. Song HY et al.: Esophagogastric neoplasms: Palliation with a modified gianturco stent. Radiology 180:349, 1991.

181. Bethge N et al.: Self-expanding metal stents for palliation of malignant esophageal obstruction—a pilot study of eight patients. Endoscopy 24:411, 1992.

182. Schaer J et al.: Treatment of malignant esophageal obstruction with silicone-coated metallic self-expanding stents. Gastrointest Endosc 38:7, 1992.

Stomach

3

Gastric Secretion in the Twentieth Century

HORACE W. DAVENPORT

The history of gastric secretion in the 20th century is the story of the application of successive new methods to answer the questions: What is gastric secretion? What does it do? How is it made? How can a physician control acid secretion?

NERVOUS CONTROL OF GASTRIC SECRETION

At the end of the 19th century, Ivan Petrovich Pavlov and his student Khizhin provided a dog with a fully innervated pouch of the acid-secreting, or *oxyntic,* area of the stomach. Pavlov believed that the pouch would behave exactly like the stomach in miniature, and when he gave the dog an esophagostomy so that the food eaten by the dog did not enter the stomach, he could study the cephalic phase of gastric secretion. He found that the sight and smell of food, the presence of food in the mouth, and the act of swallowing all caused the pouch to secrete acid juice, that the response was completely interrupted by severing the vagus nerves to the pouch or administering atropine. If Pavlov put food directly into the stomach through a gastric fistula, he could study the gastric phase of secretion, and the intestinal phase by infusing nutriments into the duodenum by means of a catheter threaded through the gastric fistula. Food in the stomach stimulated secretion by the pouch, and Pavlov, who, like all other 19th century physiologists, believed without question that all physiologic phenomena were controlled by nerves, attributed this

stimulation to a reflex. Likewise, when Pavlov's students discovered that infusing olive oil into the duodenum inhibited acid secretion by the pouch, they concluded that they had discovered an inhibitory reflex.

This doctrine of exclusive control by means of nerves, known as *nervism,* had been taught to Pavlov by his mentor Sergey Petrovich Botkyn. Pavlov, in turn, taught it to his students, one of whom, Leon Popielski, became a fervent believer in nervism. Popielski performed an elaborate series of operations on dogs to identify the nervous pathway responsible for stimulation of secretion by food in the stomach. Stimulation persisted after total extrinsic denervation of the stomach, and Popielski was driven to the conclusion that stimulation is mediated by a "peripheral reflex center" in the stomach itself.

BREAKING THE GRIP OF NERVISM

Popielski had been forced to a similar conclusion when he had sought the nervous pathway responsible for stimulation of pancreatic secretion. Another of Pavlov's students, Dolinski, had rediscovered the fact that acid in contact with the duodenal mucosa stimulates the pancreas. Dolinski had concluded that acid is a powerful stimulant of nerve endings in the duodenum that are afferent receptors for reflex excitation of the pancreas. Popielski, after another series of exhaustive denervations, concluded that stimulation is mediated through ganglion cells within the pancreas that receive afferent impulses from the intestinal mucosa. William Bayliss and his brother-in-law, Ernest Starling, tested this conclusion on the afternoon of 16 January 1901, two weeks after the beginning of the 20th century, and their experiment broke the grip of nervism on gastroenterology.

Bayliss and Starling measured the rate of secretion by the pancreas of an anesthetized dog, finding as everyone did that, when they put acid in the duodenum or upper jejunum, the pancreas responded by secreting. Then they cut, so they thought, all nerves between the upper small intestine and the pancreas, but found that, when they again put acid into the intestine, the pancreas once more secreted. Starling exclaimed: "It must be a chemical reflex!" He snipped off some jejunal mucosa, ground it with acid and sand, and injected the filtrate into the dog's veins. The pancreas secreted. Bayliss and Starling had a new concept provided by their new method: a specific stimulus acting on a specific receptor tissue liberates a specific messenger that, traveling through the blood, stimulates a specific end organ to respond in a specific manner. They called their messenger *secretin* (which they pronounced secrétin, not sécretin). Two years later, Hardy suggested that they call it a *hormone*.

Bayliss and Starling purified their hormone by the crude methods available at the time, and succeeded at least in eliminating vasodilators from the extract. It would be 50 years before methods were available to isolate that or any other gastrointestinal hormone in a pure state and determine its structure.

ACID IN GASTRIC JUICE

William Beaumont had judged by taste the concentration of the acid that he recovered from the stomach of his fistulous subject, Alexis St. Martin. None of the three professional chemists to whom Beaumont sent samples of the juice made any attempt to measure the concentration of the HCl they found in them. Throughout the 19th century, physiologists occasionally titrated samples of gastric juice, but attached little importance to the results. In the 1880s, Carl Anton Ewald and Ismar Boas invented the method of determining gastric secretory

activity by means of test meals, and introduced the concepts of *free* and *combined acid*. When Pavlov fed one of his fasting, esophagostomized dogs, he found that the concentration of acid was low as the pouch began to secrete, and that it rose to 126 to 159 mN, a concentration maintained as long as the pouch continued to secrete. Pavlov explained this by saying that, when the stomach is not secreting, the mucosa is covered with an alkaline layer, and that when secretion begins, the first acid secreted is neutralized by the alkali. When alkalinity is exhausted, secretion collected from the pouch approaches a constant composition that is characteristic of the secretion of the oxyntic cells. This is the *two-component theory*, which accounts for the relationship between the rate of secretion and the concentration of acid.

In the 1930s, Franklin Hollander was the most persuasive advocate of the two-component theory. By that time, the discovery that steady graded doses of histamine could cause steady graded rates of gastric secretion permitted Hollander to collect samples of gastric juice secreted at any desired rate, and he found that the concentration of H^+ rose with the rate of secretion. He deduced that the acid component is a pure isotonic solution of HCl secreted at variable rates, and that the second component is similar to an ultrafiltrate of plasma secreted at a constant rate. John Gray and other students of Andrew C. Ivy argued from similar data that the acid component contains about 7 mN K^+ in addition to HCl. Forty years later, Andrew Garner demonstrated that the surface epithelial cells actively secrete a bicarbonate-containing fluid in which the concentration of HCO_3^- can be as high as 50 mN and that this alkaline secretion is stimulated by acid in contact with the mucosa.

When Torsten Teorell presented his thesis at the Karolinska Institute in 1933, he gave an alternative explanation of the relationship between rate of secretion and the concentration of H^+. Teorell said that the gastric mucosa is slightly permeable to H^+ of gastric juice and to Na^+ of interstitial fluid. As juice is secreted at some constant "primary" concentration, some of its H^+ exchanges for Na^+ by diffusion through the mucosa. The resulting concentrations of H^+ and Na^+ in gastric juice can be described by differential equations relating the concentration of H^+ in the primary secretion, the rate of secretion of the primary juice, the concentration of Na^+ in interstitial fluid, and the permeability of the mucosa. Teorell and his students supported his theory by both model and animal experiments, and offered it as a substitute for the two-component theory. Most disinterested observers thought that both theories contained elements of truth. Teorell's concept of back-diffusion of H^+ became important in the 1960s, when Charles Code and I showed that back-diffusion of H^+ is greatly accelerated when permeability of the mucosa is increased by damage with aspirin or bile and that increased back-diffusion has serious pathophysiologic consequences. That story is beyond the scope of this chapter.

PEPSIN IN GASTRIC JUICE

On 14 February 1833, Beaumont deduced that digestion of meat by Alexis's gastric juice was not effected by acid but by "some principle inappreciable to the senses." He did not know that Johann Eberle, working in Germany in complete ignorance of Beaumont, was in the process of extracting that "principle" from dead gastric mucosa with acid and demonstrating that the extract digested coagulated egg yolk and cheese. The next year, Theodor Schwann, acting on the advice of his teacher, Johannes Müller, partially purified the substance responsible and named it *pepsin*. In 1870, Rudolf Heidenhain found that pepsin exists in an inactive state in what he named the *chief cells* of the oxyntic mucosa, and his Breslau colleagues, Wilhelm Ebstein and Paul Grützner, named the inactive compound *pepsinogen* and showed that it is converted to pepsin by the acid of gastric juice. Lack of methods for isolating proteins in a pure state and for determining their structure long prevented chemists from proving that pepsin is a protein. As late as 1926, a first-class chemist like Richard Willstätter could say that pepsin is not a protein but a small molecule somehow protected by adsorption on proteins.

In the 1930s, John Northrop developed a method for crystallizing a protein that he believed to be pepsin, and by means of Willard Gibbs' phase rule, demonstrated that the crystalline protein was homogeneous. Likewise, Northrop and his colleagues crystallized pepsinogen and proved its homogeneity by the same method. At the same time, Max Bergmann and his student, Joseph Fruton, showed that pepsin catalyzes hydrolysis of peptide bonds containing tyrosine or phenylalanine.

But Northrop's crystals were not really homogeneous. S. P. L. Sørensen had provided biochemists with buffers by which they could maintain solutions at some specific pH, and biochemists using buffers found several peaks in pepsin's pH-activity curve. In the 1950s, several biochemists isolated two or more different pepsins from the same starting material, and in the 1960s, Michael Samloff used the more discriminating method of electrophoresis to identify eight different pepsinogens in extracts of human gastric mucosa. Samloff also used the method of immunofluorescence to show that some pepsinogen granules are present in neck chief cells and in a few cells in the antral mucosa as well as in chief cells.

MUCUS IN GASTRIC JUICE

Beaumont knew that Alexis's gastric juice contained both ropy visible mucus and dissolved mucus. In the 19th century, histologists beginning with William Bowman used the newly invented achromatic compound microscope to show that mucus is secreted by the surface epithelial cells. Giulio Bizzozero identified neck chief cells and showed that they secrete a soluble mucus. Lack of suitable methods long delayed analysis and characterization of mucus. Throughout the second quarter of the 20th century, Boris Babkin argued that mucus protects the gastric mucosa by being secreted in response to contact with acid, by neutralizing acid, and by inhibiting pepsin. Howard Florey in Oxford showed that mucus is secreted when the vagus is stimulated, and his colleague Norman Heatly demonstrated that mucus neither delays diffusion of acid nor inhibits pepsin. The chief positive result of the study of mucus was the proof that William Castle's *intrinsic factor* binds vitamin B_{12}, is responsible for absorption of the vitamin in the terminal ileum, and in the human subject is secreted by the oxyntic cells.

Finally, beginning about 1970, Adrian Allen and his colleagues at Newcastle-upon-Tyne found methods by which they could isolate, purify, and characterize hog gastric mucus. They showed that it is composed of four subunits, each consisting of a linear protein core from which up to 19 carbohydrate side chains project like bristles on a bottle brush. The four subunits are joined by sulfhydryl bonds to a globular protein of 70,000 molecular weight. When these molecules are highly concentrated, as they are in the tips of the surface epithelial cells and in the cells' immediate secretion, the subunits interdigitate, forming a gel. When the gel is diluted in gastric juice, it is dispersed as soluble mucus.

EDKINS' GASTRIN

John S. Edkins, a teacher of physiology in St. Bartholomew's Hospital in the first decade of the 20th century, understood the current knowledge of gastric physiology. When he heard of Bayliss and Starling's discovery of secretin, he thought it possible that food in contact with the antral mucosa liberates a comparable messenger that stimulates acid secretion. Edkins extracted the antral mucosa of cats, and found that, when he injected the extract intravenously into another cat, the recipient's blood pressure fell and its stomach secreted acid. In a control experiment, Edkins prepared a similar extract of the oxyntic mucosa, and found that when he injected it, the recipient's blood pressure fell but its stomach did not secrete. Therefore, Edkins concluded, the antral extract had contained both a vasodilator and a hormone stimulating acid secretion, whereas the oxyntic extract had contained only the vasodilator. Edkins called his acid-stimulating hormone *gastrin*.

HISTAMINE

Henry Dale and his chemist colleague in the Henry Wellcome Physiological Laboratories identified the vasodilator as *histamine* in 1910, but because they did not look

for it, they failed to discover that histamine stimulates acid secretion. Upon leaving Pavlov's laboratory, Leon Popielski began to study vasodilators, and on 28 October 1916, when he was professor of Pharmacology in Lwow, Poland, Popielski discovered that histamine is a powerful stimulant of acid secretion. The report of his discovery was not published until 1920. When it became known, most physiologists thought that Edkins had made a ludicrous mistake. Histamine is present in tissue extracts; it must have been present in Edkins' antral extract; histamine stimulates acid secretion; therefore there is no such entity as gastrin. Andrew C. Ivy was the most vigorous opponent of what he called *gastreen* from the early 1920s until 1964. He said that there is no gastrin or, if there is, it is histamine. Until near the end of his life, Ivy opposed "Edkins' hypothesis" by making extracts of antral mucosa that contained or appeared to contain histamine. Only after Roderic Gregory sent Ivy a sample of *synthetic* human gastrin prepared by an organic chemist did Ivy admit there might be such an entity as gastrin. He added that he was proud of having had Gregory as his student in 1938 and 1939.

EVIDENCE FOR HORMONAL STIMULATION OF ACID SECRETION

After some grumbling, Pavlov accepted Bayliss and Starling's evidence for hormonal control of pancreatic secretion. When Pavlov read Edkins' report of his experiment, he realized how incomplete was Edkins' evidence, and applied the surgical methods, of which he was a master, to the problem. About 1904 or 1905, he provided a dog with an isolated, externally denervated pouch of the gastric antrum. He re-established continuity of the gut by making a gastroenterostomy connecting the jejunum and the remainder of the stomach. Finally, Pavlov made a gastroenterostomy so that the student to whom he assigned the dog could collect gastric juice. When the student introduced meat extract or soap into the isolated, denervated antral pouch, the oxyntic mucosa secreted acid juice. Intravenous injection of meat extract into the animal did not stimulate acid secretion, and Pavlov and his students concluded that they had confirmed "Edkins' hypothesis." At the time that work was being done, Pavlov's interest was turning toward the study of conditioned reflexes, and the Russians made no serious effort to identify the nature of gastrin.

Morton Grossman and Charlotte Robertson, working in Ivy's laboratory in 1947, provided even more rigid proof of a humoral link between the gastric antrum and the oxyntic glands. In the first of several operations on a dog, Grossman and Robertson transplanted a pouch of the oxyntic area into the mammary gland of a bitch that had recently whelped. After local blood vessels had grown into the pouch, Grossman and Robertson cut those that had originally carried blood to the pouch. Then they made an extrinsically denervated antral pouch and converted the remainder of the stomach into a vagally denervated pouch. To avoid the possibility of absorption of secretagogues, Grossman and Robertson used distention of the antral pouch as their stimulus. Both the transplanted pouch and the vagally denervated stomach responded by secreting acid.

At the same time, Lester Dragstedt and his surgical students at the University of Chicago were analyzing local control of gastrin release by equally ingenious operations upon dogs. They too demonstrated that distention of an extrinsically denervated antral pouch is followed by acid secretion by an extrinsically denervated pouch of the oxyntic area of the stomach. They added the crucial observation that, whereas irrigation of such an antral pouch with neutral liver extract stimulates secretion, irrigation with the same liver extract acidified with HCl does not. That result established the feedback nature of hormonal control of acid secretion. At the beginning of a meal, the neutral gastric contents stimulate release of gastrin from the antrum, but when the chyme in the antrum becomes acidified release of gastrin is no longer stimulated. Soon Dragstedt's students also established that irrigation of the antral pouch with neutral solutions of acetylcholine, short chain alcohols, and amino acids releases gastrin.

In the tradition of Swedish experimental physiology, where the 8 AM smell in the laboratory is a mixture of ether and cauterized cat, Björe Uvnäs showed in the 1940s that painting the antral mucosa of an anesthetized cat with a local anesthetic reduced the secretory response of the oxyntic mucosa to stimulation of the vagus. Uvnäs concluded that vagal impulses release gastrin from the antral mucosa. This was confirmed by Bryan Schofield, who constructed a mucosal dam between the oxyntic and antral areas of the stomach of a dog, thereby preventing acid secreted by the oxyntic area from inhibiting gastrin release. He also severed the gastrointestinal tract at the junction between antrum and duodenum and brought the pyloric opening onto the dog's abdominal wall as a fistula, and constructed an extrinsically denervated pouch of the oxyntic area of the stomach. He established continuity of the lower part of the digestive tract by making a gastroenterostomy, but interrupted the continuity of the upper part by making an esophagostomy. After all this, sham feeding caused the denervated oxyntic pouch to secrete, but the pouch failed to secrete in response to sham feeding after Schofield had cut the vagal fibers to the gastric antrum. Thus, Schofield proved that part of the cephalic phase of gastric secretion is mediated by vagally stimulated release of gastrin from the antrum.

HORMONAL INHIBITION OF ACID SECRETION

At the beginning of the 20th century, when Pavlov's students showed that infusion of olive oil into the duodenum inhibits secretion by a Pavlov pouch, they assumed that inhibition was mediated by a nervous reflex.

Robert K. S. Lim, the Edinburgh-educated son of Sun Yat-sen's physician and secretary, began his career in physiology by unsuccessfully attempting to show that Edkins had been right. Lim became Professor of Physiology in the newly established Peking Union Medical College in 1924, and there he showed that inhibition of secretion by fat in the duodenum occurs entirely independently of any nervous link between the stomach and duodenum. Lim prepared an "autotransplanted" stomach in a dog, the stomach removed from the animal and then replaced as a pouch with its arterial supply and venous drainage joined to the animal's blood vessels only by aluminum connectors. Secretion by the stomach was reduced when Lim introduced olive oil into the dog's duodenum. He showed that fat itself was not the inhibitory agent, for fatty lymph collected when a dog was digesting a fatty meal had no effect upon the secretory response to a meal when it was injected intravenously. Lim concluded that fat excites liberation of an inhibitory hormone, a *chalone*.

Lim had only the crude methods of separating large organic molecules available to biochemists in the 1920s, but he did succeed in extracting from the duodenal mucosa a preparation that, on intravenous injection, inhibited meal-stimulated gastric secretion. It did not stimulate flow of bile or pancreatic juice, and therefore did not contain cholecystokinin or secretin. Lim called it *enterogastrone*. Ivy began an attempt to isolate enterogastrone in 1937, and between 1945 and 1956, drug companies also made the attempt in the hope that enterogastrone would cure peptic ulcers. When it proved ineffective, work on enterogastrone was stopped, but its name and supposed function continued to be described in textbooks.

The spectrum of action of a hormone, once it has been isolated, is determined by pharmacologic means. It is given to a test animal in a wide range of doses, and the animal's reactions are cataloged. Determination of its physiologic spectrum of action is an altogether different matter.

When the structure of cholecystokinin was determined, it was found to have the same four C-terminal amino acids as gastrin. Therefore, it can be a weak stimulant of acid secretion. Because cholecystokinin can occupy gastrin receptors, denying them to the more potent gastrin, it is also a competitive inhibitor of acid secretion. These facts were determined by pharmacologic means. Cholecystokinin is liberated when fat is present in the duodenum, and its stimulation of pancreatic enzyme secretion is an authentic physiologic action of the hormone. However, the plasma concentration achieved by cholecystokinin when it is physiologically released is well below the concentration required for pharmacological inhibition of acid secretion. Consequently, cholecystokinin is not enterogastrone. A dozen or so other polypeptides, including one named *gastric inhibitory polypeptide*, have been isolated from the duodenal mucosa, and all have been found to be pharmacologic inhibitors of acid secretion. By 1990, none had been proved to be physiologic inhibitors, and the identity of enterogastrone remained in doubt.

KOMAROV'S GASTRIN

Edkins' tissue extract was as crude as could be, and because methods improved only slowly, it was not until the late 1930s that Simon Komarov could prepare an extract of antral mucosa that stimulated acid secretion but did not contain a vasodilator.

Komarov had worked alongside Boris Babkin in Pavlov's laboratory, and when Babkin became Professor of Pharmacology at McGill University, he hired Komarov to be his chemist. Komarov, with Babkin's encouragement, attempted to isolate gastrin by first extracting boiled, minced hog antral mucosa with trichloracetic acid. The active principle was in the precipitate. Komarov removed the trichloracetic acid from it with organic solvents, and after many tedious repetitions of precipitation, extraction, and salting out, Komarov obtained a powder that gave a positive color reaction for proteins but contained no choline or histamine. Komarov believed that he was justified in calling his product *gastrin,* because when he injected it into a test animal in a quantity equal to 5 g of starting material, it caused copious secretion of a highly acid juice with low peptic power. Most physiologists, but not Ivy, accepted Komarov's claim that he had prepared a histamine-free gastrin.

GREGORY AND TRACY'S GASTRIN

Roderic Gregory became Professor of Physiology at the University of Liverpool after the Second World War, and he achieved a sterling reputation as a classical gastrointestinal physiologist. In search of enterogastrone, Gregory found that extracts of the duodenal mucosa did not inhibit histamine-stimulated acid secretion. Gregory begged a sample of a crude gastrin preparation from another physiologist to see whether his duodenal extract inhibited gastrin-stimulated secretion. When Gregory found that rapid intravenous infusion of the preparation into a conscious dog did not stimulate acid secretion, he concluded that the preparation was no good, and with his assistant Hilda J. Tracy, he reluctantly undertook to prepare gastrin himself. This was 1959, and the time was at last ripe. Chromatographic methods for separating complex compounds were then commonplace. Gregory and Tracy applied the methods to 600 hog antrums a week, purchased from a Liverpool pork pie baker, and on Christmas morning of 1962, they eluted not one but two pure gastrins from a chromatographic column.

Gregory and Tracy were doubly fortunate, for George Kenner, an internationally renowned peptide chemist, was their colleague as Professor of Organic Chemistry at Liverpool. Kenner and his team needed only fractions of a milligram to determine that each of the two gastrins was a heptadecapeptide, one sulfated on a tyrosine residue and the other not. Kenner's team, supplemented by chemists from Imperial Chemical Industries (ICI), established the amino acid sequence of the gastrins and proved the structure by synthesis. The chemists also prepared synthetic fragments of the heptadecapeptide, and Gregory and Tracy used them to show that the heptadecapeptide's C-terminal tetrapeptide displays the full range of physiologic activity of gastrin. One of the ICI chemists, acting on a suggestion by Gregory that turned out to be wrong, added β-alanine to the N-terminus of the tetrapeptide, producing *pentagastrin*. Because pentagastrin is stable and soluble, it quickly replaced histamine as the stimulant of choice in clinical and laboratory studies of acid secretion.

IS HISTAMINE THE FINAL COMMON MEDIATOR OF ACID SECRETION?

In 1955, Charles Code declared that an overwhelming mass of evidence was available to show that histamine is the final common mediator of all modes of stimulation of acid secretion. He marshaled four cogent arguments: (1) histamine acts directly upon oxyntic cells, (2) histamine is present in large amounts in the oxyntic mucosa, (3) histaminase, the enzyme that catalyzes oxidation of histamine and destroys its effec-

tiveness, is absent from the mucosa, and (4) histamine is present in acid gastric juice. Code cited three additional arguments that were less cogent at the time: (5) histamine may be present in gastric venous blood during acid secretion, (6) histamine may be present in the urine during acid secretion, and (7) stimulants of acid secretion release histamine within the mucosa.

In the next 10 years, Code advanced evidence derived from study of the metabolism of histamine within the dog's stomach. He found that the nitrogen on the ethylamine side chain of histamine is methylated, producing N-methyl histamine, which is a more powerful stimulant of acid secretion than is histamine itself. In addition, histamine is converted to 1,4-methyl histamine by methylation of the imidazole ring and the product does not stimulate acid secretion. Then, in 1977, Code proposed that histamine is produced and stored within a *histaminocyte* adjacent to the oxyntic cells, that histamine is liberated from the histaminocyte by gastrin and perhaps by acetylcholine, that histamine and its N-methyl derivative stimulate the neighboring oxyntic cells, and finally, that the two active compounds are inactivated by being converted to the 1,4-methyl derivatives.

By 1990, Code's histaminocyte had been identified as an enterochromaffin-like cell (ECL) that decarboxylates histidine to produce histamine, stores histamine, and releases histamine when appropriately stimulated. Gastrin was found to have a trophic effect on the ECL cells and to stimulate both production and release of histamine. At that time, whether the ELC cells are in proximity with the oxyntic cells had not been determined.

In the meantime, Swedish physiologists succeeded in isolating almost whole gastric glands by treating the rabbit's oxyntic mucosa with collagenase. When George Sachs and his colleagues examined the glands with differential interference-contrast microscopy, they saw that, when the glands were stimulated with histamine, the canaliculi expanded, becoming filled with a fluid that took up the dye acridine orange. They proved that the fluid was acid by observing the pH-dependent fluorescence of the dye. Thus they proved what had been assumed from the time of Heidenhain, that the oxyntic cells directly secrete acid. Furthermore, when Sachs suspended the glands in a large volume of salt solution, any histamine liberated was so thoroughly diluted that it was ineffective as a stimulant for acid secretion. Those glands' oxyntic cells then failed to secrete when gastrin was added to the solution. This was taken as evidence that gastrin does not act directly upon the oxyntic cells but acts through intermediation of histamine liberated from histaminocytes. It was not conclusively established that oxyntic cells of other species do not directly respond to gastrin. At approximately the same time, other investigators found that isolated oxyntic cells have receptors for acetylcholine. Therefore, they probably respond directly to acetylcholine liberated from nerve endings in the intramural plexuses without intermediation of histamine.

APPLICATION OF IMMUNOLOGIC METHODS

Rosalyn Yalow and Solomon Berson announced in 1958 that the binding of insulin with an antibody to insulin could be used as the basis of a radioimmunologic assay for insulin, and they described the method in detail in 1960.

James McGuigan, then working at Washington University in St. Louis, developed a radioimmunologic assay for gastrin by conjugating the N-terminus of the C-terminal tetrapeptide of gastrin to bovine serum albumin and raising antibodies to the compound in guinea pigs. By 1968, McGuigan had a radioimmunoassay with which he could measure gastrin concentrations in the serum of normal persons and of patients with the Zollinger-Ellison syndrome. He found the concentration of immunoreactive gastrin in the serum of the patients to be 100 to 500 times greater than that in normal subjects.

A few years earlier, Italian workers had identified cells, called *G Cells,* in the antral mucosa that they thought were the site of gastrin synthesis and secretion. McGuigan raised antibodies in rabbits to the entire gastrin molecule coupled with bovine serum albumin, and after he had purified the antibody, he attached fluorescein isothiocyanate to it. He found that the G cells contain gastrin when he applied the fluorescing anti-

body to sections of human antral mucosa and examined them by means of a fluorescence microscope. Thereafter, others, in particular those working with A. G. Egerson Pearse at the Royal Postgraduate Medical School in London, used similar methods to locate gastrin cells in Zollinger-Ellison tumors.

In the late 1960s, both Björe Uvnäs and Morton Grossman persuaded Berson and Yalow to apply their immunoassay methods to gastrin, and Yalow continued the work after Berson's death in 1972. Yalow combined radioimmunoassay with chromatographic means of separating gastrins in serum. There were two major results. First, Yalow found, in addition to the two heptadecapeptides, corresponding gastrins composed of 34 amino acids. She called them *big gastrins.* A little later, she identified other gastrins that have the molecular weight of about 60,000, and called them *big, big gastrins.* Second, her sensitive and reasonably specific methods for identifying and quantifying serum gastrins permitted physiologists, notably those working with Morton Grossman in Los Angeles, to work out in some detail the physiology of control of gastric secretion by gastrin in both human subjects and experimental animals.

MECHANISM OF ACID SECRETION: BIOCHEMICAL METHODS

Application of biochemical methods to the problem of the mechanism of acid secretion began in 1938 and 1939 with the discovery that carbonic anhydrase is present in oxyntic cells. The enzyme reversibly catalyzes hydration of carbon dioxide to carbonic acid, H_2CO_2, which in turn ionizes to give H^+ and HCO_3^-. Anyone who thinks about it will recognize at once that those reactions cannot be responsible in themselves for secretion of H^+ at a concentration of about 150 mN, for the partial pressure of carbon dioxide driving the reaction would have to be more than 500 mm Hg. That did not stop someone from proposing a "carbonic anhydrase theory of acid secretion." When that theory was shown to be untenable, the carbon dioxide-carbonic anhydrase system was relegated to a secondary but still important role. When H^+ is secreted, OH^- is left behind to be neutralized by another H^+ produced by ionization of H_2CO_3. The simultaneously appearing HCO_3^- is excreted into plasma in exchange for the Cl^- that accompanies H^+ into the secretion. Uncatalyzed hydration of carbon dioxide does proceed at a finite rate, but F. J. W. Roughton, the discoverer of carbonic anhydrase, calculated that at high rates of acid secretion, enzymatic catalysis is required to meet the oxyntic cells' needs. The later histochemical demonstration that carbonic anhydrase is located on the canalicular membrane implies that it is closely associated with the membrane-bound enzyme responsible for H^+ secretion.

Between 1940 and 1955, several groups of biochemists in the United States and Great Britain applied biochemical methods in search of a reaction capable of generating H^+ for secretion. A favorite target was an oxidation-reduction reaction presumably situated on the canalicular membrane. If such a reaction is responsible for H^+ secretion, the electron removed from the substrate must eventually be accepted by O_2. Because one molecule of O_2 can accept only four electrons, the ratio between the quantity of H^+ secreted and O_2 consumed must be no greater than 4. There was a hot and eventually unresolved debate over the magnitude of the ratio. E. J. Conway, a Dublin biochemist distinguished for his work on electrolytes in muscle, argued forcibly for a redox reaction, and in the course of his experiments made an observation that at the time appeared not to be pertinent. Conway found that if he aerated baker's yeast for several days so that the cells used up their internal supply of succinic acid, and if he then suspended the cells in a solution of glucose and KCl, the yeast cells excreted H^+ in exchange for the K^+ they took up. In a short time, the pH of the medium fell as low as 1.4, and Conway proposed that oxyntic cells likewise secrete H^+ in exchange for K^+. No one paid much attention to Conway's proposal.

MECHANISM OF ACID SECRETION: ACTIVE TRANSPORT METHODS

Availability of radioactive isotopes after the Second World War and the development of electrophysiologic methods allowed physiologists to attack the problem of active transport in the digestive tract. In 1950, Adrian Hogben went to Copenhagen to apply the method Hans Ussing had used to show how a frog can maintain electrolyte equilibrium by actively absorbing Na^+ from a very dilute solution. Ussing had confined a sheet of frog skin in an "Ussing chamber" as a partition between two electrolyte solutions. He measured the potential difference across the frog skin and the fluxes of stable and radioactive Na^+ between the two solutions, and was able to prove that the skin actively transports Na^+ from the solution bathing its external face to that bathing its internal face. In like manner, Hogben confined a sheet of frog gastric mucosa in a similar chamber. It had long been known that the mucosal surface of the stomach is electrically negative in the external circuit with respect to the serosal surface. Hogben passed a current through the sheet of mucosa of such polarity and magnitude that the potential difference was reduced to zero. That current was equal to the current generated by the mucosa to maintain the potential difference. By use of isotopes of Cl^-, Hogben demonstrated that active secretion of Cl^- into the solution on the mucosal surface was responsible for the potential difference and for the current generated. Thus, a *chloride pump* is responsible for secretion of Cl^- into gastric juice.

A little later, Richard Durbin and Erich Heinz, using similar methods, showed that if frog gastric mucosa is held in an Ussing chamber and bathed on its serosal surface with a solution containing no Cl^-, the direction of the potential difference reverses, the mucosal surface becoming positive. Durbin and Heinz took this to be evidence that the mucosa contains a proton pump secreting the H^+ of gastric juice. How the Cl^- and H^+ pumps are coupled remained a puzzle for a long time.

MECHANISM OF ACID SECRETION: CELL BIOLOGY METHODS

After 1950, the methods of electron microscopy and cell biology began to reveal the functional organization of oxyntic cells. Electron microscopists showed that an oxyntic cell is packed with mitochondria whose function is to generate a supply of adenosine triphosphate (ATP) as the immediate source of energy used for secretion. They also showed that oxyntic cells, when not secreting, contain a large array of tubular vesicles. When the cells are stimulated, the vesicles fuse with the canalicular membrane so that the area of the membrane increases substantially. The method of differential centrifugation was used by cell biologists to isolate individual components of oxyntic cells, and a combination of enzyme chemistry and electron microscopy allowed the biologists to identify the resulting product and to estimate its homogeneity. One important preparation made from the oxyntic mucosa was composed of globular or bottle-shaped microsomes, minute vesicles bounded by a single, smooth-surfaced membrane. Those were shown to be composed of canalicular membrane turned inside out. The membrane was found to contain an enzyme catalyzing hydrolysis of ATP, an ATPase that differs from all other known ATPases in that it is stimulated by K^+, not by Na^+, and is not inhibited by ouabain. It was called (H^+, K^+)ATPase. Peter Scholes in England and George Sachs in Birmingham, Alabama, both working with colleagues, showed that if the microsomes are loaded with K^+ in their internal fluid, which corresponds to the secretion in the intact oxyntic cell, the membrane secretes one H^+ into the internal fluid in exchange for one K^+. The energy for the H^+-K^+ exchange is provided by hydrolysis of ATP catalyzed by the (H^+, K^+)ATPase. After 1980, cell biologists were able to show how the H^+-K^+ exchange is controlled by a cascade of reactions beginning with combination of histamine or acetylcholine with their respective receptors on the surface of oxyntic cells. Others using the patch-clamp method were able to show how K^+, Cl^-, and HCO_3^- channels open and close on the oxyntic cells' membrane when secretion begins and stops.

APPLICATION OF KNOWLEDGE

The object of physiological research is to be able not only to understand a physiologic function but to control it as well. As early as 1852, Friedrich Günzberg said that peptic ulceration is "the result of a quantitative anomaly of secretion of free acid as the result of inimical action of the vagus nerve." He had no evidence for his assertion, but evidence accumulated by the beginning of the 20th century. Clinicians knew that acid secretion is at least in part controlled by the vagus, and they coined the maxim: "No acid, no ulcer." Vagal stimulation could be interrupted by surgical or medical means. In 1921, André Laterjet, the Lyonnaise anatomist and surgeon after whom the nerve of Laterjet is named, described the technique and results of vagotomy in the treatment of patients with peptic ulcers. Vagotomy was popularized in the 1940s, and over the next 20 years ingenious surgeons improved the technique until highly selective vagotomy became the operation of choice. From the time of Pavlov, gastroenterologists knew that atropine in large doses blocks vagal stimulation of acid secretion, thus performing a transient chemical vagotomy. The side effects of the doses were severe. Given the problem of side effects and the adoption of in-house scientific investigation by the pharmaceutical industry early in the 20th century, it was only a matter of time before a competent chemist working for a drug company could synthesize an atropine analog that would block vagal stimulation of acid secretion with minimal side effects.

Medical intervention centered on the chemical stimulants of acid secretion, the hormones or histamine. Crude preparations of enterogastrone, the earliest known hormonal inhibitor, proved ineffective, and so did another inhibitor known as *urogastrone*. For a while, Morton Grossman thought that an analog of secretin might be the answer because secretin is both a competitive inhibitor of acid secretion and a stimulant of pancreatic bicarbonate secretion. The discovery that histamine is released from ubiquitous tissue stores spurred pharmacologists and pharmaceutical chemists to look for histamine antagonists, and by 1950 a dozen or more antihistaminics were on the market. Gastroenterologists were disappointed to learn that the drugs did not block the action of histamine on oxyntic cells. Pharmacologists said there must be two types of histamine receptors, those with which antihistaminics combine and those with which antihistaminics do not combine. They called the first class H_1 receptors, implying that oxyntic cells have H_2 receptors. Here again, it was only a matter of time before James Black and numerous colleagues, after screening more than 700 compounds, found the first antihistaminic that blocked the action of histamine on the H_2 receptors of oxyntic cells. Soon rival drug companies were marketing their own H_2 blockers which did indeed promote healing of peptic ulcers by inhibiting acid secretion.

The last step was to look beyond nerves, transmitters, and receptors to the specific intracellular machinery of oxyntic cells. Carbonic anhydrase is part of that machinery, and thiocyanate and acetazolamide inhibit both carbonic anhydrase and acid secretion. Neither is sufficiently effective to be useful. The unique part of the machinery is the (H^+, K^+)ATPase that catalyzes the last step in acid secretion, exchange of K^+ for H^+ at the canalicular membrane. In the late 1970s, pharmaceutical chemists found that a substituted benzimidazole inhibits that particular ATPase, and Swedish clinicians demonstrated that the compound, called *omeprazole,* inhibits pentagastrin-stimulated acid secretion in human subjects. When omeprazole came on the market, few persons bothered to recall that it was the end product of a long line of physiologic research that had begun with Pavlov's proof that the cephalic phase of gastric secretion is mediated by the vagus. That research had extended throughout the 20th century, first to demonstrate the humoral and hormonal control of acid secretion and then to identify the intimate chemistry of oxyntic cells. That research greatly increased understanding of the process and control of acid secretion, and it paid off handsomely in practical terms.

BIBLIOGRAPHY

Babkin BP: Secretory Mechanism of the Digestive Glands, 2nd ed. New York, Paul B. Hoeber, Inc., 1950.

Code CF (ed): Handbook of Physiology, Sec. 6. Alimentary Canal. Vol. II, Secretion. Washington, DC, American Physiological Society, 1967.

Code CF: Histamine and gastric secretion. *In* Wolstenholme G, O'Connor CM (eds): Histamine. Boston, Little, Brown, 1956, pp. 189–219.

Davenport HW: A History of Gastric Secretion and Digestion; Experimental Studies to 1975. New York, Oxford University Press, 1992.

Grossman MI (ed): Gastrin. Berkeley, University of California Press, 1966.

Harmon JW (ed): Basic Mechanisms of Gastrointestinal Mucosal Injury and Protection. Baltimore, Williams & Wilkins, 1981.

Ivy AC: Physiological significance of the effect of histamine on gastric secretion. *In* Roche e Silva M (ed): Histamine and Anti-histaminics. Handbook of Experimental Pharmacology. New York, Springer, 1966, Vol. XVII/1, 81–105.

Pavlov IP: The Work of the Digestive Glands, 2nd English ed. W. H. Thompson, trans. London, Charles Griffin & Company, 1910.

Waldum HL, Petersen H (eds): Histamine and the stomach. Scand J Gastroenterol 26:1, 1991.

Wolf S: The Stomach. New York, Oxford University Press, 1965.

4

Gastritis

WILFRED M. WEINSTEIN

The focus in this chapter is on nonerosive nonspecific gastritis, also known as chronic or chronic active gastritis. The importance of this type of gastritis is its association with peptic ulcer and adenocarcinoma. Two major developments have stimulated research in gastritis. The first came in the early 1970s, when fiberoptic endoscopy began to be used for studies of the prevalence of gastritis and also for its relationship with gastric ulcer and gastric cancer. Gastritis then reached center stage with the discovery that Helicobacter pylori (H. pylori) is the cause of most cases of chronic active gastritis and that eradication of H. pylori radically reduces the relapse rate of duodenal ulcer (1).

TECHNIQUES FOR THE STUDY OF GASTRITIS

Early studies of the gastric mucosa were done in autopsy and operative specimens (2). Magnus described the creative "Swiss roll" technique for the study of large segments of gastric mucosa from operative or autopsy specimens in one histologic section (3). A long strip of gastric mucosa was rolled in a strudel-like fashion and then histologic sections were prepared from horizontal cuts. Pioneer endoscopists such as Rudolf Schindler provided the early insight into the appearance of the gastric mucosa in ambulatory patients (4). Observations of the gastric mucosa in large numbers of military personnel were recorded by Palmer (5). The ability to obtain multiple gastric biopsies safely

came with the development of a gastric suction biopsy instrument by Wood et al. in 1949 (6). Other suction biopsy type instruments followed (7), and until the early 1970s, suction biopsy provided the bulk of the information concerning gastric mucosal diseases in ambulatory patients. Finally, the widespread availability of fiberoptic endoscopes facilitated more precise studies of gastric mucosal diseases.

THE EVOLUTION OF CLASSIFICATIONS OF GASTRITIS

In 1967, MacDonald and Rubin (7), in a review of gastritis, stated that there was as yet no satisfactory classification. The debate over classifications continues partly because knowledge of all the causes of the different patterns remains incomplete (8). An early classification of gastritis came from Schindler (4). Virtually all histologic classifications of gastritis in the past 20 years are based chiefly on the system advocated by Whitehead et al. in 1972 (9). This approach includes the mucosal type (e.g., body, antrum) and the grade according to whether glands are preserved (superficial or atrophic), the degree of inflammatory cell infiltrate, and whether or not metaplasia (intestinal or pseudopyloric) is present. A pattern of gastritis, not defined in that scheme, is that of *reactive gastritis* or *gastropathy* (10). This refers to an appearance of epithelial change without much in the way of accompanying inflammation. Clearly, histologic classifications become less important as freestanding entities as new information concerning causation evolves.

The Topography of Gastritis

A popular way to describe the topography of nonerosive gastritis came from Strickland and Mackay (11). Type A referred to the pernicious anemia type of distribution confined to fundic gland mucosa (fundus and body). Type B referred to antral gland gastritis. Many authors now use the term Type B to refer to the pattern of H. pylori gastritis, even though this is really Type AB because the fundic gland mucosa also is involved, albeit with less severe inflammation.

Multifocal atrophic gastritis is a topographic pattern that was described by Correa (12) and is seen in countries or populations with higher incidences of gastric carcinoma. It appears to begin in the region of the incisura, fanning out proximally and distally; it is commonly associated with intestinal metaplasia.

ENDOSCOPIC APPEARANCES OF NONEROSIVE NONSPECIFIC GASTRITIS

There is generally a poor correlation between the endoscopic appearance of the gastric mucosa and the presence or absence of gastritis. This is especially true for erythema, which is not only a poor predictor but is also characterized by poor inter-observer agreement (13). Nevertheless, many endoscopists for decades have instinctively applied the label of gastritis whenever red mucosa is encountered. One new endoscopic finding is that of a nodular antrum in children that signifies the presence of H. pylori commonly associated with lymphoid aggregates (14). Investigators in Japan have led the way in the use of mucosal sprays at endoscopy with Congo Red to define acid-secreting areas (blue-black color) and their reduced area in atrophic gastritis (15,16). Methylene blue has also been used to outline areas of intestinal metaplasia (16).

ASSOCIATIONS WITH NONEROSIVE NONSPECIFIC GASTRITIS

The approach here is to begin with the associations of nonerosive nonspecific gas-

Table 4–1
Nonerosive Nonspecific Gastritis: Associations*

Helicobacter pylori
Healthy aging
Duodenal ulcer
Gastric ulcer
Adenocarcinoma-Associated Reactive Gastropathy
Postgastrectomy
Adjacent to erosions and ulcers
Pernicious Anemia
Lymphocytic Gastritis
Unexplained and No Clear Disease Associations

* Modified with permission from Weinstein WM: Gastritis and gastropathies. *In* Sleisenger MH, Fordtran JS (eds): Gastrointestinal Disease. Philadelphia, WB Saunders, 1993.

tritis (Table 4-1) and trace their developments backward in time.

Helicobacter pylori Gastritis

The discovery and isolation of H. pylori were reported by Marshall and Warren in 1983 (17). Thereafter, Barry Marshall and Arthur Morris each ingested the organism and produced gastritis, one self-limited (18) and the other more persistent (19,20). H. pylori is present in almost all cases of nonerosive, chronic active gastritis and in some instances of chronic gastritis without the active component, i.e., the neutrophils.

Spiral organisms had been seen earlier in the century by several investigators (21), but their role was not recognized. In 1975, Steer and Colin-Jones reported the presence of these bacteria on the surface of the gastric mucosa and postulated that they might predispose to gastric ulceration (22).

Epidemiology of H. pylori Gastritis

Data on prevalence have come largely from serologic surveys (23). The intrafamilial clustering (24) of H. pylori probably explains in large part the familial patterns of gastritis reported earlier in population studies done in Finland by Max Siurala, Kalle Varis, and their co-workers (25). The Finnish population studies showed that serum pepsinogen measurements as developed by

Michael Samloff could be used as noninvasive predictors of gastritis (26). A low serum pepsinogen I or low pepsinogen I to II ratio can predict moderate to severe atrophic gastritis.

Effect of Aging and Different Population Groups

In North America and other "Westernized countries," H. pylori seropositivity peaks at 40 to 60% (23). In some less developed countries, the infection starts in early childhood and may reach a prevalence of 100% after the age of 40 to 50 (23). The finding of increasing H. pylori seropositivity with age paralleled the results of earlier biopsy surveys of gastritis reported from Europe, especially Finland, beginning in the 1960s (27) and also from Japan (28). Those surveys documented that nonerosive nonspecific gastritis was common in the general population, increasing in prevalence after the fourth decade, with at least 50% of the population having superficial antral and fundic gland gastritis. It also was shown that with progressive atrophic antral gastritis the fundic-antral gland border moved proximally, i.e. "antralization" (28).

H. pylori Gastritis and Peptic Ulcer

In general, the nonerosive nonspecific gastritis associated with peptic ulcer is more diffuse and severe in the antrum than in the body. Before the discovery of H. pylori, there was much greater interest in the association of gastritis with gastric ulcer (29) than with duodenal ulcer (30,31). In the 1930s and 1940s, Faber, Hebbel and Magnus suggested that the gastritis might be the primary event, with the gastric ulcer supervening (30,32,33). The observation that duodenal ulcer was also associated with antral gastritis did not gain as much attention until the H. pylori era (34), when it was shown that almost all duodenal ulcers are associated with H. pylori gastritis.

A seminal observation concerning aspirin-associated gastric ulcer and an *absence* of gastritis was reported by Walter MacDonald in 1973 (35). He demonstrated that approximately 50% of gastric ulcers in patients on chronic aspirin therapy had minimal or no associated gastritis, suggesting that their ulcers were occurring by means of some novel mechanism other than unmasking an ulcer diathesis (35). MacDonald's findings were confirmed recently by Laine et al. in relation to H. pylori, nonsteroidal anti-inflammatory drugs (NSAIDs), and nonerosive gastritis. That is, the prevalence of H. pylori was approximately 50%, in NSAID-associated gastric ulcer, whereas it was over 80% in non-NSAID associated gastric ulcer (36). Also, the severity of the gastritis was related to H. pylori status, and not to whether the patient was taking NSAIDs.

Gastric Adenocarcinoma

Adenocarcinoma of the gastric antrum and body is commonly associated with a more extensive (than in control populations) antral and fundic gland gastritis with prominent intestinal metaplasia (37). The link between intestinal metaplasia as a population risk factor for gastric cancer was reported 40 years ago (38,39). In high-risk gastric cancer areas, the nonerosive gastritis occurs at an earlier age than in lower-risk countries. This association between atrophic gastritis and carcinoma was documented in population studies from Finland, Japan, Hawaii, and Colombia (40–43). In high-risk populations, the topographic pattern may be that of multifocal atrophic gastritis, discussed previously (12). In countries with high rates of gastric cancer, H. pylori infection may develop at an earlier age, but the role of H. pylori in gastric carcinogenesis is not clear (44).

MacDonald pointed out in 1972 that there was another condition in which the *absence of gastritis* provided insight into different pathogenetic mechanisms (45). Namely, adenocarcinomas of the gastric cardia differ from carcinoma of the gastric body in that diffuse nonerosive gastritis of the fundic gland mucosa is minimal or absent. The importance of gastric cardia cancer as a distinct entity is only now being appreciated because of its dramatically rising incidence (46).

Reactive Gastropathy

Reactive gastropathy is a pattern of mucosal injury in which the dominant feature is epithelial change with minimal inflammatory cell infiltrates. The term gastropathy denotes that inflammatory cell infiltrates are not a prominent part of the reaction. The main clinical settings for reactive gastropathy are in the mucosa adjacent to erosions and ulcers, in the mucosa at or near healed gastric ulcer sites, and in the stomach after gastric surgery (47).

The most widely studied type of reactive gastropathy has been the postoperative stomach. Erythema and erosions (in 20%) are most prominent at the stoma and have been shown to bear little relationship to the histologic findings or to symptoms (48). Despite the use of the term postoperative gastritis or alkaline reflux gastritis, it is now known that the main histologic change is epithelial, with minimal to no inflammatory cell infiltrates (49,50). This *reactive gastropathy* probably was confused with dysplasia in the past and may be the main reason why some studies reported so many cases of dysplasia in the postoperative stomach (50).

H. pylori does not find the postoperative stomach hospitable, a phenomenon that has been dynamically illustrated in 12 patients, of whom 83% had H. pylori before gastrectomy, 54% after gastrectomy, and 92% after subsequent biliary diversion with a Roux-en-Y operation (51).

Pernicious Anemia

The atrophic gastritis of pernicious anemia was described at the turn of the twentieth century and was re-examined by Magnus in the 1930s (11). As mentioned previously, the term Type A gastritis originally referred to the fundic gland gastritis seen with pernicious anemia. Suction biopsy studies by Lewin et al. (52) confirmed, however, that some patients with pernicious anemia had concomitant antral gland gastritis and thus did not have pure Type A gastritis. Pernicious anemia is rare. Studies from Scandinavia established that more common than pernicious anemia is a state, usually in the elderly, in which there is diffuse severe atrophic fundic gland gastritis with achlorhydria but the residual ability to absorb vitamin B_{12} (26,53). These patients are now detected more often because of hypergastrinemia found in the course of the investigation of a variety of symptoms, especially diarrhea.

The greatest recent interest in severe atrophic fundic gland gastritis is in relation to the accompanying enterochromaffin-like (ECL) cell hyperplasia in the fundic gland mucosa. This interest is stimulated further by the theoretic possibility that long-term drug-induced achlorhydria might induce ECL cell hyperplasia and even carcinoid tumors in man. Walter Rubin characterized the endocrine cell hyperplasia at the ultrastructural level in 1969 (54). Although ECL hyperplasia is common in severe atrophic fundic gland gastritis with achlorhydria, gastric carcinoids, while increasingly recognized, are not (55). Some tumors in pernicious anemia diagnosed as small-cell adenocarcinomas in the past may actually have been gastric carcinoids (Cyrus E. Rubin, personal communication).

Lymphocytic Gastritis

In 1978, Lambert described the entity of diffuse varioliform gastritis (56), referred to sometimes in this country as chronic erosive gastritis. This condition is characterized by erosions on tiny bumps in the body of the stomach. Subsequently, it has been shown that the surrounding mucosa in this condition is typically that of *lymphocytic gastritis* (57,58). Lymphocytic gastritis is a newly recognized lesion characterized by distinctive mononuclear (primarily T cells) cell infiltrates predominantly in the surface and pit epithelium, resembling the surface epithelium of celiac disease and lymphocytic colitis. Helicobacter pylori is not a common accompaniment. Lymphocytic gastritis has now also been described in 50% of the cases of celiac disease (59) and in some instances of Menetrier's disease (60).

DOES NONEROSIVE NONSPECIFIC GASTRITIS CAUSE SYMPTOMS OF NON-ULCER DYSPEPSIA?

This debate about symptoms has continued for decades. The only change now is that the focus is on H. pylori gastritis, which of course is the most common cause of nonerosive gastritis. The pro and con views have been summarized (61,62,63). The dilemma, as it was for gastritis before the discovery of H. pylori, is that millions of asymptomatic individuals harbor gastritis and a provocative test or treatment trial efficacy is required to demonstrate that a subset of patients develop nonulcer dyspepsia on the basis of the (H. pylori) gastritis. This challenge is made more difficult by the fact that nonulcer dyspepsia probably represents a group of heterogeneous disorders.

REFERENCES

1. Hentschel E et al.: Effect of ranitidine and amoxicillin plus metronidazole on the eradication of Helicobacter pylori and the recurrence of duodenal ulcer. N Engl J Med *328*: 308, 1993.
2. Historical background. In Cheli R, Perasso A, Giacosa A (eds): Gastritis. A Critical Review, Berlin, Springer-Verlag, 1987, p 3.
3. Magnus HA, Ungley CC: The gastric lesion in pernicious anaemia. Lancet *1*:420, 1938.
4. Schindler R: Gastritis. London, Heinemann, 1947.
5. Palmer ED: Gastritis: A re-evaluation. Medicine *33*:199, 1954.
6. Wood IJ, Doig RK, Motteram B, Hughes A: Gastric biopsy. Report on fifty-five biopsies using a new flexible gastric biopsy tube. Lancet *i*:18, 1949.
7. MacDonald WC, Rubin CE: Gastric biopsy—a critical evaluation. Gastroenterology *53*:143, 1967.
8. Correa P, Yardley JH: Grading and classification of chronic gastritis: One American response to the Sydney system. Gastroenterology *102*:355, 1992.
9. Whitehead R, Truelove SC, Gear MW: The histological diagnosis of chronic gastritis in fibreoptic gastroscope biopsy specimens. J Clin Pathol *25*:1, 1972.
10. Price AB: The Sydney System: Histological division. J Gastroenterol Hepatol *6*:209, 1991.
11. Strickland RG, Mackay IR: A reappraisal of the nature and significance of chronic atrophic gastritis. Am J Dig Dis *18*:426, 1973.
12. Correa P: Chronic gastritis: A clinico-pathological classification. Am J Gastroenterol *83*: 504, 1988.
13. Sauerbruch T, Schreiber MA, Schussler P, Permanetter W: Endoscopy in the diagnosis of gastritis. Diagnostic value of endoscopic criteria in relation to histological diagnosis. Endoscopy *16*:101, 1984.
14. Hassall E, Dimmick JE: Unique features of Helicobacter pylori disease in children. Dig Dis Sci *36*:417, 1991.
15. Tatsuta M, Okuda S: Location, healing, and recurrence of gastric ulcers in relation to fundal gastritis. Gastroenterology *69*:897, 1975.
16. Tatsuta M et al.: Chromoendoscopic observations on extension and development of fundal gastritis and intestinal metaplasia. Gastroenterology *88*:70, 1985.
17. Marshall B, Warren JR: Unidentified curved bacillus on gastric epithelium in active chronic gastritis. Lancet *1*:1273, 1983.
18. Marshall BJ, Armstrong JA, McGechie DB, Glancy RJ: Attempt to fulfill Koch's postulates for pyloric Campylobacter. Med J Aust *142*:436, 1985.
19. Morris A, Nicholson G: Ingestion of Campylobacter pyloridis causes gastritis and raised fasting gastric pH. Am J Gastroenterol *82*: 192, 1987.
20. Morris AJ et al.: Long-term follow-up of voluntary ingestion of Helicobacter pylori. Ann Intern Med *114*:662, 1991.
21. Marshall BJ: History of the discovery of C. pylori. In Blaser MJ (ed): Campylobacter pylori in Gastritis and Peptic Ulcer Disease, New York, Igaku-Shoin, 1989, p 7.
22. Steer HW, Colin-Jones DG: Mucosal changes in gastric ulceration and their response to carbenoxolone sodium. Gut *16*: 590, 1975.
23. Taylor DN, Blaser MJ: The epidemiology of Helicobacter pylori infection. Epidemiol Rev *13*:42, 1991.
24. Drumm B, Perez-Perez GI, Blaser MJ, Sherman PM: Intrafamilial clustering of Helicobacter pylori infection. N Engl J Med *322*: 359, 1990.
25. Varis K et al.: Gastric morphology, function, and immunology in first-degree relatives of probands with pernicious anemia and controls. Scand J Gastroenterol *14*:129, 1979.
26. Varis K, Samloff IM, Ihamaki T, Siurala M: An appraisal of tests for severe atrophic gastritis in relatives of patients with pernicious anemia. Dig Dis Sci *24*:187, 1979.
27. Siurala M, Lehtola J, Ihamaki T: Atrophic gastritis and its sequelae. Results of 19–23 years' follow-up examinations. Scand J Gastroenterol *9*:441, 1974.
28. Kimura K: Chronological transition of the fundic-pyloric border determined by stepwise biopsy of the lesser and greater curvatures of the stomach. Gastroenterology *63*: 584, 1972.
29. Gear MWL, Truelove SC, Whitehead R: Gastric ulcer and gastritis. Gut *12*:639, 1971.
30. Hebbel R: Chronic gastritis: Its relation to gastric and duodenal ulcer and to gastric carcinoma. Am J Pathol *19*:43, 1943.
31. Aukee S: Gastritis and acid secretion in patients with gastric ulcers and duodenal ulcers. Scand J Gastroenterol *7*:567, 1972.

32. Faber K: Gastritis and its Consequences. London, Oxford University Press, 1935.

33. Magnus HA: The pathology of simple gastritis. J Pathol Bacteriol *58*:431, 1946.

34. Marshall BJ, Warren JR: Unidentified curved bacilli in the stomach of patients with gastritis and peptic ulceration. Lancet *i*: 1311, 1984.

35. MacDonald WC: Correlation of mucosal histology and aspirin intake in chronic gastric ulcer. Gastroenterology *65*:381, 1973.

36. Laine L, Marin-Sorensen M, Weinstein WM: Nonsteroidal anti-inflammatory drug-associated gastric ulcers do not require Helicobacter pylori for their development. Am J Gastroenterol *87*:1398, 1992.

37. Sipponen P, Kekki M, Siurala M: Atrophic chronic gastritis and intestinal metaplasia in gastric carcinoma. Comparison with a representative population sample. Cancer *52*: 1062, 1983.

38. Jarvi O, Lauren P: On the role of heterotopias of the intestinal epithelium in the pathogenesis of gastric cancer. Acta Pathol Microbiol Scand *29*:26, 1951.

39. Morson BC: Carcinoma arising from areas of intestinal metaplasia. Brit J Cancer *9*:377, 1955.

40. Imai T, Kubo T, Watanabe H: Chronic gastritis in Japanese with reference to high incidence of gastric carcinoma. J Natl Cancer Inst *47*:179, 1971.

41. Stemmermann G, Haenszel W, Locke F: Epidemiologic pathology of gastric ulcer and gastric carcinoma among Japanese in Hawaii. J Natl Cancer Inst *58*:13, 1977.

42. Correa P et al.: Gastric cancer in Colombia. III. Natural history of precursor lesions. J Natl Cancer Inst *57*:1027, 1976.

43. Sipponen P et al.: Gastric cancer risk in chronic atrophic gastritis: Statistical calculations of cross-sectional data. Int J Cancer *35*:173, 1985.

44. Correa P: Is gastric carcinoma an infectious disease? N Engl J Med *325*:1170, 1991.

45. MacDonald WC: Clinical and pathologic features of adenocarcinoma of the gastric cardia. Cancer *29*:724, 1972.

46. Blot WJ, Devesa SS, Kneller RW, Fraumeni JF: Rising incidence of adenocarcinoma of the esophagus and cardia. JAMA *265*:1287, 1991.

47. Lewin KJ, Riddell RH, Weinstein WM: Stomach and proximal duodenum: Inflammatory and miscellaneous disorders. In Lewin KJ, Riddell RH, Weinstein WM (eds): Gastrointestinal Pathology and its Clinical Implications. New York, Tokyo, Igaku-Shoin, 1992, p 506.

48. Hoare AM, Jones EL, Alexander Williams J, Hawkins CF: Symptomatic significance of gastric mucosal changes after surgery for peptic ulcer. Gut *18*:295, 1977.

49. Saukkonen M, Sipponen P, Varis K, Siurala M: Morphological and dynamic behavior of the gastric mucosa after partial gastrectomy with special reference to the gastroenterostomy area. Hepatogastroenterology *27*:48, 1980.

50. Weinstein WM et al.: The histology of the stomach in symptomatic patients after gastric surgery: a model to assess selective patterns of gastric mucosal injury. Scand J Gastroenterol Suppl *109*:77, 1985.

51. O'Connor HJ et al.: Effect of Roux-en-Y biliary diversion on Campylobacter pylori. Gastroenterology *97*:958, 1989.

52. Lewin KJ, Dowling F, Wright JP, Taylor KB: Gastric morphology and serum gastrin levels in pernicious anaemia. Gut *17*:551, 1976.

53. Stockbrugger R, Larsson LI, Lundqvist G, Angervall L: Antral gastrin cells and serum gastrin in achlorhydria. Scand J Gastroenterol *12*:209, 1977.

54. Rubin W: A fine structural characterization of the proliferated endocrine cells in atrophic gastric mucosa. Am J Pathol *70*:109, 1973.

55. Borch K, Renvall H, Liedberg G: Gastric endocrine cell hyperplasia and carcinoid tumors in pernicious anemia. Gastroenterology *88*:638, 1985.

56. Lambert R, Andre C, Moulinier B, Bugnon B: Diffuse varioliform gastritis. Digestion *17*:159, 1978.

57. Haot J et al.: Lymphocytic gastritis—prospective study of its relationship with varioliform gastritis. Gut *31*:282, 1990.

58. Dixon MF, Wyatt JI, Burke DA, Rathbone BJ: Lymphocytic gastritis—relationship to Campylobacter pylori infection. J Pathol *154*:125, 1988.

59. Wolber R et al.: Lymphocytic gastritis in patients with celiac sprue or spruelike intestinal disease. Gastroenterology *98*:310, 1990.

60. Wolber RA, Owen DA, Anderson FH, Freeman HJ: Lymphocytic gastritis and giant gastric folds associated with gastrointestinal protein loss. Mod Pathol *4*:13, 1991.

61. Lambert JR: The role of Helicobacter pylori in nonulcer dyspepsia. A debate for. Gastroenterol Clin North Am *22*:141, 1993.

62. Talley NJ: The role of Helicobacter pylori in nonulcer dyspepsia. A debate—against. Gastroenterol Clin North Am *22*:153, 1993.

63. Weinstein WM: Gastritis and gastropathies. *In* Sleisenger MH, Fordtran JS (eds): Gastrointestinal Disease. Philadelphia, WB Saunders, 1993.

5

History of Acid-Peptic Diseases:
From Bismuth to Billroth to Black to Bismuth

BASIL I. HIRSCHOWITZ

In a 409-page book entitled *A Treatise on Indigestion and Its Consequences [Nervous and Bilious Complaints; with Observations on the Organic Diseases, in Which They Sometimes Terminate]* by A. P. W. Phillip, third edition 1823 (1), there is no recognizable description of a peptic ulcer. One may conclude that this condition was rare and generally unrecognized as a cause of symptoms, complications, or death in the early nineteenth century.

Despite sporadic case reports of gastric or duodenal ulcer beginning in the late eighteenth century, acid peptic diseases did not become widely appreciated until the early twentieth century. In the last two or three decades of the nineteenth century, several important events began to shape the understanding and late treatment of peptic ulcer. Billroth and others from 1881 onwards pioneered gastric surgery, at first for pyloric obstruction caused by cancer and later applied to peptic ulcer. Edison invented the electric lamp and its miniaturization led to the development of early endoscopes; Roentgen discovered x-rays, and Cannon in 1897 reported the first use of contrast x-rays to study swallowing and the upper GI tract in various animals. Physiologic studies of the stomach which had their roots in much earlier investigations (1) had begun to make sense. Studies on digestion, secretion, and emptying based on direct observation and experimentation had made significant progress by the end of the century, with the discoveries by, among others, Prout,

Schwann, Beaumont on Alexis St. Martin's gastrostomy, Claude Bernard, Langley, Heidenhain and Pavlov after the turn of the century. The history of gastric secretion is described in much greater detail in the chapter by Davenport (2). In fact, by 1900, the physiology of gastric secretion was much better understood than the diseases of the upper GI tract, and it was not until the first quarter of this century that patterns of gastric acid secretion began to be related to recognizable diseases of the upper GI tract.

The first six decades of this century saw the dominance of surgery in the treatment of peptic ulcer. Debates between internists, lightly armed with generally ineffective treatment and surgeons, convinced that they had (the latest) ulcer cure in hand, generally ended in a rear-guard action by the nonsurgeons (3). Medical treatments were already being subjected to rigorous statistical analysis (4–6), but the first controlled trials of different operations only appeared in 1964 (7).

With the invention of the histamine H_2 antagonists in 1972 by Black and his colleagues (8), peptic ulcer treatment underwent a major change. The decade from 1972 to 1982 saw the rise of the controlled trial and the retreat of surgery which had reached its refined best in the use of the fundic vagotomy. After cimetidine was generally introduced in 1974, the intense studies of the many and various medical treatments now were bound by the combined requirements of science and the regulatory agencies that demanded proof of both efficacy and safety. Only fiberoptic endoscopy could provide the definition of disease and the endpoints required of such studies.

In the last decade or two, the pathophysiology of acid peptic disease and of injury and repair of cells, and integrated physiology and science in general have accelerated and broadened the field of inquiry to a level only dimly perceived 100 or even 50 years ago (9,10).

The literature of acid peptic diseases is large and complex. The subjects are dealt with in many excellent chapters and monographs, including the comprehensive mid-century review by Ivy, Grossman, and Bachrach (10). This chapter highlights the perception of acid peptic diseases at various stages in the past century and the source of the concepts and discoveries that have influenced present day knowledge.

DIAGNOSIS

In 1912, Perry (11) published a well-written and well-reasoned review of the diagnosis of gastric and duodenal ulcer. These were "considered collectively inasmuch as their symptomatology, etiology and treatment are almost identical."

The diagnosis of peptic ulcer was made therefore on clinical grounds, largely on the basis of postprandial pain, early in gastric ulcer and 2 to 5 hours postprandial in duodenal ulcer. Half the cases of gastric ulcer presented with hemorrhage; other symptoms being vomiting, epigastric pain, tenderness, pyrosis, and "hyperacidity." Spontaneous recovery was expected, but in many, vomiting and decreased food intake led to weakness, anemia, and emaciation. Perry gives the differential diagnosis as gastric cancer, gastritis, neurotic affections of the stomach, cholelithiasis, and gastroptosis (a new diagnosis based on the recently introduced radiology). Obstruction of the pylorus was recognized by the retention of a test meal, and more currently (in 1912) by x-rays.

Duodenal ulcer symptoms were recognized as being cyclical, with burning and gnawing, sometimes reaching the intensity of biliary colic. Relief by food, drink, alkalis, vomiting, or irrigation provided additional evidence for DU. Perforation was well recognized clinically and hemorrhage was felt to be much less frequent in duodenal than in gastric ulcer.

Other methods then used included inspection of the abdominal wall, palpation, percussion (especially if the stomach could be distended with gas to give an accurate outline). Examination of gastric contents by test meals, and blood counts were considered of little value. In selected cases, contrast (bismuth subcarbonate) x-rays were used to diagnose pyloric stenosis and gastric motility by fluoroscopy. Perry (11) states that "the use of the x-ray has brought about a wonderful change in the minds of the medical profession as to the actual functions of the stomach and the best method of treating same."

Also in 1912, Friedenwald (12) published a clinical study of 1000 cases of ulcer of the stomach and duodenum. He claimed to have exercised the greatest care to eliminate all cases in which there had been the slightest question of the diagnosis, but he did not provide any of the diagnostic criteria as to how he distinguished duodenal (529 cases) from gastric ulcer (409 cases) or peptic ulcer from the pool of 12,600 patients with dyspepsia. In this population of 1000 ulcers, he reported alcoholism in 214, syphilis in 54 (in only 5 was the ulcer caused by syphilis). Gastric secretion (i.e., acid concentrations with a test meal) was measured in 810 cases: 46% were normal, 30% high, and 23% low; 94% had pain, 91% had epigastric tenderness, and vomiting occurred in 68%; 230 had current or prior hematemesis and melena, and 287 had melena without hematemesis. 90% had positive tests for occult blood in the stool. "Atony of the stomach" was present in 321 and "enteroptosis" in 411. The cases were analyzed by age, sex, and duration of symptoms (average 12 years): seventy-one patients had surgery. Of these, 7 died and 64 were "cured." Of 794 patients treated medically, 521 had the "rest cure treatment" in bed for 6 to 8 weeks using a liquid diet (13). The remainder were ambulatory. Of these, 153 were treated with silver nitrate and 110 with bismuth subnitrate; 50% in each group were cured.

After the more general use of x-rays in diagnosis, the validity of the pain patterns in making a diagnosis of gastric or duodenal ulcer was re-examined. Only 45% of GU and 70% of DU patients had relief of pain by food or antacids (10). Vomiting was reported in 75% of gastric ulcer and 60% of duodenal ulcer patients, belching in from 60 to 80% of peptic ulcer patients, and constipation in the greatest majority—data that are clearly different today. It is thus not certain whether the disease has changed or the patients included under the diagnosis have changed.

By 1925, the fractional test meal described by Rehfuss (14) in 1914 had become widely used in the diagnosis of ulcer and various dyspepsias. In his book on gastric function in health and disease, Ryle (in London) reports that the Rehfuss gruel test meal (14) had supplanted the Ewald test meal which used starch. His results were based on tests in 100 normal subjects in whom he measured the "free" and "total" acidity at 15-minute intervals for 2 hours after a test meal of gruel, as well as the starch content to determine gastric emptying. With these figures, he enlisted the help of the famous statistician Karl Pearson to define normal status, hypochlorhydria, and hypo- or achlorhydria. By applying formal statistics to experimental data, Ryle (15) established a standard for all future studies of this kind. By the use of x-rays, he also described gastric tonus and divided his subjects into sthenic, hyposthenic, and hypersthenic. Peptic ulcers were still considered to be a subset of dyspepsia, and Ryle in 1925 presented the following:

Classification of the Dyspepsias

Group 1. Habit Dyspepsias. Dyspepsias resulting from faulty physical habits.

Examples: Overeating, undereating, overwork, lack of occupation and exercise, insufficient mastication, constipation, or some combination of these factors.

Group 2. Nervous or Psychogenic Dyspepsias. Dyspepsias due to faulty mental or nervous adjustment.

Examples: Nervous traits such as aerophagy, nervous exhaustion, worry and anxiety states, hysteria, hypochondriasis, and refusal of food.

Group 3. Toxic and Infective Dyspepsias. Dyspepsias due to (a) tissue poisons and (b) general or local infective disease, and other and more obscure conditions interfering with general health and nutrition.

Examples: (a) Alcohol or tobacco; (b) pulmonary tuberculosis, oral sepsis, severe anemias, states of general debility associated with auto-intoxication, muscular hypotonus, loss of fatty deposits, and visceroptosis.

Group 4. Irritative Dyspepsias. Dyspepsias due to stimuli originating in a local or distal organ lesion.

Examples: Gastric and duodenal ulcer, gastrojejunal ulcer, chronic infections of the appendix and gallbladder, special sense disturbances such as astigmatism, and central nervous lesions such as tabes dorsalis.

Group 5. Mechanical Dyspepsias. Dyspepsias due to gross structural disease or surgical modifications of the anatomy of the stomach.

Examples: Pyloric stenosis, hourglass stomach, chronic extensive ulceration, certain complications and sequelae of gastrojejunostomy, and carcinoma ventriculi. *(Cited verbatim from Ryle (15))*

This type of classification of dyspepsias and the supposed or observed causes are reminiscent of the descriptions of indigestion and its causes presented 100 years previously by Phillip (1), whose book on indigestion never once mentions gastric or duodenal ulcer. Using these criteria, Ryle classified 267 consecutive patients with dyspepsia seen in consultation into groups: (1) 12%, (2) 24%, (3) 12%, (4 and 5) 52%, the distribution being weighted because groups 4 and 5 were the more resistant to treatment and thus more likely to be referred to a specialist. He noted that two or more of these could coexist and that there was much overlap. It was only group 4 and 5 that exhibited hyperchlorhydria in about 70% of patients, a finding he considered pathognomonic of duodenal ulcer. In such cases, he also reported rapid emptying and prolonged "aftersecretion" in the test meal, both of which are still considered today major abnormalities in the control of acid secretion in duodenal ulcer. He reported also that no hypo- or achlorhydria was found in this group. In gastric ulcer, secretion was found to be normal, but in gastrojejunal ulcer following gastroenterostomy, he typically found high secretion, in some instances higher than before surgery. He recommended that gastrojejunostomy not be done in patients with high secretion who did not need the operation for pyloric stenosis.

His clinical description of duodenal ulcer, however, is compatible with what we would use today, the x-rays described as showing exaggerated tonus and peristalsis, and sometimes rapid evacuation of the meal. Postsurgical gastrojejunal ulcer was well recognized and closely resembled duodenal ulcer. Gastric ulcer, he conceded, was less typical in its clinical presentation, with a non-diagnostic gastric analysis and an inconstant but diagnostic finding of an incisura and hourglass stomach.

Radiology

In 1897, Cannon first used bismuth subnitrate as a contrast material to study swallowing by fluoroscopy in various animals (16). Bismuth subcarbonate was incorporated in a food paste, which was used for the next 20 or more years. Barium sulfate was first used in 1910 by Bachem and Gunther (17). However, because of the inadvertent use of barium sulfide, resulting in deaths, barium sulfate was not routinely used until it could be guaranteed safe. What Gelfand (18) called the pioneer era in GI radiology lasted from 1896 to about 1925. During the pioneer era, fluoroscopy, spot films, barium sulfate suspensions, cinefluoroscopy, and double-contrast studies were proposed and some brought into common use (18). Standardized serial contrast studies were generally used by 1925. The second era of GI radiology from 1925 to 1950 brought better equipment, and technique and most pathologic entities were already described by 1950.

In 1914, George and Gerber (19) laid down some rules by which to make a "direct method of diagnosis of duodenal ulcer by means of the Roentgen ray." They offered the concept of making a positive or direct diagnosis, rather than using symptom complexes which provided only inferential evidence. Based on their experience of serial x-ray studies in 600 patients, they point out that (1) 95% of duodenal ulcers occur in the first portion of the duodenum; (2) the first part of the duodenum is a constant entity; (3) if normal, a smooth outline in various positions will always be shown on a plate; (4) a constant defect means a pathologic condition, which included ulcer, adhesions, cholecystitis, or anatomic or accidental variation; (5) any duodenal ulcer other than a simple mucosal erosion will deform the outline of the bismuth mass; and (6) a normal bulb or cap rules out an indurated or "surgical" duodenal ulcer. Mayo (20) in 1914 placed roentgen rays second only to history and physical examination in the diagnosis of duodenal ulcer.

Improvements in technique and experience, better barium suspension, longer fluoroscopy time, shorter exposure times to get better radiographs, and duodenal compression raised the number of niches found from 15% in the mid-20s to as much as 60 to 70% of ulcers found at subsequent surgery or autopsy. By 1925, standardized serial contrast studies were in general use (19). However, the intervals between x-ray studies and the anatomic diagnosis were not always short enough to rule out healing or relapse of the ulcer. Summerville (21), a surgeon working in India, reported in 1942 that he had operated on 500 patients in whom duodenal deformity had been found on x-ray and found ulcer disease in 497. The absence of reliable reference standards rendered many such early claims of radiologic diagnosis of duodenal ulcer uncertain (10).

The third quarter-century of radiology, 1950 through 1975, saw extremely active technical advancements, including image amplification, television imaging, major improvements of barium suspensions, photo time spot films, powerful generators and tubes, and remote control fluoroscopic tables (18). The number of contrast studies peaked in the U.S. in 1975 and has declined by approximately 25% as endoscopy has grown.

Evolution of radiologic technique and skill has clearly depended on interaction with and feedback from other objective means such as autopsy, surgery, gastroscopy, and in the last 30 years flexible fiberoptic or electronic endoscopy with further histologic and photographic documentation. At present, between 75 and 85% of duodenal ulcers over 5 mm are discoverable by x-ray (22,23) and about 92% by endoscopy (23).

The diagnosis and treatment of *gastric ulcer* was caught up from the beginning in the problem of gastric cancer. Haudek, in 1910 (24), first described the gastric ulcer niche, and over the next 20 years or so, the diagnosis of gastric ulcer was made by steadily improving radiologic techniques. However, many cancers were not diagnosed, leading to the insistence of surgeons that gastric ulcer required surgical treatment regardless of other considerations (3). Despite the addition of semiflexible gastroscopy in the 1930s and the claims of Schindler (25) that it was possible to correctly classify gastric ulcer and cancer in 90% of cases, diagnosis remained difficult. It is hard to imagine today, with all the tools at our disposal, the intensity of debate that went on up to the late 60s on the fine points of making a radiologic differential diagnosis between benign and malignant gastric ulcer (10,26).

By 1950, Ivy, Grossman, and Bachrach (10) concluded that, using both x-rays and the endoscopy then available, the diagnosis would be wrong in 5 to 10% of cases and indeterminate in another 15%. Small wonder that, as late as 1966 (3), surgeons would argue that a 20 to 25% uncertainty in diagnosis *required* surgical treatment for all gastric ulcers. It was conceded, however, that a trial of two weeks' treatment with x-ray evidence of healing would be reasonable before invoking surgery (3). X-ray remained the dominant technique in making the diagnosis of gastric ulcer/cancer. The impact of endoscopy is dealt with below.

The role of radiology in gastroesophageal *reflux disease* (GERD) has been defined by comparison with other tests of mucosal disease (endoscopy) and reflux (pH) and motility (manometry). Radiography is insensitive (22%) in mild degrees of inflammation but better for severe esophagitis including ulceration and stricture (90% sensitive) (27). Reflux at fluoroscopy has 40% sensitivity and 85% specificity (28). Radiology and manometry are complementary in diagnosis of motility disorders (28).

Endoscopy

The understanding and management of acid peptic upper GI diseases has been immeasurably altered by the development of fully flexible fiberoptic endoscopes in 1957 (29–32). Fiberoptic endoscopy was introduced into clinical practice by 1961 (30,33, 34) and, modified and improved by the mid to late 1960s, soon achieved almost universal use in gastroenterology (31,32,35–40). The ability to visualize the esophagus, stomach, and first and second parts of the duodenum routinely, and to supplement this capacity with biopsy and cytology, have totally transformed the study, understanding and treatment of acid peptic diseases. Endoscopy has become the benchmark for radiologic and other diagnoses and the key to determining the results of treatment.

From 1963 onward (40), it was possible to diagnose degrees of esophagitis accurately and with ease and safety, to confirm these histologically, and to observe the natural history of these disorders through repeated examinations.

The 50 years of gastroscopy from Elsner's 1910 instrument, modified and made semiflexible by Schindler in 1932 (25,29, 31,32), remained an awkward and inadequate procedure for understanding the nature and natural history of gastric ulcer.

After 1961, gastric ulcer soon lost the overbearing aura of possible malignancy. Not only did frequent use enlarge the experience of each endoscopist in visual diagnosis, but the addition of cytology and biopsies and the ease of serial endoscopic follow-up provided a level of assurance in making the differential diagnosis. GI pathologists became more experienced and confident of making diagnoses, not only of cancer but of other histopathology as well. These capabilities have greatly reduced the need for elective surgery (3). Whether there has been any significant improvement in gastric cancer therapy or survival is less certain, but fewer patients with gastric ulcer are being subjected to unnecessary surgery. The state of an ulcer that has recently bled and the capacity to control bleeding or to preempt rebleeding represents a major advance in managing gastric ulcer. The range of the lesions of the stomach amenable to diagnosis by endoscopy but not x-ray includes erosive gastritis, whether it is caused by aspirin (41) or NSAIDS (42) or by the stress of serious illness or burns (43,44).

Although it is theoretically possible to see 100% of duodenal ulcers—some 10% are overlooked through inability to see the bulb due to pyloric stenosis or deformity enough to hide the ulcer, endoscopy provides the standard by which duodenal ulcers are diagnosed and their natural history studied. We can now relate ulcers to symptoms and follow asymptomatic (silent) ulcers (45,46) and their behavior. Duodenitis is no longer a hypothetic diagnosis made by radiologists on the basis of an "irritable" duodenal cap without crater, and pseudodiverticula can be distinguished from ulcers. The ability to diagnose duodenal ulcer with such ease and certainty contrasts with the findings of Wilkie (47) in 1914 that only 6 of 41 cases of duodenal ulcer found at autopsy had been diagnosed antemortem and then had been diagnosed in life only at surgery.

The postsurgical upper GI tract presented particular difficulties in diagnosis of the cause of symptoms. Because of altered anatomy, radiology was at a disadvantage, and much postgastrectomy pathology, including ulcers, was undiagnosed or misdiagnosed (48). What struck me in the early 1960s was not that surgery was successful in many patients, but that so many patients who had had surgery for ulcer had simply exchanged one set of problems for another. In less than 10 years, at the University of Alabama, I had examined and endoscoped almost 600 symptomatic postgastrectomy patients (48). Endoscopy revealed a high prevalence of mucosal or anatomic disease, which when added to the metabolic and functional impairments, painted a much worse picture of the results of ulcer surgery than claimed by the surgeons or uncovered by radiologists. Endoscopy was central to this investigation.

With the explosive development of effective new treatments for peptic ulcer came the need for better objective standards by which to judge efficacy and outcome. Because peptic ulcer is mostly nonfatal, survival statistics were not applicable. It was also clear that symptoms alone were not reliable enough to make the diagnosis of gastric or duodenal ulcer (50) or as an objective measure of healing or of relapse. The insensitivity of x-rays in diagnosing DU and of determining healing was recognized early (10) and led to the adoption by the late 1970s of endoscopy as the sole criterion of ulcer diagnosis (23), healing and relapse in the multitude of clinical trials of ulcer treatment since then. In this way, the natural history of duodenal and gastric ulcer has been gradually revealed (5,49,51).

Laboratory Diagnosis

By the late 1920s and early 1930s, the value of radiologic techniques in the diagnosis of gastric or duodenal ulcer and of complications such as pyloric stenosis had become evident. The differential diagnosis had been improved, although the gastric ulcer/cancer differential remained a difficult problem. A process of cross-learning between physicians, surgeons, radiologists and pathologists was expanded by the introduction of the semiflexible gastroscope by Schindler in 1932 (25).

Gastric analysis by the fractional test meal (14,15) was widely performed and a large experience analyzed by age and sex was accumulated at the Mayo Clinic (52) by 1932. Polland and others (53,54) developed the criteria for a histamine test, using the middle 80% as normal measuring acid concentration as Ryle had done. Other stimuli included alcohol, beef bouillon, and caffeine, but in many cases tests lacked standardization.

Gradually, over the next 20 years to 1950, when Ivy et al. (10) and Babkin (9) reviewed gastric secretion in both diagnosis and the study of pathophysiology, studies of overnight acid output and basal secretion (53) had been added and acid output, rather than the previously used concentration studies, was being used to measure responses. In all studies, hypersecretion by any measure (volume, acid concentration, or acid output) was noted in a significant proportion of DU patients, although in many results were in the normal range. Little has changed up to today, despite an enormous amount of effort in the intervening 40 years (55). Studies of *pepsin* secretion had been rare and by inadequate methods such as egg white digestion, using so-called "Mett's tubes," which yielded little reliable information. The same may be said of studies of gastric mucin which had been found to be either decreased or normal in DU (10).

By 1950, a considerable effort had been invested in studying gastric motility (16) largely by x-ray and balloon kymography. No conclusive results dealing with duodenal ulcer had been reached. Secretion and motility were studied in much greater detail after vagotomy became established in the treatment of ulcer in the mid-60s to mid-70s.

The study of gastric secretion in the last 40 years has continued at an accelerated rate. For example, in 1991 over 250 papers were published on the subject. Pentagastrin has replaced histamine as the preferred stimulus, and the study of basal and maximal acid outputs is now considered the minimum necessary to describe secretion patterns. In 1953, Kay (56) used graded doses of histamine [rather than the standard 0.1 mg introduced by Polland in 1933 (53)] to establish a maximum rate of acid secretion. This value was shown to represent the parietal cell mass as determined by histologic means (57). The parietal cell mass was found to have the same distribution as maximum acid output in DU and GU and controls (58). Variations of the graded dose studies have used pentagastrin or gastrin. These have made it possible to describe the gastric response to stimulation in mathematical terms (59–61).

Despite many attempts to define secretion in terms of weight or body habitus, or by the stimulus used or the product measured (acid, pepsin) (55), gastric analysis today is still considered to have too much overlap between DU and normal to be useful for diagnosis (43,69). Gastric secretion studies are still important in the diagnosis of hypersecretion states (62,63) and of achlorhydria of pernicious anemia (PA) and in the differential diagnosis of hypergastrinemia (64).

For a number of years, gastric analysis was studied as a possible predictor of success of gastric surgery (65,66). With the decline of surgery, the futility of the earlier studies remains evident. However, Ryle's (15) conclusion that gastric secretion always be studied before surgery still holds to rule out Zollinger-Ellison syndrome (62).

In 1860, Brucke reported the presence of pepsinogen in the urine (uropepsin). Uropepsin excretion was studied extensively as a method for diagnosing upper GI disease. It was high in a significant number of patients with DU, absent in PA, and low in gastric cancer. It was felt to have value in predicting the development of DU in Army recruits. Most of all, many hoped that it could replace gastric analysis (67). Measurement of pepsinogen in serum found that the distribution mirrored the urine values in DU and PA. Although the subtypes of pepsinogen in serum or urine were found useful in genetic studies (68), little was added to the laboratory diagnosis of duodenal or gastric ulcer or cancer. An apparent pedigree of hyperpepsinogenemic patients with a high predictability of development of DU (43,69) was found later to represent H. pylori infection.

The history of gastric secretion studies described by Davenport (2) provides insight into the eventual development of highly effective acid-suppressing drugs.

Present Perspectives on Diagnosis

The means available to us today still begin with a medical history, which leads to further evaluation for diagnosis. However, the not unreasonable approach to "treat first and ask later" (70) has brought the ulcer field back to the status of 80 years ago, when Friedenwald (5) described 1000 cases of peptic ulcer, all presumably clinically diagnosed with such certainty that he excluded all cases in which "there was the slightest doubt." Today we find any and all "dyspepsias" and "abdominal pain" being treated, sometimes interminably, with H_2 antagonists. Are we back to the purely clinical diagnosis of peptic ulcer despite having readily available highly sensitive, specific, and simple tools for making definitive diagnoses of esophagitis or gastric and duodenal ulcer?

TREATMENT

Surgical Treatment

For almost 100 years, the history of peptic ulcer was defined by its surgery. Abdominal surgery had slow beginnings in the mid-19th century, becoming feasible for the first time after the demonstration of ether anesthesia by Morton in 1846 at the Massachusetts General Hospital for a major operation by Dr. Warren (71). In 1865, Joseph Lister developed the principles of antisepsis, making it possible to anticipate successful abdominal surgery. The earliest gastric operations were performed for perforated ulcer and pyloric obstruction. The first successful surgical gastrostomy was by Sidney Jones in London in 1875 (71). In 1881, Billroth performed the first successful partial gastrectomy for pyloric cancer, and in the same year, Wolfler in Vienna performed a gastroenterostomy for obstructive cancer. In 1883, Kocher (71) performed the first successful suture of a gunshot wound of the stomach. However, the first successful closure of a gastric ulcer perforation was not accomplished until 1892 by Heusner, operating in a patient's home (72). Two years later, Dean (72) was the first to successfully close a perforated duodenal ulcer. In 1901, Moynihan (73) collected 51 cases operated on for perforated duodenal ulcer with only nine (17%) surviving. Loreta dilated the pylorus through a gastrostomy (see 72); pylorectomy and excision of a gastric ulcer in 1882 by Rydygier were followed by pyloroplasty (Heineke and Mikulicz) and later by gastroenterostomy (72).

From these early beginnings, gastric surgery developed rapidly, and with the elimination of the bad and dissemination of the good, it gradually came to assume a recognized approach by the end of the 19th century (71,74). Posterior gastrojejunostomy (von Hacker, 1885) became the preferred operation and was championed later by Moynihan for the treatment of all duodenal ulcers (73). Jaboulay in 1894 (71) recommended gastroduodenostomy instead.

The surgical treatment of uncomplicated duodenal ulcer by gastroenterostomy was first reported in 1898 by Codivilla, who additionally transected the distal antrum and oversewed both ends to "rest the duodenum." Occlusion of the pylorus was performed at surgery with gastroenterostomy to prevent passage of gastric contents. Mayo in 1915 (20) felt that "the evidence as to the necessity of this procedure is not clear."

In the early days of gastric surgery, the choice of operation was dictated above all by whether the patient would survive. Partial gastrectomy was gradually being performed more commonly, although with uncertain benefit, and by 1893 a review in the Annals of Surgery recorded a mortality of 41% (71). In otherwise fatal conditions, such as gastric cancer, surgeons were willing to take risks and extended the limits of

resection gradually to total gastrectomy despite the punishing mortality statistics (71).

By the beginning of this century, the techniques of gastric surgery had been sufficiently improved and mortality reduced to such a level that the debate as to feasibility in the 1880s and permissibility in the 1890s shifted to the logical application of the diseases at hand. In 1900, Mayo Robson claimed that gastric ulcers not responding to medical therapy should have surgery and W. J. Mayo declared gastric cancer a surgical disease. Duodenal ulcer in the 19th century became either more common or more commonly recognized and thoughts turned to treating this disorder by surgery.

Ogilvie, reviewing this period in 1947 (71), wrote: "for ulcer, a distressing but not mortal malady, the attempt to find an operation which would give permanent relief at small risk led to the adoption of a number of procedures which varied as views on the etiology of ulceration changed." At first performed for pyloric obstruction caused by cancer or ulcer, gastroenterostomy produced such good results that it was soon applied to all ulcers, even those with no stenosis (71,73).

In 1905, Moynihan published his first book on surgical treatment of gastric and duodenal ulcers and Mayo in 1904 reported a series of 58 cases treated by gastrojejunostomy (75). At that time, however, physicians were laboring under the handicap of inadequate diagnosis. Wilkie (47,76), for example, reported that only 15% of duodenal ulcers found at autopsy had been diagnosed in life, and these only in operated patients.

With time, the clinical diagnosis of typical duodenal ulcer became better established and was based on the appearance of pain 2 to 4 hours after food and further relief by food. Few surgical papers in the period from 1900 to 1915 mentioned the use of x-ray, although Mayo (20) does place x-rays second in diagnostic worth behind history and the physical examination. Surgery therefore was applied only to the most typical cases. It was not stated in any of these papers how many were misdiagnosed before surgery.

Moynihan (73) was the most enthusiastic proponent of surgery for chronic duodenal ulcer: ". . . cases are within the experience of all in which prolonged medical treatment . . . is powerless to ward off the recurrence of dyspepsia—. I do not know of any operation in surgery which gives better results, which gives more complete satisfaction both to the patient and his surgeon than gastroenterostomy for chronic ulcer of the stomach.'' He reported 7 years later in 1910 a 2% mortality and no failures in 186 patients. There was no report of new ulceration in any of these patients. Mayo (1915) (20), who was equally impressed with surgery for duodenal ulcer, ascribed recurrent ulcer symptoms to poor technique and "stitch" ulcers. "In those rare cases in which true jejunal ulcers form after gastroenterostomy, the jejunal ulcer should be excised—and a Finney [pyloroplasty] done—.'' Following surgery, he recommended that the patient be under "good medical advice until permanent cure is assured." His excellent article on duodenal ulcer ends on this high note. His recommendations on good medical advice could not be seriously undertaken for another 60 years.

Complications of gastroenterostomy were few at first. In 1899, Braun described a jejunal ulcer, and in 1905 Mayo Robson felt that it was a rare complication (71). However, as gastroenterostomy became more widely applied, stomal ulceration became an obvious problem. In the average case, a lag time of years between surgery and relapse obscured the problem. At first, failure was ascribed to technique (20) (clamps, suture extrusion), but it became apparent in the early 1920s that the fault lay in the disease being treated (15,77). In 1929, Finney (78) reported a 59% marginal ulcer rate after gastroenterostomy, and after noting the high rate of recurrence and the failure to reduce acidity, suggested some strict rules for performing this operation. Gastroenterostomy dominated the field from 1900 to about 1925. The complications not reported by the early enthusiasts included afferent limb obstruction, gastrojejunocolic fistula, dumping, diarrhea, and bilious vomiting (72). The Roux-en-Y gastrojejunostomy (Roux 1902) (see 71) is now used to remedy the bilious vomiting (79), but in 1947 Ogilvie described it as a "technique which now has a historic interest only," because of the high frequency of jejunal ulceration. This outcome is very reminiscent of the experimental Mann-Williamson marginal ulcer of the 30s (80).

Surgery now turned to a group of operations on the pylorus—gastroduodenostomy (Jaboulay 1894), pyloroplasty, various gastroduodenal anastomoses to treat pyloric stenosis and to hasten emptying into the duodenum to promote rapid neutralization. However, these operations shared the fate of the gastroenterostomy, with recurrent ulceration, dumping, and bilious vomiting.

Mayo (20) recognized that alkalis, diet restriction and milk and cream could heal ulcers, but not cure them. He therefore used the failure of medical treatment as an indication for surgery but despite his sharp insights into the natural history of duodenal ulcer, did not aim at reducing acid. Surgeons began to realize that the immediate fall of acidity after the various short circuiting operations were shortlived and when tested a year later all had returned to high preoperative levels. It was becoming evident that duodenal ulcer was, if not caused by, at least was maintained by acid and that reduction or elimination of acid was the key to treatment (71). In 1947, Ogilvie (71) mentions four approaches to reduce acid—gastrectomy (Fig. 5–1), short circuiting operation (Fig. 5–2), vasoligation of the gastric arteries, and vagal section (Fig. 5– 3). To this must be added the rather curious operation of cholecystgastrostomy to alkalinize the stomach.

Rokitansky, 1841–1846 (cited by Jordan, 72) stated that the "proximate cause of duodenal ulcer may be looked for in diseased innervation of the stomach owing to a morbid condition of the vagus and to extreme acidification of the gastric juice." The oft-quoted dictum of Schwarz (81) in 1910, "No acid, no ulcer," and the excellent results of acid neutralization first enthusiastically demonstrated by Sippy in 1913 (82) led to a surgical reappraisal. At the same time, the increasing safety of larger operations, in skilled hands, which resulted in permanent reduction of acid secretion, led to abandonment of bypass operations in favor of gastrectomy. Like earlier operations, partial gastrectomy went through a period of intensive testing, with good results of low ulcer recurrence balanced against the undesirable side effects. In 1918, Finsterer (cited by Jordan, 71) recommended two-thirds gastric resection. By the mid-1930s, gastrectomy was dominant in Europe, and by 1940 was

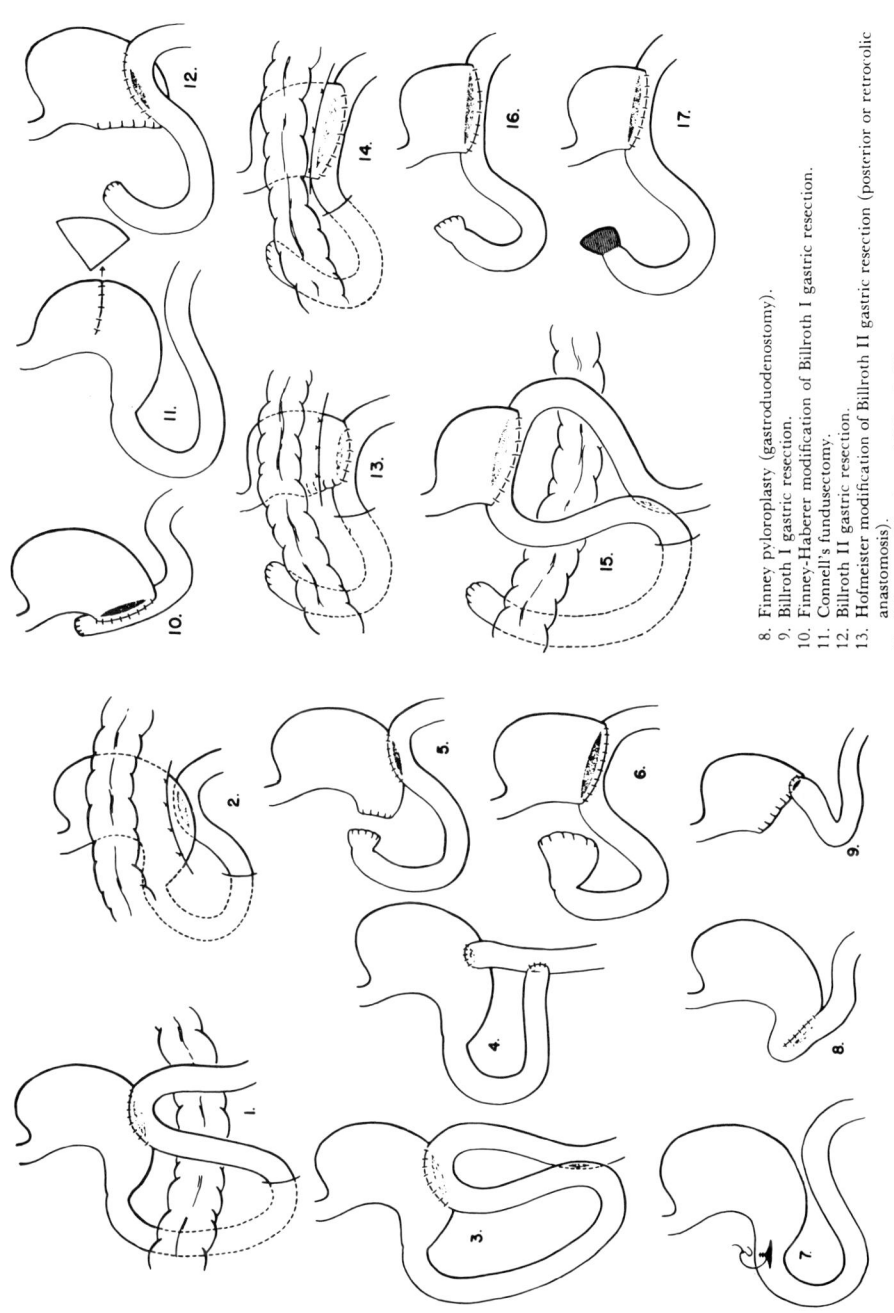

1. Anterior gastrojejunostomy (gastroenterostomy).
2. Posterior gastrojejunostomy (gastroenterostomy).
3. Gastroenterostomy with (Braun's) enteroenterostomy.
4. Gastroenterostomy with Roux-en-Y anastomosis.
5. Gastroenterostomy with pyloric exclusion (von Eiselsberg).
6. Devine's pyloric exclusion operation (no stomach is resected).
7. Heineke-Mikulicz pyloroplasty.
8. Finney pyloroplasty (gastroduodenostomy).
9. Billroth I gastric resection.
10. Finney-Haberer modification of Billroth I gastric resection.
11. Connell's fundusectomy.
12. Billroth II gastric resection.
13. Hofmeister modification of Billroth II gastric resection (posterior or retrocolic anastomosis).
14. Pólya modification of Billroth II gastric resection (posterior or retrocolic anastomosis).
15. Pólya type gastric resection with anterior (antecolic) anastomosis and entero-enterostomy.
16. Finsterer's resection with pyloric exclusion (the remnant of the pars pylorica is not resected).
17. Finsterer's resection with pyloric exclusion and excision of the pyloric mucosa (the mucous membrane of the excluded pyloric remnant is excised).

Fig. 5–1. Seventeen of the many dozens of operations and modifications that were in use and developed between 1881 and about 1950 for the treatment of peptic ulcer. Reproduced with permission from Ivy AC, Grossman M, Bachrach WH: Peptic Ulcer. Philadelphia, The Blakiston Company, 1950, p. 1144.

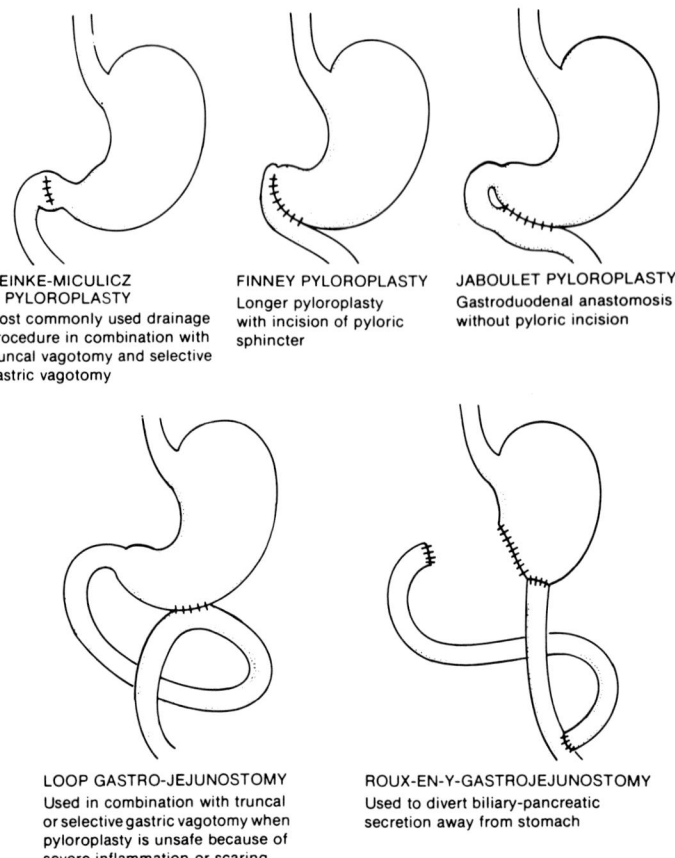

Fig. 5–2. Various drainage operations developed over the years, many for use with vagotomy. Reproduced with permission from Yamada T et al.: Textbook of Gastroenterology, Vol. 1. Philadelphia, JB Lippincott Co., 1991, pp. 1382–1383.

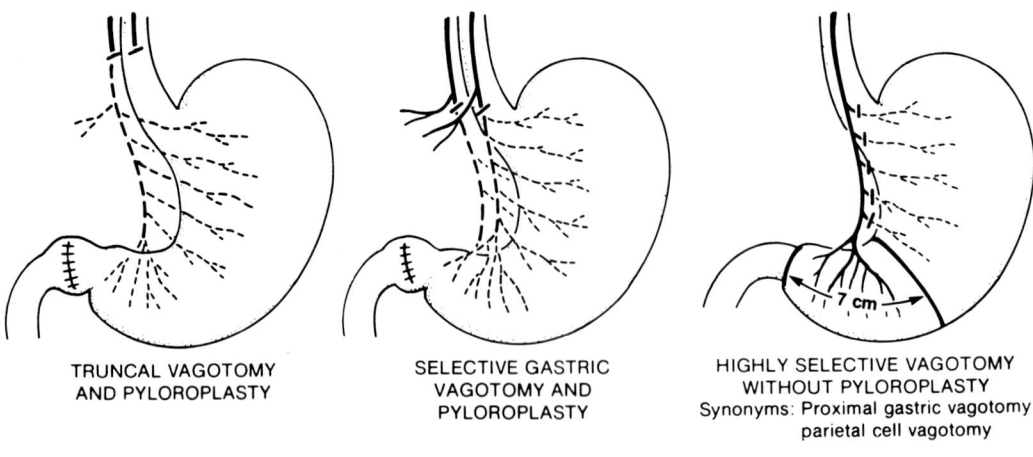

Fig. 5–3. Illustrations of vagotomy options, first proposed by Latarjet in 1922[87] and popularized by Dragstedt.[85] Reproduced with permission from Yamada T et al.: Textbook of Gastroenterology, Vol. 1. Philadelphia, JB Lippincott Co., 1991, pp. 1382–1383.

becoming the worldwide standard for surgical treatment of ulcer. However, the reaction to these high resections was not always very favorable. Rodman (71), commenting on a presentation by Finney, remarked that "the cure is worse than the disease."

One of the many variants of gastric resection is that of antral exclusion, which left a portion of the antrum in situ when the duodenum was difficult to close. Finsterer and Cunha (83), who also practiced this operation, recognized the high rate of ulcer recurrence and excised the remaining antrum to cure the problem. It was not until later that experiments on antral exclusion in dogs by Dragstedt and his colleagues (84) demonstrated that uncontrolled gastrin release caused the high secretion leading to recurrence.

At the height of popularity of gastrectomy, Ogilvie in 1947 (71) in addressing the centenary of the American Medical Association on 100 years of gastric surgery described radical gastrectomy in experienced hands as a satisfactory ulcer operation with mortality of 2%, a cure rate for ulcer of over 90% and a recurrence rate of at most 1%. In the average clinic, he described risks as being perhaps 4 or 5 times as high, with the prospects of cure less assured. He clearly outlined the physiology of the control of acid secretion and felt that hormonic (sic), rather than vagal mechanisms were at fault. He described Dragstedt's pioneer work in dogs and the introduction of supradiaphragmatic vagotomy into clinical practice in 1943 (85) with strikingly successful results. Ogilvie (71) followed this, however, with the comment that "It is odious to criticize the darling of the moment, whether in films, sport or surgical technique, but it would be well before rushing into the operation wholesale, to ask whether it has drawbacks as well as advantages, whether it is indeed the answer to the gastric surgeons prayer?" He criticized the procedure because he said it would not affect "hormonic" secretion, did not remove stricture, and delayed gastric emptying. He saw no reason to abandon radical gastrectomy, in which he saw all good and no negative effects, especially if by removing the lesser curve he also removed half of the vagal innervation. In fact, it was to be Dragstedt's day and not, as Ogilvie predicted, "a passing fancy." Gastrec-tomy was ultimately abandoned precisely because of its undesirable side effects, which its proponents, dazzled by the low ulcer recurrence rate, minimized or rationalized. Surgeons sought to overcome the illogicality of treating a small ulcer in one organ by removing seven eighths of its neighbor (86), by searching for lesser procedures.

Up to this point, the debate on ulcer treatment involved mostly surgeons. The aggressive neutralization with antacids and food pioneered by Sippy in 1913 (82) had remained the mainstay of medical treatment; the addition of anticholinergics and phenobarbital had done little to alter the course of duodenal or gastric ulcer.

The history of vagotomy goes back to the "ancients." Phillip in 1823 (1) reported extensive experiments in rabbits in which cutting the "eighth pair of nerves in the neck" resulted in gastric retention of undigested food. He cited similar studies by Paracelsus in the 16th century (Opus Chirurgicum, 1565). He concluded that the vagus nerves controlled both secretion and emptying. He also reported an interesting observation that galvanic current applied to the distal vagus reversed the acute effects of vagotomy in rabbits. This kind of knowledge was further developed by the physiologists of the late 19th and early 20th centuries—Heindenhain (1879), who constructed denervated pouches of canine stomachs, and Pavlov, who made vagally innervated pouches and numerous physiological experiments (9,55). The response of the stomach to food and sham feeding were known to be vagally mediated and insulin hypoglycemia was shown in 1926 to stimulate gastric secretion via the vagus (9). This technique was later to become the standard means of testing for completeness of vagotomy (2,9).

In 1922, Latarjet (87) described in detail the vagal innervation of the stomach and reported successfully treating six patients with gastric and pyloric ulcer with vagotomy and gastroenterostomy. ". . . . in all our cases, gastroenteroanastomosis was done at the same time as denervation, ... to avoid the possibility of an aggravated ulcer evolution as a consequence of prolonged journey of food in a stomach which had been rendered hypotonic by denervation." This lesson, as well as that of experiments by Phillip (1), had not been remembered when vagotomy without drainage was later reintroduced. Several surgeons had tried vagotomy with mixed results. Klein in 1929 cut the left vagus nerves in patients for persistent hyperacidity after resection, and Berg in 1930 (71) incorporated left vagotomy into his partial gastrectomy operations as well. The combination later became popular. Dragstedt and Owens (85) in 1943 reported supradiaphragmatic vagotomy for duodenal ulcer with good results. Vagotomy met considerable resistance from the many proponents of gastrectomy from Ogilvie (71), from the Mayo Clinic and from Wangensteen among others (71). The AGA undertook a review of gastric surgery that showed results of vagotomy and gastroenterostomy to be the same as gastrectomy (71). Ochsner predicted in 1970 that vagotomy would eventually have the same bad results as gastroenterostomy (71).

It was found early that truncal vagotomy caused unpleasant gastric retention. Soon subdiaphragmatic vagotomy was the preferred route and drainage by pyloroplasty or gastroenterostomy was added (72). In his last paper, published posthumously, Dragstedt (89) attributed the development of a gastric ulcer in patients after transthoracic vagotomy to stasis. It is possible that, in using the statement "the success of drugs such as Alka-Seltzer in relieving distress. . . ," Dr. Dragstedt may in fact have pinpointed the culprit, aspirin, in the development of gastric ulcer in his patients. To avoid denervating all the intestinal organs by truncal vagotomy, selective vagotomy was proposed, but because it was not conclusively shown to be superior (71) and was a more tedious operation, it was not very popular and, within the decade, was overtaken by highly selective vagotomy.

The monumental 1950 monograph by Ivy, Grossman, and Bachrach (10) is an encyclopedic description of peptic ulcer at the mid-century. Chapter 23 reviews surgery of various types developed until then (Fig. 5–1). The differences in attitudes in various places may be illustrated by the frequency of referrals to surgery. Between 1930 and 1945, Brown referred 10.6% of 1500 patients for surgery; the Lahey Clinic did the same for 6.1% of 7844 duodenal ulcers and 19.3% of gastric ulcers; and at the Mayo Clinic,

where gastric ulcer was considered to be a surgical disease, 45 to 65% of patients with gastric ulcer between 1935 and 1944 were sent to surgery each year (10). However, for duodenal ulcer, the rate fell from 26% in 1930 to 12% in 1944. Others reported from 14 to 29% of duodenal ulcer patients referred to surgery (10). The referral for complicated ulcer was higher than that for pain alone, although ultimately many more patients were operated on for intractability than for complications (obstruction, bleeding, perforation) (10).

By the 1940s, gastric surgery still had a significant mortality (about 5% for elective surgery (10) and considerably higher for emergency surgery). Also, postoperative problems were recognized with increasing frequency, leading to abandonment of one group of operations after another (86). Yet there was still a great deal of debate about the "best operation" for duodenal ulcer. Many dozens of operations had been proposed (Fig. 5–1) and improvements in technique of the most popular, i.e., gastrectomy, were being made all the time (86). By about 1950, gastrectomy was dominant and vagotomy was still under review (71,90).

By combining vagotomy with partial gastric resection (71) in the early 1950s, surgeons felt that they had achieved an almost perfect ulcer operation—elimination of the vagal, nervous control and the "hormonic"(sic) influence of the antrum, which by this time was well understood (71,84,85).

Although the clinical results of various operations by the late 1950s were perceived as being equally good, several attempts were made to individualize surgery according to preoperative acid studies (55). Bruce and Card in Edinburgh (66) were major proponents of matching the resection to the acid output. Andrew Kay (56) standardized the histamine test and, with the correlation between parietal cell counts and maximal acid output (57), it was felt that "tailored gastrectomy" was the scientific way to guide surgery for duodenal ulcer (65,66). Failures of surgery were laid to inadequate reduction in acid secretion. This approach was the basis for many later gastric secretion studies in cases of relapse after vagal denervation (55).

The concept of randomized clinical trials pioneered by Doll (5) in evaluation of medical treatment for gastric and duodenal ulcer was applied to surgical treatments for duodenal ulcer. In a landmark article, Goligher et al. (7) reported that in such a trial subtotal gastrectomy, truncal vagotomy and gastroenterostomy and vagotomy and hemigastrectomy, all performed by experienced surgeons under the same conditions, were essentially equally successful and with similar adverse effects except for an increased number of recurrent ulcers after gastroenterostomy and vagotomy, although far fewer than before the combination with vagotomy. By 1960, the enthusiasm for radical gastrectomy for duodenal ulcer had begun to wane and the lesser gastrectomy with vagotomy had in turn begun to yield to the vagotomy and pyloroplasty (Figs. 5–2, 5–3), although older surgeons still clung to gastroenterostomy as the preferred drainage operation (86,89).

In the 1960s, the magnitude of the problems of radical gastrectomy began to be evident (91). It was no longer forbidden to talk of gastric cripples (79). Over 100 remedial operations or modifications were devised (79) for the problems of afferent loop, efferent loop obstruction, dumping syndrome, reactive hypoglycemia, small pouch syndrome, bile gastritis, recurrent ulcer, diarrhea, weight loss, anemia, and various postgastrectomy pain syndromes.

In the end, even when a specific problem could be identified and an apparently rational approach applied, the problem was seldom solved (48). Many patients had multiple operations. It is easy to sympathize with Johnstone et al. (92), who described postgastrectomy patients or perhaps their surgeons as suffering from the albatross syndrome.

Because of such problems, all those concerned with treating ulcer welcomed the clinical application of the important studies on highly selective vagotomy by Griffith and Harkins (93). Johnson and Williamson (95) and Amdrup and Jensen (94) in 1970 reported the results of highly selective vagotomy, which denervated the body and fundus of the stomach (Fig. 5–3), leaving the antrum innervated by the nerves of Latarjet, whose contribution to gastric surgery and vagal anatomy had been made some 50 years before (87,88).

At last there was an operation that appeared to be ideal. It was effective in reducing acid sufficiently to heal and prevent relapse in the great majority of duodenal ulcers; it preserved the integrity of the upper GI tract, including the neurohormonal control of digestion; it could be performed with minimal mortality and could be performed well by most surgeons; and most important, when done properly it had no morbidity. Retention, bilious vomiting, weight loss, anemia, diarrhea, dumping, and reactive hypoglycemia had, to all intents and purposes, been avoided. This left conventional surgery to be used only for obstruction, perforation, and control of bleeding.

In 1984, Jordan (72) reported a 5-year cumulative recurrence rate of 8% in 100 patients, only 1 of whom required reoperation. Although relapse of ulcer was less in antrectomy with vagotomy and Billroth-I, at the same time, side effects were greater. Jordan favored highly selective vagotomy. The recurrence of ulcer after highly selective vagotomy between 5 and 30%, although generally below 10%, continued to concern surgeons. Elaborate studies of gastric secretion before and after surgery attempted to anticipate or explain the relapses (55). For the most part, relapses were more common after incomplete vagotomy, but that was apparently only part of the explanation (65,66).

Even as the apparently ideal operation established its credentials and had lived up to its promise, events overtook it. H_2 receptor antagonists were described in 1972 (8) and widely used clinically after 1974 (96). The number of operations for duodenal ulcer fell precipitously as the indication "unresponsive to good medical management" began to take on a new meaning because of a new definition of "good medical management." There are now far fewer such cases and, as will be detailed elsewhere, even the acid inhibitors as virtually ideal treatments for duodenal ulcer are facing up to the possible role of Helicobacter pylori in ulcer healing and relapse, and of ASA and NSAIDs as possible causes of intractability before surgery and of recurrence of marginal or pyloric ulcer after surgery (97). Because it may now be possible to perform highly selective vagotomy by laparoscopy, we may yet reassess the role of surgery in treating duodenal ulcer.

Gastric Ulcer

The almost obsessive fear of missing the diagnosis of gastric cancer clouded every rational debate on the proper role of surgery for many decades. A tabulation of malignancies discovered in over 2200 cases of gastric ulcer studied between 1927 and 1943 showed 12.7% to be malignant (10). Despite the improving experience and skill of the radiologists, this kind of statistic made a good case for surgery.

The state of controversy evoked by gastric ulcer is illustrated in a debate between a gastroenterologist and two surgeons in a 1966 book entitled *Controversy in Internal Medicine* (3). Tumen (3) considered gastric ulcers to be different from duodenal ulcer in their propensity for chronicity, complications and overlooked malignancy. It was a common perception that gastric ulcers were prone to bleed much more than duodenal ulcers and thus required prompt and early curative surgery. Tumen made the argument that surgery for all would include the 60 to 70% of cases that healed and never recurred and, as for the cancer argument, he believed that benign gastric ulcers did not undergo malignant degeneration. He also anticipated the present view that if a reliable diagnosis of malignancy could be made, there would be less need for controversy. "The problem of management of gastric ulcer therefore, is to a large extent a problem of differential diagnosis." The practice of the day then, in cases that did not initially suggest malignancy, was a trial of strict diet treatment plus hourly antacids, preferably in hospital for 2 weeks (the early 1960s were leisurely days) expecting a reduction in ulcer size of 50%. Failure to respond meant surgery; a response allowed continued observation to complete healing.

The application of his principles illustrated the dilemma: 16 of 80 (20%) "probably malignant" ulcers were in fact benign, whereas 1 (4%) of 20 patients "probably benign" was malignant at surgery, and of the 152 patients not operated on, 10 were later found to be malignant.

Kinsey and Zollinger (3) admitted the surgical tendency to operate on all gastric ulcers, but recognized that this approach was valid only for complications and for strong indications of malignancy—x-ray, positive cytology, failure to heal, and achlorhydria. They had only misdiagnosed 5% of benign ulcers in 495 such patients. Moreover, they found no evidence that prompt surgery improved survival among gastric cancer patients, and "cannot honestly say the possibility of cancer in gastric ulceration justifies immediate operative intervention." They also pointed out that most gastric ulcers in the over-50-years age group had the largest number of drug-induced (ASA, steroids, phenylbutazone, reserpine, and tobacco smoking) lesions. These drugs were reported by 104 of 514 (25%) of their cases; in those they avoided surgery. Nevertheless, in the remainder, "gastric ulcer should be considered primarily a surgical lesion," not from fear of cancer but from poor results of nonsurgical management of benign ulcers. Because of lower mortality and morbidity and a very low rate of recurrent ulcer, Kinsey and Zollinger (3) recommended an antrectomy and vagotomy with intraoperative biopsy of the ulcer. Vagotomy was recommended because 20% of their patients had coexistent duodenal ulcer disease.

Claude Welch (3) still felt that three quarters of gastric ulcers should be treated surgically for the same reasons—possible malignancy and poor medical and surgical outcome. He noted a decline in gastric cancer in the U.S., but still felt that 8 to 10% of ulcers were malignant. He supported his approach by citing a mortality of 1 to 3% and results of surgery as 95% excellent with only 1 to 2% recurrent marginal ulcer. He also avoided excessive resection. As for results of medical therapy, he cited Cain from the Mayo Clinic (6), who found only 20% of 414 patients with small gastric ulcer treated between 1940 and 1945 to be free of symptoms 5 years later, whereas 10.4% had cancer and 140 had undergone surgery. For gastric ulcer, the picture changed radically in the next decade with the universal use of endoscopy and biopsy and the introduction of H_2 antagonists. It is difficult today to understand the intensity of debate and even confrontation between internists and surgeons that raged until the late 1970s, or the often petty but endless arguments as to which operation was "best" (86).

Surgery for Esophageal Reflux

Hiatal hernia was not diagnosed in life before the introduction of contrast radiology. At the Mayo Clinic, only 30 cases were diagnosed between 1900 and 1925 and 211 between 1925 and 1937 (100). Hiatal hernia was considered an anatomic abnormality, analogous to an inguinal hernia and thus deserving of anatomic repair in its own right. The first recorded repair of hiatal hernia was in 1919 by the Italian surgeon Soresi (101). To improve the operation of repair by crural approximation, phrenic nerve crush or division (100,102) was added to allow the diaphragm to rise and thereby change the pressure relationship between the stomach and the esophagus.

Winkelstein in 1935 (103) first defined the essential clinical picture of reflux and suggested that the esophagitis resulted from the action of digestive gastric juice. This concept did not gain wide understanding until the classic publications of Allison (104) and Barrett (105), who concluded that reflux esophagitis was common and could cause ulceration and stricture. Although it was recognized that a mechanism existed for preventing reflux, it was not until manometric studies that the anatomically inconspicuous sphincter was found to be a functioning reality (98,107) and most surgical repair procedures aimed at reducing the hernia and reconstructing the hiatus. Eventually, the high recurrence rate of the Allison operation (106) led to a search for newer surgical methods in the late 1960s. Barrett's "short esophagus" (105), felt to be a congenitally short esophagus with acid and pepsin-secreting mucosa, was understood to be a cause of esophagitis, ulceration, stricture and susceptible to malignant degeneration (107). Resection with jejunal substitution was also recommended for those with complications.

Failure of repair of hiatal hernia as hernia by the Allison and similar operations (106) led to the operations of fundal plication by Belsey (108) and by Nissen (109), in which the gastric fundus is wrapped around the lower esophagus in two thirds or complete circle. The Hill posterior gastropexy repair was introduced in 1967 (110) and, like the former two, was also modified by later experience. All three procedures have had satisfactory results confirmed by manometry and in recent years 24 hours pH probe of reflux. However, they are not without problems in 10 to 15% of patients (111), including relapse, dysphagia, and difficulty in belching.

Today, highly effective medical therapy can eliminate acid and treat virtually every case of reflux esophagitis and its complications (28). This has sharply reduced the need for surgery and redefined its indications (111,28).

Medical Therapy

The foundations of ulcer therapy were laid in ancient times when powdered coral, seashell, or chalk ($CaCO_3$, calcium carbonate) was used to relieve dyspepsia, long before it was realized that peptic ulcer was responsible for the pain. The very complicated regimens of the late 18th and early 19th centuries (1,112) reflected the primitive state of medical knowledge and included changing of environment, illogical diets, mercury, silver or bismuth salts, alkalies, purging, vomiting, and blood letting. Leeches were applied to the upper abdomen to treat dyspepsia (1,112). Johnson (cited by 10) in 1831 recommended soda, magnesia, and chalk for pain in the stomach due to acidity. The concept of "resting the bowel" introduced by Leube in 1876 (13) was used extensively for ulcer and was gradually displaced by the frequent-feeding regimen of Sippy in 1915 (82). The Leube regimen consisted of bed rest from 1 to 3 and even up to 8 weeks with nothing by mouth for up to 7 days, moist compresses to the epigastrium, rectal administration of alcohol and glucose in saline four times daily; oral feedings of gruel and magnesium oxide were begun on the third to the seventh day and opium or belladonna given for pain (10). The "rest," i.e., starvation treatment was most deleterious when applied to bleeding peptic ulcer, resulting in many deaths due to dehydration and acute renal failure (99). It was not until the early 1930s that Meulengracht's (113) principle of early feeding after GI bleeding replaced Leube's ill-conceived treatment (98,99).

Bland diets which avoided "rough" and spicy foods were based on the ideas that white foods (e.g., milk, porridge, mashed potatoes) were more benign. These held sway until the late 1960s (3). Wangensteen (74) credits William Hunter in 1784 as the first to advise the use of milk in the treatment of peptic ulcer. The disciplinarian regimens that prescribed not only diets and the accompanying antacids, but the strict timing and progression were first fully formulated by Sippy in 1915 (82), who clearly enunciated the principles of strict acid neutralization. He also advocated testing the gastric contents for acid and removing them by stomach tube before bedtime. The rigid requirements of this therapy for as long as 12 to 18 months (82) led to Kinsey and Zollinger's (3) recommendation in 1966 for surgery to free the patient from "the abstemious existence required by strict medical therapy."

A large variety of antacids ($NaHCO_3$, and salts of calcium, magnesium and aluminum) were tested both in vitro and in vivo (10,98), and prescribed for symptoms to be taken with hourly feedings between 7:00 a.m. and 9:00 p.m. The milk/alkali drip of Winkelstein (103) applied the principle of continuous neutralization for initial treatment of symptomatic ulcer.

Other therapies included synthetic resins, gastric mucin, vegetable mucins ("Okrin"), cabbage juice, vitamin C, high-fat diets, protein hydrolysates, pectin, powdered duodenal mucosa, and a number of parenteral agents. Various non-specific protein products were injected in the 1920s and early 1930s to evoke an "immune reaction." Pepsin injections to provoke pepsin antibodies; pituitary extract, histidine ("Larostidine"), parathormone, insulin and even histamine were administered for ulcer. These are detailed by Ivy et al. (10). Avery Jones (98) in 1952 counted 56 different regimens, 89 drug preparations, and 19 non-pharmaceutical remedies, each with a "brief flowering of popularity." One (114) even used injections of distilled water and encouraged smoking, achieving 95% healing in 4 to 8 weeks.

The principles of a controlled clinical trial had not yet been established, and were introduced by Doll (5,49) in the early 1950s. Spontaneous healing (placebo responses) and the rapid subsidence of symptoms were to confuse interpretation of all the uncritical open trials of ulcer treatment.

Bed rest, often in hospital, was considered essential to remove the patient from the environment in which the ulcer occurred or relapsed, adding emotional to physical rest (5,10,107). Anticholinergics (antispasmodics) were used to reduce pain and make acid easier to control. Phenobarbital was widely used, especially in Europe (107) in the treatment of many disorders felt to have a psychologic component, as ulcer disease was (98,115). Its role in treatment was summarized in 1944 (115): "the most important single drug in the management of peptic ulcer is phenobarbital, given in sufficient doses to have the desired effect of sedation." Psychotherapy became popular in the 40s and 50s, as it did for many other illnesses, including ulcerative colitis (10,98,107).

One study anticipated late discovery of EGF and its possible role in repair of GI ulcers (see Restitution and Repair). An extract of gastrointestinal mucosa containing "enterogastrone" was injected 3 to 6 times weekly in 46 patients with chronic ulcer by Ivy et al. (10).

With the introduction of the randomized clinical trial (5,49), it became possible to examine various treatments for gastric and duodenal ulcer. Although they lacked sharp endpoints, improved radiologic techniques provided the objective evidence for adequate statistical analysis. Doll and Friedlander (5) concluded that diet did not significantly affect healing but that bed rest did.

The power of appropriately designed clinical trials was shown in a study that examined the treatment with diet, phenobarbital and stilbestrol (4) and found clear benefit only from estrogen. Its feminizing effects were considered a significant disadvantage and stilbestrol never reached general use for peptic ulcer. Of interest, 75% of their patients relapsed in 5 years and 48% required surgery. A later controlled trial (116) showed benefit from antacids in healing duodenal ulcer. Antacids remained the mainstay of ulcer treatment until cimetidine.

Anticholinergics or antispasmodics were mentioned only briefly by Ivy et al. in 1950 (10), although belladonna had been used in clinical practice for many decades for control of "stomach spasms" (115). In the 1950s, with the introduction of synthetic anticholinergics, there was a large surge of interest in this treatment. Because of individual variation in response, it was necessary to titrate the dose of belladonna to just below the dry-mouth level. However, efficacy in healing was not uniformly shown, and use of anticholinergics fell, at first gradually and then rapidly after cimetidine. When cholinergic receptor subtypes were first demonstrated by Hammer et al. (117) and the subtype-specific drug, pirenzepine was developed, there was a brief revival of interest (118). However, efficacy was generally less than the H_2 antagonists (24), and pirenzepine never licensed in the U.S. faded from clinical use in peptic ulcer (119). Although thoughtful practitioners recognized that control of acid secretion was the key to controlling ulcer symptoms and to healing peptic ulcers, the multitude of (generally ineffective) treatments (119,120) reflected groping for the goal, which was not achieved until the introduction of H_2 antagonists (119,121). Other treatment unrelated to acid suppression also came and went (10,98,120,121) most frequently for lack of a scientific base.

Among the interesting nonsurgical treatments were *gastric irradiation* and gastric freezing. Irradiation of the stomach was first used by Bruegel in 1917 (122), and numerous studies of radiation injury and specific experiments on gastric irradiation showed a decrease in acid secretion (10). Ricketts et al. (123) reported that 90% of gastric ulcers healed with medical treatment plus radiation versus 60% without radiation. Similar results were obtained in duodenal ulcer. Recurrences of gastric ulcer in a 1-to-10-year follow-up were reduced from 70 to 33%. Similar effects were seen with duodenal ulcer. Gastric irradiation was used until about 1970 for patients with "surgical" ulcers who were poor surgical risks.

Gastric Freezing

In 1962 Wangensteen (74) delivered the Moynihan lecture at the Royal College of Surgeons on the topic "The stomach since the Hunters—gastric temperature and peptic ulcer." He discussed Moynihan's contribution to gastric surgery and outlined the history of gastric secretion and the progression of knowledge of acid peptic diseases. He then presented the case for and the

methodology of gastric freezing using a specially designed balloon and a coolant pump for "the control of the peptic ulcer diathesis." Gastric freezing was widely practiced for a few years throughout the U.S. until endoscopy began to reveal the extent of the serious mucosal damage with its inevitable complications, as well as its lack of benefit.

Bettarello in 1985 (119) felt that five events defined the present treatment of acid peptic disease: (1) fiberoptic endoscopy, which enabled routine examination and precise assessment of therapeutic results, (2) prospective double blind trials, (3) continuous pH monitoring to assess efficacy of acid suppression, (4) new drugs such as H_2 blockers, proton pump inhibitors, sucralfate, prostaglandins, bismuth preparations, pirenzepine, and (5) reduction of relapse by long term therapy.

H_2 Blockers

A new era of ulcer treatment was initiated by the development of histamine H_2 receptor antagonists by James Black and his colleagues (8). Within a short time, metiamide, the first H_2 blocker used clinically, had caused agranulocytosis, and the new drug seemed doomed to extinction by this potentially fatal side effect (124). However, cimetidine was fortunately available from Smith Kline & French, and soon a huge body of evidence on its biochemical, pharmacological and therapeutic actions became available. Several symposia (96) in the late 1970s documented its mode of action and its efficacy at a surprisingly low risk, making it one of the safest and most widely used drugs in the world. Nevertheless, some questions remained regarding antiandrogenic effects, CNS effects and drug interactions (43,69). Not all H_2 antagonists, however, were safe, e.g., tiotidine produced gastric carcinoma; oxmetidine, liver toxicity; and metiamide, agranulocytosis (43). By 1981, Wyllie et al. (125,126) were able to document a sharp (38%) decline in the number of operations for duodenal ulcer in the United Kingdom within 2 years after the introduction of cimetidine.

Many clinical trials confirmed these findings and defined the pharmacology for cimetidine and the other H_2 receptor antagonists ranitidine, famotidine, and nizatidine. The similar range of healing rates for various regimens and doses of H_2 antagonists are summarized in various tables (43, 69). While H_2-antagonists were recording healing rates for duodenal ulcer of 80 to 95% at 6 weeks, placebo healing rates of 20 to 60% were also being documented using the precise assessment provided by endoscopy.

Other Drugs

Antacids, at first shown to be as effective as cimetidine when used in high doses (116), have been shown to be effective in progressively smaller doses even suggesting the possibility of an action different from reducing acid to "healing levels" (127), but better drugs have largely relegated antacids to a supporting role for symptoms only in peptic ulcer disease.

Carbenoxolone, an extract of licorice, was shown in the early 1960s to promote healing of gastric ulcers without affecting pH (121). Because of aldosterone-like side effects and lower efficacy, carbenoxolone was finally abandoned for ulcer therapy.

Sucralfate, another drug without effect on acid, was developed in Japan and introduced into clinical practice around 1980 (128,129). It was shown to have efficacy equal to that of other effective agents in ulcer healing. No thoroughly satisfactory explanation of its mode of action has been presented.

Bismuth (colloidal bismuth suspension), like sucralfate and carbenoxolone and perhaps even the small-dose antacids in promoting ulcer healing by non-acid effects, has claimed a place as an effective ulcer-healing drug (130). Bismuth had been used for dyspepsia for over 200 years (112), and first claimed interest in the 1970s, not only because it was effective, but because of apparently lower relapse rates (43,69). In recent years, a possible explanation of the latter findings might be suppression of H. pylori, which is sensitive to bismuth.

Cytoprotection was a term coined to explain why (rat) stomachs exposed to various agents like boiling water and absolute ethanol failed to develop visible erosions and hemorrhages if the rat had been pretreated with prostaglandins. However, when such preparations were examined histologically, denudation of mucosa appeared regardless of treatment. Silen (131) has thus raised serious questions as to the definition and existence of cytoprotection. Prostaglandins seem to act on vessels rather than the epithelium.

Prostaglandins have been particularly studied in relation to the gastroduodenal damage caused by NSAIDs (132). In the 20 or more years during which these agents have been studied, no mode of action in healing ulcer other than by acid suppression has been clearly defined. Among the many candidate prostaglandin analogs, only misoprostol has become commercially available. However, misoprostol does not heal ulcers as well as H_2 antagonists or omeprazole and, although it appears to prevent NSAID lesions in 3-month studies, it has not been fully evaluated in patients who have had prior ulcers. Walt (132) concludes that its routine use for prophylaxis is not yet justified. Side effects, especially diarrhea prevent use in doses that inhibit gastric secretion to a degree that would allow it to compete with other acid-inhibiting drugs such as H_2 antagonists.

Omeprazole was described by Davenport (2) in the background studies which elucidated the ATPase-dependent ion pumps of the parietal cell and led to the invention of a specific class of inhibitors (substituted benzomidazoles) of the proton pump, a K^+-dependent H^+ ATPase.

Omeprazole was found to be free of the undesirable side effects of the first drug H149/94 (picoprazole), developed by Hässle in Sweden. The most striking demonstration of the greater potency of omeprazole than the H_2 antagonist in suppressing acid secretion was measured by 24-hour pH profiles (133). Not only was omeprazole highly effective, with close to 100% healing at 4 weeks in early European studies, but for the first time we had a reliable and specific medical treatment for the hypersecretion of the Zollinger-Ellison syndrome (62). We were now capable of controlling acid secretion completely, and other treatment-resistant acid-peptic diseases began to yield, e.g., severe reflux esophagitis (134), NSAIDs-induced ulcers (135), and cimetidine or H_2 antagonist-resistant duodenal and gastric ulcers (135,136).

The use of omeprazole was restricted for

a while by the finding of the investigators at Hässle that the achlorhydria produced by omeprazole in rats led to the development of gastric carcinoids late in life (137). This led to a moratorium on clinical use of omeprazole except in Zollinger-Ellison (ZE) patients, in whom it was life-saving. Extensive studies have shown that the ECL hyperplasia and carcinoids were in fact due solely to hypergastrinemia produced by several means of causing achlorhydria other than omeprazole and were reversible (137). A clinical counterpart of gastric carcinoids in humans with pernicious anemia was also reversible by antrectomy and normalization of serum gastrin levels (64). Despite experimental evidence to the contrary, considerable opposition to the use of such a potent acid-suppressing drug was led by Wormsley (138), who believes that omeprazole is a genotoxic drug. Continuous use of omeprazole for almost 10 years in ZE syndrome produced further evidence of safety (43,62,135).

Omeprazole has now become the benchmark for determining whether acid is responsible for a symptom or even a disease. Evidence from high effectiveness in healing duodenal ulcer and esophagitis and in wholly reversing the effects of acid in ZE syndrome (135) seems to have finally vindicated the predictions of Sippy in 1915 (82) and his successors that ulcer healing is dependent upon tight control of acid.

Treating Complicated Ulcer

In the 19th and early 20th centuries, peptic ulcer was largely recognized in life only on presentation with complications—hemorrhage, perforation and pyloric obstruction. Because perhaps as many as half the cases of GI hemorrhage arise from nonulcer sources (139), a misdiagnosis of ulcer was not infrequent; pyloric obstruction carried the differential diagnosis of gastric cancer. The surgical treatment for these complications carried a very high risk.

The management of acute bleeding was at first dominated by fear of restarting bleeding by feeding. Accordingly, bleeders were treated with sips of water and no food for up to a week or more (13). Not surprisingly, a number of deaths were attributed to azotemia (99). In 1935, Meulengracht in Denmark (113) recommended feeding rather than fasting. Avery Jones (46), managing 171 patients with upper GI bleeding between 1940 and 1942 with early transfusions and early feeding, reported a reduction in mortality of 50% over that of Cullinan and Price, who studied ulcers between 1926 and 1930 (98,99). Avery Jones also advocated aggressive endoscopy, although it was seldom performed in less than 1 week after admission. However, only four patients underwent surgery, citing mortality in other series of over 25% in surgery for bleeding ulcer. He also pointed out the rising risk with age, with repeat bleeding and associated disease. In the next 10 years at the same hospital, experience in over 1000 cases showed a mortality of 19% of bleeders with gastric ulcer, 8% with duodenal ulcer, and 27% for bleeding varices (107).

The principles laid down in the period from 1940 to 1960 for the management of upper GI bleeding have remained valid even after the introduction of H_2 antagonists, although these agents are now almost universally used in all patients admitted to intensive care units (ICUs) for the prevention of secondary hemorrhage. The progressive improvement in management of acute GI bleeding by the rapid transport to hospital, emergency care, early transfusion, and other supportive care in ICUs has been balanced by the increase in average age of bleeders, who since Avery Jones' report in 1947 (99) have been known to be particularly vulnerable. The massive recent increase in use of NSAIDs, which underlies as many as 90% of bleeders (139), makes GI bleeding a persistent danger despite effective treatments now available for ulcer.

NATURAL HISTORY

Factors Affecting Healing

Understanding the natural history of peptic ulcer, or any disease for that matter, depends on the accuracy with which the disease can be defined or measured. In diseases of vital organs, e.g., kidneys, lungs, liver, and heart, function generally serves to define the course of the disease. In peptic ulcer disease, including reflux in which the symptoms are subjective, frequently not directly linked to disease activity, and often nonspecific; in which function is rarely impaired unless complicated by stricture; when physical examination and measurements of gastric secretion are of little value, much depended on objective evidence of the presence and status of ulcer crater or esophagitis.

In the purely clinical years, i.e., before radiology of ulcer became refined and routine, perhaps until 1925 or 1930, diagnosis of gastric or duodenal ulcer in life was made on clinical grounds (12,20) and healing and relapse on the presence of symptoms. Confirmation of diagnosis came from surgery performed for complications, and autopsy studies (47) showed a poor record of diagnosis in life. Therefore data on healing and relapse rates before the widespread use of fiberoptic endoscopy and controlled clinical trials from 1975 onward are not totally reliable.

By 1950, estimates of recurrence of peptic ulcer varied widely, depending on the means of assessing recurrence—largely symptomatic but also by x-ray. Outcome was graded from "clinically satisfactory to incapacitating." A range of studies, many by eminent U.S. gastroenterologists (Crohn, Flood, Jordan and Kiefer, Kirsner, Palmer, Sandweiss, Ivy) using various regimens and starting points (e.g., healed, unhealed) gave a wide range of recurrence. At 1 year, the range of relapse was from 9% on a strict Sippy regimen to 92% on no treatment, with an average relapse rate of 20% at 6 months, 42% at 1 year, 55% at 2 years, and 75% at 4 and 5 years (10).

Factors leading to recurrence included a long history, short remissions, more than one prior hemorrhage, resistance to initial treatment, obstruction, acid resistance to neutralization, smoking, tension, and alcohol, although no one factor stood out (10).

By contrast, in the last 20 years—the era of placebo controlled, endoscopically monitored studies of ulcer—more precise information is available (140). When one adds asymptomatic relapses of ulcer crater to the symptomatic, as many as 80 to 90% of ulcers relapse in one year (43,69). Moreover, the much lower rate of complications of asymptomatic duodenal ulcers under treatment with cimetidine than on placebo (141) underscores the importance of endoscopy in understanding the natural history of peptic ulcer. Subgroup analysis shows much higher figures of relapse for smokers than for nonsmokers (43,51,141).

Improved statistical analyses have also made it possible to examine subgroups. Thus placebo healing was found to be widely different (from 20 to 60% in one month) in various countries (140), possibly related to factors having nothing to do with geography, e.g., earlier endoscopy for symptoms may diagnose ulcers that would be healed if the patients were examined perhaps 4 or 6 weeks later, after the onset of symptoms (140).

Factors favoring healing include female sex and acid suppression, with healing rate inversely related to the placebo healing rate (141) and moderate alcohol consumption (140). Unfavorable conditions include smoking, age, male sex (in some countries only) and NSAIDs. Whereas until about 1970, patients resistant to treatment would have been referred for surgery, today more potent acid suppression is attempted, together with the elimination of smoking and NSAIDs.

Relapse

It has always been understood that peptic ulcer is a relapsing disorder with a potential for serious and even fatal complications in as many as 10 or 20% of patients (10,142).

The factors examined by 1950 in the tendency to relapse were clearly different from the questions asked today. Ivy et al. (10) list (1) a long history, (2) previous short remissions (<7 months), (3) more than one bleed, (4) nocturnal distress, (5) epigastric tenderness, (6) slow or inadequate response to bed rest or "strict management," (a) within 2 weeks, (b) intolerance to alkalis, (c) persistent obstruction for longer than 3 weeks, (4) occult blood in the stool more than one week, (5) persistent duodenal deformity, (6) resistance to neutralization (Zollinger-Ellison syndrome had not yet been described), (7) age of onset over 40. Sex did not appear to be a factor. Smoking and aspirin were not discussed. In short, a "bad track record" was used to predict future behavior.

By 1978, a conference (143) on peptic ulcer examined and rejected treatment with bed rest and diet, confirmed the ill effects of smoking and coffee, and reported the early results of healing with cimetidine and treatment with antacids, anticholinergics, and prostglandins. In this conference appeared the first report (144) of the effect of substituted benzimidazoles on gastric secretion. This conference represented the watershed years (1973 to 1978) in the treatment of peptic ulcer.

The last 20 years have produced a huge number of statistically analyzed studies confirming the efficacy of H_2 antagonists and omeprazole (43,69,140,141) and other agents including carafate. In recognizing the factors that promote relapse, there has been a rationalization of the selection of cases for long term treatment. In the last 8 to 10 years, the recognition of H. pylori as a possible major factor in ulcer recurrence has received wide attention. In a field that has seen many claims for cure of ulcer, there is still a watchful skepticism regarding H. pylori. It may well be that the cure of peptic ulcer is indeed now at hand and that the 1990s may see the end of the history of peptic ulcer, but we have to remember Moynihan thought the same of gastroenterostomy almost 90 years ago (73,75).

EPIDEMIOLOGY

The Changing Face of Ulcer

In the 19th century, peptic ulcer, so named by Quincke in 1882 (cited by 10), which had been quite rare, began to be seen sporadically, presenting largely by its complications of bleeding and perforation and showing a remarkable predilection for perforation of gastric ulcers in young women (145). The low prevalence might be ascribed to the inability to diagnose uncomplicated gastric or duodenal ulcer in life (76); statistics on peptic ulcer came largely from autopsy studies (45,47,120,140).

Susser (146), using perforation as the most useful indicator of peptic ulcer (145), described three syndromes. The first, hematemesis from or perforation of acute fundic gastric ulcers in young women, began before 1850, became common in the latter half of the century, and disappeared by 1920 (146). Second, beginning in the early 1900s, perforation of chronic juxtapyloric ulcers began to appear in older women (146) and

middle-aged men, peaking in incidence by the first World War and declining since the end of the second World War in 1946. Third, chronic duodenal ulcers, which were rare in the 1800s (147), began to appear in young and later in middle-aged men, exceeding gastric ulcer in prevalence by 1900 (140) and becoming what Avery Jones (121) has described as "an epidemic during this century." This epidemic apparently began receding in the 1960s (142), even before the introduction of present therapy in the last 20 years (72,121,125,140,146–149). The complexity of the decline in various age groups in different countries has been analyzed by cohort analysis (146,149), which follows each group as it ages. Since 1850, the risks of peptic ulcer in Europe increased for each successive generation with impressive regularity to a peak and then declined (146,149,150), suggesting an unknown environmental influence during childhood (149). The dramatic changes in the sex- and age-related prevalence, complications, and ulcer type in various countries and regions from 1950 until the present (69,142,147,148) has led to speculation of the role of race and genetic predisposition, industrialization, urbanization, social class, diet, smoking, and drugs (e.g., aspirin) (146). Prevalence and incidence data of uncomplicated peptic ulcer for the period before the standardization and general use of reliable radiologic techniques before 1940 must be considered imprecise.

Despite misgivings about the validity of demographic and epidemiologic data (140,145–149), several large trends can be distinguished over the last 100 years. Two major uniform trends have emerged in Europe—duodenal ulcer, which was much less common than gastric ulcer, equaled and exceeded gastric ulcer progressively since 1920, and the ratio of male to female followed the same pattern (142). By midcentury, a detailed analysis of duodenal ulcer prevalence by Doll (151) showed gastric ulcer 2 to 3 times more common and duodenal ulcer 6 to 12 times more common in men than in women aged from 25 to 65. Peptic ulcer was present in 10% of men aged 45 to 54 years and commoner in towns than in rural areas. In the U.S., male-to-female ulcer rates, which were 22 and 8 per 1000 in 1957 to 1959, gradually equalized by about 1979 to about 18 to 20 each per 1000 because of a rise in peptic ulcer rates in women and a small decline in men (69,152). By 1987, gastric ulcer to duodenal ulcer rates (GU:DU) in men was 7:10 and the reverse in females (153). There are also large geographic differences (14,154,155), even within regions of the same country. Thus, although DU:GU in Europe and the U.S. has a 2:1 ratio, in Japan the rate is 1:5 (140). Regional differences exist in north and south India (121); in Scotland perforation was much higher than in England (121,147); and gastric ulcer exceeded duodenal ulcer in northern Norway (156). Similar wide differences were found in mortality, e.g., 30 per 100,000 for GU in Japan versus 3 in Israel; 10 per 100,000 for male DU in Scotland versus 0.5 in France (146).

A decrease in peptic ulcer prevalence, hospitalizations, operations, and mortality has been apparent since about 1960 in the U.S. and Europe, although the reverse may be true in the developing countries (140,147). Between 1947 and 1965, duodenal ulcer declined 40% among British physicians, and between 1960 and 1972 a similar decline was noted in the U.S. (148). Patient visits to physicians for duodenal ulcer in the U.S. peaked in 1963 and then declined fivefold in men and threefold in women, to about 800 to 1000 visits per 100,000 by 1984. For gastric ulcer over this 25-year period, the rate for men fell and that for women rose by about 50%, each by about 1000 visits per 100,000 population (156). In 1991, hospital discharges listed 74,000 admissions for gastric ulcer with hemorrhage and 54,000 duodenal ulcer with hemorrhage, indicating the stubborn persistence of complicated peptic ulcer (153). Hospitalization has shown a steady decline from 1970 to 1985 from 105 to 30 per 100,000 for uncomplicated peptic ulcer, a decrease from 40 to 30 for hemorrhage but no change for perforation admissions (148). The meaning of hospitalization data differs today from 50 years ago, when Doll (5) showed the value of hospital bed rest above all other therapies.

Elective operations, which also had been falling steadily since about 1968, fell steeply for 1 to 2 years after cimetidine (125) but rebounded and resumed the original slope of decline from about 60 per 100,000 in 1970 to 30 per 100,000 population in 1985 to 1986

(126). Other figures show no change in the number of emergency operations performed between 1974 and 1984, most of the decline being caused by elective operations. Death rates from ulcer had begun to fall after 1960 (148). Between 1962 and 1978, deaths from GU fell 58% and for DU 68% or from 42 to 27 per 100,000 cases for all peptic ulcers (−36%) (148). For men under 85, death rates have continued to fall; the trend for women is less evident (148). After a gradual decrease in patients over age 85 for both men and women since 1978, there has been a steep increase in deaths from peptic ulcer in this age group despite the introduction of H_2 antagonists (153). In 1979, 5900 deaths in the U.S. were attributed to peptic ulcer; in 1982, 6700; and in 1991, 6400 (153) despite widespread availability of effective ulcer therapy. Most of the deaths were caused by bleeding, which in turn is caused largely by the increased intake of NSAIDs (139).

Epidemiology has been used to study not only the time trends and general utilization of treatment and outcome, but also to uncover possible etiologic or pathogenetic associations. Susser (146) in 1967 could not discern an influence of geography, urbanization, climate, season, time, social class and occupation, race, inheritance, diet, alcohol, psychogenic factors, or personality. Kurata (152), using similar tools in 1991, found evidence to support an association of cigarette smoking, aspirin, and NSAIDs. Equivocal results were obtained for long-term steroid use and genetic and psychologic factors. Diet and alcohol could not be associated.

PATHOGENESIS OF PEPTIC ULCER

In 1950, Ivy, Grossman and Bachrach (10) devoted over 600 pages (Part II) to systematic examination of the published data on etiology and pathogenesis of peptic ulcer (Table 5–1). Each of these theories of ulcer genesis had been put forward in the preceding 50 or so years.

Ivy et al. (10) assumed that chronic lesions developed from acute lesions. Summarizing the literature of almost 100 years from pathologists and experimentalists, Ivy et al. presented a number of possible causes of the acute initial lesion (10). Various infec-

Table 5–1
Theories of Ulcer Genesis by 1950*

I. Intragastric or Intraduodenal
  A. MUCOSAL DISTURBANCES
    1. Excessive secretion of acid-pepsin and a deficiency of normal neutralizing secretions
    2. Mechanical factors
      a. Rough food
      b. Internal and external pressure of organs and clothing
      c. Peristalsis
      d. Spasm
    3. Irritants in foods and drinks
    4. Gastritis and duodenitis
    5. Inadequate production of mucus
    6. Natural differences in mucosal susceptibility to acid-pepsin
  B. VASCULAR DISTURBANCES
    1. Anatomic vascular defects
      a. Relatively poor blood supply to ulcer-susceptible sites
      b. Tugging on blood vessels
      c. Abnormal capillaries
      d. Infarction
      e. Arteriosclerosis
    2. Physiologic disturbances
      a. Vasomotor spasm due to nerves or toxic substances
II. Extragastric and Extraduodenal
  A. CONSTITUTIONAL PREDISPOSITION
    1. Tendency to excessive secretion
    2. Tendency to spasm of musculature
    3. Tendency to vasomotor spasm
    4. Tendency for stomach and duodenum to be affected deleteriously by emotogenic stimuli
	B. PSYCHOGENIC
	    1. Certain emotogenic stimuli causing excessive secretion, excessive motor activity, or vascular spasm
	    2. Vagotonia or vegetative nervous system imbalance
	C. INFECTIOUS OR TOXIC
	    1. Oral sepsis
	    2. Foci of infection
	    3. Specific streptococci
	    4. Bacterial toxins
	    5. Tobacco
	    6. Skin burns
	    7. Lymph folliculitis
	D. ALLERGIC
	E. NUTRITIONAL DEFICIENCY
	    1. Protein
	    2. Vitamin
	    3. Amino acid
	    4. Mineral
	F. ENDOCRINE GLANDS
	    1. Pituitary, sex glands
	    2. Gastrointestinal—enterogastrone and urogastrone
	G. NEUROPATHIC
	    1. Analogous to the buccal aphthous ulcer or canker sore, which may be vasoneurotic, infectious, or allergic in origin
	H. CHRONICITY FACTORS
	    1. Mechanical
	    2. Chemical
	    3. Mucosal susceptibility
	    4. Nutritional or reparative

* Reproduced with permission from Ivy AC, Grossman M, Bachrach WH: Peptic Ulcer. Philadelphia, The Blakiston Company, 1950, p. 1144.

tious theories, such as the streptococcal theory of Rosenow (157), were proposed at a time (1916) when bacterial toxins were the subject of intense interest. In more recent years, herpes was proposed and later rejected (158) as a cause of duodenal ulcer. Vascular disturbances and localized anoxia were candidates for the cause of the initial lesion, as was a nervous effect on gastric or duodenal secretion.

On the role of gastric and duodenal secretions, experimental evidence indicated that the perfusion of the duodenum of dogs with 0.1 M HCl produced chronic DU, not diffuse mucosal erosion, and that lesser concentrations did not (10). This led to the cal-culation that the dog duodenum could neutralize 1800 mL of 140 mM HCl per day (10). Histamine had been used to stimulate secretion, and when injected subcutaneously every 2 hours for over 2 months, produced no ulcers (10). However, Code and Varco (159) in 1940 described the gastroduodenal ulcerogenic effect of histamine in beeswax injected into dogs and other animals. This effect was ascribed to the hypersecretion, although an angiotoxic action was considered. Indeed, intramucosal hemorrhages were often seen in such experiments. An observation that ultimately led to the concept of histamine receptor subtypes and the search for the parietal cell histamine receptor was the report that the newly discovered antihistamine diphenhydramine (Benadryl) did not block either gastric secretion or the ulceration induced by histamine (160).

Ivy et al. (10) and Lambert (161) summarized systematically more than 1000 papers before 1960 on the experimental production of peptic ulcer in relation to mucosal susceptibility and damage that could initiate and sustain mucosal ulceration, whether by increased acid, trauma, x-rays, or irritants. The principal models of experimental ulcer used to any extent after 1950 included the histamine-beeswax model of Code and Varco (159); the pylorus-ligated rat introduced by Latzel in 1913 (cited by 10) and Friedman in 1914 (162) and popularized by Shay in 1945(163). Although the ulceration of the pylorus-ligated "Shay" rat bears little resemblance to chronic peptic ulcer, this model became the most extensively used experimental ulcer for the testing of anti-ulcer drugs into recent times.

Cincophen caused chronic antral ulcers in dogs, but extensive studies failed to establish a mechanism (10), and the model was discarded. Studies with immunizations which produced acute lesions and various nutritional and endocrine interventions failed to yield any usable model or data. More recent models include the cysteamine-induced duodenal ulcer in rats (164).

Surgical models of peptic ulcer, mostly variants of the Mann-Williamson model (80), included diversion or exclusion of bile from the duodenum, which led to ulcers in over 50% of dogs (bile duct ligation) and 25 to 35% with bile diversion, internal or external (10). Pancreatic secretion diversion was much less ulcerogenic (7%) (10). These lesions were felt to be caused at least partly by interference with nutrition.

Gastrojejunostomy had become a popular and indeed the standard operation for peptic ulcer. By 1920, a significant number of patients had been reported to have developed jejunal ulcer. Yet gastroenterostomy in dogs did not often lead to ulceration. Mann and Williamson (80) diverted the distal duodenum to the ileum and anastomosed the jejunum to the stomach end on. Practically 100% of dogs then developed a chronic jejunal ulcer just beyond the gastrojejunostomy. In clinical practice, the Roux-en-Y

operation before vagotomy was introduced and also led to a very high incidence of jejunal ulceration (71). The Mann-Williamson model was the subject of intense study until the 1950s, but interest faded thereafter.

It was natural to examine the effects of nicotine, alcohol, and caffeine on gastric secretion, because all had been reported to increase acid secretion. It had also been reported that acid secretion responded abnormally to caffeine in duodenal ulcer compared to controls. However, the conclusion was that nicotine had little effect on experimental ulcer and that, although alcohol and caffeine could stimulate secretion, no connection to ulcer etiology could be established. Today it is clear that smoking promotes recurrence and may delay healing (132,51), although the subject is still not entirely settled. An effect on gastric circulation remained to be studied. The idea that the 20th century epidemic of duodenal ulcer (98) could be caused by H. pylori infection is now being evaluated (see subsequent text).

Psychosomatic Aspects

The two decades from 1920 to 1940 saw a great interest in the psychosomatic and psychoanalytic approach to disease. Alexander in 1934 (165) analyzed six patients with duodenal ulcer and formulated a narrowly defined hypothesis of dependency conflict in the development of peptic ulcer. His untested hypothesis dominated for many years, and even now still lingers in the models of pathogenesis (69,166). Studies in Army recruits led Wolff (160) and Mirsky (167) to define an apparent personality profile associated with hypersecretion or increased urinary pepsinogen excretion in the prediction of peptic ulcer. Stewart Wolf and H. G. Wolff examined the effects of emotional stress on gastric mucosa in five patients with gastrostomy, especially their subject Tom (168), confirming many of the observations of Beaumont on the gastric fistula of Alexis St. Martin more than a century earlier.

Some blamed emotional stress for the increase in complications of peptic ulcer, especially perforations during air raids in Britain in World War II (169). However, the physical stress, irregular meals, and increase in smoking and drinking could not be separated from other stresses of the wartime bombing in cities of Britain. Other periods of stress, such as the Great Depression or World War I, did not show the same trends. More recent studies in large numbers of patients (170) have failed to support a psychogenic basis for duodenal ulcer.

However, a major reappraisal of the brain-gut interaction at some stage will probably rediscover a basis for integrating the behavioral with the pathogenetic mechanisms of peptic ulcer.

Helicobacter pylori

In 1983, Warren and Marshall (176) in Australia reported finding unidentified curved bacteria in gastric biopsies, and in 1984 Marshall and Warren (177) extended the observation to link the bacteria to both gastritis and ulcer. Marshall infected himself with a culture of the bacteria and reproduced symptomatic gastritis, from which he fortunately spontaneously recovered. The H. pylori organism now occupies its own genus and is called Helicobacter pylori, and its immunology, toxins, enzymology, and cell wall lectins are now known. Its worldwide distribution is well defined, and its causal relationship to type B gastritis appears to be established (43,69).

Not so clear is the connection to DU or GU with which H. pylori is found associated in 90 to 100% of cases; elimination of H. pylori by antibiotics can promote ulcer healing and appears to delay or prevent relapse of DU. Yet ulcers heal as well with H_2 antagonists without changing H. pylori infection, and many persons who do not have DU are infected at a rate roughly equal to the age decade and much higher in some underdeveloped countries. Patients with hypersecretion, e.g., ZE, get ulcers but few have H. pylori.

There is no clear explanation of how H. pylori might cause DU or delay healing or how its eradication prevents duodenal ulcer recurrence, at least for 1 year (178). Recent publications (179), with similar results, indicate that eradication of H. pylori greatly reduces relapse of duodenal ulcer. If so, this treatment would provide a strong clue to direct research toward the etiology and pathogenesis.

NSAIDs

Aspirin, introduced before the turn of the century, has long been known to cause dyspepsia. In 1938, Barbour and Dickinson (171) reported that ASA, given orally or subcutaneously, produced dose-related gastric ulcers in rats. In the same year, Douthwaite (41) reported a gastroscopic study that showed acute hemorrhages in volunteers given ASA and also the induction of melena by aspirin (172).

Recent years have seen the introduction of NSAIDs other than aspirin, first indomethacin, and since then a large number of agents having in common inhibition of arachidonic acid metabolism. Without exception (42,173), all have the potential to cause acute and chronic peptic ulcer, especially GU. Because of the very extensive prescribed and nonprescribed use in the U.S. (in 1986 70 million NSAID prescriptions were written (174)), NSAIDs have come to play a major role in the epidemiology of present day peptic ulcer. NSAIDs, especially aspirin, may be responsible for as many as 90% of the estimated 250,000 cases of GI bleeding per year in the U.S. Although patients on treatment with H_2 antagonists are much less likely to bleed (131), many of those who bled, at least because of NSAIDs, had no warning of impending bleeding and were not being treated for ulcer (137). NSAID use may explain the unexpected rise of mortality in elderly patients since the introduction of H_2 antagonists.

The acute lesions seen at endoscopy after taking aspirin and first described in 1938 by Douthwaite (41) are not the forerunners of chronic lesions (42,174). Shallow antral erosions, commonly seen in NSAID users are also felt to be relatively insignificant, but may coexist with significant deep chronic ulcers. Perhaps as many as 10 to 15% of NSAID users develop chronic ulcers (42,173). In a nonulcer population, taking 1 g of ASA per day for cardiovascular prophylaxis for 4 years, the progressive risk of developing gastric or duodenal ulcers was increased tenfold (175).

Not only do NSAIDs contribute to new ulcer formation, they also interfere with healing. In an ongoing study, I have found that most, if not all, recurrent peptic ulcers after surgery for gastric or duodenal ulcer were related to the chronic intake of ASA, often surreptitiously (97). One wonders how many of the refractory ulcers of years gone by may have been caused by aspirin, especially disguised in the form of Alka-Seltzer.

The mechanism whereby NSAIDs cause or delay healing of peptic ulcer has not been established, and its prophylaxis (133) and treatment other than withdrawal of the NSAID (42) are still unclear.

PATHOPHYSIOLOGY

It is an uncomfortable fact that even today, 100 years after the emergence of duodenal ulcer as a major disease, there is no satisfactory model of the pathophysiology of peptic ulcer. Today we know about neurohormonal, biochemical, and cellular controls of secretion and motility and can measure their components and fluctuations; we know the parameters of secretion of acid, pepsin, and mucins; we understand more of the mucosal defenses and cell population dynamics; we know what some agents such as tobacco, NSAIDs, or H. pylori do to healing and relapse but not how they do it; we can look at and biopsy ulcers at will; and above all, we can heal ulcers, but yet not cure the disease.

Foremost in our present state, active ulcers can be healed by effective reduction of acid. It has been known for most of the century that acid was increased and that peptic ulcer did not occur in the absence of acid (81), and duodenal ulcer was rare with hypochlorhydria (15). It was recognized early that most DU patients (70%) secreted acid above the normal range, but that in gastric ulcer, except that associated with duodenal ulcer, secretion was almost invariably in the normal range (15,52,55). This applies to concentrations of acid (15,52) or to BAO (53), MAO (56), nocturnal secretion, 24-hour output, or parietal cell counts (57,58). Pepsin secretion measured directly or indirectly by means of uropepsin output or serum pepsinogen followed the same pattern as acid (43,55,69).

Women with DU secrete less than men (10,55,59) and develop duodenal ulcer at lower levels of secretion; non-ZE hypersecretors are almost exclusively men (55,64). In patients secreting in the upper two thirds of the DU range, several possible defects in the control of secretion have been proposed. These have included overactivity of the vagus and an increase in circulating gastrin (89). A response of such hypersecreting subjects to anticholinergics and vagotomy seems to confirm a role for vagal overreactivity. The isolation of gastrin by Gregory and Tracy (180) in 1960 and the development of a reliable RIA for gastrin by McGuigan (181) and others provided data on the role of gastrin. In fact, circulating gastrin was found to be not sufficiently elevated to account for all the instances of elevated BAO (43,69). It was also suggested that the prolonged acid secretory response to a meal (182) may (183) or may not (184) be caused by the failure of the acid feedback inhibition of gastrin release. It is also accepted that the increased parietal cell mass first described 40 years ago by Cox (58) was caused by the prolonged increased postprandial gastrin levels (43,69).

In many, if not most, patients with DU, gastrin levels are in the normal range, but acid output is elevated. For these, the concept of increased sensitivity to exogenous (185) and endogenous gastrin (186) was proposed, but a closer look failed to show hypersensitivity to either exogenous (59) or endogenous (60) gastrin in DU with hypersecretion. Other inhibitory mechanisms examined in DU have included fat in the intestine, distention of the stomach, and a possible defect in the release of somatostatin. None has been firmly established (43). Isenberg (43) has given an estimate of the influence of various physiologic abnormalities in DU, although the denominators have not been well defined. He lists decreased duodenal HCO_3 and increased nocturnal acid output with an increased duodenal acid load in about 75% of DU; increased daytime acid, MAO and increased sensitivity to gastrin in 50 to 60% of DU; elevated gastrin, increased gastric emptying, and defective pH inhibition of gastrin release in 25 to 40%. This leaves a number of patients with normal or low output in whom the only possible explanation is diminished mucosal resistance.

Mucosal protection and resistance to acid digestion have been a question for over 150 years. The concept of a mucosal barrier (2) has been developed to include the mucous layer into which HCO_3 is secreted, creating a pH gradient (43). Additional resistance was provided by the tight-junction barrier of the underlying surface mucosa (2). A decrease in amount or quality of mucin might predispose to ulceration (187,188).

Zollinger-Ellison Syndrome

The effect of an excess of acid is best illustrated by the experiment in nature of hypergastrinemia in which the gastrin stimulated excessive gastric secretion. In 1955, Zollinger and Ellison (189) reported a new syndrome, with fulminating and intractable gastrointestinal ulceration, associated with islet cell adenomas of the pancreas. They reported two patients with jejunal ulceration and reviewed the evidence from seven others. They proposed that the new syndrome had a diagnostic triad of gigantic gastric hypersecretion, ulceration in unusual sites or recurrence after surgery, and a non-insulin-secreting tumor of the pancreas. The authors postulated that a hormone produced by the adenoma was responsible for the hypersecretion. Its identification by Gregory et al. (180) as gastrin-like was reported in 1960, and the identification of amino acid sequence followed in 1967 (190). Because these tumors contained gastrin, they were called gastronomas.

A year before the Zollinger and Ellison paper, a report from the Mayo Clinic (191) on patients with multiple endocrine adenomas showed a prevalence of peptic ulcer of 50%. Another paper in 1954 (192) showed the strong association of peptic ulcer in one family with multiple endocrine adenomas, comprising a father and four children, all with MEA and peptic ulcer. It has been found since that 20% of ZEs were of the MEN I type and 80% the isolated or sporadic types (162).

In the almost 40 years since Zollinger and Ellison, the syndrome has been widely recognized and intensively studied (62). Diagnosis was made possible by a reliable RIA (181) and the serendipitous findings that secretin elevated serum gastrin, as did calcium (62). In the 20 years before 1975, the only choices for effective treatment were removal of the tumor where possible and, where not possible, total gastrectomy. It was soon recognized that in MEA it was not possible to remove the gastrinoma, and it was in fact quite uncertain that even sporadic gastrinomas could be removed, so that the conservative choice generally ended with total gastrectomy. When tumors could be successfully removed, the patient was cured (62), leading to the understanding that duodenal ulcer could be ascribed to a single cause—an excessive gastric acid and pepsin load on the duodenum. After the introduction of H_2 antagonists, most patients with ZE could be controlled, albeit with very large doses, in some cases up to 10 g of cimetidine per day, and in a few even that was not enough (62). Pirenzepine was used to supplement the inhibition by H_2 antagonists in resistant cases, with some benefit (62). In others, vagotomy was tried, also with some benefit.

By 1983, omeprazole was first reported to inhibit acid secretion in ZE syndrome, and rapidly proved effective in every case. For the first time, it was possible to predictably lower acid output below 5 or even 2 mEq/hr, and all cases of ZE responded. Those with esophagitis—40% of the total ZE population—and postgastrectomy patients with marginal ulcer represented the most vulnerable ZE patients who required the greatest suppression of acid to between zero and 2 mEq/hr BAO (62). Newer techniques—CT, endoscopic ultrasound, arteriography, and careful search at surgery—have led to improved yield of tumor diagnosis, so that a proportion of patients can be cured (62). Because of the relatively small number of cases, recurrence rates and tumor spread and death rate from tumor have not yet been fully established. No effective medical therapy for the malignancy has yet been found.

Restitution and Repair

Even as the process by which an ulcer develops and becomes chronic is poorly understood, the process by which an ulcer heals also is not well enough understood to have produced specific therapy. By 1950, much work had been done on skin wound healing and the process observed in detail, as described by Arey in 1936 (193). As early as 1927, Burrows (194) had named an extract of embryonic cells that promoted cell growth "archusia." Such substances were later called wound hormones (195), predicting the multitude of growth factors currently being discovered. In superficial lesions caused by application of alcohol or acetic acid, Grant in 1943 to 1945 (196) reported complete restitution of surface cells by migration evident by 1 hour and complete by 4 to 6 hours. This process has been amply confirmed but is still not completely understood (131). Acute shallow ulcers were known to heal in 3 days (169). Ivy et al. (10) concluded that acid, gastric retention, and rough foods were the only factors that might delay healing. In the 40 years since, NSAIDs and smoking may be added to the factors delaying healing of ulcer (155). The temporal integration of steps in repair have not been defined for peptic ulcer, but involvement of various blood elements (platelets, macrophages) and fibroblasts, as well as mucosal stem cells and integrated and sequential production of growth factors, is likely in the repair of ulcers (197).

One interesting recent finding has been reported by Nick Wright of London. Gastrointestinal ulcers, however formed, developed de novo branched EGF-producing glands that grow from the base into the edges of the ulcer. This EGF presumably plays an important part in ulcer healing (198).

CONCLUSION

Peptic ulcer as we know it today is a disease of the 20th century. It has been the nursery and training ground for abdominal surgeons, has engaged the attention of many scientists, and has led to the understanding of some of the fundamental functions of secretory cells and neurohormonal control of organ function. Ulcer diseases have provided much impetus to the development of radiology and spurred the revolution in endoscopy from lens to fibers to CCD.

Acid-peptic diseases have spawned hundreds of theories, treatments, and operations. Just when, by 1970, we thought that the latest in a long tradition of surgical "cures" was the ultimate, H_2 antagonists began the era of acid suppression; and just as omeprazole seemed to provide the ultimate in treatment of acid-peptic disease, H. pylori has emerged as a possible cause for peptic ulcer and has led to a recommendation that peptic ulcer be treated as an infection, with promise of cure by eradication of the cause (200). If this is truly so, then indeed peptic ulcer, which arose so mysteriously to epidemic proportions in this century and which has in fact been declining already (199), may be largely eradicated by the end of the century. There is speculation that this goal might be brought about by (universal) vaccination against H. pylori, leaving only sporadic cases caused by gastrinoma and the minor epidemic of iatrogenic NSAID-induced ulcers, with the promise that this too shall be conquered. As we contemplate not only discovery of the cause, but also the cure of this slippery disease of peptic ulcer, it would be well to remember Stolley and Lasky's admonition (201): "as to the many blind alleys down which science must wander in search of the truth. . . with hindsight, we can spot the blind alleys of yesteryear, but who can say which are the blind alleys of today?" The history of peptic ulcer of this century provides many examples of "the ease with which intelligent and educated scientists can mistake illusion for truth." We may or may not be ready to write the last word of this chapter.

ACKNOWLEDGMENTS

I am most grateful to Rhonda Harris for tirelessly typing and retyping this manuscript and to Marian Royal and other members of the Lister Hill Library of the University of Alabama at Birmingham for providing invaluable bibliographic support.

REFERENCES

1. Phillip APW: A Treatise on Indigestion and its Consequences. 3rd ed. London, Thos & Geo Underwood, 1823, p. 409.
2. Davenport HW: A History of Gastric Secretion and Digestion. Oxford, Oxford University Press, 1992, p. 414.
3. Ingelfinger FJ, Relman AS, Finland M: Controversy in Internal Medicine. Philadelphia, WB Saunders, 1966, p. 679.
   a. Roth JL, Ingelfinger FJ, Finland M: Dietary treatment of duodenal ulcer. *In* Ingelfinger FJ et al. (eds): Controversy in Inter-

nal Medicine. Philadelphia, WB Saunders, 1966, p. 679.

b. Tumen HJ et al.: Management of gastric ulcer. *In* Ingelfinger FJ et al. (eds): Controversy in Internal Medicine. Philadelphia, WB Saunders, 1966, p. 181.

4. Truelove SC: Stilbestrol, phenobarbitone and diet in chronic duodenal ulcer: A factorial therapeutic trial. Br Med J *ii*:559, 1960.

5. Doll R, Friedlander P, Pygott F: Dietetic treatment of peptic ulcer. Lancet *i*:5, 1956.

6. Cain JC, Jordan GL, Comfort MW, Gray HK: Medically treated small gastric ulcers. Five year followup study of 414 patients. JAMA *150*:481, 1952.

7. Goligher JC, Pulverfaft CW, Watkinson G: Controlled trial of vagotomy and gastroenterostomy, vagotomy and antrectomy and subtotal gastrectomy in elective treatment of duodenal ulcer. Interim report. Br Med J *i*:455, 1964.

8. Black JW et al.: Definition and antagonisms of histamine H_2 receptors. Nature *236*:385, 1972.

9. Babkin BP: Secretory Mechanisms of the Digestive Glands. New York, Paul B. Hoeber, Inc., 1950, p. 1027.

10. Ivy AC, Grossman M, Bachrach WH: Peptic Ulcer. Philadelphia, The Blakiston Co., 1950, p. 1144.

11. Cummins AJ, Perry PE: Annotated reprint: Gastric and duodenal ulcer. South Med J *76*:827, 1983.

12. Friedenwald J: A clinical study of a thousand cases of ulcer of the stomach and duodenum. Am J Med Sci *144*:157, 1912.

13. Leube WO: Bemerkungen ueber die Abloesung der Magenschleimhaut durch die Magensonde und ihre Folgen. Deutsches Arch f klin Med *18*:496, 1876. *In* Ziemssen: Handbuch Spec Pathol., cited by 10.

14. Rehfuss ME, Bergeim O, Hawk PB: Gastro-intestinal studies: II. The fractional study of gastric digestion with a description of normal and pathological curves. JAMA *63*:909, 1914.

15. Ryle JA: Gastric Function in Health and Disease. Oxford, Oxford University Press, 1926, p. 152.

16. Davenport HW: Gastrointestinal physiology, 1895–1945: Motility. *In* Handbook of Physiology. The Gastrointestinal System, Bethesda, American Physiological Society, 1989, Chapter 1, p. 1.

17. Bachem D, Guenther H: Bariumsulfat als schattenbildenes Kontrastmittel bei Roentgenuntersuchungen. Z Roentgenk *12*:369, 1910. The warning is Bachem C: Baryumsulfate als Diagnosticum in der Roentgenkunde. Ber Klin Wochenschr *49*:1425, 1912. Cited by Davenport (16).

18. Gelfand DW: Gastrointestinal radiology: A short history and predictions for the future. Am J Roentgen *150*:727, 1988.

19. George AW, Gerber I. The direct method of diagnosis of duodenal ulcer by means of the Roentgen ray. Am J Roentgenol *1*:287, 1914.

20. Mayo WJ: Chronic duodenal ulcer. JAMA *64*:2036, 1915.

21. Somerville TH: Further contributions to the causation and treatment of duodenal ulcer and its complications. Br J Surg *30*:133, 1942.

22. Brown P et al.: The endoscopic, radiologic and surgical findings in chronic duodenal ulceration. Scand J Gastroenterol *13*:557, 1978.

23. Dooley CP, Larsen AW, Stace NH: Double contrast barium meal and upper GI endoscopy: A comparative study. Ann Intern Med *101*:538, 1984.

24. Haudek M: Zur Roentgenologischen Diagnose der ulzerationen in der Pars Media des Magens. Munich Med Wchschr 57:1587, 1910.

25. Schindler R: Gastroscopy. The Endoscopic Study of Gastric Pathology. 2nd ed. Chicago, Chicago University Press, 1950.

26. Richardson CT: Gastric ulcer. Chapter 18; in Gastrointestinal Disease. 4th ed. Sleisinger MH and Fordtran JS, (eds). Philadelphia, WB Saunders, 1989, p. 2023.

27. Ott DJ, Wu WC, Gelfand DW: Reflux esophagitis revisited: Prospective analysis of radiologic accuracy. Gastrointest Radiol 6:1, 1981.

28. Marks RD and Richter JE: Gastroesophageal reflux disease. *In* D Zakim and AJ Dannenberg (eds). Peptic Ulcer Disease and Other Acid Related Disorders. New York, Academic Research Assoc Inc, 1991.

29. Hirschowitz BI, Curtiss LE, Peters CW, Pollard HM: Demonstration of a new gastroscope, the "Fiberscope." Gastroenterology *35*:50, 1958.

30. Hirschowitz BI: A personal history of the fiberscope. Gastroenterology 76:864, 1979.

31. Edmonson JM: History of the instruments for gastrointestinal endoscopy. Gastrointest Endosc *37*:S27, 1991.

32. Gerstner P: The American Society for Gastrointestinal Endoscopy: A History. Gastrointest Endosc *37*:S1, 1991.

33. Stein ST: Das Photo-Endoskop. Berl Klin Wchschr, January 1874, p. 31.

34. Morrissey JF, Tanaka Y, Thorsen WB: Gastroscopy. A review of the English and Japanese literature. Gastroenterology *53*:456, 1967.

35. Hirschowitz BI: Development and applica-

tion of endoscopy. Gastroenterology *104*: 337, 1993.

36. Hopkins HH, Kapany NS: A flexible fiber-scope using static scanning. Nature *173*:39, 1954.

37. Van Heel ACS: A new method of transporting optical images without aberrations. Nature *173*:39, 1954.

38. Hirschowitz BI: Endoscopic examination of the stomach and duodenal cap with the fiberscope. Lancet *i*:1074, 1961.

39. Hirschowitz BI: Photography through the fiber gastroscope. Am J Dig Dis *8*:389, 1963.

40. Hirschowitz BI: A fibre optic flexible oesophagoscope. Lancet *2*:388, 1963.

41. Douthwaite AH, Lintott GAM: Effect of aspirin and certain other substances on the stomach. Lancet *267*:917, 1954.

42. McCarthy DM: Nonsteroidal anti-inflammatory drug-induced ulcers: Management by traditional therapies. Gastroenterology *96*:662, 1989.

43. Skillman JJ, Silen W: Acute gastroduodenal "stress" ulceration: Barrier disruption of varied pathogenesis. Gastroenterology *59*:478, 1970.

44. Martin P, Dudnick R, Friedman LS. Management of complicated peptic ulcer disease. *In* Zakim D and Dannenberg AJ (eds): Peptic Ulcer Disease and Other Acid-related Disorders. New York, Academic Research Assoc Inc, 1991.

45. Penston JG, Wormsley KG: Asymptomatic duodenal ulcer—implication of heterogeneity. Aliment Pharmacol Therap *4*:557, 1990.

46. Pounder R: Silent peptic ulceration: Deadly silence or golden silence? Gastroenterol *96*: 626, 1989.

47. Wilkie R: Observations on the pathology and etiology of duodenal ulcer. Edinburgh Med J *13*:196, 1941.

48. Hirschowitz BI: Classification of the post gastrectomy syndromes based on observation of 580 patients. Ala J Med Sci *8*:50, 1971.

49. Doll R, Jones FA, Pygott F: Effect of smoking on the production and maintenance of gastric and duodenal ulcers. Lancet *i*:657, 1958.

50. Ivy AC: The problem of peptic ulcer. JAMA *132*:1053, 1948.

51. Guslandi M: How does smoking harm the duodenum? Br Med J (Clin Res Ed) *296*: 311, 1988.

52. Vanzant FR et al.: The normal range of gastric acidity from youth to old age. Arch Intern Med *49*:345, 1932.

53. Polland WAS: Histamine test meals. Arch Intern Med *49*:345, 1932.

54. Bloomfield AL, Chen CK, French LR: Basal gastric secretion as a clinical test for gastric function with special reference to peptic ulcer. J Clin Invest *19*:864, 1940.

55. Baron JH: Clinical Tests of Gastric Secretion. London, The McMillan Press, 1978.

56. Kay AW: Effects of large doses of histamine in gastric secretion of hydrochloric acid. An augmented histamine test. Br Med J *ii*:77, 1953.

57. Card WI, Marks IN: The relationship between the acid output of the stomach following "maximal" histamine stimulation and the parietal cell mass. Clin Sci *19*:147, 1960.

58. Cox AJ: Stomach size and its relation to chronic peptic ulcer. JAMA *54*:407, 1952.

59. Hirschowitz BI: Apparent and intrinsic sensitivity to pentagastrin of acid and pepsin secretion in peptic ulcer. Gastroenterology *86*:843, 1984.

60. Hirschowitz BI, Ou Tim L, Helman CA, Molina E: Bombesin and G-17 dose responses in duodenal ulcer and controls. Dig Dis Sci *30*:1092, 1985.

61. Makhlouf GM, McManus JPA, Card WI: The action of pentagastrin (ICI^{50}, 123) on gastric secretion in man. Gastroenterology *51*:455, 1966.

62. Jensen RT, Gardner JD: Zollinger-Ellison syndrome: Clinical presentation, pathology, diagnosis and treatment. *In* Zakim D, Dannenberg AJ, (eds). Peptic Ulcer Disease and Other Acid Related Disorders. New York, Acad Res Assoc Inc, 1991.

63. Feldman M: Gastric secretion in health and disease. *In* Sleisinger MH, Fordtran JS (eds): Gastrointestinal Disease. 4th ed. Philadelphia, WB Saunders, 1989, pp. 731–735.

64. Hirschowitz BI: Pathobiology and management of hypergastrinemia in the Zollinger-Ellison syndrome. Yale J Biol Med *65*:1, 1992.

65. Marks IN: The augmented histamine test. Gastroenterology *41*:599, 1961.

66. Bruce J, Card WI, Marks IN, Sircus W: The rationale of selective surgery in the treatment of duodenal ulcer. J Roy Coll Surg Edinb *4*:85, 1959.

67. Hirschowitz BI: Pepsinogen: An update. Postgrad Med J *60*:715, 1984.

68. Kreunig J et al.: Pepsinogen in man: Clinical and genetic advance. Prog Clin Biol Res, Vol. 173. New York, Alan R Liss, 1985, p. 312.

69. Soll AH: Duodenal ulcer and drug therapy. *In* Sleisinger MH, Fordtran JS (eds). Gastrointestinal Disease, 4th ed. Philadelphia, WB Saunders, 1989, pp. 814–878.

70. Endoscopy in the evaluation of dyspepsia. Health and Public Policy Committee, American College of Physicians. Ann Intern Med *102*:266, 1985.
71. Ogilvie H: A hundred years of gastric surgery. Ann Roy Coll Surg *1*:37, 1947.
72. Jordan PH: Duodenal ulcers and their surgical treatment: Where did they come from? Am J Surg *149*:1, 1985.
73. Moynihan BGA: Duodenal Ulcer. 2nd ed. Philadelphia and London, WB Saunders, 1912.
74. Wangensteen OH. The stomach since the Hunters: Gastric temperature and peptic ulcer. Ann Roy Coll Surg *31*:143, 1962.
75. Mayo WJ: Duodenal ulcer, a clinical review of fifty-eight operated cases with some remarks on gastroenterology. Ann Surg *90*:900, 1904.
76. Wilkie R: Observations on the pathology and etiology of duodenal ulcer. Edinburgh Med J *13*:196, 1914.
77. Ryle JA: The natural history of duodenal ulcer. Lancet *i*:327, 1932.
78. Finney JMT: Surgical treatment of duodenal ulcer. Ann Surg *90*:904, 1920.
79. Herrington JL: Remedial operations for postgastrectomy syndromes. Chicago, Yearbook Medical Publishers, 1970, p. 63.
80. Mann FC, Williamson CS: The experimental production of peptic ulcer. Ann Surg *77*:409, 1923.
81. Schwarz K: Ueber pentrierdende magen- und jejunal geschwüre. Beitr Klin Chir *67*:96, 1910.
82. Sippy BW: Gastric and duodenal ulcer: Medical cure by an efficient removal of gastric juice corrosion. JAMA *64*:1625, 1915.
83. Finsterer H, Cunha F: The surgical treatment of duodenal ulcer. SGO *52*:1099, 1931.
84. Dragstedt LR et al.: Effect of transplantation of antrum of stomach on gastric secretion in experimental animals. Am J Physiol 165:386, 1951.
85. Dragstedt LR, Owens FM: Supradiaphragmatic section of the vagus nerve in treatment of duodenal ulcer. Proc Soc Exp Biol Med *53*:152, 1943.
86. Editorial: Fashions in duodenal ulcer surgery. Br Med J *i*:563, 1973.
87. Latarjet MA: Résection des nerfs de l'estomach. Technique operatoire. Bull Acad Med (Paris) *87*:681, 1922.
88. Weinberg HA et al.: Vagotomy and pyloroplasty in the treatment of duodenal ulcer. Am J Surg *92*:202, 1956.
89. Dragstedt LR: Some comments on the cause of gastric and duodenal ulcers. Dig Dis *21*:197, 1976.

90. Tanner NC: Peptic ulcer: Elective surgery. *In* Jones FA (ed): Modern Trends. Gastroenterology. London, Butterworths Med Pub., 1952, p. 399.
91. Fromm D: Complications of gastric surgery. New York, John Wiley and Sons, 1977, p. 162.
92. Johnstone FRC, Holubitsky IB, Debas HT: Postgastrectomy problems in patients with personality defects: "The albatross syndrome." Canad Med Ass J *96*:1559, 1967.
93. Griffith CA, Harkins HN: Partial gastric vagotomy: An experimental study. Gastroenterology *32*:96, 1957.
94. Amdrup E, Jensen HE: Selective vagotomy of the parietal cell mass preserving innervation of the undrained antrum. Gastroenterology *59*:522, 1970.
95. Johnston D, Wilkinson AP: Highly selective vagotomy without a drainage procedure in the treatment of duodenal ulcer. Br J Surg *57*:289, 1970.
96. Wastell C, Lance P (eds): Cimetidine: The Westminster Symposium. Edinburgh, Churchill Livingston, 1978, p. 307.
97. Hirschowitz BI, Lanas A: Intractable and recurrent postsurgical peptic ulceration due to aspirin (ASA) abuse, much of it surreptitious. Gastroenterology *102*:A84, 1922.
98. Doll R et al.: Peptic ulcer. *In* Jones FA (ed): Modern Trends in Gastroenterology. London, Butterworths Medical Publications, 1952, p. 361.
99. Jones FA: Haematemesis and melaena with special reference to bleeding peptic ulcers. Br Med J *ii*:441, 1947.
100. a. Harrington SW: Phrenicotomy in treatment of diaphragmatic hernia and of tumors of the chest wall. Arch Surg *18*:561, 1929.
     b. Various types of hiatal hernia and anatomy of repair. SGO *86*:735, 1948.
101. Soresi AL: Diaphragmatic hernia: Its unsuspected frequency. Diagnosis and technique to radical cure. Ann Surg *69*:254, 1919.
102. Drake EH: Phrenicotomy for esophageal hiatus hernia. N Engl J Med *256*:487, 1957.
103. Winkelstein A: Peptic esophagitis. A new clinical study. JAMA *104*:906, 1935.
104. Allison PR: Reflux esophagitis, sliding hiatal hernia and the anatomy of repair. SGOT *92*:419, 1951.
105. Barrett NR: Chronic peptic ulcer of the esophagus and esophagitis. Br J Surg *38*:175, 1952.
106. Allison PR: Hiatus hernia: A 20-year retrospective survey. Ann Surg *178*:273, 1973.
107. Jones FA, Gummer JWP: Clinical Gastroenterology. Oxford, Blackwell, 1960, p. 652.

108. Skinner DB, Belsey RHR: Surgical management of esophageal reflux and hiatus hernia: Long term results with 1,030 patients. J Thoracic Cardiovasc Surg 53:33, 1967.

109. Nissen R: Gastropexy and "fundoplication" in surgical treatment of hiatal hernia. Am J Dig Dis 6:954, 1961.

110. Russell CO and Hill LD: Gastroesophageal reflux. Curr Prob Surg 20:205, 1983.

111. Zakim D, Dannenberg NJ (eds): Peptic Ulcer Disease and Other Acid Related Disorders. New York, Acad Res Ass Inc, 1991.

112. Thomas R: The Modern Practice of Physic. 6th ed. London, Longman Hurst, 1819, p. 914.

113. Meulengracht E: Treatment of hematemesis and melena with food. Lancet ii:1220, 1935.

114. Hunt T: Treatment and prognosis of peptic ulcer. *In* Jones FA: Modern Trend in Gastroenterology. New York, PB Hoeber Inc, 1952, p. 395.

115. Jones FA. The management of acute dyspepsia: With special reference to gastric and duodenal ulcer. Br Med J ii:1463, 1949.

116. Peterson WL, Sturdevant RAL, Frankl HD: Healing of duodenal ulcer with an antacid regimen. N Engl J Med 297:341, 1977.

117. Hammer R et al.: Pirenzepine distinguishes between different subclasses of muscarinic receptors. Nature (Lond) 283:90, 1980.

118. Londong W: Review: Anticholinergics for peptic ulcer—A Renaissance? Hepatogastroenterology 29:40, 1982.

119. Bettarello A: Anti-ulcer therapy: Past to present. Dig Dis Sci 30:365, 1985.

120. Pollard HM, Augur NA: Peptic ulcer over past one hundred years. Practitioner 201:139, 1968.

121. Jones FA: Annual oration on peptic ulcer—in perspective. Trans Med Soci Lond 107:101, 1986.

122. Bruegel C: Die beeinflussingdes magenschemismis dürch Rontgestrahler Munch Med Wchschr 64:379, 1917.

123. Ricketts WE, Palmer WL, Kirsner JB, Harman A: Radiation therapy in peptic ulcer: An analysis of the results. Gastroenterology 11:789, 1948.

124. Schunack W: What are the differences between H$_2$ receptor antagonists? Aliment Pharmacol Ther 1:493S, 1987.

125. a. Wylie CM: The complex wane of peptic ulcer. I. Recent national trends in deaths and hospital care in the United States. J Clin Gastroenterol 2:327, 1981. b. Wylie CM: The complex wane of peptic ulcer. II. Trends in duodenal and gastric ulcer admissions to 790 hospitals, 1974–1979. J Clin Gastroenterol 3:333, 1981.

126. Wyllie JH et al.: Effect of cimetidine on surgery for duodenal ulcer. Lancet i:1307, 1981.

127. Halter F (ed): Antacids in the eighties. Baltimore, Urban and Schwarzenberg, 1982, p. 153.

128. Richardson CT: Sucralfate (editorial). Ann Intern Med 92:269, 1982.

129. Brogden RN et al.: Sucralfate: A review of its pharmacodynamic properties and therapeutic use in peptic ulcer disease. Drugs 27:194, 1984.

130. Wagstaff AP, Benfield P, Monk JP: Colloidal bismuth subnitrate. A review of its pharmacodynamic and pharmocokinetic properties and its therapeutic use in peptic ulcer disease. Drugs 36:122, 1988.

131. Silen W: What is cytoprotection of the gastric mucosa. Gastroenterology 94:232, 1988.

132. Walt RP: Misoprostol for the treatment of peptic ulcer and anti-inflammatory-drug-induced gastroduodenal ulceration. N Engl J Med 327:1575, 1992.

133. Walt RP et al.: Effect of daily oral omeprazole on 24 hour intragastric acidity. Br Med J ii:12, 1983.

134. Bell NJV, Hunt RH: Role of gastric acid suppression in the treatment of gastro-oesophageal reflux disease. Gut 33:118, 1992.

135. McTavis D, Buckley M, Heel RC: Omeprazole: An updated review of its pharmacology and therapeutic use in acid-related disorders. Drugs 42:138, 1991.

136. Brunner G, Creutzfeldt W: Omeprazole in the long-term management of patients with acid-related diseases resistant to ranitidine. Scand J Gastroenterol 166:101, 1989.

137. Larsson H et al.: Time course of development and reversal of gastric endocrine cell hyperplasia after inhibition of acid secretion. Studies with omeprazole and ranitidine in antrectomized rats. Gastroenterology 95:1477, 1988.

138. Penston J, Wormsley K: Achlorhydria: Hypergastrinemia: Carcinoids. A flawed hypothesis? Gut 28:488, 1987.

139. Lanas A, Sekar C, Hirschowitz BI: Objective evidence of aspirin use in both ulcer and non-ulcer upper and lower gastrointestinal bleeding. Gastroenterology 103:862, 1992.

140. Sonnenberg A: Geographic and temporal variations in the occurrence of peptic ulcer disease. Scand J Gastroenterol 110:11, 1985.

141. Bianchi Porro G, Petrillo M: Natural history of peptic ulcer disease: The influence

of H₂ antagonist treatment. Scand J Gastroenterol *21*:4, 1986.

142. Bonnevie O: a. The incidence of gastric ulcer in Copenhagen County. b. The incidence of duodenal ulcer in Copenhagen County. Scand J Gastroenterol *10*:231 and 385, 1975.

143. Walan A (ed): Peptic ulcer and its treatment—present situation and future prospects. Scand J Gastroenterol *14*:1, 1978.

144. Olbe L et al.: Properties of a new class of gastric acid inhibitors. Scand J Gastroenterol *14*:131, 1979.

145. Jennings D: Perforated peptic ulcer. Changes in age-incidence and sex-distribution in the last 150 years. Lancet *395*:198, 1940.

146. Susser M: Causes of peptic ulcer: A selective epidemiologic review. J Chron Dis *20*:435, 1967.

147. Bonnevie O: Changing demographics of peptic ulcer disease. Dig Dis Sci *30*:8S, 1985.

148. Mendeloff AL: What has been happening to duodenal ulcer. Gastroenterology *67*:1020, 1974.

149. Sonnenberg A: Birth cohort analysis of peptic ulcer mortality. J Chronic Dis *38*:309, 1985.

150. Pflanz M: Epidemiological and sociocultural factors in the etiology of duodenal ulcer. Adv Psychosom Med 6:121, 1971.

151. Doll R: Peptic ulcer. Section I Epidemiology. *In* Jones FA (ed): Modern Trends in Gastroenterology. London, Butterworth, 1952, p. 831.

152. Kurata JH: Epidemiology of peptic ulcer disease. *In* Swabb and Szabo S (eds): Ulcer Disease: Investigation and Basis for Therapy. New York, Marcel Dekker, Inc. 1991.

153. Monthly vital statistics report. Advanced report of final mortality statistics 1990. National Center for Health Statistics *41*: Suppl 7, January 7, 1993.

154. Ostensen H, Burhol PG, Bonnevie O, Bolz KD: Changes in the pattern of peptic ulcer disease in the northern part of Norway between 1946 and 1981. Scand J Gastroenterol *17*:1073, 1987.

155. Sonnenberg A: Factors which influence the incidence and course of peptic ulcer. Scand J Gastroenterol *8*:119, 1988.

156. Sonnenberg A: Changes in physician visits for gastric ulcer and duodenal ulcer in the United States during 1958–1984 as shown by National Disease and Therapeutic Index (NDTI). Dig Dis Sci *32*:1, 1987.

157. Rosenow EC: The causation of gastric and duodenal ulcer by streptococci. J Inf Dis *19*:333, 1916.

158. Rune SJ et al.: Acyclovir in the prevention of duodenal ulcer recurrence. Gut *31*:151, 1990.

159. Code CF, Varco RL: Chronic histamine action. Proc Soc Exp Biol *44*:475, 1940.

160. Friesen SF, Baronofsky ID, Wangensteen OH: Benadryl fails to protect against the histamine provoked ulcer. Proc Soc Exp Biol *63*:23, 1946.

161. Lambert R: Les aspects récents de l'ulcère expérimental. Librairie Arnette Paris, 1958, p. 480.

162. Friedman JC, Hamburger WW: Experimental chronic gastric ulcer: A second contribution to the experimental pathology of the stomach. JAMA *63*:380, 1914.

163. Shay H et al.: A simple method for the uniform production of gastric ulceration in the rat. Gastroenterology *5*:43, 1945.

164. Szabo S et al.: Duodenal ulcerogens; effect of FGF on cysteamine-induced duodenal ulcer. Halter F, Garner A, Tygat GNJ: Mechanisms of peptic ulcer healing. Dasdrecht, Kluner Acad Publishers, 1990.

165. Alexander F: The influence of psychologic factors upon gastrointestinal disturbances, a symposium. I. General principles, objectives and preliminary results. Psychoanalytic Quart *3*:501, 1934.

166. Mittleman B, Wolff HG: Emotions and gastroduodenal function: Experimental studies in patients with gastritis, duodenitis and peptic ulcer. Psychosom Med *4*:5, 1942.

167. Mirsky IA: Physiologic, psychologic and social determinants in the etiology of duodenal ulcer. Am J Dig Dis *3*:285, 1958.

168. Wolf S: The stomach. London, Oxford University Press, 1965, p. 321.

169. Spicer CE, Stewart DN, Winser DM: Perforated peptic ulcer during period of heavy air raids. Lancet *i*:14, 1944.

170. Talley NJ et al.: Suppression of emotions in essential dyspepsia and chronic duodenal ulcer. A case control study. Scand J Gastroenterol *23*:337, 1988.

171. Barbour HA, Dickerson VS: Gastric ulceration produced in rats by oral and subcutaneous aspirin. Arch Int Pharmacodyn Ther *58*:78, 1938.

172. Douthwaite AH: Some recent advances in medical diagnosis and treatment. Br Med J *i*:1143, 1938.

173. Soll A, Kurata J: Ulcers, NSAIDs and related matters. Gastroenterology *96*:561, 1989.

174. Barrier CH, Hirschowitz BI: Controversies in the detection and management of nonsteroidal anti-inflammatory drug-induced side effects of the upper gastrointestinal tract. Am J Rheum *32*:926, 1989.

175. Kurata JH, Abbey DE: The effect of chronic aspirin use on duodenal and gastric ulcer hospitalization. J Clin Gastroenterol *12*:260, 1990.

176. Warren JR, Marshall BJ: Unidentified curved bacilli on gastric epithelium in active chronic gastritis. Lancet *i*:1273, 1983.

177. Marshall BJ, Warren JR: Unidentified curved bacilli in the stomach of patients with gastritis and peptic ulcer. Lancet *1*: 1311, 1984.

178. Rauws EA, Tytgat GN: Cure of duodenal ulcer associated with eradication of Helicobacter pylori. Lancet *335*:1233, 1990.

179. Hentschell E et al.: Effect of ranitidine and amoxicillin plus metronidazole on the eradication of Helicobacter pylori and the recurrence of duodenal ulcer. N Engl J Med *328*:308, 1993.

180. Gregory RA, Tracy H, French JM, Sircus W: Extraction of a gastrin like substance from a pancreatic tumor in a case of Zollinger-Ellison syndrome. Lancet *i*:1045, 1960.

181. McGuigan JE, Trudeau WL: Immunochemical measurement of elevated levels of gastrin in serum of patients with pancreatic tumor of the ZE variety. N Engl J Med *27*: 1308, 1968.

182. Malagelada JR et al.: Gastric secretion and emptying after ordinary meals in duodenal ulcer. Gastroenterology *73*:989, 1977.

183. Walsh JH: Gastrointestinal peptide hormones. *In*: Sleisenger MH, Fordtran JS (eds): Gastrointestinal Disease, ed. 4. Philadelphia, WB Saunders, 1989, p. 78.

184. Cooper RQ, Dockray GJ, Calan J, Walker R: Acid and gastrin responses during intragastric titration in normal subjects and duodenal ulcer patients with G-cell hyperfunction. Gut *26*:232, 1985.

185. Isenberg JI et al.: Increased sensitivity to stimulation of acid secretion by pentagastrin in duodenal ulcer. J Clin Invest *55*:330, 1975.

186. Lam SK et al.: Gastric acid secretion is abnormally sensitive to endogenous gastrin released after peptone test meals in duodenal ulcer patients. J Clin Invest *65*:555, 1980.

187. Bhaskar KR et al.: Viscous fingering of HCl through gastric mucin. Nature (London) *360*:458, 1992.

188. Hirschowitz BI, Streeten DHP, Pollard HM, Boldt, HA Jr: Role of gastric secretions in activation of peptic ulcers by corticotropin (ACTH). JAMA *158*:27, 1955.

189. Zollinger RA, Ellison EH: Primary peptic ulcerations of the jejunum associated with islet cell tumors of the pancreas. Ann Surg *142*:709, 1955.

190. Gregory RA, Grossman MI, Tracy H, Bentley PH: Nature of the gastric secretagogue in ZE tumors. Lancet *2*:543, 1967.

191. Moldawer MP, Nardi GL, Raker JW: Concomitance of multiple adenomas of the parathyroids and pancreatic islets with tumor of the pituitary: A syndrome with familial incidence. Am J Med Sci *228*:190, 1954.

192. Wermer P: Genetic aspects of adenomatosis of endocrine glands. Am J Med *16*:363, 1954.

193. Arey LB: Wound healing. Physiol Rev *16*: 327, 1936.

194. Burrows MT: The mechanisms of cell division. Am J Anat *39*:83, 1927.

195. Davidson JW: Wound hormones. Edinb Med J *50*:70, 1943.

196. Grant R: Rate of replacement of the surface epithelial cells of gastric mucosa. Anat Res *91*:175, 1945.

197. Halter F, Garner A, Tytgat GNJ: Mechanisms of peptic ulcer healing. Dasdrecht, Kluwer Acad Publishers, 1990.

198. Wright NA, Pike C, Elra G: Induction of a novel epidermal growth factor-secreting cell lineage by mucosal ulceration in gastrointestinal stem cells. Nature *343*:82, 1990.

199. Bloom BS: Cross-national changes in the effects of peptic ulcer disease. Ann Intern Med *114*:558, 1991.

200. Graham DY: Treatment of peptic ulcers caused by H. pylori. N Engl J Med *328*:349, 1993.

201. Stolley PD, Lasky T: Johannes Fibiger and his Nobel Prize for the hypothesis that a worm causes stomach cancer. Ann Intern Med *116*:765, 1992.

Small Intestine

6

Digestion, Absorption, and Malabsorption in the Small Intestine

SIDNEY F. PHILLIPS AND MICHAEL CAMILLERI

The title of this chapter establishes the scope of this review of the physiology, pathophysiology, and diseases of the small intestine. The first section summarizes, in temporal sequence, the major advances in our understanding of the small intestine and its functions generally, without direct reference to specific diseases. These form the foundations needed for clinical scientists to expand the data base on which the prevention, diagnosis and treatment of the digestion/absorptive diseases can be based. The second section presents, in chronologic terms, three prototypic examples of small bowel disease. In describing what is now possible, we hope to illustrate by example the benefits for medical management that have accrued from a greater understanding of fundamental processes.

We shall emphasize the advances that are most relevant to the science of gastroenterology, that is, the useful application of the knowledge that relates to the management of patients with intestinal disease. Since our focus is the 20th century, a logical starting point is the body of information available to physiologists and clinicians in the late 19th and early 20th centuries. For this, we turned to a small selection of well-recognized texts (1–4).

HISTORICAL PERSPECTIVE

The Late 19th Century

As a starting point, a text for students and practitioners of medicine, written by a Pro-fessor of Physiology and Microscopic Anatomy at the Columbia College of Physicians and Surgeons, was examined (1). The date was 1864; Beaumont's observations on Alexis St. Martin were 30 years old and Claude Bernard's fundamental studies were acknowledged and much quoted. Salivary digestion by ptyalin was recognized, the role of pepsin was known, and the concept was stated that "different elements of the food are digested in different parts of the alimentary canal by the agency of different fluids."

Beyond these rudimentary beliefs, little was understood. Digestion and rapid absorption of starch in the small intestine was recognized, and it was suspected that the digestion of fats was primarily by pancreatic juices. Overall, the message to the student was that digestion and absorption could be localized to regions of the upper gut, but the underlying chemical processes were only just being probed. Not surprisingly, no clinical associations with disease could be described. It will be clear to clinical historians that the malabsorption syndromes had been already described, and that clinicians and basic scientists shared little common ground or communication.

The Turn of the Century

If the 19th century can be viewed as a time when the science of gastroenterology was rudimentary at best, progress was more obvious by the beginning of the 20th century. In retrospect, even though the contributions of Bernard, Beaumont, and others now may be seen as seminal, the clinical base of knowledge as applied to diagnosis and treatment had not expanded much, and it encompassed little that was new scientifically. For this next era, texts of 1896 from the U.S. (2) and of 1915 from England (3) were consulted.

In an 800-page book, Howell (2) devoted almost 100 pages to the chemistry of digestion and nutrition. Clearly, what had happened since Dalton's text, 32 years earlier, was a tremendous advance in the science of chemistry. The Law of Mass Action was now well known, and its concepts were integrated into the digestive process. The term "enzyme" was used, and considerable space was devoted to proteolytic, amylolytic, fat-splitting and inverting (disaccharidase) enzymes. The concept of catalysis was accepted, as was the bidirectional nature of enzymic action. Experiments with isolated loops of small bowel had established that the gut contained no lipase or proteolytic activity, but that disaccharidases were present in the small bowel. The mechanisms of absorption were discussed rather more crudely: diffusion, osmosis and dialysis were considered, as was the presence of an active, or "vital" process, for the absorption of salt and water.

By 1915, Bayliss included a full chapter on catalysts and enzymes. Mass action now had been characterized mathematically and the appropriate formulae were given in detail. "Zymogens" was a new word in the vocabulary and, although pro-enzymes were not named as such, "coenzymes" were; trypsin and enterokinase were described as phenomena. However, although the basic biochemical base had progressed importantly, clinical science had not. A system of pathophysiology was not recognized; nevertheless, the hydrogen ion concentrations necessary for adequate peptic and tryptic digestion were well established and "erepsin" (oligopeptidase) was recognized as a component of succus entericus. Lipolysis also was well accepted, as was the role of bile as an "emulsifier." Re-synthesis of neutral fat in enterocytes and the lacteal route for the assimilation of fat were described, but these were still based on Bernard's work half a century before. An active mechanism for the absorption of salt and

water was now widely held. Interestingly, Bayliss placed great emphasis on the role of smooth muscle function ("motility") in the overall process of digestion. The movement of food, secretions, and chyme along the gut was discussed in detail. Attention also was directed to the control of gut function and, perhaps not surprisingly, humoral mechanisms were preferred. While granting the enteric nervous system a role in peristalsis, Bayliss opined that "nerves probably do not play any normal role in the case of the pancreas, liver and small intestine." Integrative physiology received little real attention; in this 800-page text, the chapter on digestion received only 12 pages!

The Early 20th Century

The book authored by Best and Taylor (4) and published in 1937 was entitled *The Physiological Basis of Medical Practice*. Digestion represented about 10% of the text, and the organization of the material began to approach the integrative concepts widely accepted today. Of note, though, is that the chapter entitled "Digestion in the Intestine" included all aspects of pancreatic function as well as those of the small bowel. In retrospect, this combination of luminal and mucosal digestion exemplified the fact that specific defects of pancreatic enzyme secretion were not recognized clinically. The role of pancreatic disease in leading to deficiencies of hydrolytic enzymes was not appreciated. In the section on intestinal digestion, it was not accepted that disaccharidases (specifically lactase) and oligopeptidases ("erepsin") were located in mucosal tissues. On the other hand, the mechanisms of absorption received scant attention, and "vital forces" (active transport) were still extolled in no further detail (and somewhat in a 19th century context) as an important process for salt and water uptake by the gut.

Given the pathophysiologic focus of this particular text, it is noteworthy that gallbladder function, cholelithiasis, and jaundice were discussed in some detail, but no comment was made on maldigestion or malabsorption. Steatorrhea, pancreatic enzyme deficiency, and diarrheal disease were not even mentioned. One must conclude from this text that, up to the mid-20th century, there was little scientific basis for the clinical discipline of gastroenterology. Best and Taylor briefly discussed the early experiments of Florey and Wright at Oxford; these had begun to revive interest in the role of the nervous system in the control of small bowel secretion. By inference, therefore, the nervous system also might be implicated in the general processes of digestion and absorption.

It is also apparent from a broader review of the literature, however, that much important basic science had not reached the clinical arena. Work of the Coris, Czaky, and others, which had begun to explore the active absorption of simple sugars, was not mentioned; the absorptive advances provided by the digestion of sugars at the brush border were unknown. The experiments of Sperber, Verzar, Bloor, Frazer, and others that had begun to prove the complex processes of fat absorption and the origin of fecal fat were not included by Best and Taylor. We must conclude that, by the time of the scientific hiatus created by World War II, systematic gastroenterology had a relatively poor infrastructure on which to build a rational approach to clinical problems. The status of knowledge available to most gastroenterologists up to 1937 is summarized in Table 6-1.

The Modern Era: 1950–1990s

The emergency pressures of World War II accelerated to breakneck speed certain initiatives, such as the development of the first antibiotics, new vaccines, blood replacement therapy, and heroic surgical procedures, to name a few. Thereafter, what reinvigorated biomedical research after 1950 is not clear. However, after 1950 increasing scientific attention was directed toward human disease, human experimentation, and the clinical sciences. In the U.S., this post-war re-emphasis on human disease was nurtured by the establishment of the National Institutes of Health. This greater focus on human experimentation, in the laboratory as well as at the bedside, extended to the science of gastroenterology. We wish to discuss these advances under two main headings:

1. The development of more precise methods for human experimentation.

2. Important hypotheses that arose from systematic and well-documented clinical observations.

Table 6–1
Digestion, Absorption, and the Science of Gastroenterology, 1860–1940

Reference	Date	Digestion	Absorption
Dalton (1)	1864	Salivary digestion recognized. Action of pepsin known. Role of pancreatic lipase appreciated (Bernard).	Regional absorption suspected No clinical correlates
Howell (2)	1896	Enzymes described (proteolytic, lipolytic, amylolytic and invertase). Digestive activity known to reside in the small bowel epithelium.	Active absorption ("vital processes") had been demonstrated
Bayliss (3)	1915	Enzymic action well characterized biochemically and mathematically. Role of bile as an emulsifier well recognized.	Little detail given
Best and Taylor (4)	1937	Epithelial digestion recognized. Role of pancreatic enzymes not well described.	Few clinical correlates No description of basic observations on fat and carbohydrate absorption

NEW METHODS FOR THE STUDY OF HUMANS

Up to 1940, the history of gastrointestinal physiology in humans was largely comprised of scientific reports of experiments on individual subjects. These often were performed on patients with fistulas or surgical operations whereby access to the gut was facilitated; sometimes these were merely chance observations. Planned studies with humans as the test species were virtually nonexistent. Beginning in the 1950s, experimenters were able to gain simple and reliable access to the normal human small intestine. These approaches revolutionized human experimentation on digestion and absorption.

Transintestinal Intubation

Important to the beginning of this era were advances in the plastics industry. New technologies permitted the manufacture of thin, soft, polyethylene tubing; thereafter, comfortable and predictable intubation of the human gut became feasible. The first attempts were with the various systems used by Miller and Abbott, which often used a series of balloons to isolate segments of intestine (5). Thinner, even more flexible systems became popular after the report of Blankenhorn, Hirsch and Ahrens (6), which described transintestinal intubation in man (Fig. 6–1). Subsequently, other groups used this approach successfully (7) in qualitative observations, but true quantification of luminal events needed another step.

Marker-dilution Techniques for the Quantitative Recovery of Intestinal Aspirates

Bengt Borgström (Fig. 6–2) and his Swedish collaborators at Lundh and the Karolinska Institute brought these to our attention. In 1953, Sperber, Hyden, and Eckman first used polyethylene glycol 4000 (PEG) as a reference substance for the study of digestion by ruminants (8). Subsequently, in their classic paper of 1957 (9), Borgström, Dahlquist, Lundh, and Sjövall used PEG in man to show clearly that humans digest and absorb in the proximal jejunum (Fig. 6–3) virtually all carbohydrate, fat, and protein delivered as a liquid meal ("milkshake").

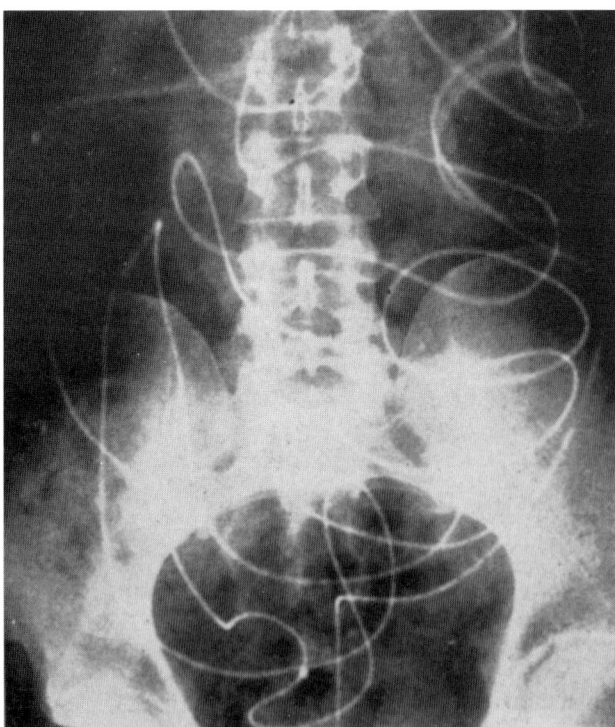

Fig. 6–1. Radiograph of transintestinal tube as described by Blankenhorn, Hirsch and Ahrens. Reproduced with permission from Blankenhorn DH, Hirsch J, Ahrens EH Jr: Transintestinal intubation; technic for measurement of gut length and physiological sampling at known loci. Proc Soc Exper Biol Med *88*:356, 1955.

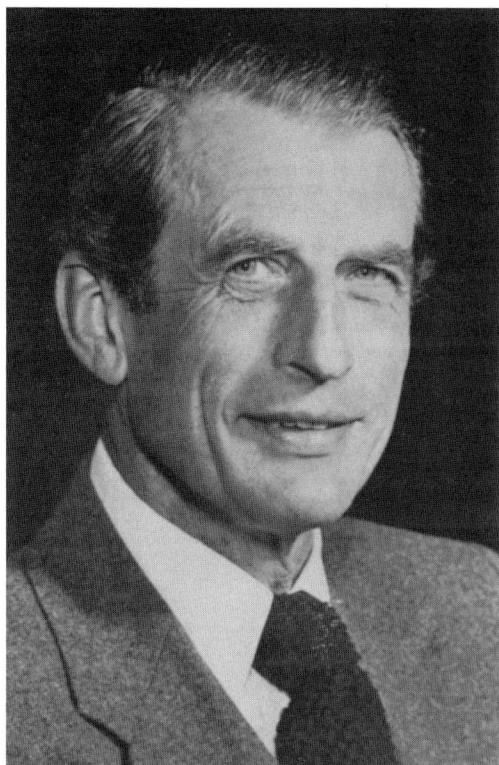

Fig. 6–2. Bengt Borgström. Reproduced with permission from Borgström B, Hofman AF: Acceptance remarks. Beaumont Prize 1979. Gastroenterology 77:952, 1979.

These experiments integrated many of the experimental data that had been waiting to be focused on human physiology and disease. To quote from Borgström, ''. . . intraluminal digestion is digestion by pancreatic enzymes. The enzymes formerly ascribed to the intestinal juice such as lactase, maltase and dipeptidase were localized and functioning in the brush border'' (10). Even more importantly, these techniques nurtured inquiry and led to experiments in several new directions. Dahlquist used it to explore disaccharidases in the brush border of enterocytes (11), Lundh (12) exploited marker dilution of the Lundh Test Meal to measure enzyme output in response to food as an index of pancreatic function, and Lindquist described the malabsorption of monosaccharides (13). The Lundh meal became the basis of a clinical test for pancreatic disease that was widely used for two decades. In the present context, these

workers opened up the human physiology of intestinal digestion and absorption by establishing new and rational experimental and diagnostic approaches. Indeed, they firmly moved scientific gastroenterology into a new era, in which safe investigation of humans allowed man to be used as the ultimate experimental model.

Extension of Marker-dilution Techniques to the Study of Active and Passive Absorption

Ingelfinger, Fordtran, and their collaborators in Boston and Dallas were quick to recognize the potential of PEG for use as a volume marker in more specific studies of nutrient absorption (14,15). Rather than evaluating the gut's handling of a test meal as an index of digestion or absorption, they used artificial solutions introduced into various segments of intestine to quantify absorption in intact humans. As these methods became more refined, sophisticated experiments could be designed; these examined in vivo the specific transport processes that underlie the active and passive uptake of electrolytes, water, sugars, other carbohydrates and vitamins. Indeed, the studies of Turnberg and Fordtran described clearly the transport characteristics of the human jejunum and ileum, in ways that had previously been approached only by studies in vitro (16,17). These methods were expanded and utilized to examine the abnormalities of absorption in disease states (18,19). The spectrum of maldigestion and malabsorption of carbohydrates was described (20,21), as were fat absorption and malabsorption (22) and normal bile acid reabsorption in humans (23). Thus, the ultimate expression of these methods was to explore the physiologic phenomena in humans that accompanied maldigestion or malabsorption of nutrients.

The era of intestinal perfusion flourished into the mid-1970s, during which data from human experimentation were able, at the very least, to confirm parallel observations that were being made in other species. In the past decade, investigators have used intestinal intubation and nonabsorbable marker techniques somewhat less; fewer problems are still accessible solely to these approaches.

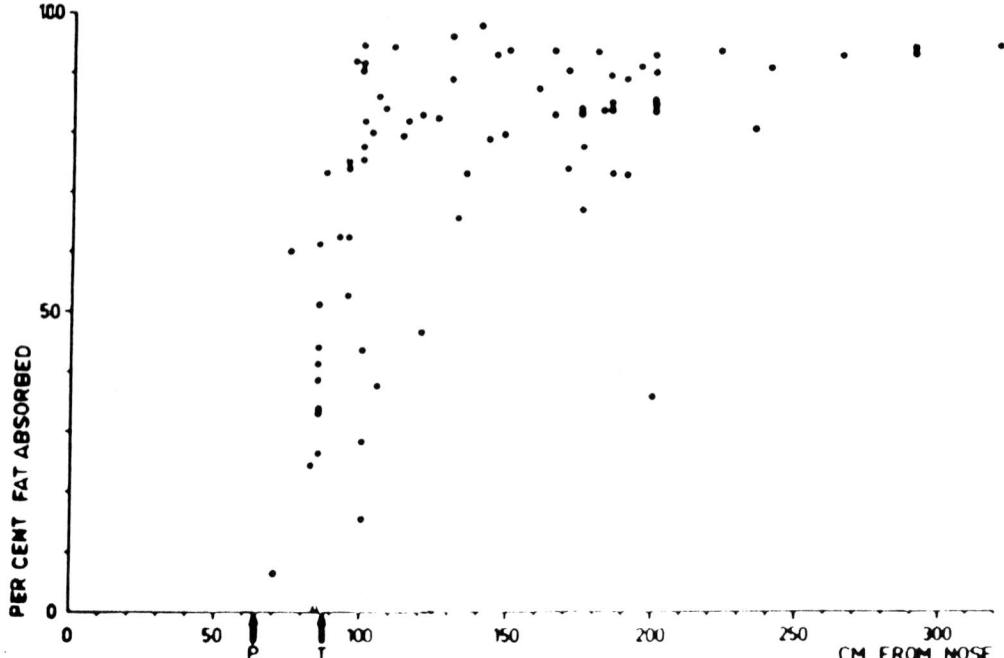

Fig. 6–3. Percentage of fat absorbed from a liquified test meal, samples retrieved at different lengths of tubing from the nose; p is the site of the pylorus and T the angle of Treitz. The methodology used polyethylene glycol as a recovery marker for aspirates. Reproduced with permission from Borgström B, Dahlquist A, Lundh G, Sjovall J: Studies of intestinal digestion and absorption in the human. J Clin Invest *36*:1521, 1957.

Small Bowel Biopsy

Reports in the 1930s had drawn attention to an anatomical abnormality, villous atrophy, in the clinical syndrome of sprue (24). However, the observations of Thaysen (25), who injected formalin into recently deceased patients with sprue, appeared to reject the presence of a structural abnormality in malabsorption syndromes. What was needed if this subject was to be explored in greater detail was a simple and safe means of obtaining fresh tissue from the intestinal mucosa. The need for an intubation technique became even more critical when, in 1954, Paulley reported on surgical jejunal biopsies from two patients with steatorrhea (26); the villi were broad, clubbed and the site of an inflammatory infiltrate (Fig. 6–4A).

Meanwhile, Wood and his colleagues in Melbourne had devised and used a flexible gastric biopsy tube (27), which they subsequently used safely many hundreds of times. Lengthening the tube and increasing its flexibility enabled the duodenum or proximal jejunum to be reached (28); mucosal changes in patients with sprue were confirmed (Fig. 6-4B). There followed a profusion of modified "Wood tubes" (e.g., Shiner tube, Rubin multipurpose tube, etc.) and a variety of spring-operated capsules (Crosby, Carey capsules, etc.) for obtaining biopsies from one or more duodenal and jejunal sites. Eventually, multiple retrieving systems were developed; these allowed biopsies to be obtained and retrieved at the time of intubation from multiple loci (29). Thus, the extent of morphologic lesions along the length of the small bowel in sprue could be localized (e.g., by the Flick tube, Baker and Hughes tube, etc.). These multiple biopsy systems, in fact, were discarded rather quickly when patients were found to develop a "postbiopsy syndrome" of abdominal pain and fever. Peritoneal irritation (i.e., subclinical perforation) was strongly suspected. However, the multipurpose

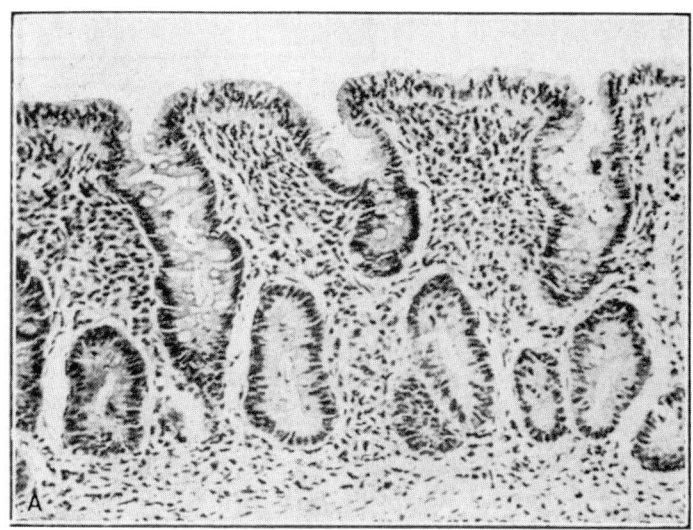

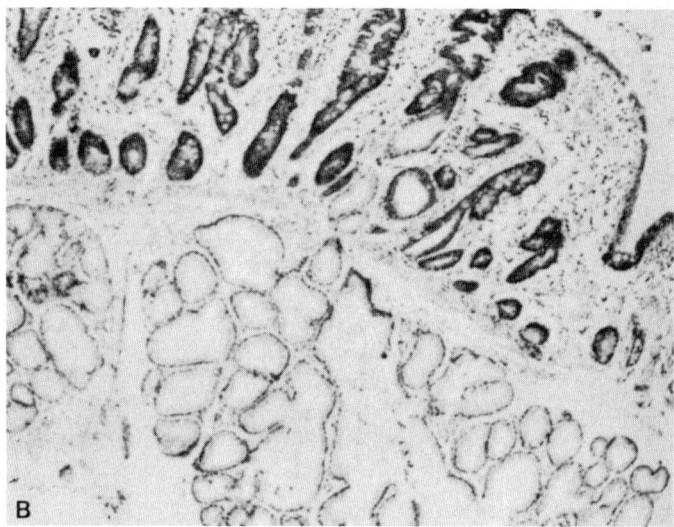

Fig. 6–4. A. Surgical biopsy of small intestine from a patient with sprue (idiopathic steatorrhea). Reproduced with permission from Paulley JW: Observations on the etiology of idiopathic steatorrhea. Br Med J 2:1318, 1954. **B.** Peroral biopsy from small intestine from a patient with sprue (celiac disease). Reproduced with permission from Sakula J, Shiner M: Coeliac disease with atrophy of the small intestine mucosa. Lancet 2:876, 1957. Note the blunting and atrophy of villi in both photomicrographs and prominent Brunner's glands in **B** (duodenal biopsy).

tubes and the Crosby capsule have remained in the diagnostic armamentarium. The availability of a safe and simple system for mucosal biopsy was a major technologic advance that allowed the clinical investigation of maldigestion and malabsorption to proceed.

Schilling Test

Vitamin B_{12}'s interactions with intrinsic factor (IF) and its uptake by the intestine are described later in this chapter, as are pernicious anemia and its response to treatment. However, the development by Schilling in 1953 of a simple and logical test for the secretion of intrinsic factor by the stomach and the absorption of the vitamin B_{12}/IF complex by the ileum prompted extensive investigations in humans and experimental animals (30,31). Indeed, this was the first well-documented example of a test of regional absorption (i.e., vitamin B_{12}/IF in the ileum). Thus, Schilling opened up the subject of the regional specialization of absorption by the small intestine.

Breath Tests for Carbohydrate Malabsorption

Levitt, first working in Ingelfinger's department, opened a new door with his re-

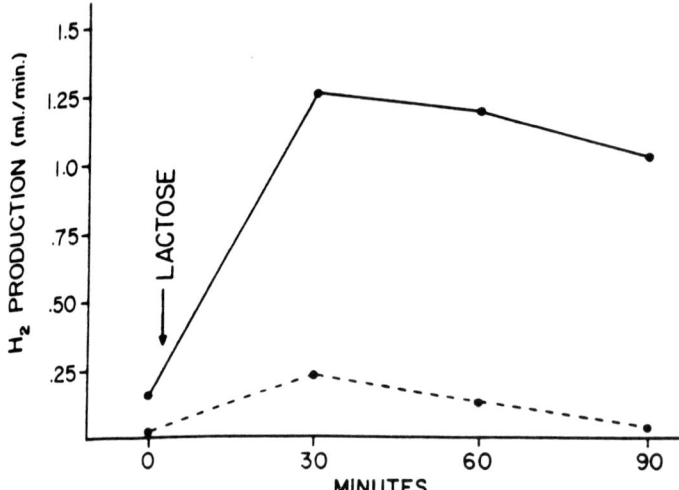

Fig. 6–5. Production of H_2 in the small intestine (dotted line) and large intestine (solid line) in a patient with bacterial overgrowth of the small bowel. Fasting levels of H_2 production (at zero time) and the increase after lactose instillation are shown. Reproduced with permission from Levitt MD: Production and excretion of hydrogen gas in man. N Engl J Med *281*:122, 1969.

ports of the breath hydrogen test (Fig. 6-5) (32). Most important was a new concept, that material that had escaped absorption could be used as a "signal" of malabsorption (33). The general principle has proved to be reproducible, at least in semiquantitative terms. Thus, the magnitude of breath hydrogen excretion after an oral dose can be used as a measure of the relative absorbability of different carbohydrate substrates. Levitt subsequently refined and extended the method to an index of gut transit which is now widely used (34). Unabsorbed carbohydrate generates a "signal" of breath hydrogen only when it reaches the colonic flora; thus, the timing of hydrogen excretion after ingestion of a substrate is an index of mouth-to-cecal transit time in health.

HYPOTHESES GENERATED FROM CLINICAL OBSERVATIONS

Gluten-sensitive Enteropathy

In 1888, Samuel Gee described a diarrheal disease in children which he called the "coeliac affection" (35). The condition was well recognized and expanded upon up to the 1930s (24,25). Moreover, Gee was aware that a comparable problem may occur in adults. Whether or not malabsorptive diarrhea was associated with a structural lesion

was uncertain (24–26), and the answer to this important question would require the development of a new technique, small bowel biopsy. However, a major breakthrough came from the clinical observations of Dicke in the early 1950s (36,37). He compared the incidence of celiac disease in Holland during World War II with that noted in other parts of Northern Europe. During this period, the prevalence of the disease decreased in Holland, and Dicke proposed that this was caused by a lack of cereals in the diet. The group subsequently showed that fecal fat excretion (measured by the method of van de Kamer, a member of the group) was increased when children were challenged with cereal fractions (38). These key observations and the concepts they embodied set the stage for an explosion of clinical research on the maldigestion-malabsorption of fat that lasted two decades and that forms the basis of our current understanding. Celiac disease is considered in detail later in the chapter.

Chronic Pancreatitis, Pancreatic Exocrine Insufficiency, Fat Balance Studies

The observations of Comfort and his coworkers from Mayo (39) first established the clinical syndrome of chronic pancreatitis in the absence of associated disease of the biliary tree or intestine. As part of the natural sequelae of chronic pancreatic inflammation, enzyme deficiency was presumed to occur, and steatorrhea, the prime digestive consequence of pancreatic enzyme failure, was well described. As a direct consequence of these descriptions, Wollaeger and his colleagues performed meticulous studies of fecal fat excretion and fat balance under a variety of physiologic and pathologic circumstances. Eric Wollaeger's observations supported the concepts of an endogenous source for fecal fat and an upper limit to the fecal excretion of fat in health, one that was essentially constant regardless of the pattern of defecation (40). The quantitative fecal fat test thus emerged as the most appropriate "gold standard" for steatorrhea. The perceived inconvenience of the fecal fat quantification as a clinical test led to four decades in which "simpler tests" for steatorrhea were sought. Some of these have survived, but most were not of comparable specificity, sensitivity or reliability (41).

Gastric Resection and Postgastrectomy Malabsorption/Maldigestion

The prevalence of peptic ulcer disease was high, and indeed may have peaked, in the mid-20th century. Facilitated by the technical advances in anesthesia and surgery that were encouraged by trauma surgery in World War II, surgical treatment for complicated peptic ulcer disease became extremely fashionable in the period from 1950 to 1975. The advent of pharmacological blockade of histamine type 2 receptors brought this need to a natural finale. The initial operative approaches utilized subtotal gastric resection for removal of the parietal cell mass, with gastrointestinal continuity being restored by a variety of anastomoses. The postoperative problems that followed were of two sorts: (1) recurrent stomal ulceration and (2) nutritional deficiencies. Thus, one surgical approach was to remove increasingly large amounts of the parietal cell mass (to protect against stomal ulceration), or to add a vagotomy. Unfortunately, vagotomy merely tended to accentuate the digestive and nutritional deficiencies that followed gastric resection. Vagotomy without gastric resection (but with an associated "drainage procedure") came into fashion as an alternative. Lesser degrees of gastric resection were better tolerated nutri-

tionally, but appeared to increase the risk of postoperative (stomal) ulceration. Ultimately, these dilemmas led to major clinical comparisons (42) of several different surgical procedures. The overall results of the various procedures were not much different, although impaired nutrition and weight loss were more frequent after gastric resection.

However, these disturbances of digestion and absorption engendered by resective surgery and vagotomy for duodenal ulcer stimulated great interest in postoperative pathophysiology (43). Several principles emerged from the study of the "postgastric surgery" syndromes; moreover, these observations in patients were supplemented by extensive experiments on animal models.

Uncontrolled gastric emptying allowed large amounts of disaccharides to reach the small intestine; these were often sufficient to overwhelm the hydrolytic activity of brush border enzymes (44). Indeed, "dumping" had been recognized for many years as a consequence of gastric surgery. However, the specific "unmasking" by rapid gastric emptying of lactase deficiency that previously had been merely a subclinical disorder established a new concept. Thus, it became accepted that mucosal digestion was a balance between the substrate load and the available digestive potential.

Similarly, rerouting of the flow of food led to subtle disturbances as to how digestive enzymes mixed with chyme; impaired intraluminal digestion led predictably to low grade steatorrhea (43). The ways in which digestive secretions come in contact with chyme, in a temporal and anatomic sense, stress the subtle balance needed for normal digestion, emphasizing the integrated response of the upper gut to food. This disease model pointed out that gastric, pancreatic and hepaticobiliary components all needed to mix optimally with the meal. As another example of the way in which an alteration of the anatomy placed a "stress" on the gut, sprue syndromes that had been asymptomatic were also "unmasked" by vagotomy (45).

Stasis in the afferent loop of a Billroth II type anastomosis could allow bacteria to populate the upper small bowel. Although the "blind loop syndrome" (46,47) had been recognized as a sequel of other anatomic abnormalities (jejunal diverticula, entero-enteric fistulas, strictures, etc.), postgastrectomy steatorrhea soon became another example (48). Indeed, study of such patients helped establish the pathophysiology of blind loop syndrome. The details need to be consulted elsewhere, but the hypothesis emerged that bacterial enzymes in the proximal gut were also able to disturb the fine balance of functions needed for proper digestion and absorption, particularly the deconjugation of bile acids.

Zollinger-Ellison Syndrome

First described in 1955 (49), gastric hypersecretion of mammoth proportions captured attention as a cause of severe or atypical peptic ulcer disease, often involving the esophagus and/or postbulbar duodenum. Soon afterwards, diarrhea was recognized as an accompanying or occasionally sole manifestation. The diarrhea was sometimes watery and voluminous, but malabsorption and steatorrhea also were described.

Patients with the Zollinger-Ellison syndrome may have steatorrhea as a result of several mechanisms (50). Pancreatic lipase is inactivated by the enormous amounts of acid in the lumen of the upper small intestine. Pancreatic lipase is exquisitely susceptible to irreversible denaturation by acidification, rendering the lipase molecule inactive. Inactivation of lipase results in a failure to hydrolyze intraluminal triglycerides to diglycerides, monoglycerides, and fatty acids. Hypersecretion of gastric acid also may produce steatorrhea by the direct effects of a low pH on bile acids. The acid environment of the small intestine renders primary bile acids less soluble, reducing their ability to form micelles, which are necessary for fatty acid and monoglyceride absorption. Duodenitis and jejunitis may be present, and vitamin B_{12} malabsorption also was described (50).

Asiatic Cholera

Although the pathophysiology of cholera was predicted by John Snow in 1854 ("withdraws fluid from the blood"), there was much uncertainty and controversy for the next 100 years as to whether ulceration and exudation contributed to the voluminous, "rice water" stools so characteristic of the established disease. Soon after World War II, the U.S. Navy Medical Research Unit in Southeast Asia reported several key clinical observations (51).

Using methods developed in the early 1950s (see previous text), a series of seminal studies showed that (1) the small bowel mucosa was histologically normal in established cholera, (2) cholera fluids were not exudates, (3) the composition of fecal water was relatively fixed, reflecting a secretory fluid arising from the small intestine, and (4) absorption of glucose continued in the face of massive fluid secretion, i.e. the pathophysiology was one of secretion, not an abnormality of absorption. Further discussion of this area is beyond the present scope, but the cholera story prompted decades of basic and clinical research into absorption/secretion of electrolytes and water by the small intestine (52), and is another important example of systematic clinical observations that lead to a renewed interest in a basic process.

It should be apparent from this brief summary that during the 10 to 20 years after 1945, interest in digestion/absorption accelerated, especially from the standpoint of human physiology and pathophysiology. Most of these initiatives followed directly from systematic clinical observations and human experimentation that was facilitated by novel experimental methods. We shall now consider the important overall advances in knowledge of the digestion, absorption and malabsorption of fat, carbohydrate, and protein.

DIGESTION AND ABSORPTION OF MAJOR NUTRIENTS

Fat

The lacteal route for fat absorption was well described in Claude Bernard's classic experiment in the rabbit that also demonstrated that both bile and pancreatic juice were required for fat to be absorbed. These principles were never seriously challenged into the mid-20th century, although the ideas of Frazer (53) raised much controversy. Frazer's thesis was that mono-, di-, and triglycerides were largely absorbed without the need for complete hydrolysis to glycerol and fatty acids. Although he did not deny the occurrence of lipolysis, Frazer thought that the products of lipolysis merely facilitated emulsification. Subsequently, the specific hydrolytic properties of pancreatic lipase (which acts on the 1-monoglyceride bond only) were described by Mattson (54). Thereafter, the roles of bile acids, 2-monoglyceride (the residue of triglyceride that was unhydrolyzed by lipase) and free fatty acids in forming mixed micelles were recognized and the micellar route for absorption substantiated (55).

The advent of radiobiology and the availability of ^{14}C-labeled fats opened another era. Isotopic studies allowed fatty acid molecules to be followed through the intestinal wall and into lymph (56); reacylation of monoglyceride was shown and incorporation of resynthesized triglycerides into chylomicrons was elucidated. Moreover, Borgström had developed the methods needed to demonstrate rapid and complete absorption from the human duodenum and jejunum of fat that was ingested as a liquid test meal (9). By the mid-1960s, the major elements of the story were in place; they seemed to be correct scientifically and were ready to be applied to clinical problems. Indeed, it was now possible to review and classify the malabsorptive diseases on a logical basis of the known pathophysiology. In an important review, Sleisenger (57) subdivided fat malabsorption into abnormalities of (1) the intraluminal phase of digestion, (2) mucosal cell transport of lipolytic products, and (3) lymphatic transport of absorbed fat. In the next two decades, clinically relevant concepts of pathophysiology have extended very little upon these ideas.

One interesting byway that attracted considerable interest was provided by the advent of medium-chain triglycerides (MCT). These mixed triglycerides are made up of fatty acids with chain lengths between 6 and 10 carbons, and the theoretical lessons learned from their study are worth noting. Because of their different molecular configuration, MCTs are more rapidly and completely hydrolyzed by pancreatic enzymes, do not require bile acids for their absorption, do not form chylomicrons, exit from the intestine through the portal venous system, and are more rapidly and completely

metabolized than are long-chain fats. Despite these impressive physiological credentials, and despite their use during the late 60s and early 70s for almost every form of malabsorption (58), MCTs have not continued as a major weapon in the gastroenterologist's armamenterium. Their initial formulations, as "full dietary supplements," contained dextrose and milk protein; these were often hypertonic and poorly tolerated. MCT oil alone is best tolerated, but only to a maximum of about 400 calories (50 g MCT) daily. Although the digestive/absorptive phenomena exemplified by MCTs are still of considerable interest, they have now become something of a physiologic curiosity.

Although syndromes of fat maldigestion/malabsorption after gastric resection and in small bowel diseases such as sprue were the initial stimuli of clinical research in these areas, ileal resection provided one of the cleanest clinical examples of pathophysiology, with salutary lessons. The important studies of Alan Hofmann integrated a number of concepts. Evolving knowledge of the enterohepatic cycling of bile acids implied that the greater the degree of ileal dysfunction or resection, the greater would be the wastage of bile acids from the body. Hofmann and Poley (59) showed that when fecal losses of bile acids were only moderate, hepatic synthesis was able to compensate for wastage from the enterohepatic circulation, and steatorrhea was modest. These conditions occurred after short resections of the ileum. Moreover, a specific consequence of bile wastage was a diarrheal state caused by the secretory effects of bile acids on the colon (60). When more ileal function was lost (as with more extensive resections), fecal losses of bile acid were greater, and the liver was unable to compensate for the loss. Severe steatorrhea ensued and, in this instance, the accompanying diarrhea was caused more by the effects of excess fatty acids on the colon (Fig. 6–6) (60). Treatment of bile acid deficiency after ileal resection has been complicated by lack of a bile acid replacement that was not secretory and that facilitated micelle formation; Alan Hofmann's description of cholyl sarcosine is a very promising lead (62).

Recognition of those absorptive functions localized to the ileum, bile acids, and vitamin B$_{12}$ (61,63), were part of a more general

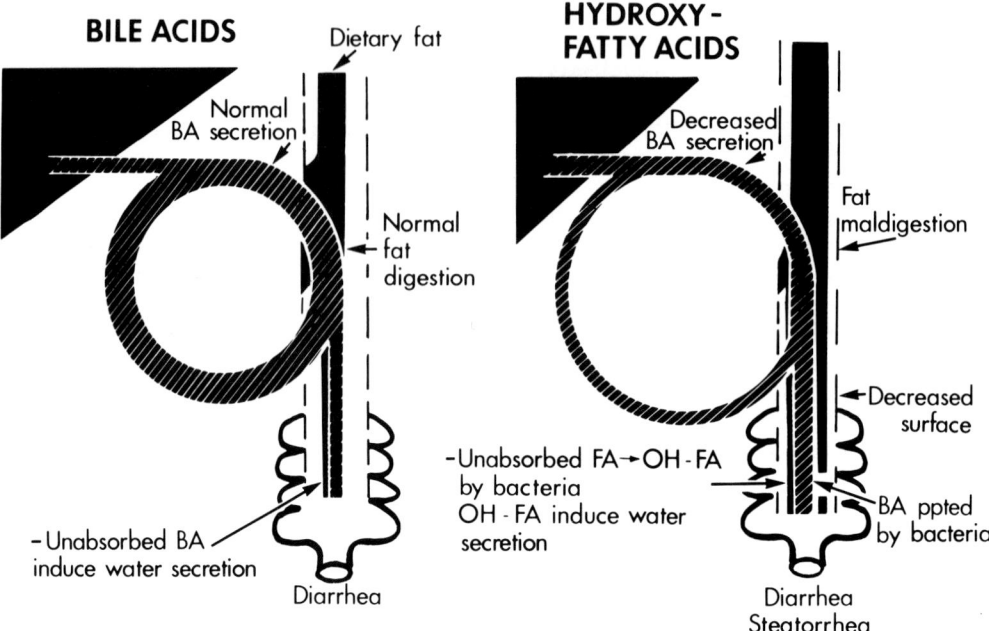

Fig. 6–6. Diagrammatic representation of the enterohepatic cycling of bile acids after ileal resection. On the left, after a short resection, the bile acid pool is maintained, steatorrhea is minimal, and diarrhea results from bile acids colonic secretion. On the right, after more extensive resection, the bile acid pool is depleted, steatorrhea is pronounced, and diarrhea is caused by fatty acids in the colon. Reproduced with permission from Borgström B, Hofmann AF: Acceptance remarks. Beaumont Prize 1979. Gastroenterology 77:952, 1979.

appreciation that small bowel function varied regionally. During the 1960s and 1970s, many clinical observations on persons after resections of small intestine led to parallel, animal studies that contrasted the normal functions of the jejunum to those of the ileum. The work of the Hammersmith group (63,64) is noteworthy. The concepts that emerged were that the jejunum normally digested and absorbed most dietary nutrients, particularly those ingested as a homogenized meal. The role of the jejunum in the absorption of certain micronutrients also was proven. Although the jejunum could maintain nutrition adequately, the proximal gut did not compensate well after ileal resection. Lacking active transport mechanisms for bile acids, the jejunum was unable to maintain the enterohepatic circulation of bile acids; the human ileum was demonstrated to be the only site for active reabsorption of bile acids (23). On the other hand, after jejunal resection, the ileum was able to assume many of the absorptive functions of the proximal bowel; nutrition was better preserved and diarrhea usually was less severe. These principles became increasingly important. The later development of enteral feedings in persons with impaired small bowel function, with or without resection, continued to rely on these concepts.

A major, though tangential, advance was the description by Dudrick that the role of the small bowel as a digestive/absorptive organ could be replaced entirely by total parenteral nutrition (TPN). Thus, although the idea had been developed that most functions of the small intestine could be replaced by adequate nutritional replacement, the demonstration that TPN allowed normal growth and development in young patients who essentially lacked small bowel function was required to prove this key point.

Carbohydrates

As discussed previously, techniques for the safe recovery of small intestinal mucosal tissue made available biopsies upon which assays of digestive enzymes could be performed. In parallel, a clinical syndrome in children, attributable phenomenologically to lactase deficiency, had been described in the early 1960s (65,66). Dahlquist, who had worked with Borgström in Sweden on disaccharidase activity (11), reported from Chicago the clinical features of lactose intolerance and intestinal lactase deficiency (65). At the same time, the Zurich group, using Dahlquist's assay for lactase activity in mucosal tissues, reported the same finding (66). These seminal observations can be followed in several directions.

The next important chapter in the story of lactase deficiency suggested incorrectly that lactase deficiency could be blamed for abdominal symptoms and diarrhea in many varied circumstances; these ranged from the irritable bowel syndrome to inflammatory bowel disease (67,68). On the other hand, secondary lactase deficiency as a consequence of any severe mucosal disease (such as sprue) came to be recognized. Moreover, the ontogeny of lactase activity and its obligatory loss in the postweaning phase of humans and most other mammals also received much attention. Thus, it became clear that lactase was an enzyme that was utilized by most mammals during suckling only; it then regressed after weaning. At the same time, data were being accumulated that not all the human races experienced a similar prevalence of adult lactase deficiency (69). The facts were reviewed and hypotheses were generated in 1969–70 by Simoons (70). He postulated that longstanding ethnic habits of diet, notably the availability of milk as a dietary component after weaning, determined the racial prevalence of lactase deficiency. Importantly, the pulling together of results from many racial groups and geographic regions placed in perspective the frequency with which lactase deficiency should be expected in any mixed population. The African and Oriental races generally lose lactase activity soon after weaning; races with a background in Northern Europe and Scandinavia remain tolerant of lactose in adult life. It then became apparent that the description of lactase deficiency as a presumably important factor in a variety of gastrointestinal diseases merely reflected the normal regression of lactase activity in many adult populations.

Another direction opened up by the "lactase story" was the description of deficiencies of other disaccharidases (e.g., sucrase-isomaltase, see subsequent text) and rare congenital defects of monosaccharide absorption (13). More recently came the recognition that a definite threshold exists in most persons for the absorption of other monosaccharides. Thus fructose, when ingested as a disaccharide in the form of sucrose, is well absorbed. We now believe that this is because of the spatial-metabolic advantages afforded when high concentrations of the hydrolytic products (glucose, fructose) are elaborated at the brush border by the action of mucosal sucrase. The uptake of the digestive products by active transport is therefore favored. However, malabsorption of fructose (when taken in large amounts as the monosaccharide) is now well recognized (71). The clinical importance of this phenomenon stems from the use of fructose as a sweetening agent in many foods and drinks. The monosaccharide is not so well absorbed as is fructose that is generated by the brush border digestion of sucrose (71). An inherited form of fructose intolerance also has been described (72). The principles of carbohydrate tolerance in relation to ingested doses have been applied not only to fructose but also to sugar alcohols (73) used as artificial sweeteners (e.g., sorbitol, mannitol).

The third general direction in which the lactase story moved was clarification of the mechanisms by which mucosal disaccharidase activity is controlled, as will be discussed for sucrase-isomaltase. Regional distributions of disaccharidases along the intestine were established; lactase activity is most pronounced in the proximal small bowel, other disaccharidases are distributed more generally (74). Dietary control of disaccharidase activity is important (75), as is the phenomenon of end-product inhibition (76). The disaccharidase enzymes are known to turn over rapidly and to be modified by pancreatic proteinases, which influence, at the luminal level, the final expression of several brush border proteins (77). Biosynthesis of the disaccharidases is modified at the post-translational level, including, for lactase, cleavage of the protein into two subunits immediately prior to insertion into the membrane (78).

Turning to monosaccharide uptake, the concept of a combined sodium-glucose active transport mechanism was first developed in the early 1960s, largely because of the work of Robert Crane and his coworkers (79). Their model of a cotransporter has helped explain many subsequent observations. The biochemistry of the glucose transporter proved difficult to finalize; the protein represents only a very small proportion of total membrane protein and its biochemistry has been bedeviled by its sensitivity to a variety of standard laboratory approaches. For instance, the protein was inactivated by most of the detergent solvents used in standard extraction procedures.

The sodium/glucose cotransporter was eventually cloned from human ileal tissue in 1989 by E. M. Wright and his colleagues; the protein, whose physiologic functions had been studied so carefully by so many groups, could now be scrutinized precisely (80). The next exciting step was not far behind. The same group described a single base change at position 92, in two children with glucose-galactose malabsorption; the parents were heterozygotes (81). The authors described this as the first membrane transport protein to be associated with a specific molecular defect that caused a genetic disorder. Thirty years were required for this molecular solution to be found, following the first clinical description of glucose-galactose malabsorption in 1962 (13).

A final comment is needed on dietary fiber, which can best be categorized as those dietary carbohydrates that are resistant to digestion by mammalian enzymes in the small bowel. Fiber, or "unavailable carbohydrate," passes through the small bowel largely unaltered; its interaction with fecal bacterial enzymes has provided many important new insights into new avenues of pathophysiology and treatment (82–84).

Interest in dietary fiber was established by Hugh Trowell (85), who defined it as "plant cell wall material that was resistant to the intestinal secretions of the host." Much dietary fiber is broken down only in the colon, as a result of bacterial metabolism. Fiber comprises structural plant cell walls, composed mainly of polysaccharides and lignins. Fiber was proposed by Burkitt (86) as a major factor in many diseases of man. Although all these initial claims have not been substantiated, fiber certainly modifies bowel function.

Fiber is extensively degraded in the colon to volatile (short-chain) fatty acids (SCFAs) and other metabolic products. SCFAs are absorbed from the colon and some (e.g., butyrate) are utilized as fuel by the colonic mucosa. Residual fiber, some of the metabolic products, and bacteria make up the bulk of the feces. Concepts have therefore developed that (1) the products of fiber digestion may be important nutrients of colonocytes, and it has been suggested that lack of SCFAs contributes to colitis, (2) some bulking agents may have important metabolic benefits (on hyperlipidemia, diabetes mellitus) and (3) fiber provides bulk for the feces, and is needed if colonic excretory function is to be normal.

Proteins

Digestion of protein by pepsin and pancreatic trypsin was well understood in the early 20th century; moreover, enzymes thought to reside in the small intestine (erepsins) and the role of enterokinase in the activation of trypsinogen were well described by Bayliss in 1915 (3). Major advances in our understanding came later in three main directions. First, the existence of a major enterosystemic turnover of proteins and amino acids was recognized. Thus, an endogenous secretion of proteins and amino acids into the gut existed normally. Pancreatic and intestinal secretions provided the major normal input, and, in pathologic states, the exudation of protein ("protein-losing enteropathies") added to this. Second, it was recognized that the range of peptidase activities in the mucosa was very broad. Third, *specific transport defects* were recognized for oligopeptides and amino acids. These abnormalities of amino-acid transport often were shared between enterocytes and renal tubular cells, expressed most dramatically by the aminoaciduria. Although of little nutritional consequence, these deficiencies of renal transport mechanisms had great theoretic significance, pointing to more generalized defects in transport proteins.

Exploration of the enteral flux of endogenous proteins was possible only when techniques of intestinal intubation in man were developed and quantitative observations were possible. The details are beyond the scope of this chapter, but Alpers has summarized them in a review (87). Along other lines, techniques were developed in clinical research whereby exudation of protein into the lumen of diseased intestine could be quantified. The principle was that a labeled protein molecule, or an inert chemical equivalent (e.g., polyvinyl pyrolidine), was delivered to the circulation and then recovered quantitatively from the stools (88). Thus, "clearance" into stools could be calculated. Currently the endogenous protein, α-1 anti-trypsin, is most often used (89). At one time, almost every mucosal and transmural disease of the gut was reported as having an element of protein loss in its pathophysiology (88). A more mature view restricts the importance of protein-losing enteropathies to a few conditions, such as Ménétrier's disease, intestinal lymphangiectasia, and some examples of inflammatory bowel disease.

The final steps of protein digestion and absorption now are known to depend on the wide variety of peptidases that reside in the brush border and cytoplasm of enterocytes. In contrast to the disaccharidases, however, deficiencies of small intestinal peptidases are probably of little clinical significance. Perhaps this is because of the multiple mechanisms available for absorption of peptides and amino acids. Further evidence of this functional redundancy in peptide/amino acid uptake comes from study of the disorders of amino acid uptake. There are numerous examples in which the defect for transport of an amino acid is shared between the kidney and the gut (e.g., Hartnup's disease for neutral amino acids, cystinuria), but amino acid deficiencies do not develop as a result of impaired gut uptake.

EXAMPLES OF SPECIFIC DISEASES

Knowledge of human pathophysiology blossomed in the 1950s, when technical advances permitted the study of patients by tolerable and increasingly less invasive techniques. To provide additional insights on the growth of knowledge in gastroenterology, several prototypic diseases are discussed chronologically. These are celiac sprue, sucrose-isomaltase deficiency, and vitamin B_{12} deficiency. In this last segment, we wish to place in historic perspective knowledge of three disorders of gastrointestinal digestion and absorption.

Celiac Sprue (Table 6–2)

Although the celiac diathesis was first recognized by the Roman physician Aretaeus, the definitive description of celiac disease is attributed to Samuel Gee in 1888 (35). The sprue syndrome thereafter became an established clinical entity, but there was considerable controversy during the 1930s (24,25) as to whether or not sprue was associated with a mucosal lesion (see previous text). However, the most significant milestone in this field stemmed from the careful observations of Dutch physicians during the Second World War, when it was noted that patients with celiac disease appeared to improve at times of food scarcity, especially of products derived from wheat. The Utrecht School also was responsible for the introduction of quantitative approaches to assess malabsorption including van de Kamer's test for stool fat (38). Soon after the epidemiologic observations of Dicke and his colleagues regarding the deleterious effects of wheat flour, Frazer (90) showed that peptic-tryptic digests of wheat flour also were capable of damaging the small bowel mucosa. A few years later, detailed descriptions of the small bowel lesions came from tissue obtained at laparotomy (26) and subsequently by means of jejunal biopsy (28). Documentation of small bowel mucosal damage, its improvement on withdrawal of gluten from the diet, and relapse on gluten challenge established the diagnostic criteria for celiac sprue. These were essential criteria by which the natural history and complications of the disease could be studied more formally.

A better understanding of the subcellular biochemistry of enterocytes was crucial for clarification of the role of intestinal peptidases in celiac sprue. In the mid-1950s, Frazer (90,91) proposed that peptidase deficiency was an essential component of the

Table 6–2
Annotated Historical Milestones: Celiac Sprue

Discipline	Author	Year	Contribution	Reference
	Gee	1888	First description	35
Clinical epidemiology	Dicke	1950	Deleterious effect of wheat flour	36
Clinical chemistry	Frazer et al.	1952	Peptides derived from peptic tryptic digest of wheat flour damage mucosa	90, 91
Pathophysiology	van de Kamer et al.	1953	Deleterious effect of gluten, gliadin on steatorrhea	38
Histopathology	Paulley	1954	First detailed description of small bowel tissue obtained at laparotomy	26
	Sakula & Shiner	1957	Peroral small bowel biopsies	28
Biochemistry/cell biology	Booth and Douglas	1970	Subcellular biochemistry of enterocytes; normalization of intestinal peptidases with restoration of normal mucosa with GFD	92, 93
Immunology	Falchuk et al.	1972	Association with HLA-A8	94
	Keuning et al.	1976	Association with HLA-DW3	95
	Betuel et al.	1980	Association with HLA-DRW3 and DRW7	96
Population genetics	Alper et al.	1983	Recessive inheritance of MHC-linked susceptibility gene for gluten-sensitive enteropathy	97, 98
Molecular genetics	Ehrlich et al.	1989	Specific structurally normal allelic variants in the DP and DQ/DR subregions contribute to disease susceptibility	99

syndrome. The hypothesis was that a deficiency of peptidases exposed the mucosa to toxic, unhydrolyzed proteins or polypeptides. However, intestinal peptidase levels returned to normal when the mucosa was removed from contact with gluten, proving that peptidase deficiency was secondary to mucosal damage rather than a primary defect (92,93).

With the peptidase hypothesis regated, other proposals needed to be considered. The association of the sprue with certain HLA-A haplotypes, such as A8, DRW3 and DRW7, which also are commonly seen in other diseases of immune etiology (94–96), led to further explorations of immunologic mechanisms for mucosal damage. These observations helped to explain the previous clinical observations of familial clustering of and racial predispositions to celiac sprue. In fact, population genetic studies subse-

quently showed that there is a recessive inheritance of an MHC-linked susceptibility gene among patients who subsequently develop gluten-sensitive enteropathy (97). Thus, after almost two decades of reports on interesting immunologic phenomena in celiac disease, population and molecular genetic studies have led to a novel concept in which the enterocyte itself is the bystander that is injured by the underlying abnormal immune response triggered by a specific chemical structure of a dietary antigen in genetically susceptible individuals.

Current thinking is that sequences of wheat, rye, and barley prolamins contain recurring tetrapeptide motifs that are predicted to have beta-reverse-turn secondary structures. Structural polymorphisms of subloci in the major histocompatibility complex identify codon switches in the beta chain and set up the cell-mediated response

(98). Disease susceptibility is recessively inherited and appears to be multigenic, with specific but structurally normal, allelic variants in the DP and DQ/DR regions (99).

With these advances in the understanding of disease susceptibility, it may be possible in the future to define gluten sensitivity without qualitative assessment of small bowel morphology (100). Such studies also may provide a noninvasive method to screen populations for disease susceptibility and provide clues to early, even asymptomatic diagnosis.

Sucrase-Isomaltase Deficiency (Table 6–3)

Disaccharidase activity ("invertase") was known to 19th-century physiologists, but the enzyme was first thought to be contained in small intestinal, or even pancreatic, secretions. By the late 1930s it was known that lactase was present in the mucosa of the small intestine, but further study of membrane digestion in man had to await the development of techniques for safe and simple mucosal biopsy.

Table 6–3
Annotated Historical Milestones: Sucrase-Isomaltose Deficiency

Discipline	Author	Year	Contribution	Reference
Physiology	Miller and Crane	1960–62	Brush border hydrolysis and carrier-mediated transport of sugars	101
Clinical	Weijers et al.	1960	First description	102
Epidemiology	Peterson and Herber	1967	Rare in adults, 0.2% in North America	103
	McNair et al.	1972	10% of Greenland Eskimos	104
	Ament et al.	1973	Commoner problem in children	105
Pathophysiology	Gray and Ingelfinger	1965	Calculation of absorption rate	20
	Alper	1975	Dynamic equilibrium of brush border hydrolases: synthesis and degradation	98
Cell biology	Miller and Crane	1961	Hybrid of 2 subunits linked by a disulfide bond: large	106, 107
	Brunner et al.	1979	hydrophilic (catalytic) site oriented to lumen; hydrophobic site anchored into brush border	
Molecular genetics and biology	Hunziker et al.	1986	Complete primary structure of pro-sucrase-isomaltose described	108
	Naim et al.	1988	Different phenotypes of SI deficiency: enzyme is functionally altered or cannot be transported intracellularly	109
	Fransen et al.	1991	(a) Intracellular transport defect: lack of terminal glycosylation in Golgi results in missorting of pro-SI to basolateral membrane; (b) Two structural variants of pro-SI precursors result in transport of isomaltose alone to brush border and intracellular degradation of sucrose	110

Advances in the physiology and biochemistry of brush border hydrolysis and carrier-mediated transport of sugars across several epithelia, including the renal tubule and gastrointestinal tract (11,101), immediately preceded the first clinical description of sucrase-isomaltose deficiency by Weijers, van de Kamer and colleagues in 1960 (102). During the next decade, the epidemiology of this relatively rare condition (103) was described and, although it is seldom seen among adults in North America (0.2%), it was documented that almost 10% of Greenland Eskimos are deficient in this enzyme (104). In pediatric populations, sucrase-isomaltose deficiency appears to be a common, albeit transient, consequence of viral enteritis (105).

Understanding of the pathophysiology of sucrose and maltose malabsorption was facilitated by the development of methods to calculate the absorption rates for dietary substrates (20), and it was later shown that the brush border hydrolases such as sucrase-isomaltose were in a dynamic equilibrium of synthesis and degradation (77). The biochemical studies of Miller and Crane had shown earlier that the enzyme consisted of a hybrid of two subunits linked by a disulfide bond (106). Subsequently, Brunner documented the topography of the two subunits, with a large hydrophilic (catalytic) site being oriented towards the lumen, and the hydrophobic site being anchored into the brush border (107).

Molecular biology has provided fundamental insights into the primary structure, membrane orientation, and anchoring of this hybrid molecule (108). Phenotypic variants have been identified in patients in whom a deficiency state results from missense mutations either preventing intracellular transport or allowing intracellular degradation of the sucrase moiety (109–110). Thus, Hunziker described the complete primary structure of pro-sucrase-isomaltose in 1986, and Naim et al. (109) identified phenotypically different variants of the mutant enzyme which are either functionally altered or cannot be transported intracellularly. The latter group subsequently demonstrated an intracellular transport defect, with lack of terminal glycosylation in the Golgi, resulting in misdirection of the pro-sucrase-isomaltose molecule to the basolateral rather than to the apical membrane. Two other structural variants of the precursors result in transport of isomaltose alone to the brush border or intracellular degradation of the sucrase moiety.

Pernicious Anemia (Table 6–4)

Addison first described pernicious anemia in the mid-19th century (111). From his description came the therapeutic recommendation of "use of a bracing air and a nutrient and stimulating diet" (112). For almost 100 years, the only significant advance was the contribution of Castle, who demonstrated the association of pernicious anemia with gastric achlorhydria. He proposed that an intrinsic factor (IF) arising in the stomach was needed for the vitamin's assimilation (113). Almost 100 years after the original description of the condition, vitamin B_{12} was purified (114,115), and West demonstrated its therapeutic efficacy (116). The availability of radiolabeled vitamin B_{12} allowed the effects of normal gastric juice on the absorption of vitamin B_{12} to be proven by Schilling (30), who subsequently developed the Schilling test for vitamin B_{12} absorption. Later refinements allowed this robust test of small bowel and gastric function to distinguish between defects at the gastric and ileal levels, as well as to demonstrate the consequences of bacterial overgrowth in the small bowel (31).

During the period from 1950 to 1970, several clinical disciplines contributed important insights into pernicious anemia. These included the description of the gastric mucosal lesion (117), with particular emphasis on the atrophic nature of the gastritis by Siurala (118) and the use of immunologic techniques to measure intrinsic factor in gastric juices, leading to clarification of the autoimmune nature of pernicious anemia, especially the significance of antibodies to intrinsic factor (119–121). From a practical standpoint, the observations of hematologists and gastroenterologists at Hammersmith Hospital had perhaps the greatest clinical impact. Baker and Mollin in 1955 observed a stoichiometric relationship between vitamin B_{12} absorption and IF secretion (122), and Booth demonstrated clearly, in man (61) and rats (123), that the ileum was the site of absorption of vitamin B_{12}.

Table 6–4
Annotated Historical Milestones: Pernicious Anemia

Discipline	Author	Year	Contribution	Reference
Clinical	Addison	1856	First description	111
	Habershon	1863	Treatment with "a bracing air, and a nutrient and stimulating diet"	112
	Castle et al.	1930	Association with achlorhydria and a gastric intrinsic factor (IF)	113
Clinical chemistry and therapeutics	Rickes, Smith and Parker	1948	Purification of vitamin B_{12}	114, 115
	West	1948	Activity of vitamin B_{12}	116
Experimental and applied physiology	Schilling	1953	Use of radioisotopic B_{12} to demonstrate effects of normal gastric juice on B_{12} absorption	30
	Klayman and Brandborg	1955	Development of "Schilling test"	31
Histopathology	Magnus and Ungley	1938	Gastric lesion	117
	Siurala	1955	Atrophic gastritis	118
Immunology	Jeffries and Sleisenger	1963	Immunologic quantitation of intrinsic factor in gastric juices	119
	Glass et al.	1963	Association with other autoimmune diseases	120
	Doniach and Raitt	1964	Significance of antibodies to IF	121
Pathophysiology and biochemistry	Baker and Mollin	1955	Stoichiometric relationship between B_{12} absorption and IF	122
	Booth et al.	1957	Ileum is site of B_{12} absorption	123
	Boass and Wilson	1964	B_{12}-IF complex absorbed by enterocyte and converted to B_{12}-protein complex	124
	Donaldson et al.	1967	IF mediates attachment of B_{12} to brush border	125
	Toskes et al.	1973	Pancreatic protease involved in B_{12} cleavage to binding proteins, including "R" protein	126
	Allen	1973–74	Characterization of B_{12} binding proteins, including "R" protein	127
	Allen et al.	1978	Effects of proteolytic enzymes on binding of B_{12} to R protein and IF	128
	Chanarin et al.	1978	Transcobalamin II derived from ileal enterocyte	129
Cell biology	Gräsbeck	1977	Isolation of porcine receptor in ileal brush border and initial characterization of α and β subunits	130
	Kouvonen and Gräsbeck	1981	Topology of receptor: α subunit binds IF and faces outwards; β subunit (hydrophobic) faces inwards	131
	Seetharam and Alpers	1981	Purification, amino acid and sugar composition of canine ileal receptor	132
Molecular biology	Alpers	1991	IF gene is localized to human chromosome 11; patients with congenital pernicious anemia do not have a sizable gene deletion	133

Almost a decade later, in the mid 1960s, it was shown that IF mediates the attachment of vitamin B_{12} to the brush border of the ileal enterocytes (124) and that the B_{12}-IF complex is absorbed by the enterocyte and subsequently converted to a B_{12}-protein complex (125). During the 1970s, the importance of cofactors that bind to vitamin B_{12}

during its passage through the gastrointestinal tract was recognized. Toskes and Allen and their colleagues (126–128) showed that pancreatic proteases were involved in cleaving vitamin B_{12} from binding proteins, including the "R" protein, which was subsequently characterized further. In 1978, Chanarin provided evidence that the protein to which B_{12} was complexed within the ileal enterocytes was a carrier protein, transcobalamin II (129).

Cellular and molecular biologic approaches since the late 1970s have focused on isolating and characterizing the ileal brush border receptor. Alpha and beta subunits were described by Marcoullis and Gräsbeck in 1977 (130); the same group subsequently showed that the alpha subunit binds IF and faces towards the lumen, whereas the beta subunit, which is hydrophobic, faces towards the cell (131). Alpers and colleagues, during the 1980s and early 1990s (132–133), purified the canine ileal receptor, characterized its amino acid and sugar composition, and localized the IF gene to human chromosome 11. Now that the intrinsic factor gene has been localized, it is anticipated that gene alterations leading to failure of IF synthesis will be described in the near future. It is already known that patients with congenital pernicious anemia do not have a sizable gene deletion because gene patterns assessed by restriction analysis are normal (133).

Thus, about 30 years after Jerzy Glass (134) commented that "the intrinsic factor has eluded definition," few mysteries regarding pernicious anemia and the factors involved in its absorption remain to be solved. Although Glass commented that the search for IF "added a certain romance and Sherlock Holmes quality to its investigation," one might anticipate that the end of the 20th century will find this mystery entirely solved.

In summary, knowledge has accumulated on digestion, absorption, and malabsorption within several categories. First, some advances were determined by the gathering of information in the basic sciences that underlie these processes; second, the recognition of human pathophysiology, often by simple though systematic clinical observations, sparked curiosity and led to new hypotheses; and last, the development of methods that allowed digestive/absorptive processes to be studied in intact man was sine qua non. We choose to address the historical process this way because our focus has been "gastroenterology," with its clear clinical context. Any of the fundamental processes, involving ultimately the cell and molecular biology of a single digestive or absorptive function, also could be followed chronologically. Much has been accomplished; nevertheless, in the 1990s, many questions still remain. The integrative role of the neurohumoral biology that controls these processes in man is still largely unknown.

REFERENCES

1. Dalton JC Jr: A Treatise on Human Physiology Designed for the Use of Students and Practitioners of Medicine. Philadelphia, Blanchard and Lea, 1864.
2. Howell WH (ed): An American Textbook of Physiology. Philadelphia, WB Saunders, 1896.
3. Bayliss WM: Principles of General Physiology. London, Langmans, Green and Co., 1915.
4. Best CH, Taylor NB: The Physiological Basis of Medical Practice. Baltimore, William Wood and Co., 1937.
5. Abbott WO, Miller TG: Intubation studies of the human small intestine III. A technic for the collection of pure intestinal secretion and for the study of intestinal absorption. JAMA *106*:16, 1936.
6. Blankenhorn DH, Hirsch J, Ahrens EH Jr: Transintestinal intubation; technic for measurement of gut length and physiological sampling at known loci. Proc Soc Exper Biol Med *88*:356, 1955.
7. Schedl HP, Clifton JA: Solute and water absorption by the human small intestine. Nature *199*:1264, 1963.
8. Sperber I, Hyden S, Ekman J: The use of polyethylene glycol as a reference substance in the study of ruminant digestion. Ann R Agric Coll Sweden *20*:337, 1953.
9. Borgström B, Dahlquist A, Lundh G, Sjövall J: Studies of intestinal digestion and absorption in the human. J Clin Invest *36*:1521, 1957.
10. Borgström B, Hofmann AF: Acceptance remarks: Beaumont Prize 1979. Gastroenterology *77*:952, 1979.
11. Dahlquist A, Borgström B: Digestion and absorption of disaccharides in man. Biochem J *81*:411, 1961.

12. Lundh G: Pancreatic exocrine function in neoplastic and inflammatory disease; a simple and reliable new test. Gastroenterology *42*:275, 1962.

13. Lindquist B, Meeuwisse GW: Chronic diarrhea caused by monosaccharide malabsorption. Acta Pediatr Scand *51*:674, 1962.

14. Fordtran JS et al.: The kinetics of water absorption in the human intestine. Trans A Am Phys *74*:195, 1961.

15. Cooper H, Levitan R, Fordtran JS, Ingelfinger FJ: A method for studying absorption of water and solute from the human small intestine. Gastroenterology *50*:1, 1966.

16. Turnberg LA, Fordtran JS, Carter NW, Rector FC Jr: Mechanism of bicarbonate absorption and its relationship to sodium transport in the human jejunum. J Clin Invest *49*:548, 1970.

17. Turnberg LA, Bieberdorf FA, Morawski SG, Fordtran JS: Inter-relationships of chloride, bicarbonate, sodium and hydrogen transport in the human ileum. J Clin Invest *49*:557, 1970.

18. Fordtran JS, Rector FC, Locklear TW, Ewton MF: Water and solute movement in the small intestine of patients with sprue. J Clin Invest *46*:287, 1967.

19. Phillips SF, Schmid WC: Jejunal transport of electrolytes and water in intestinal disease. Gut *10*:990, 1969.

20. Gray GM, Ingelfinger FJ: Intestinal absorption of sucrose in man: The site of hydrolysis and absorption. J Clin Invest *44*:390, 1965.

21. Gray GM, Santiago NA: Disaccharide absorption in normal and diseased human intestine. Gastroenterology *51*:489, 1966.

22. Simmonds WJ, Hofmann AF, Theodore E: Absorption of cholesterol from a micellar solution: Intestinal perfusion studies in man. J Clin Invest *46*:874, 1967.

23. Krag E, Phillips SF: Active and passive bile acid absorption in man: Perfusion studies of the ileum and jejunum. J Clin Invest *53*:1686, 1974.

24. Mackie FP, Fairley NH: The morbid anatomy of sprue. Ind J Med Res *16*:799, 1928.

25. Thaysen TEH: Pathological anatomy of the intestinal tract in tropical sprue. Tr Rog Soc Trop Med *24*:529, 1931.

26. Paulley JW: Observations on the etiology of idiopathic steatorrhea. Br Med J *ii*:1318, 1954.

27. Wood IJ, Doig RK, Motteram R, Hughes A: Gastric biopsy—report on fifty-five biopsies using a new flexible gastric biopsy tube. Lancet *i*:18, 1949.

28. Sakula J, Shiner M: Coeliac disease with atrophy of the small intestine mucosa. Lancet *ii*:876, 1957.

29. Flick AL, Quinton WE, Rubin CE: A peroral hydraulic biopsy tube for multiple sampling at any level of the gastrointestinal tract. Gastroenterology *40*:120, 1961.

30. Schilling RF: Intrinsic factor studies. II. The effect of gastric juice on the urinary excretion of radioactivity after the oral administration of radioactive vitamin B_{12}. J Lab Clin Med *42*:860, 1953.

31. Klayman MI, Brandborg L: Clinical application of cobalt[60]-labeled vitamin B_{12} urine test. N Engl J Med *253*:808, 1955.

32. Levitt MD: Production and excretion of hydrogen gas in man. N Engl J Med *281*:122, 1969.

33. Bond JH, Levitt MD: Quantitative measurement of lactose absorption. Gastroenterology *70*:1058, 1976.

34. Bond JH, Levitt MD: Investigation of small bowel transit time in normal subjects utilizing pulmonary hydrogen measurements. J Lab Clin Med *85*:546, 1974.

35. Gee S: On the celiac affection. St. Bartholomews Hosp Rep *24*:17, 1888.

36. Dicke WK: Coeliac disease. Investigation of the harmful effects of certain types of cereal on patients with coeliac disease. Thesis, University of Utrecht, 1950.

37. Dicke WK, Weijers HA, van de Kamer JH: Coeliac disease. II. The presence in wheat of a factor having a deleterious effect in cases of coeliac disease. Acta Paediatrica *42*:34, 1953.

38. van de Kamer JH, Weijers HA, Dicke WK: Coeliac disease. IV. An investigation into the injurious constituents of wheat in connection with their action on patients with coeliac disease. Acta Paediatrica *42*:223, 1953.

39. Comfort MW, Gambill EE, Baggenstoss AH: Chronic relapsing pancreatitis, an analysis of twenty-nine cases without associated disease of the biliary or gastrointestinal tract. Gastroenterology *6*:239, 1946.

40. Wollaeger EE, Lundberg WO, Chipault JR, Mason HL: Fecal and plasma lipids. A study of two normal human adults taking (1) a diet free of lipid and (2) a diet containing triolein as the only lipid. Gastroenterology *24*:422, 1953.

41. DiMagno EP, Clain JE: Chronic pancreatitis. In Go VLW et al. (eds): The Exocrine Pancreas. New York, Raven Press, 1986.

42. Goligher JC: The comparative results of different operations in the elective treatment of duodenal ulcer. Br J Surg *57*:780, 1970.

43. Meyer JH: Chronic morbidity after ulcer

surgery. *In* Sleisenger MH, Fordtran JS (eds): Gastrointestinal Disease, 4th Ed. Philadelphia, WB Saunders Co., 1989.

44. Bank S, Barbezat GO, Marks IN: Postgastrectomy steatorrhea due to intestinal lactase deficiency. S Afr Med J *40*:597, 1966.

45. Binder HJ: Celiac sprue-unmasking after vagotomy and hiatal hernia repair. N Engl J Med *283*:520, 1970.

46. Barber WH, Hummell LE: Macrocytic anemia in association with intestinal strictures and anastomoses. Bull Johns Hopkins Hosp *46*:215, 1939.

47. Kinsella VJ, Hennessy WB: Gastrectomy and the blind loop syndrome. Lancet *ii*:1205, 1960.

48. Wirts CW, Goldstein F: Studies of the mechanism of postgastrectomy steatorrhea. Ann Intern Med *58*:25, 1963.

49. Zollinger RM, Ellison EH: Primary peptic ulcerations of the jejunum associated with islet cell tumors of the pancreas. Ann Surg *142*:709, 1955.

50. Shimoda SS, Saunders DR, Rubin CE: The Zollinger-Ellison syndrome with steatorrhea. Mechanisms of fat and vitamin B_{12} malabsorption. Gastroenterology *55*:705, 1968.

51. Phillips RA: Cholera in the perspective of 1966. Ann Intern Med *65*:922, 1966.

52. Field M: Cholera toxin, adenylate cyclase and the process of active secretion in the small intestine; the pathogenesis of diarrhea of cholera. *In* Andrioli TE, Hoffman JF, Fanestil DD (eds): Physiology of Membrane Disorders. New York, Plenum Medical Books, 1978.

53. Frazer AC, Sammons HF: The formation of mono and diglycerides during the hydrolysis of triglyceride by pancreatic lipase. Biochem J *39*:122, 1945.

54. Mattson FH, Beck LW: The digestion *in vitro* of triglycerides by pancreatic lipase. J Biol Chem *214*:115, 1955.

55. Hofmann AF, Borgström B: The intraluminal phase of fat digestion in man; the lipid content of the micellar and oil phases of intestinal content obtained during fat digestion and absorption. J Clin Invest *43*:247, 1964.

56. Bergström S, Borgström B, Carlsten A: On the mechanism of intestinal fat absorption in the cat. Acta Physiol Scand *32*:94, 1954.

57. Sleisenger MH: Malabsorption syndrome. N Engl J Med *281*:111, 1969.

58. Holt PR: Medium chain triglycerides. A useful adjunct in nutritional therapy. Gastroenterology *53*:961, 1967.

59. Hofmann AF, Poley JR: Role of bile acid malabsorption in pathogenesis of diarrhea

and steatorrhea in patients with ileal resection I. Response to cholestyramine or replacement of dietary long-chain triglycerides by medium chain triglyceride. Gastroenterology *62*:918, 1972.

60. Mekhjian HS, Phillips SF, Hofmann AF: Colonic secretion of water and electrolytes induced by bile acids: Perfusion studies in man. J Clin Invest *50*:1577, 1971.

61. Ammon HV, Phillips SF: Inhibition of colonic water and electrolyte absorption by fatty acids in man. Gastroenterology *65*:744, 1973.

62. Longmire-Cook SJ et al.: Effect of replacement therapy with cholyl sarcosine on fat malabsorption associated with severe bile acid malabsorption. Dig Dis Sci *37*:1217, 1992.

63. Booth CC, Mollin DL: The site of absorption of vitamin B_{12} in man. Lancet *i*:18, 1959.

64. Dowling RH, Booth CC: Structural and functional changes following small bowel resection in the rat. Clin Sci *32*:139, 1967.

65. Dahlquist A et al.: Intestinal lactase deficiency and lactose intolerance in adults. Gastroenterology *45*:488, 1963.

66. Auricchio S et al.: Isolated intestinal lactase deficiency in an adult. Lancet *ii*:324, 1963.

67. Ferguson A: Diagnosis and treatment of lactose intolerance. Br Med J *283*:1423, 1981.

68. Struthers JE, Singleton JW, Kern F: Intestinal lactase deficiency in ulcerative colitis and regional enteritis. Ann Intern Med *63*:221, 1965.

69. Bayless TM, Rosensweig NS: A racial difference in incidence of lactase deficiency; a survey of milk intolerance and lactase deficiency in healthy adult males. JAMA *197*:968, 1966.

70. Simoons FJ: Primary adult lactose intolerance and the milking habit; a problem in biologic and cultural inter-relations II. A cultural historical hypothesis. Am J Dig Dis *15*:695, 1970.

71. Rumessen JJ, Gudmand-Hoyer E: Absorption capacity of fructose in healthy adults. Comparison with sucrose and its constituent monosaccharides. Gut *27*:1161, 1986.

72. Cornblath M et al.: Hereditary fructose intolerance. N Engl J Med *269*:1271, 1963.

73. Hyams JS: Sorbitol intolerance: An unappreciated cause of functional gastrointestinal complaint. Gastroenterology *84*:30, 1983.

74. Newcomer AD, McGill DB: Distribution of disaccharidases in the small bowel of normal and lactase deficient subjects. Gastroenterology *51*:481, 1966.

75. Rosensweig NS, Herman RH: Timed responses of jejunal sucrase and maltase activity to a high sucrose diet in normal man. Gastroenterology *56*:500, 1969.

76. Alpers DH, Cote MN: Inhibition of lactose hydrolysis by dietary sugars. Am J Physiol *221*:865, 1971.

77. Alpers DH, Tedesco FJ: The possible role of pancreatic proteases in the turnover of intestinal brush border proteins. Biochim Biophys Acta *401*:28, 1975.

78. Danielsen EM, Skovbjerg H, Noren O, Sjostrom H: Biosynthesis of intestinal microcellular proteins. Intracellular processing of lactase-phlorigin hydrolase. Biochem Biophys Res Commun *122*:82, 1984.

79. Crane RK, Miller D, Behler I: The restrictions on possible mechanisms of intestinal active transport of sugars. *In* Kleinzeller A, Kotyk A (eds): Membrane Transport and Metabolism. London, Academic Press, 1961.

80. Hediger MA, Turk E, Wright, EM: Homology of the human intestinal Na+/glucose and Escherichia coli Na+/proline cotransporters. Proc Natl Acad Sci USA *86*:5748, 1989.

81. Turk E et al.: Glucose/galactose malabsorption caused by a defect in the sodium/glucose co-transporter. Nature *350*:354, 1991.

82. Spiller GA, Amen RJ (eds): Fiber in Human Nutrition. New York, Plenum Press, 1976.

83. Spiller GA, Kay RM (eds): Medical Aspects of Dietary Fiber. New York, Plenum Press, 1980.

84. Vahouny GV, Kritchevsky D (eds): Dietary Fiber in Health and Disease. New York, Plenum Press, 1982.

85. Trowell HC: Definition of dietary fiber and hypotheses that it is a protective factor in certain diseases. Am J Clin Nutr *29*:417, 1976.

86. Burkitt DP, Trowell HC: Refined Carbohydrate Foods and Disease. Some Implications of Dietary Fiber. London, Academic Press, 1975.

87. Alpers DH: Digestion and absorption of carbohydrates and proteins. *In* Johnson LR (ed): Physiology of the Gastrointestinal Tract. 2nd Edition. New York, Raven Press, 1987.

88. Waldmann TA: Protein losing enteropathy. Gastroenterology *50*:422, 1966.

89. Florent C et al.: Gastric clearance of alpha-1-antitrypsin under cimetidine perfusion. New test to detect protein losing enteropathy? Dig Dis Sci *31*:12, 1986.

90. Anderson CM et al.: Coeliac disease: Gastrointestinal studies and the effect of dietary wheat flour. Lancet *i*:836, 1952.

91. Frazer AC et al.: Gluten-induced enteropathy. The effect of partially digested gluten. Lancet *ii*:252, 1959.

92. Booth CC: Enterocyte in coeliac disease. I. Br Med J *iv*:725, 1970.

93. Douglas AP, Booth CC: Digestion of gluten peptides by normal human jejunal mucosa and by mucosa from patients with adult coeliac disease. Clin Sci *38*:11, 1970.

94. Falchuk ZM, Rogentine GN, Strober W: Predominance of histocompatibility antigen HL-A8 in patients with gluten-sensitive enteropathy. J Clin Invest *51*:1602, 1972.

95. Keuning JJ et al.: HLA-DW3 associated with coeliac disease. Lancet *i*:506, 1976.

96. Betuel H et al.: Adult celiac disease associated with HLA-DRw3 and -DRw7. Tissue Antigens *15*:231, 1980.

97. Greenberg DA, Hodge SE, Rotter JI: Evidence for recessive and against dominant inheritance at the HLA-"linked" locus in coeliac disease. Am J Hum Genet *34*:263, 1982.

98. Alpers CA et al.: Extended major histocompatibility complex haplotypes in patients with gluten-sensitive enteropathy. J Clin Invest *79*:251, 1987.

99. Kagnoff MF, Harwood JI, Bugawan TL, Ehrlich HA: Structural analysis of the HLA-DR, -DQ, and -DP alleles on the celiac disease-associated HLA-DR3(DRw17) haplotype. Proc Natl Acad Sci USA *86*: 6274, 1989.

100. Marsh MN: Gluten, major histocompatibility complex, and the small intestine. Gastroenterology *102*:330, 1992.

101. Miller D, Crane RK: The digestive function of the epithelium of the small intestine. I. An intracellular locus of disaccharide and sugar phosphate ester hydrolysis. Biochim Biophys Acta *52*:281, 1961.

102. Weijers HA, van de Kamer JH, Dicke WK, Ijsseling J: Diarrhoea caused by deficiency of sugar splitting enzymes. I. Acta Paediatrica *50*:55, 1961.

103. Peterson ML, Herber R: Intestinal sucrase deficiency. Trans Am Assoc Physicians *80*: 275, 1967.

104. McNair A, Gudmand-Hoyer E, Jarnum S, Orrild L: Sucrose malabsorption in Greenland. Br Med J *ii*:19, 1972.

105. Ament ME, Perera DR, Esther LJ: Sucrase-isomaltase deficiency—a frequently misdiagnosed disease. J Pediatr *83*:721, 1973.

106. Miller D, Crane RK: The digestive function of the epithelium of the small intestine. II. Localization of disaccharide hydrolysis in the isolated brush border portion of intestinal epithelial cells. Biochim Biophys Acta *52*:293, 1961.

107. Brunner J et al.: The mode of association of the enzyme complex sucrase-isomaltase with the intestinal brush-border membrane. J Biol Chem *254*:1821, 1979.

108. Hunziker W, Spiess M, Semenza G, Lodish HF: The sucrase-isomaltase complex: Primary structure, membrane-orientation, and evolution of a stalked, intrinsic brush border protein. Cell *46*:227, 1986.

109. Naim HY et al.: Sucrase-isomaltase deficiency in humans. Different mutations disrupt intracellular transport, processing, and function of an intestinal brush border enzyme. J Clin Invest *82*:667, 1988.

110. Fransen JA, Hauri HP, Ginsel LA, Naim HY: Naturally occurring mutations in intestinal sucrase-isomaltase provide evidence for the existence of an intracellular sorting signal in the isomaltase subunit. J Cell Biol *115*:45, 1991.

111. Addison T: Anemia: Disease of suprarenal capsules. Lond Med Gaz *8*:517, 1849.

112. Habershon SO: On idiopathic anemia. Lancet *i*:518, 1863.

113. Castle WB, Townsend WC, Heath CW: Observations on the etiologic relationship of achylia gastrica to pernicious anemia. III. The nature of the reaction between normal human gastric juice and beef muscle leading to clinical improvement and increased blood formation similar to the effect of liver feeding. Am J Med Sci *180*:305, 1930.

114. Rickes EL et al.: Crystalline vitamin B_{12}. Science *107*:396, 1948.

115. Smith EL, Parker LFJ: Purification of antipernicious anaemia factor. Biochem J *43*:viii, 1948.

116. West R: Activity of vitamin B_{12} in Addisonian pernicious anemia. Science *107*:398, 1948.

117. Magnus HA, Ungley CC: Gastric lesion in pernicious anaemia. Lancet *i*:420, 1938.

118. Siurala M: Gastric lesion in some megaloblastic anemias. Results of follow-up examinations. Acta Med Scand *154*:337, 1956.

119. Jeffries GH, Sleisenger MH: The immunologic identification and quantitation of human intrinsic factor in gastric secretions. J Clin Invest *42*:442, 1963.

120. McIntyre PA, Hahn R, Conley CL, Glass B: Genetic factors in predisposition to pernicious anemia. Bull Johns Hopkins Hosp *104*:309, 1959.

121. Doniach D, Roitt IM: An evaluation of gastric and thyroid autoimmunity in relation to hematologic disorders. Semin Hematol *7*:313, 1964.

122. Baker SJ, Mollin DL: The relationship between intrinsic factor and the intestinal absorption of vitamin B_{12}. Br J Haematol *1*:46, 1955.

123. Booth CC, Chanarin I, Anderson BB, Mollin DL: The site of absorption and tissue distribution of orally administered ^{56}Co-labelled vitamin B_{12} in the rat. Br J Haematol *3*:253, 1957.

124. Boass A, Wilson TH: Intestinal absorption of intrinsic factor complex. Am J Physiol *207*:27, 1964.

125. Donaldson RM, Mackenzie IL, Trier JS: Intrinsic factor mediated attachment of vitamin B_{12} to brush borders and microvillus membranes of hamster intestine. J Clin Invest *46*:1215, 1967.

126. Toskes PP, Deren JJ, Conrad ME: Trypsin-like nature of the pancreatic factor that corrects vitamin B_{12} malabsorption associated with pancreatic dysfunction. J Clin Invest *52*:1660, 1973.

127. Allen RH: Human vitamin B_{12} transports proteins. Prog Hematol *9*:57, 1975.

128. Allen RH, Seetharam B, Podell E, Alpers DH: Effect of proteolytic enzymes on the binding of cobalamin to R protein and intrinsic factor. J Clin Invest *61*:47, 1978.

129. Chanarin I, Muir M, Hughes A, Hoffbrand AV: Evidence for intestinal origin of transcobalamin II during vitamin B_{12} absorption. Br Med J *i*:1453, 1978.

130. Marcoullis G, Gräsbeck R: Isolation of the porcine ileal intrinsic factor receptor by sequential affinity chromatography. Biochim Biophys Acta *499*:309, 1977.

131. Kouvonen I, Gräsbeck R: Topology of the hog intrinsic factor receptor in the intestine. J Biol Chem *256*:154, 1981.

132. Seetharam B, Alpers DH: Isolation and characterization of the ileal receptor for intrinsic factor-cobalamin. J Biol Chem *256*:3785, 1981.

133. Hewitt JE et al.: Human gastric intrinsic factor: Characterization of cDNA and genomic clones and localization to human chromosome 11. Genomics *10*:432, 1991.

134. Glass GBJ: Gastric intrinsic factor and its function in the metabolism of vitamin B_{12}. Physiol Rev *43*:529, 1963.

7

The Evolution of Studies of Intestinal Electrolyte Absorption and Secretion

HENRY J. BINDER

Study of intestinal fluid and electrolyte transport during the past three decades has been vitally important in the development of present understanding of the pathogenesis and pathophysiology of diarrhea and in revealing new approaches to the treatment of diarrheal disorders. Such a close relationship between the physiology of water and electrolyte transport and the clinical problem of diarrhea had not always been so evident. This chapter highlights several important landmarks that have established the *science* of both the physiology of the intestinal fluid and electrolyte movement and the mechanisms of diarrhea. The "modern" era began in the 1960s, when intestinal fluid and electrolyte secretion was "rediscovered" after 25 years of inactivity. Subsequently, there has been an explosive increase in information, and the scientific basis for diarrhea rapidly evolved from the "physiology of diarrhea" to the "cell biology of diarrhea" and soon will become the "molecular biology of diarrhea." Most of this latter information is beyond the scope of the present discussion.

This presentation focuses on (1) the use of the term *secretion* in intestinal physiology and (2) the introduction of two different methods to study (fluid and) electrolyte movement in the small and large intestines. During most of this time, the development of concepts of intestinal ion transport lagged behind the evolution of similar concepts of renal electrolyte physiology: a trend reflected also in the much fewer members of

the American Physiological Society who indicated a primary interest in gastrointestinal physiology (including the study of gut muscle, splanchnic circulation, and gastric secretion) compared with those whose primary area of interest was renal physiology (especially renal tubular electrolyte transport). Potential explanations include the early realization that understanding of the processes responsible for urine formation in health and disease required detailed knowledge of renal tubular function. Only since the 1960s has evidence accumulated that the genesis of diarrhea involved comparable changes in intestinal fluid and electrolyte movement. Fortunately, the close relationships between jejunal transport and proximal renal tubular transport and between colonic and distal tubular transport function have facilitated the recent expansion of knowledge of intestinal ion transport.

Intestinal secretion was a legitimate area for physiologic investigation during the first four decades of this century. Much of the knowledge obtained during this period was summarized in a review entitled "The Secretions of the Intestine" by H. W. Florey, R. D. Wright, and M. A. Jennings, published in The Physiological Reviews in 1941 (1). Harold Florey, an Australian scientist at Oxford, is better known as a Nobel Prize winner in medicine and physiology for his co-discovery of penicillin. For reasons that are not clear, the field of intestinal secretion ceased to exist for the next 25 years. For example, the first edition of the *Handbook of Physiology,* a five-volume treatise published in 1967–1968, did not contain a single chapter on intestinal secretion, nor did the index of the volume on intestinal absorption include a single entry on "secretion" (2). In contrast, intestinal secretion was well represented in the second edition of the *Handbook of Physiology* published 20 years later (3).

This scarcity of information about secretion has been followed by increasing knowledge of intestinal secretion of all types. What was responsible for this renaissance, which began in the 1960s? The initial phenomenon that renewed awareness of secretion as a physiologic process and also its importance as a pathophysiologic mechanism for diarrhea was the demonstration that cholera was associated with net fluid secretion caused by an exotoxin that induced massive intestinal fluid and electrolyte secretion, i.e., an enterotoxin (4,5) (Fig. 7–1). During this period, Powell and colleagues, then at the Walter Reed Army Institute of Research, observed that net fluid and electrolyte secretion was normally present in the guinea pig small intestine (but not in the guinea pig colon or in the rat small or large intestine) (6,7). Hendrix and Bayless of Johns Hopkins University (1970) summarized the emerging evidence that intestinal secretion was an important physiologic and pathophysiologic process (8).

An appropriate methodology often facilitates and parallels the evolution of fundamental knowledge, and this relationship is exemplified in the improved understanding of intestinal fluid and electrolyte movement and the pathophysiology of diarrhea. Parsons' encyclopedic historical summary of "Methods for Investigation of Intestinal Absorption" that appeared in the *Handbook of Physiology* (1968) (9) lists primary methods of study as: luminal perfusion of isolated segments of intestine of experimental animals and modifications of Thiry fistulae and/or Thiry-Vella loops, usually in dogs (10,11). These loops represented transected segments of intestine that had been exteriorized, and the studies most often were performed in dogs. Florey et al. commented on the potential problem associated with partial denervation that would undoubtedly occur following transection and described studies that, in retrospect, clearly provide

evidence for opposing neurally-mediated effects on intestinal absorption and secretion (1). Understanding of the important role that the enteric nervous system plays in the regulation of fluid and electrolyte movement only now is being established (see Chapter 10).

Florey et al. also noted that most previous investigations (i.e., before 1941) almost exclusively had studied the canine intestine (1). This species exclusivity undoubtedly was an additional contributing factor in the delayed recognition of intestinal secretion as an important physiologic process. The term *secretion* actually describes *two* different phenomena (12). In one process, fluid and electrolytes are added to intestinal luminal contents; that is, when plasma-to-lumen movement exceeds lumen-to-plasma movement. Thus, net secretion under these circumstances also can be referred to as net fluid accumulation (the opposite of net absorption) and does not imply that a specific transport mechanism is responsible. The term secretion also is used to refer to an active secretory process, e.g., that which is stimulated by cholera enterotoxin. Net secretion may not necessarily result from an active secretory process (because an increase in luminal osmolality also can produce net secretion) and stimulation of an active secretory process may not necessarily result in net secretion. The magnitude of the existing basal absorptive process largely determines whether stimulation of an active secretory process results in net secretion or, alternatively, where it will be observed merely as a decrease in net absorption. On a relative scale among experimental animals, the magnitude of absorptive processes in the intestine is greater in the dog than in most other experimental animals (e.g., the rat). Similarly, the magnitude of colonic absorption is greater than that in the small intestine. Thus, a greater stimulation of secretion is required to produce net secretion in the canine jejunum than in the rat jejunum or in the colon than in the jejunum. Similarly, stimulation of active secretion of the same magnitude in the dog and rat results in a decrease in net absorption in the dog but an increase in net secretion in the rat. Hence, the performance of many of the initial studies of intestinal fluid and electrolyte

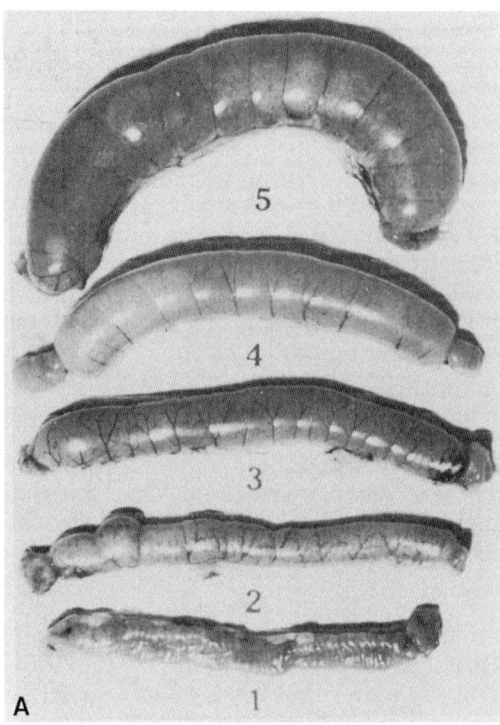

Fig. 7–1. Effect of cholera toxin in an experimental model (A) and in man (B). **A.** Cholera toxin induces fluid secretion in a ligated rabbit ileal loop during 18-hour incubation. Bottom loop (1) is negative control and top loop (5) shows fluid secretion following injection of toxin. Remaining loops (2–4) had intermediate responses. Reproduced with permission from Burrows W, Musteikis GM: Cholera infection and toxin in the rabbit ileal loop. J Infect Dis *116*: 183, 1966. **B.** Patient who had recovered from clinical cholera in Phillipines, surrounded by all the intravenous fluid bottles that were required to correct volume repletion and metabolic acidosis. This case provides evidence that cholera is self-limiting and treatable if sufficient fluid and electrolytes can be provided to replace stool losses caused by cholera toxin-induced active intestinal secretion. Reproduced with permission from Phillips RA: Water and electrolyte losses in cholera. Fed Proc *23*:705, 1964.

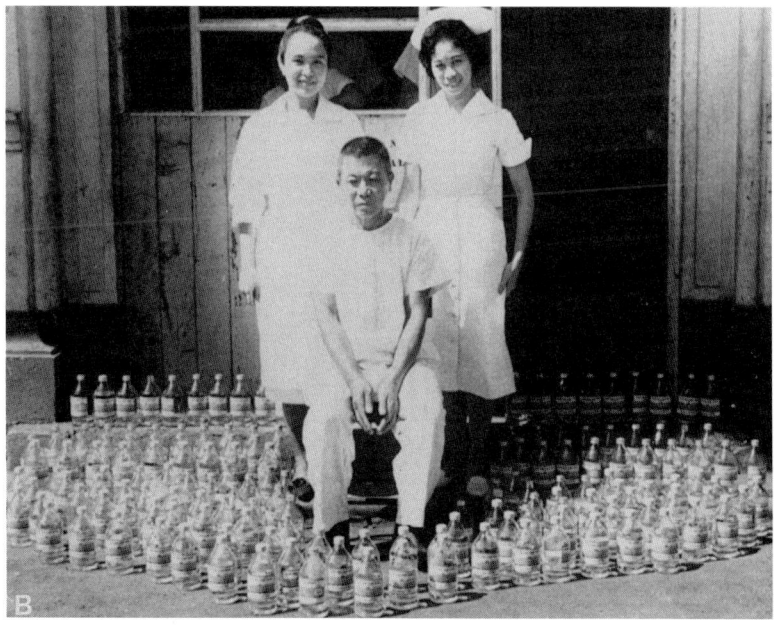

movement in the canine intestine probably delayed recognition of the process of intestinal secretion. Not surprisingly, secretory stimuli of similar magnitude result in net secretion in the small intestine but not in the colon, and for a substantial period of time, cholera was thought not to influence colonic fluid and electrolyte movement (13,14).

METHODS TO STUDY ION MOVEMENT

The development and application of two experimental methods to study different aspects of intestinal electrolyte movement have been vitally important in establishing our present state of knowledge. These methods include an in-vivo approach used extensively in humans: luminal perfusion with nonabsorbable markers (Fig. 7–2) and an in-vitro method that has been used with tissue from both humans and experimental animals: ion flux determinations across isolated mucosa under voltage clamp conditions (Fig. 7–3).

The present method of luminal perfusion to study segmental rates of fluid, electrolyte and nutrient absorption, and secretion evolved from initial studies performed by Miller and Abbott at the University of Pennsylvania. They developed methods to intubate the small intestine with multi-lumen tubes and with occluding balloons to permit study of localized segments of intestine (15). The results of 10 years of these studies were summarized by Miller in 1944 (16). However, the scientific basis for the study of water and electrolyte movement in the intestine actually was provided by a series of experiments that had been performed by Maurice Visscher and colleagues at the University of Minnesota beginning in the late 1930s (17).

John Fordtran, as a fellow in Franz Ingelfinger's laboratory at Boston University, adapted this approach and initiated studies of intestinal electrolyte movement in normal subjects and patients with a variety of diarrheal disorders, now spanning three decades. The initial presentation of these studies was at the annual meeting of the Association of American Physicians in 1961 (18). Luminal perfusion methodology in man also was performed at approximately the same time by Schedl and Clifton (University of Iowa) and by Dawson and colleagues (London) (19,20). The essential advances included the introduction of nonabsorbable markers that permitted aliquot sampling of luminal contents without the need for complete aspiration or the use of occluding balloons. With such markers, it was necessary to establish the fact that luminal contents were in steady-state equilibrium before initiation of sampling. Polyethylene glycol (PEG) 4000, originally used to study fluid movement in ruminants by Swedish veterinary scientists, was rapidly adopted as the nonabsorbable markers of choice despite problems with its assay (21). The initial studies employed two tubes: an infusion port for introduction of the perfusate and a distal aspiration port. It was referred to as "double lumen perfusion method" (22).

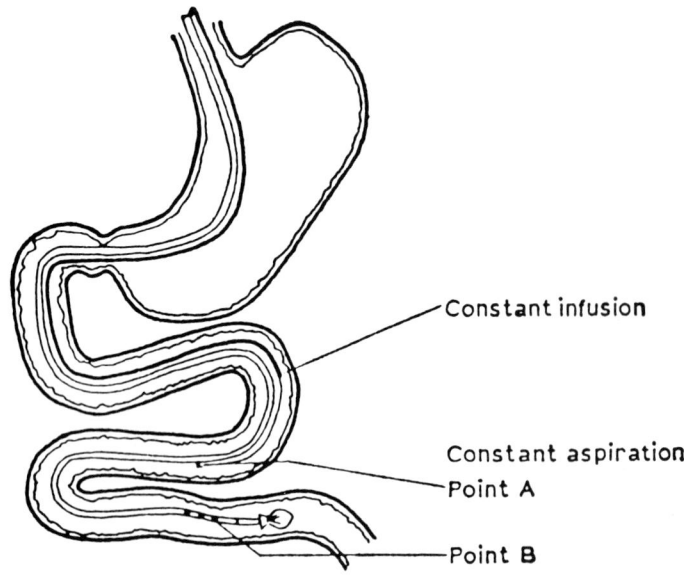

Constant infusion

Constant aspiration

Point A

Point B

Fig. 7–2. Diagram depicting the details of luminal segmental perfusion methodology with nonabsorbable markers. The mixing segment is between the infusion site and point A, and the study segment is between points A and B. Reproduced with permission from Cooper H, Levitan R, Fordtran JS, Ingelfinger FJ: A method for studying absorption of water and solute from the Herman small intestine. Gastroenterology *50*:1, 1966.

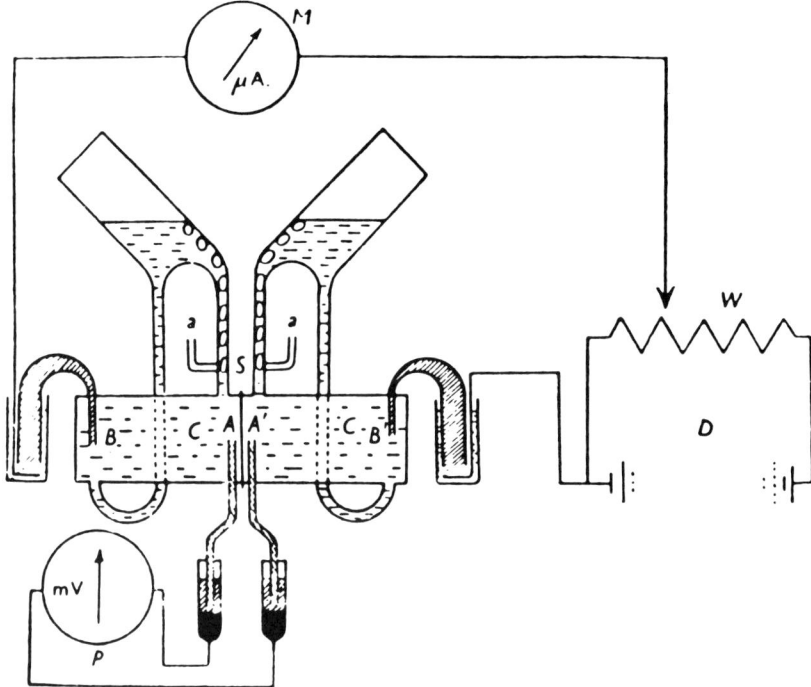

Fig. 7–3. Schematic diagram depicting details of studies in an Ussing flux chamber under voltage clamp conditions. Reproduced with permission from Ussing HH, Zerahan K: Active transport of sodium as the source of electric current in the short circuited isolated frog skin. Acta Physiol Scand 23:110, 1951.

The rate of absorption represented the difference between that which was infused and the calculated amount of material passing the collection port. It soon became apparent that this arrangement required modification. A high rate of fasting intestinal contents (which would certainly occur during a secretory state) resulted in the need to infuse material approximately 10 to 15 cm upstream from the sampling site. As a result, these types of studies now employ three lumens. This is referred to as the "triple lumen perfusion method:" a proximal infusion site and two distal sampling ports, usually 15 cm and 45 cm downstream resulting in a relatively short mixing segment and a 30 cm study segment (see Fig. 7–2). Although there have been several variations of this general method, the same overall methodologic approach has been followed during the ensuing 30 or more years.

Using this general method, Fordtran and his colleagues in Dallas, as well as several other groups, established that net fluid and electrolyte secretion occur in several different diarrheal disorders including celiac sprue, tropical sprue, watery diarrheal syndrome, microscopic colitis, carcinoid syndrome, and cholera (23); and that in normal subjects luminal glucose stimulates fluid and electrolyte absorption. This latter finding provided some of the experimental basis for the use of oral glucose in the treatment of diarrhea in children; so-called oral rehydration solution (ORS) (24,25). Fordtran's experiments established the importance of solvent drag, in addition to glucose-sodium co-transport (see subsequent text), as the mechanism whereby glucose enhances sodium absorption (26). This subject has been reopened recently with important implications for the cell biology of enterocytes (27).

USSING CHAMBER TECHNIQUE

A second important method utilized to better understand fluid and electrolyte secretion has been the determination of unidirectional fluxes across isolated intestinal mucosa under voltage clamp conditions, i.e., under short-circuit conditions. This method often is referred to as the "Ussing chamber" technique after Hans Ussing, a Danish physiologist, who initially developed this approach in 1951 to investigate active Na transport in frog skin (28) (Fig. 7–3). This method permits measurements of oppositely directed ion fluxes across isolated mucosa and emphasizes investigation of active ion absorption and secretion. Ussing established in the frog skin that the so-called short-circuit current was completely accounted for by electrogenic Na absorption. This observation resulted in the rapid acquisition of important new information on Na transport in frog skin and other "tight" epithelia (e.g., toad bladder). During this period, Ussing presented preliminary studies on the guinea pig cecum indicating that active Na absorption also occurred in this epithelium (29).

The adaptation of this method to intestinal epithelia was accomplished by Stanley Schultz in 1964 in studies with rabbit ileum. These initial studies were performed at the Air Force School of Aerospace Medicine in San Antonio by Schultz and Zalusky, who made several important observations (30–32). They demonstrated that active Na absorption is present in the rabbit ileum; active Na absorption is completely electrogenic; glucose stimulates active Na absorption as a result of a glucose-Na cotransport process (not as a result of glucose metabolism); and active Cl transport is not present. Schultz, subsequently at the Harvard Biophysical Laboratory with the late Peter Curran, initiated studies of the interaction of glucose and amino acids with Na at the apical membrane of the rabbit ileum (33). Curran (who did not consider himself an intestinal physiologist but rather a biophysicist who at times studied intestinal epithelia) previously had made two important findings: the model establishing the coupling of solute and water across epithelia and the initial demonstration of the relationship between Na and water absorption in the rat ileum (34,35). These observations by Curran and Schultz provided substantial support for the Na gradient hypothesis that had been initially proposed by Crane and provided an elegant explanation for glucose/amino acid stimulation of Na absorption and

for the Na-dependent glucose/amino acid absorption (36). These studies provided a biophysical basis for ORS.

Since the studies of Schultz and Zalusky, there have been multiple applications of the Ussing chamber/voltage clamp technique to all segments of the intestinal tract in both health and disease and in isolated cell lines grown in culture to form monolayers. During at least the first half of this period, almost all investigators who used the Ussing chamber/voltage clamp technique had received a portion of their training either in the laboratories of Curran or Schultz or with one of Curran-Schultz' initial fellows, who included Powell, Binder, Field, and Frizzel.

In contrast to frog skin, intestinal epithelia have low resistances and, therefore, to accomplish "true short-circuiting" requires a more sophisticated voltage clamp (to adjust for fluid resistance more or less automatically) than the simple battery-voltmeter setup that may be used in studies of frog skin and other "tight" epithelia. (This is not to deny that fluid resistance cannot be adjusted by "hand.") the initial voltage clamps that were used for intestinal studies often were difficult to maintain. Although there have been several small manufacturers of voltage clamps (almost all have evolved from academic physiology department electronic shops), WPI, originally a New Haven-based manufacturer of physiologic electronic equipment, has supplied a substantial number of dependable automatic voltage clamps. These instruments have been vitally important in facilitating the increased knowledge of intestinal ion transport.

Although the nature of Na transport is considerably more complicated than originally described, this in-vitro approach has helped to clarify both normal physiology and the pathophysiology of diarrhea. Undoubtedly, during the last decade of the 20th century and into the 21st century, knowledge of intestinal absorption and secretion will continue to increase and further clarify the pathophysiology of diarrheal disorders and identify more effective treatment.

REFERENCES

1. Florey HW, Wright RD, Jennings MA: The secretion of the intestine. Physiol Rev *21*:36, 1941.

2. Code CF (ed): Handbook of Physiology. Section 6: Alimentary Canal. Volumes I-V. Baltimore, Waverly Press, 1967–1968.
3. Schultz SG (ed): Handbook of Physiology. The Gastrointestinal System. Vol. I-IV. Bethesda, American Physiology Society, 1989–1991.
4. Burrows W, Musteikis GM: Cholera infection and toxin in the rabbit ileal loop. J Infect Diseases *116*:183, 1966.
5. Banwell JG et al.: Intestinal fluid and electrolyte transport in human cholera. J Clin Invest *49*:183, 1970.
6. Powell DW, Malawer SJ, Plotkin GR: Secretion of electrolytes and water by the guinea pig small intestine in vivo. Am J Physiol *215*: 1226, 1968.
7. Powell DW, Malawer SJ: Relationship between water and solute transport from isogmatic solutions by rat intestine in vivo. Am J Physiol *215*:49, 1968.
8. Hendrix TR, Bayless TM: Digestion: Intestinal secretion. Ann Rev Physiol *32*:139, 1970.
9. Parsons DS: Methods for investigation of intestinal absorption. *In* Code CF (ed): Handbook of Physiology. Section 6. Alimentary Canal. Volume III: Intestinal Absorption. Baltimore, Waverly Press, 1968.
10. Thiry L: Uber eine neue Methode, den dunndarm zu isolieren. Sitzber. Akad. Wiss. Wein. Math. Naturw. Kl. I *50*:77, 1864.
11. Vella L: Neues Verfahren zue Gewinnung reinen Darmsaftes und Feststellung seiner physiologischen Eigenschaften. Moleshott's Untersuch Naturl Mensch Thiere *13*:40, 1888.
12. Binder HJ: Net fluid and electrolyte secretion: The pathophysiologic basis of diarrhea. *In* Binder HJ (ed): Mechanisms of Intestinal Secretion. New York, Alan R. Liss, Inc., 1979, p. 1.
13. Donowitz M, Binder HJ: Effect of bacterial enterotoxins on fluid and electrolyte transport in the colon. J Infect Dis *134*:135, 1976.
14. Speelman P et al.: Colonic dysfunction during cholera infection. Gastroenterology *91*: 1164, 1986.
15. Abbott WO, Miller TG: Intubation studies of the human small intestine. III. A technic for the collection of pure intestinal secretion and for the study of intestinal absorption. JAMA *106*:16, 1936.
16. Miller TG: Intubation studies of the human small intestine. XXIV. A review of a ten year experience. Gastroenterology *3*:141, 1944.
17. Visscher M et al.: Sodium ion movement between the intestinal lumen and the blood. Am J Physiol *141*:488, 1944.
18. Fordtran JS et al.: The kinetics of water absorption in the human intestine. Trans Assoc Am Physicians *74*:195, 1961.
19. Schedl HP, Clifton J: Solute and water absorption by the Herman small intestine. Nature (London) *199*:1264, 1963.
20. Holdsworth CD, Dawson AM: The absorption of monosaccharides in man. Clin Sci *27*: 371, 1964.
21. Sperber I, Hyden S, Edman NJ: The use of polyethylene glycol as a reference substance in the study of ruminant digestion. Ann Agr Coll Sweden *20*:337, 1953.
22. Cooper H, Levitan R, Fordtran JS, Ingelfinger FJ: A method for studying absorption of water and solute from the Herman small intestine. Gastroenterology *50*:1, 1966.
23. Fine KD, Krejs GJ, Fordtran JS: *In* Sleisenger M, Fordtran J (eds): Gastrointestinal Diseases. 4th Ed. Philadelphia, WB Saunders, 1989, p. 290.
24. Phillips RA: Water and electrolyte losses in cholera. Fed. Proc. *23*:705, 1964.
25. Greenough WB III, Khin-Maung U: Oral rehydration therapy. *In* Field M (ed): Diarrheal Diseases. New York, Elsevier Science Publishing Company, 1991, p. 485.
26. Fordtran JS: Stimulation of active and passive sodium absorption by sugars in the human jejunum. J Clin Invest *55*:728, 1975.
27. Pappenheimer JR, Reiss KZ: Contribution of solvent drag through intercellular junctions to absorption of nutrients by the small intestine of the rat. J Membrane Biol *100*: 123, 1987.
28. Ussing HH, Zerahn K: Active transport of sodium as the source of electric current in the short circuited isolated frog skin. Acta Physiol Scand *23*:110, 1951.
29. Ussing HH, Anderson B: The relation between solvent drag and active transport of ions. Proc Intern Congr Biochem p. 434, 1956.
30. Schultz SG, Zalusky R: Ion transport in isolated rabbit ileum. I. Short-circuit current and Na fluxes. J Gen Physiol *47*:567, 1964.
31. Schultz SG, Zalusky R: Ion transport in isolated rabbit ileum. II. The interaction between active sodium and active sugar transport. J Gen Physiol *47*:1043, 1964.
32. Schultz SG, Zalusky R, Gass AE Jr: Ion transport in isolated rabbit ileum. III. Chloride fluxes. J Gen Physiol *48*:275, 1964.
33. Schultz SG, Curran PF: Coupled transport of sodium and organic solutes. Physiol Rev *50*:637, 1970.
34. Curran PF, MacIntosh JR: A model system for biological water transport. Nature (London) *193*:347, 1962.
35. Curran PF, Solomon AK: Ions and water fluxes in the ileum of rats. J Gen Physiol *41*: 143, 1957.
36. Crane RK: Hypothesis of mechanism of intestinal active transport of sugars. Fed Proc *21*:891, 1962.

8

The History of Gastrointestinal Hormones

ANDREA TODISCO AND TADATAKA YAMADA

The history of gastrointestinal hormones begins with the discovery of secretin by Bayliss and Starling in 1902 (1). Before this discovery, the physiology of the gastrointestinal system was dominated by the theories of Pavlov and his pupils, who considered nervous reflexes as the only mediators of the secretory functions of the gastrointestinal tract (2). For his theories on "nervism" and for his many contributions to gastrointestinal physiology, Pavlov was to receive the Nobel Prize for Medicine or Physiology in 1904 despite the remarkable reports of Bayliss and Starling that a humoral factor may be responsible for the control of pancreatic secretion. These reports derived from a series of experiments that began on January 16, 1901 at the University College of London. According to the account of this experiment by an eyewitness, Charles Martin, the events unfolded as follows.

In an anesthetized dog a loop of jejunum was tied at both ends and the nerve supplying it dissected out and divided so that it was connected with the rest of the body only by its blood vessels. On the introduction of some weak HCl into the duodenum secretion from the pancreas occurred and continued for some minutes. After this had subsided, a few cubic centimeters of acid were introduced into the ennervated loop of jejunum. To our surprise, a similarly marked secretion was produced. I remember Starling saying: "Then it must be a chemical reflex." Rapidly cutting off a further piece of jejunum he rubbed its mucous membrane with sand in weak HCl, filtered and injected it into the jugular vein of the animal. After a few moments the pancreas responded by much greater secretion than had occurred before. It was a great afternoon (3).

Thus, in a single day, in a single experiment, Bayliss and Starling were able to demonstrate that acid in the intestine stimulated the pancreas, that the effects continued to persist after the nerves were cut, and that the effect could be reproduced by injecting an acid extract of the jejunal mucosa. They concluded that acid must stimulate the release of a chemical messenger from the intestine that traverses through the bloodstream to the pancreas, stimulating it to secrete. They termed this substance "secretin." Later the authors, at the suggestion of William Hardy, created the term "hormone" from the Greek "I excite" to describe a chemical messenger by which one organ exercises an influence on another (4). This series of observations marked the birth of the science of endocrinology in general, but most particularly of the endocrinology of the gut.

Since the discovery of gastrointestinal hormones, there has been a remarkable progression of the field of gastroenterology. This progression has occurred in five recognizable phases, although there is considerable overlap between them. The first phase was that of whole-animal physiology. In these earlier experiments, a variety of other hormonal substances were identified by their physiologic properties. Following the discovery of secretin, John Edkins proposed the existence of a gastric antral hormone that was responsible for stimulating acid secretion, which he called gastrin (5).

Later, other biological activities were defined, identified by their physiologic properties, such as cholecystokinin, incretin, enterogastrone, villikinin, duokinin, enterokinin, gastrone, urogastrone, antrochalone, and bulbogastrone. Some of these substances since have been purified and their chemical structures determined. Others exist only as biologic activities still in search of the substance that is responsible for them.

The second phase of gastrointestinal hormone research was that of biochemical purification. The famous teams of Jorpes and Mutt from Stockholm on the one hand and Gregory, Tracy, and Kenner from Liverpool on the other capitalized on the development of modern protein extraction techniques and coupled them with advances in protein separation methodology to isolate and purify the first gastrointestinal hormones, cholecystokinin (6), secretin (7), and gastrin (8,9). Mutt continued his purification efforts long after others had ceased their efforts and, in collaboration with numerous scientists from all over the world who served as fellows, contributed the structures of a wide variety of peptide hormones including vasoactive intestinal peptide, gastrin-releasing peptide, and motilin. In an important series of studies conducted with Tatemoto, Mutt took advantage of the observation that many peptide hormones contained a carboxyl terminal amide moiety and developed a method for identifying and purifying peptides on the basis of this single property. With this technique, he was able to characterize a number of additional peptide hormones including PHI, PYY, NPY, and galanin (10–17).

The availability of purified or synthetic peptide hormones ushered in the third phase of gastrointestinal endocrinology, the era of pharmacology. In this era, peptides were injected into animals and into human subjects to examine their effects on a variety of physiologic functions. This created the problem of identifying which of the effects were physiologic as opposed to artifactual pharmacological events. In this dilemma, scientists were greatly aided by the remarkable discovery of the technique of radioimmunoassay by Berson and Yalow in 1959 (18,19). This technique permitted the measurement of the tiniest quantities of peptide hormones in the circulation for the first time under normal physiologic conditions. Thus, the issue of physiologic function of hormones could be answered if intravenous injection of the putative hormone produced a functional effect and this effect was achieved by injection of the hormone in quantities sufficient to reproduce its normal circulating concentrations elicited by a physiological stimulus. Surprisingly, with this strict definition, the true physiologic function of only a small handful of hormones, such as gastrin and cholecystokinin, has been confirmed.

Knowledge of the biochemical structure of hormones also provided the entree into the fourth phase of gastrointestinal endocrinology, that of molecular biology. Amino acid sequence information shed insight into the nucleotide sequence that encoded them. Using these nucleotide sequences, it was possible to derive the structures of the complete genes that encoded the peptides. The structure of the gene provided insight into the precursor-product relationship between multiple molecular forms of peptide hormones and, furthermore, shed light on the derivation of different peptides, such as VIP and PHI, or calcitonin and calcitonin gene-related peptide (CGRP) from the same gene (20,21). Moreover, the availability of the gene provided the means by which to understand how expression of peptide hormones was regulated by physiologic events.

The age of molecular biology has helped to usher in the fifth phase of gastrointestinal endocrinology, that of cell and molecular physiology. The advancement of cell isolation and culture techniques has provided models for the study of the direct action of hormones at their receptors and the intracellular events that follow. Preparations of gastric parietal cells (22–26), D-cells (27), and G-cells (28) have helped to elucidate the interaction between hormones and their target organs to regulate acid secretion. Through biochemical means, the receptors and the postreceptor signal transduction events have been characterized and, more recently, the application of molecular biologic methodologies has led to the cloning and expression of a variety of peptide hormone receptors. These receptors can be used for in-depth characterization of receptor binding properties and linkages to intracellular pathways. Most importantly, the use of molecular biologic tools has helped to lead the field of gastrointestinal endocrinology back to the whole animal once again through the creation of transgenic mice for the study of gene regulation in specific sites in the body.

Thus, through a series of phases punctuated by the advancement of scientific methodologies, gastrointestinal endocrinology as a field of inquiry has come full circle from the original animal studies that defined their existence back to the whole animal. Hopefully, this time there are better tools to understand the true physiologic relevance of these important chemical messengers that regulate organ function. To bring into focus the developments that have characterized the history of gastrointestinal endocrinology, we will examine in depth the events that have contributed to the evolution of current knowledge on gastrin.

EDKINS AND THE DISCOVERY OF GASTRIN

One of the major physiologic questions at the turn of the century was the issue of gastric acid secretory regulation. The presumption, on the basis of Pavlov's theories of nervism, was that gastric distention stimulated a neural reflex that resulted in acid secretion. However, experiments by a number of investigators, including a physiologist at St. Bartholomew's Hospital Medical School in London, John Edkins, indicated that mechanical irritation such as that caused by gastric distention resulted in only a minute amount of acid secretion when compared to that elicited by food. The publication of the reports of Bayliss and Starling no doubt contributed to Edkins' conviction that there must be a chemical messenger that can account for the secretion of acid in response to a meal. To confirm this hypothesis, he extracted antral mucosa of cats and pigs and injected these extracts into the jugular vein of an anesthetized cat. The extracts of the pyloric mucosa stimulated acid secretion and also reduced systolic blood pressure. Comparable extracts from the oxyntic mucosa had the same effect on blood pressure but did not stimulate acid secretion. Edkins concluded from these experiments that there was a gastric secretin, or

"gastrin," in the antral mucosa (5). From the beginning of this discovery there was controversy about the existence of such a hormone, and following the rapid developments surrounding the physiology of histamine (29) in the early 1920s, the work of Edkins was thought to have been a mistake because, like histamine itself, the antral extracts resulted in reduced blood pressure. The presumption was that the extracts contained histamine and not an antral hormone counterpart to secretin. The important control experiments with the extracts of the oxyntic mucosa were conveniently forgotten.

PROOF OF THE GASTRIN HYPOTHESIS

Over the next three decades, numerous investigators attempted with difficulty to prove the gastrin hypothesis. The final proof was left to the experiments of Morton Grossman, who at the time was a young postdoctoral fellow working in the laboratory of A. C. Ivy, the legendary Professor of Physiology at Northwestern University Medical School. In a series of experiments, Grossman, Ivy, and another colleague, Charlotte Robertson, proved the existence of an antral hormone responsible for acid secretion (30). For these experiments Grossman considered two important problems with prior experiments that aspired to prove or disprove the gastrin hypothesis. The first was that there was no clear demonstration that the acid-secreting portion of the stomach was completely denervated. The second was that the stimulus used for acid secretion, generally a liver extract, might be absorbed into the circulation and have an acid stimulatory effect independent of an intermediary hormone. To circumvent these problems, Grossman and his colleagues created three separate pouches by surgical means in a set of dogs. The first pouch consisted of a completely denervated gastric antrum. A second pouch consisting of a portion of the body of the stomach was transplanted into the mammary gland, and after allowing the gland to develop a local blood supply, the vessels that presumably carried both blood and neural fibers to the pouch were severed. Thus, these pouches unquestionably had no remaining neural connections to the stomach. Finally, the remaining portion of the gastric body was vagally denervated. To circumvent the problem with the liver extracts, Grossman inflated a condom balloon in the antral pouch to serve as a secretory stimulus. In this elegant preparation, he and his colleagues were able to demonstrate that distention of the antral pyloric pouch was sufficient to induce acid secretion in both the denervated oxyntic mucosa transplanted to the mammary gland and the remnant of the gastric body. Grossman's words describe best the impact of these experiments:

> The question of whether substances or distention of the antrum stimulated acid secretion, and, if so, whether it did so through hormonal or nonhormonal mechanisms, and if by hormonal mechanisms, what the nature of the hormone was were all very much in the air. There were very disparate results, some showing completely negative results, saying that the antrum played no special role, and others showing that it was a special receptor region.
>
> Then there was the quite separate area as to whether or not one could extract from the antrum a substance which would stimulate acid secretion, and there the controversy revolved around whether histamine accounted for the stimulatory effect or whether there was a separate substance. So that there was just a mass of contradictory information, and one of the problems on the physiological side was the question of whether, if one put substances such as liver extract into the antral portion of the stomach, and if one did get positive results and saw acid secretion, whether that wasn't simply due to the absorption of the liver extract itself. There have been studies showing that liver extract given intravenously would stimulate acid secretion, and that turned out to be due to contamination with histamine. So the reason that this particular paper was felt to be decisive was that it gave clear-cut positive results that eliminated the possibility of nervous pathways, and it eliminated the question of absorption of substances, because distention was a stimulus. For that reason, it was believed to be a landmark paper (31).

Grossman went on to characterize the mechanisms of gastrin-stimulated acid secretion much further. A very important point that he recognized very early was a potentiating interaction between various agents that stimulated acid secretion. He defined the potentiated response as one in which "two stimuli acting together give a response greater than the sum of the responses of the individual stimuli." He demonstrated in dogs with vagotomized fundic pouches that the acid secretory response to a combination of urecholine and histamine greatly exceeds the maximal response to gastrin histamine and urecholine alone (Fig. 8–1) (32). On the basis of such studies, some 15 years before the pioneering work of Andrew Soll with isolated canine gastric parietal cells, Grossman predicted that there were interactions between separate receptors for histamine, gastrin, and acetylcholine on the gastric parietal cell. Because of these interactions, it is impossible to predict the relative importance of any single secretagogue on the basis of individual stimulation or inhibition studies in vivo.

These important experiments were not the end of Grossman's contributions to gastrointestinal endocrinology. Through his laboratory at the Veterans Administration Wadsworth Medical Center in Los Angeles and the Center for Ulcer Research and Education that he established there, he had a major role in the development of the academic careers of countless investigators who have served as the vanguard for gastrointestinal endocrinology research throughout the world (Table 8–1).

PURIFICATION OF GASTRIN

Despite the controversy surrounding Edkins' proposed antral hormone, gastrin, by the late 1930s the general consensus was that such a hormone surely must exist. A scientist, Simon Komarov, who had trained in Pavlov's laboratory from 1910 to 1913, found himself a research assistant to Boris Babkin, another former Pavlov trainee who became Professor of Physiology at McGill University. Komarov undertook the isolation of gastrin, a project that had been attempted by numerous investigators without success. He reasoned that gastrin must be a protein and, therefore, extractable by precipitation with trichloroacetic acid. This crucial step separates the active ingredient in antral extracts from histamine, and thus

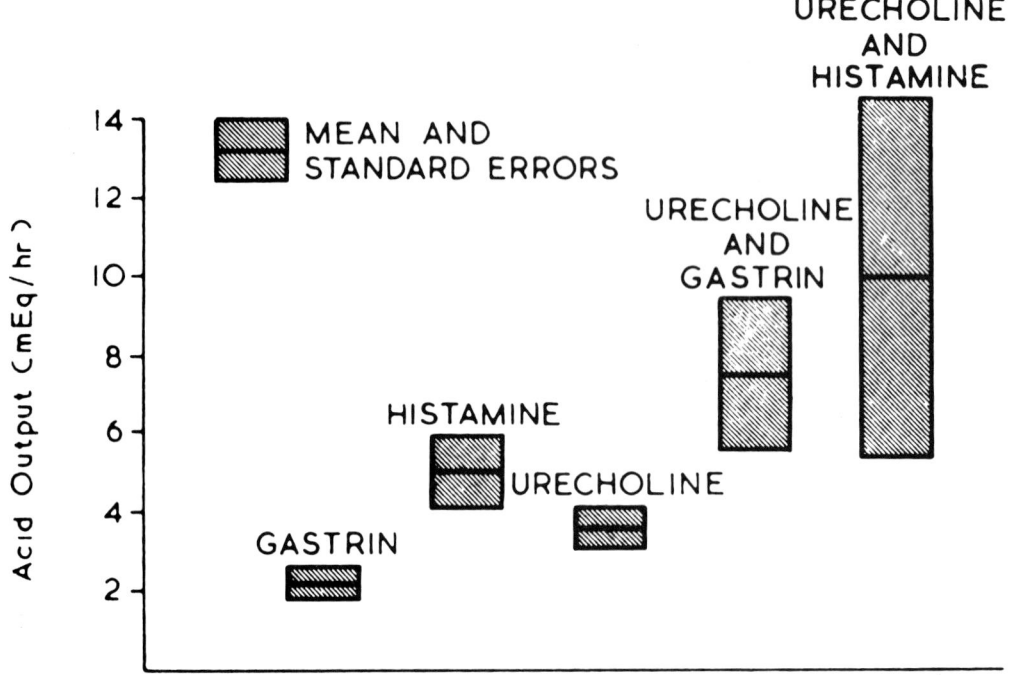

Fig. 8–1. Maximal acid responses of Heidenhain pouches to gastrin extract, histamine, and urecholine, alone and in combination. Reproduced with permission from Gillespie JE, Grossman MI: Potentiation between urecholine and gastrin extract and between urecholine and histamine in the stimulation of Heidenhain pouches. Gut 5:71, 1964.

extracts subjected to this treatment were able to stimulate gastric acid secretion without lowering the blood pressure of an anesthetized cat. These observations, which were made in 1938, were not published in detail until 4 years later in the *Reviews of Canadian Biology* (33,34). It is said that the reason for the tardiness of the publication and the obscurity of the journal was the result of A. C. Ivy's unwillingness to accept Komarov's findings.

Some 20 years later, in their Liverpool laboratory, Roderick Gregory and his collaborator, Hilda Tracy, undertook the purification of gastrin beginning with an improved method for trichloroacetic acid precipitation of the gastrin biologic activity. Efforts at purification were greatly facilitated by the availability of new methods for protein purification such as cellulose and Sephadex chromatography. After determining that gastrin was a heptadecapeptide with a molecular weight of around 2,114 daltons (35), Gregory and Tracy collaborated with George Kenner, the renowned Chairman of

the Department of Organic Chemistry at Liverpool, to obtain the amino acid sequence. In the process of the purification, the investigators discovered that there were two gastrins that could be separated on aminoethyl cellulose chromatography. They called these gastrin I and II (9). Ultimately, the difference between the two gastrins was determined to be the sulfation of a tyrosine residue in gastrin II. Amino acid sequencing in those days was not by automated Edman degradation but by sequential digestion with various peptidases. As shown in Figure 8–2, the sequence was deduced on the fragments obtained by digestion with the enzymes chymotrypsin, papain, and subtilisin and by reaction with cyanogen bromide. The accuracy of the sequence was confirmed by synthesizing the deduced molecule and demonstrating its biologic activity. The initial peptide isolated was from hog stomachs because of their availability from a Liverpool company that specialized in making pork pies. Two years after the amino acid sequence of porcine gastrin 17 I and II were

Table 8–1
Chronological List of Fellows of M. I. Grossman*

R. Roback	B. Fox	A. M. Brooks
W. Sangster	E. Strub	R. S. Jones
G. M. Cummins	G. H. Becker	J. Isenberg
R. Sonnenschein	M. Kalser	L. Way
I. F. Stein	T. M. Lin	J. Spenser
C. Robertson	L. Pevsner	J. Meyer
M. Hanson	H. Moeller	A. Dinbar
K. Hwang	S. Tuttle	L. Spingola
C. C. Wang	K. Matsumoto	G. Barbezat
H. Janowitz	A. Bettarello	H. Trout
E. Hale	F. Rufin	J. Walsh
M. Fogelman	E. Castro	A. Csendes
S. Krasnow	D. Pelot	H. Debas
A. Littman	L. Ventzke	J. Karen
E. Newman	I. Gillespie	H. Verine
K. J. Wang	R. Mitchell	G. Slaff
D. Blickenstaff	K. Adashek	M. Impicciatore
D. Fainer	E. Passaro	O. Farooq
Z. Maratka	K. G. Wormsley	G. Dockray
K. Hartiala	R. Preshaw	J. Valenzuela
C. E. Rosiere	S. Andersson	R. Bugat
F. Benjamin	A. Cooke	R. Sturdevant
K. Langlois	E. Jacobson	U. Strunz
C. Martin	K. Swan	H. Peterson
G. Slezak	S. Zaterka	M. Thompson
D. Magee	M. Eisenberg	D. Hansen
H. Kobrin	D. Nahrwold	T. Solomon
F. Antia	S. Emas	A. Soll
E. Kammerling	D. Bloom	D. Carter
A. L. de Almeida	M. Vagne	G. Kauffman
I. A. Share	F. Stening	I. Taylor
R. Villarreal	L. R. Johnson	T. Yamada

* Adapted with permission from Boyle JD, Morton I, Grossman MD: An oral history. Gastroenterology *83*:285, 1982.

reported, Gregory and Tracy were able to determine the structure of human gastrin I and II and found that the only difference between it and porcine gastrin was the substitution of a leucine for methionine at position five (36).

Simultaneously with the purification of gastrin, two scientists at the VA Hospital in the Bronx, New York, Solomon Berson and Rosalyn Yalow, developed a methodology for using antibodies to quantify small amounts of insulin in bodily fluids. This method, which was reported in *Advances in Biological and Medical Physics* as a short addendum to a larger study on the binding of insulin to anti-insulin antibody in patients who were sensitized to bovine insulin, used a small amount of anti-insulin antisera, a minute quantity of ^{125}I-labeled beef insulin, and crystalline insulin standard (18). Berson and Yalow observed that when the labeled insulin was incubated with the antisera, the ratio of bound to free radioactivity varied with the amount of unlabeled insulin standard added to the mixture. The details of the methodology were published 2 years

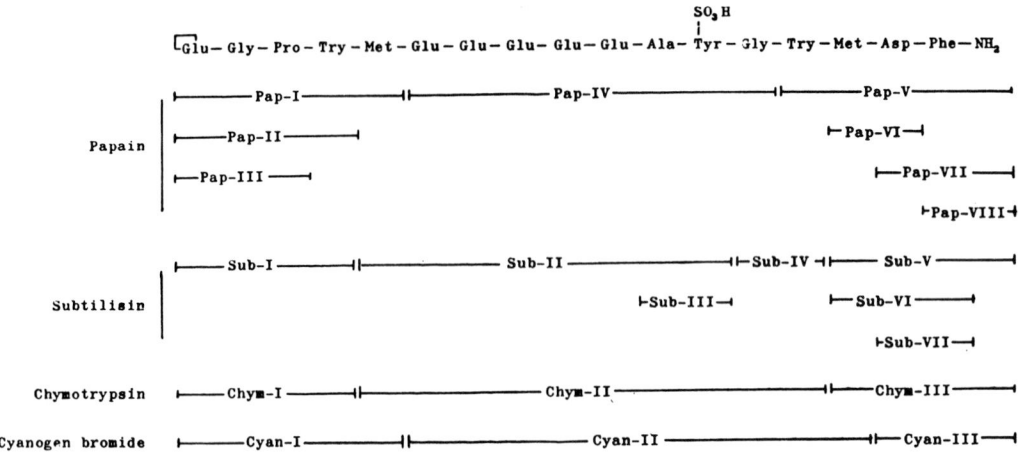

Fig. 8–2. Peptides obtained by degradation of gastrin II. Reproduced with permission from Gregory RA et al.: Structure of gastrin. Nature *204*:931, 1964.

later (19). When the structure of gastrin became known, numerous investigators throughout the world, including James McGuigan, James Thompson, Jack Hansky, and Berson and Yalow themselves, with the assistance of John Walsh, developed radioimmunoassays for gastrin and explored the biochemistry and physiology of the hormone (37–41).

The introduction of the gastrin radioimmunoassay was crucial for the understanding of the role that gastrin plays in human disease. In 1955, two surgeons from Ohio State University, Robert Zollinger and Edwin Ellison, described a syndrome of peptic ulcerations of the jejunum associated with islet cell tumors of the pancreas (42). The pathophysiology of this syndrome remained unknown until Gregory and Tracy obtained an extract from a Zollinger-Ellison tumor and demonstrated its ability to stimulate gastric acid secretion when injected into conscious dogs. Secretagogue activity also was demonstrated in extracts from metastatic lesions in the liver and lymph nodes. It was clear from these observations that the active principle present in the tumor was similar in nature to the hormone gastrin. In 1967 Gregory was able to isolate from one of these pancreatic tumors a product that had a quantitative amino acid constitution very similar to that of human gastrin (43). Finally, in 1968 McGuigan and Trudeau measured by radioimmunoassay gastrin levels in patients with Zollinger-Ellison tu-

mors. They found values ranging from 3550 to 21000 μμg of gastrin per milliliter as compared to the mean serum gastrin level of 425 μμg per ml in the control population (44,45). Radioimmunoassay since has become an important tool for the diagnosis of these tumors.

One of the early observations made by Berson and Yalow was that, aside from the different gastrins defined by the presence of a sulfated tyrosine moiety, there were multiple molecular forms of gastrin on gel filtration of Zollinger-Ellison tumor extracts. They noticed an immunoreactive form of gastrin that eluted as a much larger molecule than human gastrin 17. They called this form "big" gastrin as opposed to gastrin-17, which was called "little" gastrin (46). They noted the presence of this form of gastrin, not only in the tumors but also in extracts of human antrum, duodenum, and proximal jejunum, with larger amounts of big gastrin present in the intestine. Subsequently, Jens Rehfield and his colleagues in Copenhagen identified four "components" of gastrin immunoreactivity on Sephadex gel chromatography (47). Components II and III corresponded to big and little gastrins. Component IV represented a very small form of gastrin, and component I a much larger form of gastrin than big gastrin. This component was smaller, however, than another large gastrin molecular form that Berson and Yalow identified, which they called "big, big" gastrin (48,49). Although there is considerable doubt as to the existence of "big, big" gastrin, the amino acid sequences of big gastrin and component I gastrin have been determined. The amino acid sequence of human big gastrin was initially reported in a lecture at a symposium on gastrointestinal hormones organized by James Thompson in Galveston in 1974 (50). The impediments to the determination of the structure of big gastrin were the paucity of available tissues, the blockage of the amino terminus with a pyroglutamyl residue and the difficulty in determining the structure of a peptide of such large size by peptide digest analysis. Each of these problems was overcome in sequence. First, in September of 1972, Dr. Edward Passaro, a general surgeon at the VA Wadsworth Medical Center where Morton Grossman worked, obtained a very large amount of gastrinoma tissue from a hepatic metastasis of a patient with Zollinger-Ellison syndrome. This tissue was reported to Grossman, who then promptly had the sample shipped to Liverpool. In addition, Grossman obtained from Professor R. F. Doolittle of the University of California, San Diego, a large supply of the enzyme pyrrolidone carboxypeptidase, which has the capability of specifically cleaving amino terminal pyroglutamyl residues. And finally, Professor George Kenner secured the collaboration of Dr. Ieuan Harris of the Molecular Biology Laboratory in Cambridge, who was familiar with the Edman degradation technique for protein sequencing. This combination of events resulted in Gregory's ability to obtain the sequence of both human and porcine big gastrin (Fig. 8–3). The results were presented to the audience of the Symposium on Gastrointestinal Hormones and published in a chapter of the proceedings of the meeting with the notation, "We are grateful to Dr. Harris and Professor Kenner for their permission to reproduce the sequences in advance of their account of the structural studies, which will be published in full elsewhere."

It is ironic that this structure ultimately was not published as such because, in fact, there was an error in the sequence. This error was suspected in experiments conducted by one of Gregory's trainees, Graham Dockray in the mid-1970s as he developed a variety of antisera to regions of the synthetic big gastrin (now known to be gastrin 34). What was surprising was that some of the antisera that clearly recognized synthetic gastrin 34 constructed on the basis of its sequence as reported by Gregory was unable to recognize natural human gastrin 34 obtained from antral and Zollinger-Ellison tumor extracts. A careful analysis of this information ensued and resulted in the determination of the correct amino acid sequence of human big gastrin by both standard biochemical and molecular biological means (about which more will be discussed below). This finding, which should have been a happy discovery for scientists in the field, turned out to be tragic. Kenner, who was said to have been already somewhat depressed, became despondent upon learning that his initial sequencing of big gastrin had been incorrect. Despite the fact that the sequence was never published under his authorship as a full manuscript, he assumed

A.

Glp*-Leu-Gly-Pro-Gln-Gly-***His-Pro-Ser***-Leu-Val-Ala-Asp-Pro-Ser-Lys-Lys-Gln-Gly-Pro-Trp-Leu-Glu-Glu-Glu-Glu-Glu-Ala-Tyr-Gly-Trp-Met-Asp-Phe-NH$_2$

* Pyroglutamyl

B.

Glp*-Leu-Gly-Pro-Gln-Gly-***Pro-Pro-His***-Leu-Val-Ala-Asp-Pro-Ser-Lys-Lys-Gln-Gly-Pro-Trp-Leu-Glu-Glu-Glu-Glu-Glu-Ala-Tyr-Gly-Trp-Met-Asp-Phe-NH$_2$

* Pyroglutamyl

Fig. 8–3. Comparison of the initial amino acid sequence of human G34 *(A)* with the revised correct sequence *(B)*. The incorrect sequence is in italic characters.

complete responsibility for the error. Shortly after being informed of the corrected sequence, Kenner committed suicide by ingestion of ethylene glycol. Ironically, Kenner's collaborator in the sequencing of human big gastrin, Ieuan Harris, had died a few months before in a tragic accident. He and his family were at a holiday home in South Wales, and a malfunctioning gas heater claimed the lives of Harris and two of his daughters, although his wife and an additional daughter survived.

THE ADVENT OF
MOLECULAR BIOLOGY

At the exact moment when the error in the structure of gastrin 34 was recognized, a new era began, not only in gastrointestinal endocrinology, but in the broad field of science. The rapidly developing field of molecular biology was to have a major effect on peptide hormone research. Kan Agarwal, a biochemist of East Indian origin who trained under the guidance of George Kenner, was intimately involved in much of the early gastrin sequencing work. After training with Kenner, Agarwal partook in a postdoctoral fellowship with Gobin Khorana and in his laboratory was responsible for the construction of synthetic oligonucleotides in the study of transfer RNA for which Khorana was to receive a Nobel Prize. Agarwal later accepted an appointment as an Assistant Professor in the Departments of Biochemistry, Biophysics, and Theoretical Biology at the University of Chicago. There he combined his interest in gastrin with his talents in oligonucleotide synthesis to construct a plan for the application of molecular biology to the study of the structure of the gastrin gene.

Agarwal reasoned that if an amino acid sequence were known, one could deduce the nucleotides that encoded that sequence on the basis of the genetic code. By constructing a synthetic oligonucleotide that was the exact complement of the deduced messenger RNA sequence that encoded a specific portion of a peptide such as gastrin, one could utilize it both to identify gastrin mRNA and to prime the synthesis of a complementary DNA strand from the messenger RNA by means of the action of the enzyme reverse transcriptase. This novel idea required two special levels of expertise. The first was the ability to make oligonucleotides, no easy matter in the days before oligonucleotide synthesis machines. Because of Agarwal's previous experience in Khorana's laboratory, he was highly skilled at the synthesis of oligonucleotide, using the complex diester technique. The other required level of expertise was provided through an unique circumstance that brought Barbara Noyes to Agarwal's laboratory. She had previous experience in the nucleotide hybridization studies from her postdoctoral fellowship in George Stark's laboratory at Stanford University. Her arrival at Chicago when her husband went there for a psychiatry residency provided exactly the molecular biologic expertise that Agarwal needed to conduct his studies. For the selection of the oligonucleotide to be used as a primer for the synthesis of a complementary DNA to gastrin RNA, Agarwal selected the sequence 5'-d (CTCCTCCATCCA) -3', which was specific for the unique amino acid sequence Trp-Met-Glu-Glu. This was a highly advantageous sequence because both tryptophan and methionine each have only single codons and glutamic acid only has two. The experiment worked and the result was the determination not only of the correct sequence of the first 17 amino acids of gastrin 34, but also of several amino acids in the structure of the precursor to gastrin, which were amino terminal to the first amino acid of gastrin 34 (Fig. 8–4) (51,52,53).

The profound implications of these experiments extended far beyond their importance in the field of gastrointestinal endocrinology. Before these experiments, investigators working in the field of molecular biology only could work with high abundance mRNAs. For example, people were relegated to studying albumin gene expression in hepatocytes or globin gene expression in reticulocytes. Low-abundance messages such as gastrin in the antrum mucosa could not be studied without the application of oligonucleotide probes such as those used by Agarwal and his colleagues. In a sense, then, these experiments opened up the entire field of molecular biology to the "masses." With the development of the triester technique for oligonucleotide synthe-

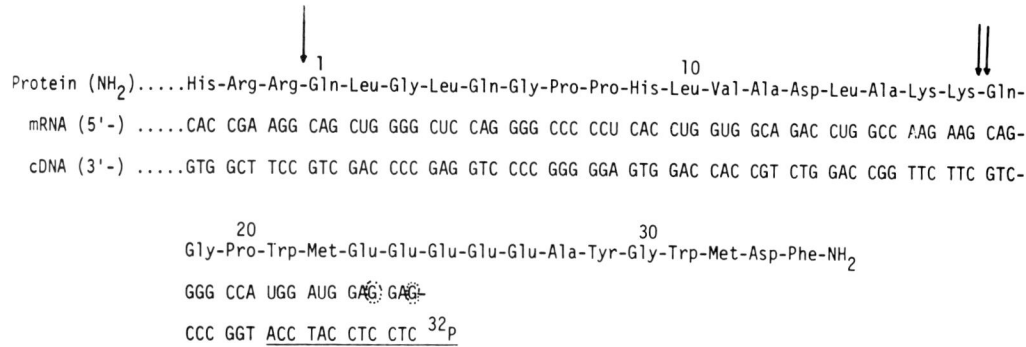

Fig. 8–4. Comparison of the amino acid sequence of hog progastrin with the nucleotide sequence of its mRNA. The lower line indicates the nucleotide sequence of cDNA derived from hog antral RNA using [^{32}P]dodecanucleotide as a primer for reverse transcription. The dodecanucleotide sequence is underlined. The mRNA sequence corresponding to this cDNA is given above the actual sequence determined. The circled nucleotides are tentative and represent positions of possible mismatch between the primer and the mRNA. The amino acid sequence derived from the mRNA is depicted in the upper line and corresponds to that previously determined for progastrin. On the basis of the nucleotide sequence, three additional amino acids of a preprogastrin are deducted at the amino terminus of progastrin. An arrow indicates the proposed site for trypsin-like cleavage that would generate progastrin from a longer prepropeptide. The cleavage site for conversion of progastrin to gastrin, indicated by double arrows, is similar. Reproduced with permission from Noyes BE et al.: Detection and partial sequence analysis of gastrin mRNA by using an oligodeoxynucleotide probe. Proc Natl Acad Sci USA 76:4;1770, 1979.

sis and the automated synthesis of oligonucleotides, work in molecular biology was greatly simplified, as evidenced by the enormous explosion of the use of this technology in all fields of biomedical science.

As a follow-up to their initial experiments, Agarwal's group extended its studies to the use of oligonucleotides as hybridization probes to detect and quantify gastrin specific mRNAs. In the studies conducted by Moshe Mevarech, RNA separated by gel electrophoresis was transferred to Whatman's filter paper that had been diazotized, then ^{32}P-labeled gastrin oligonucleotides were hybridized to the paper (Fig. 8–5) (54). The amount of hybridized radioactivity was directly proportional to the amount of RNA that was added to the paper. This provided the first useful application of the Northern blot technique for quantifying protein specific messenger RNA in tissues. The technique has been put to great use in recent years to assess the regulation of gastrin messenger RNA content in varying conditions. In the laboratories of John Walsh, Michael Wolf, and Stephen Brand, studies have been conducted to demonstrate that gastrin gene expression, as quantified by steady state mRNA levels, is induced by feeding and achlorhydria and inhibited by starvation and somatostatin (55–57).

The availability of the sequence of the gastrin precursor (preprogastrin) from the complete sequence of its mRNA revealed that the structures of big and little gastrin are contained within a central core of a larger molecule with carboxyl and amino terminal extensions. The sites at which the cleavages occur to form G34 and G17 are punctuated by the presence of paired amino acid residues (Fig. 8–6). A particularly important sequence is the presence of a Gly-Arg-Arg moiety following the carboxyl terminal phenylalanine of gastrin that is amidated in the biologically active form of the molecule. Careful analysis of the precursors for other amidated peptide hormones revealed a similar carboxyl terminal structure consisting of glycine followed by two or more basic amino acids. The sequence of the reactions that occur at the site was determined in part by the findings of Kentaro Sugano and his colleagues in Tadataka Yamada's laboratory, who developed a radio-

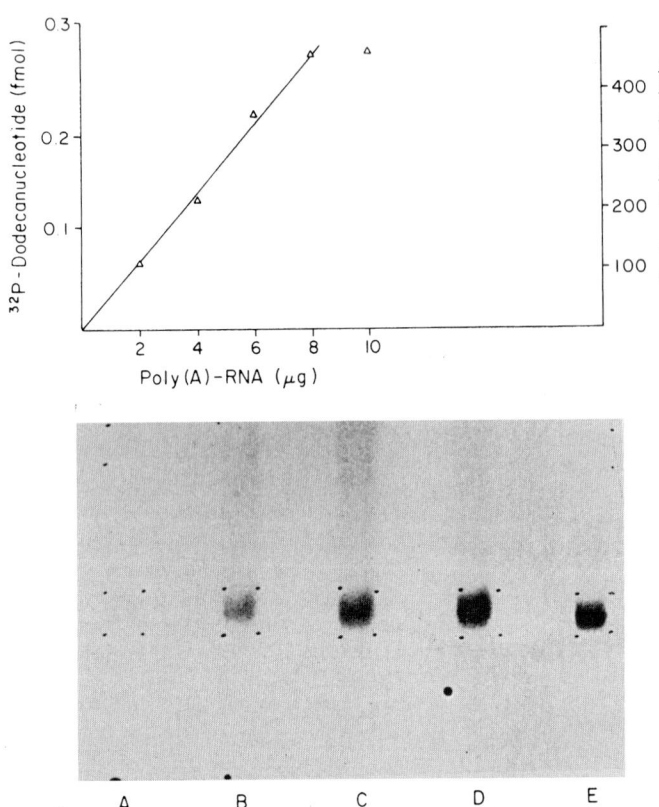

Fig. 8–5. Hybridization of ^{32}P-dodecanucleotide with increasing amounts of hog antral poly (A)-RNA. Different amounts of poly (A)-RNA from hog antrums, (A) 2 μg, (B) 4 μg, (C) 6 μg, (D) 8 μg, and (E) 10 μg were separated by agarose gel electrophoresis, immobilized on DBM paper, and hybridized with ^{32}P-dodecanucleotide-II (2.56 × 106 cpm/pmol) for 48 h at 23°C. Following autoradiography, the radioactive spots were cut out and counted. The data are plotted in the upper portion of the figure. Reproduced with permission from Mevarech M, Noyes B, Agarwal KL: Detection of gastric-specific mRNA using oligodeoxynucleotide probes of defined sequence. Biol Chem 254:7472, 1979.

immunoassay for glycine-extended gastrin processing intermediates and determined their presence in relatively high concentrations in both tissues and in the circulation (58,59). It appeared that the dibasic residues are cleaved by specific enzymes and then glycine-extended processing intermediates of gastrin are formed. In other experiments previously conducted by Derek Smythe and by Elizabeth Eipper and Richard Mains, the nature of the reaction that forms a carboxyl-terminal amide residue from the glycine moiety was determined to be a two-step reaction involving copper and molecular oxygen as co-factors in a mono-oxygenase type reaction (60). The substrate specificities for these reactions relative to gastrin were determined in a series of experiments conducted by Chris Dickinson and Toshiyuki Takeuchi in Yamada's laboratory (61–63).

The significance of the post-translational reactions appears to be that it is another means by which hormonal expression and action can be regulated. Different molecular

forms of peptide hormones may have different biological activities at various sites. Thus, the production of the numerous gastrin molecular forms in varying concentrations may influence the site specific effects of the circulating peptides. Both John DelValle, in Yamada's laboratory, and investigators in Jens Rehfield's laboratory have confirmed that there may be defects in post-translational processing in Zollinger-Ellison tumors that may account for different ratios of the processing intermediates in the circulation and in tumor tissues (64,65).

The availability of the gastrin cDNA has permitted numerous investigators to study the regulation of gastrin gene expression. Initial studies focused on the measurement of gastrin mRNA content by various physiologic stimuli as noted previously. Stephen Brand capitalized on the cloning of the rat gastrin gene in his laboratory to characterize the regulatory elements controlling gastrin gene transcription. He observed that a developmentally regulated transfactor

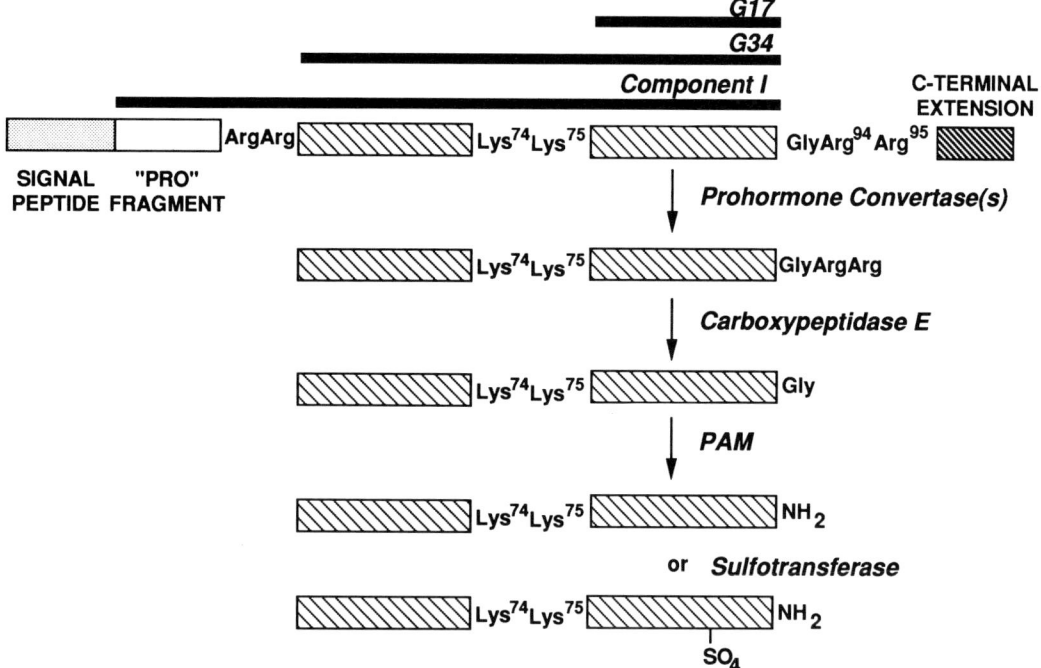

Fig. 8–6. Schematic representation of gastrin processing. The signal peptide that directs preprogastrin to the endoplasmic reticulum is depicted as a stippled box. Three dibasic cleavage sites are shown. GLY^{93} is the carboxyl-terminal amino acid remaining after carboxypeptidase removal of Arg^{94} and Arg^{95} and serves as the precursor for formation of the biologically active Phe^{92}-amidated gastrins.

binds to a specific portion of the gastrin gene regulatory element (66,67). He and his colleagues have gone on to define elements on the gastrin gene promoter/enhancer region that respond to epidermal growth factor and somatostatin (68,69). These experiments have been carried on by one of his former fellows, Timothy Wang, to transgenic animal studies. In his experiments, Wang determined that the evolution and development of islets of Langerhans in the pancreas was determined by the combination of gastrin and TGFα expression in the pancreas. These studies have provided the first insight into the functional importance of fetal pancreatic gastrin expression (70).

THE GOLDEN AGE OF GASTRIN CELL BIOLOGY

Grossman, who pioneered much of the early work on the physiology of gastrin in the stomach, postulated on the basis of in vivo dog studies the existence of multiple interactive receptors for secretagogues on gastric parietal cells. Numerous other investigators across the country had different ideas. In particular, Charles Code, the legendary physiologist at the Mayo Clinic, proposed the hypothesis that histamine was the final common mediator of acid secretion. According to his theory, if gastrin were to stimulate acid secretion, it did so by acting on an intermediary cell that secreted histamine (71). The confirmation of the hypothesis of either Grossman or Code depended upon the isolation of gastric parietal cells and the demonstration of the various receptors on them.

In the mid-1970s, a young physician-scientist, Andrew Soll, arrived in Morton Grossman's laboratory from the National Institutes of Health, where he had worked with Jessie Roth on the insulin receptor. Soll's goal was to isolate gastric parietal cells and to characterize the gastrin receptors on them. This process was a long and arduous one and involved multiple failed experiments. Finally, by using the new technique of counterflow elutriation, Soll was able to develop a parietal cell preparation of sufficient purity to determine function (22–25). Initially, he examined parietal cell activity by measuring oxygen consumption by these cells, but later he developed a technique to measure acid production by quantifying the uptake of a radiolabeled weak base, aminopyrine (26). This preparation provided gastrointestinal physiology with its first tool to examine events at a cellular level. Using it, Soll demonstrated first that parietal cells responded to histamine, carbachol, and gastrin as single agents. He further confirmed Grossman's potentiation hypothesis by demonstrating that the effects of histamine plus gastrin and histamine plus carbachol greatly exceeded the effects of the sum of the individual agents acting alone (Fig. 8–7).

These experiments provided evidence that gastrin acted directly on parietal cells

to stimulate acid secretion. Soll later went on to characterize the binding of radiolabeled gastrin canine parietal cells (72) and Masahiro Matsumoto in Yamada's laboratory demonstrated in crosslinking experiments that the receptor was a single subunit protein of 72 kilodaltons in size (73). Despite the findings Soll obtained using canine gastric parietal cells, there was still considerable controversy over whether gastrin acted directly or indirectly to stimulate acid secretion. Thomas Berglindh in Sweden, almost simultaneously with Soll, had used another preparation, that of isolated rabbit gastric glands, to demonstrate that histamine stimulated aminopyrine uptake by parietal cells; however, he was unable to observe any effect with gastrin (74). This led him to conclude that gastrin had no direct effect on acid secretion. The controversy has persisted for well over 10 years at this point, and there is still no clear resolution. The general consensus is that there might be a species difference between the dog and the rabbit, although there are some concerns that the gastric gland preparation is relatively impure and may contain inhibitors of acid secretion that might be stimulated by gastrin at the same time that gastrin stimulates acid secretion from the parietal cell. Tsutomu Chiba (75), in Yamada's laboratory at Michigan, and Catherine Chew, at the Morehouse School of Medicine in Atlanta, Georgia (76) conducted a series of experiments to indicate that gastrin induces the turnover of membrane in inositol phospholipids and activates a calcium signal in gastric parietal cells. John DelValle took these experiments one step further by demonstrating the mobilization of intracellular calcium and the influx of extracellular calcium by gastrin in single isolated parietal cells from both dogs and rabbits (Fig. 8–8) (77). Thus, there was proof that gastrin has a direct effect on parietal cells and that species differences could not account for the differences of the observations of Soll and Berglindh. The controversy that remains is whether this effect of gastrin accounts for all of the acid secretion stimulated by gastrin. The evidence to suggest that gastrin's actions are mediated in large part by the effects of histamine derive from studies in both man and dogs that gastrin-stimulated acid secretion can be inhibited virtually

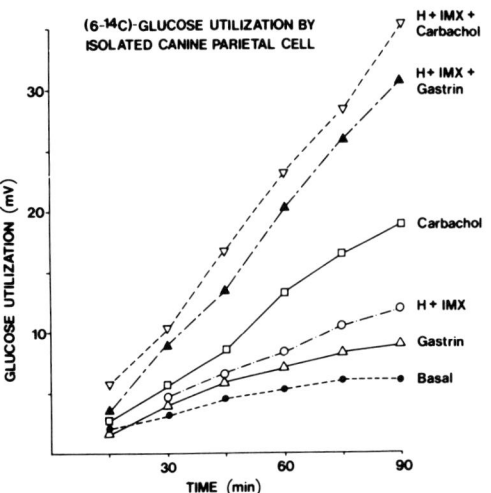

Fig. 8–7. Glucose oxidation by isolated canine parietal cells. Parital cells were incubated in presence of 10 μm histamine (H) = 100 μm isobutylmethylxanthine (IMX), 10 nm gastrin, or 100 μm carbachol, as indicated. The oxidation of [^{14}C]glucose was continuously monitored using a vibrating reed ionization chamber technique. Reproduced with permission from Soll AH, Davidson W. *In* Johnson LR (ed): Physiology of the Gastrointestinal Tract. 2nd ed. New York, Raven Press, 1987.

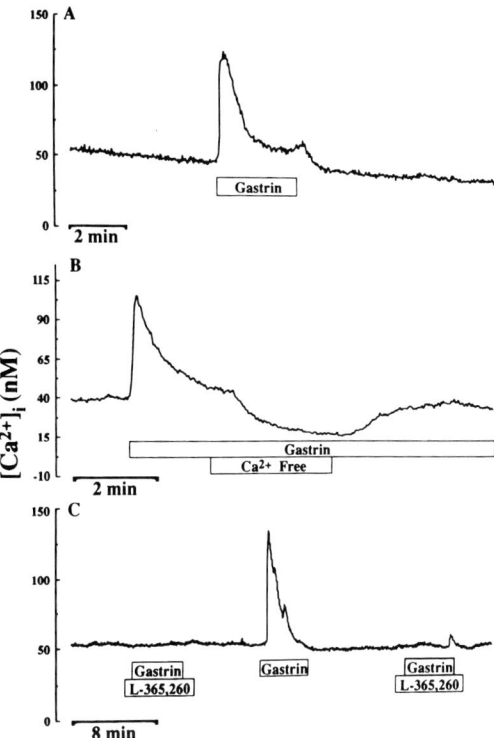

Fig. 8–8. Characterization of gastrin (10^{-9} M)-mediated mobilization of $[Ca^{2+}]i$ in single isolated canine parietal cells. A: biphasic effect of gastrin on parietal cell $[Ca^{2+}]_i$. B: sustained rise in $[Ca^{2+}]_i$ is reversibly abolished by removal of extracellular Ca^{2+}. C: gastrin's effect on parietal cell $[Ca^{2+}]_i$ was inhibited by the selective cholecystokinin-gastrin receptor antagonist L 365260 (10^{-7} M). Data shown are representative of 5 separate experiments obtained from 3 animal preparations. Reproduced with permission from DelValle J, Tsunoda Y, Williams JA, Yamada T: Regulation of $[Ca^{2a}]i$ by secretagogue stimulation of canine gastric parietal cells. Am J Physiol 262:G240, 1992.

completely by the application of H2 histamine receptor antagonists. On the other hand, if the potentiation hypothesis put forward by Soll and Grossman is correct, one would expect that blockade of one limb of a potentiating interaction would be sufficient to have a far greater inhibitory effect than might be expected. This controversy cannot be resolved without further experimentation in whole animals.

Major recent developments have focused on the isolation and characterization of the gastrin receptor structure. Once gastrin receptors were identified on parietal cells, numerous groups throughout the world focused on an effort to isolate the gene encoding it. One approach taken by Ira Gantz, a surgeon working in Yamada's laboratory, was to capitalize on the structural homology between members of the family of receptors that appear to be coupled to guanine nucleotide binding proteins (G-proteins). These G protein-linked receptors have a common structural theme in that they consist of a single long protein that traverses the plasma membrane seven times. There is remarkable homology between members of the family, particularly in their transmembrane regions. Gantz's approach towards isolation of the gastrin receptor gene was to construct oligonucleotides specific for regions of homology between G protein-linked receptors in their third and sixth transmembranes. He then used these degenerate oligonucleotides, in a technique first described by Vassart and colleagues in Belgium (78), to prime a polymerase chain reaction using cDNA obtained from messenger RNA of isolated canine gastric parietal cells. Much to the investigators' dismay, they were unsuccessful in obtaining the gastrin receptor gene. As a consolation, they were delighted to have discovered the gene encoding the H2 histamine receptor (79). Another group of investigators headed by Alan Kopin at Tufts University used a completely different method to clone the gastrin receptor gene (80). Their approach was to screen with a radiolabeled gastrin ligand a library of complementary DNA from dog stomachs that was expressed in COS cells (a kidney cell line derived from monkeys). The presumption was that the expressed receptor would be detectable by autoradiography once the ligand bound to it. After screening several hundred thousand clones, Kopin and his colleagues were successful in their search for a single clone that encoded a gastrin receptor (Fig. 8–9). Having obtained the receptor, they proved by biochemical and pharmacologic analysis that the receptor they had expressed was identical to the parietal cell gastrin receptor so well characterized by others. Il Song, in Yamada's laboratory, has since cloned the gene encoding the gastrin receptor and determined that, unlike most other genes en-

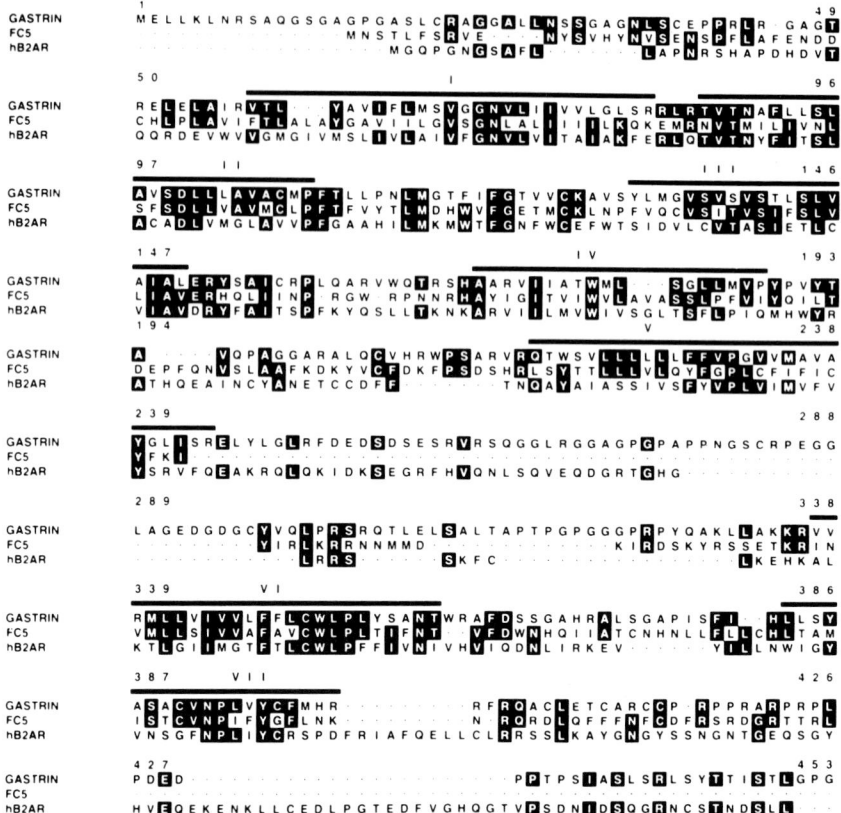

Fig. 8–9. Primary structure of the canine parietal cell gastrin receptor and alignment with known G protein-coupled receptors. Shaded amino acids are identical in at least two of the three receptors. Bars over sequences represent transmembrane segments predicted by the Klein-Kanehisa-DeLisi algorithm. Numbering corresponds to amino acids in the gastrin receptor. FC5, neuropeptide Y-Y1 receptor: hB2AR, human β_2-adrenergic receptor. Reproduced with permission from Kopin AS et al.: Expression cloning and characterization of the canine parietal cell gastrin receptor. Proc Natl Acad Sci USA *89*:3605, 1992.

coding seven transmembrane G protein-linked receptors, the gastrin receptor gene has numerous introns (81). The gene consists of six exons and five introns and has been localized on a region of chromosome 11 (chromosome 11p15.4). Most interestingly, it appears that the gene produces two different receptor proteins as a result of alternative RNA splicing. The functional differences of the two receptors have yet to be established.

CONCLUSION

Peptide hormones of the gut, the very chemical messengers that signal information from one part of the body to the other, play a critical role in the physiology of the gastrointestinal tract in health and disease. The history of gastrointestinal hormones, as exemplified by the history of gastrin, is intimately intertwined with the evolution of biomedical science in general. Each key concept and technology that has had enormous importance in biomedical science also has had an impact on the field of gastrointestinal endocrinology. Although the story of gastrin provided is not meant to be complete, it indicates how the combination of the right people at the right time has resulted in our current state of knowledge on the subject. As in all subjects of history, the story of the events as they unfolded is fascinating to those people who are involved in the field. Hopefully, they will provide insight on the background from which gastroenterologists treat their patients today.

ACKNOWLEDGMENTS

We are grateful to D. Hall for assistance in typing the manuscript. The valuable insights and advice of Drs. Horace Davenport and Graham Dockray are gratefully acknowledged. This work was supported by NIH grants RO1-DK34306 and RO1-DK33500, as well as funds from the University of Michigan Gastrointestinal Peptide Research Center (NIH grant P30-DK34933). Dr. Todisco is a recipient of a Senior Research Fellowship Award from the American Gastroenterological Association.

REFERENCES

1. Bayliss WM, Starling EH: The mechanism of pancreatic secretion. J Physiol 28:325, 1902.
2. Pavlov IP: The Work of the Digestive Glands. 2nd English Ed. London, Chas. Griffin & Co., Ltd., 1910.
3. Davenport HW: A History of Gastric Secretion and Digestion. Experimental Studies to 1975. New York, Oxford University Press, 1992.
4. Starling EH: The chemical correlation of the functions of the body. Lancet ii:339, 1905.
5. Edkins JS: On the chemical mechanisms of gastric secretion. Proc Roy Soc 76:376, 1905.
6. Mutt V, Jorpes J: Structure of porcine cholecystokinin-pancreozymin. Eur J Biochem 6:156, 1968.
7. Mutt V, Jorpes JE, Magnusson S: Structure of porcine secretin. Eur J Biochem 15:513, 1970.
8. Gregory RA, Tracy HJ: The constitution and properties of two gastrins extracted from hog antral mucosa. Gut 5:103, 1964.
9. Gregory H et al.: Structure of gastrin. Nature 204:931, 1964.
10. Tatemoto K: Isolation and characterization of peptide YY (PYY), a candidate gut hormone that inhibits pancreatic exocrine secretion. Proc Natl Acad Sci USA 79:2514, 1982.
11. Tatemoto K, Mutt V: Isolation of two novel candidate hormones using a chemical method for finding naturally occurring polypeptides. Nature 285:417, 1980.
12. Tatemoto K: Neuropeptide Y: Complete amino acid sequence of the brain peptide. Proc Natl Acad Sci USA 79:5485, 1982.
13. Tatemoto K, Carlquist M, Mutt V: Neuropeptide Y—a novel brain peptide with structural similarities to peptide YY and pancreatic polypeptide. Nature 296:659, 1982.
14. Tatemoto K, Mutt V: Chemical determination of polypeptide hormones. Proc Natl Acad Sci USA 75:4115, 1978.
15. Tatemoto K, Mutt V: Isolation of two novel candidate hormones using a chemical method for finding naturally occurring polypeptides. Nature 285:417, 1980.
16. Tatemoto K, Mutt V: Isolation and characterization of the intestinal peptide porcine PHI (PHI-27), a new member of the glucagon-secretin family. Proc Natl Acad Sci USA 78:6603, 1981.
17. Tatemoto K et al.: Galanin—a novel biologically active peptide from porcine intestine. FEBS Lett 164:124, 1983.
18. Berson SA, Yalow RS: Isotopic tracers in the study of diabetes. In Lawrence JH, Tobias CA (eds): Advances in Biological and Medical Physics. New York, Academic Press Inc, 1958.
19. Yalow RS, Berson SA: Assay of plasma insulin in human subjects by immunological methods. Nature 184:1648, 1959.
20. Itoh N, Obata K, Yanaihara N, Okamoto H: Human preprovasoactive intestinal polypeptide contains a novel PHI-27 like peptide, PHM-27. Nature 304:547, 1983.
21. Rosenfeld MG et al.: Production of a novel neuropeptide encoded by the calcitonin gene via tissue-specific RNA processing. Nature 304:129, 1983.
22. Soll AH: The isolated mammalian parietal cell: Actions and interactions of secretagogues. Gastroenterology 70:794, 1976.
23. Soll AH: Isolated mammalian parietal cells: Effects of atropine (A) and metiamide (M) on the actions and instructions of secretagogues. Gastroenterology 72:824, 1976.
24. Soll AH: The actions of secretagogues on oxygen uptake by isolated mammalian parietal cells. J Clin Invest 61:370, 1978.

25. Soll AH: The interaction of histamine with gastrin and carbamylcholine on oxygen uptake by isolated mammalian parietal cells. J Clin Invest *61*:381, 1978.

26. Soll AH: Secretagogue stimulation of ^{14}C-aminopyrine accumulation by isolated canine parietal cells. Am J Physiol *238*:G366, 1980.

27. Soll AH, Yamada T, Park J, Thomas LP: Release of somatostatin-like immunoreactivity from canine fundic mucosal cells in primary culture. Am J Physiol *247*:G-558, 1984.

28. Sugano K, Park J, Soll AH, Yamada T: Stimulation of gastrin release by bombesin and canine gastrin-releasing peptides. J Clin Invest *79*:935, 1987.

29. Davenport HW: A History of Gastric Secretion and Digestion. Experimental studies to 1975. New York, Oxford University Press, 1992, p. 153.

30. Grossman MI, Robertson CR, Ivy AC: Proof of a hormonal mechanism for gastric secretion. The humoral transmission of the distention stimulus. Am J Physiol *153*:1, 1948.

31. Boyle JD, Grossman MI: An oral history. Gastroenterology *83*:285, 1982.

32. Gillespie IE, Grossman MI: Potentiation between urecholine and gastrin extract and between urecholine and histamine in the stimulations of Heidenhain pouches. Gut *5*:71, 1964.

33. Komarov SA: Gastrin. Proc Soc Exp Biol Med *38*:514, 1938.

34. Komarov SA: Methods of isolation of a specific gastric secretagogue from the pyloric mucous membrane and its chemical properties. Rev Canad Biol *I*:191, 1942.

35. Davenport HW: A History of Gastric Secretion and Digestion. Experimental studies to 1975. New York, Oxford University Press, 1992, p. 222.

36. Gregory RA et al.: Human gastrin: Isolation, structure and synthesis. Nature *209*:583, 1966.

37. McGuigan JE: Immunochemical studies with synthetic human gastrin. Gastroenterology *54*:1005, 1968.

38. Hansky J, Cain HJ: Radioimmunoassay of gastrin in human serum. Lancet *ii*:1388, 1969.

39. Charters AC et al.: Gastrin: Immunochemical properties and measurement by radioimmunoassay. Surgery *66*:104, 1969.

40. Yalow RS, Berson SA: Radioimmunoassay of gastrin. Gastroenterology *58*:1, 1970.

41. Yalow RS, Berson SA: Further studies on the nature of immunoreactive gastrin in human plasma. Gastroenterology *60*:203, 1971.

42. Zollinger RM, Ellison EH: Primary peptic ulcerations of the jejunum associated with islet cell tumors of the pancreas. Ann Surg *142*:4, 709, 1955.

43. Gregory RA: Gastrin—The natural history of a peptide hormone. Harvey Lectures *64*: 121, 1968.

44. McGuigan JE, Trudeau WL: Immunochemical measurement of elevated levels of gastrin in the serum of patients with pancreatic tumors of the Zollinger-Ellison variety. N Engl J Med *278*:1308, 1968.

45. McGuigan JE: The Zollinger-Ellison Syndrome. *In* Sleisenger MH, Fordtran JS (eds): Gastrointestinal Disease, 4th Ed. Philadelphia, WB Saunders Co., 1989.

46. Berson SA, Yalow RS: Nature of immunoreactive gastrin extracted from tissues of the gastrointestinal tract. Gastroenterology *60*: 215, 1971.

47. Rehfeld JF, Stadil F, Vikelsoe J: Immunoreactive gastrin components in human serum. Gut *15*:102, 1975.

48. Yalow RS, Berson SA: And now, big big gastrin. Biochem Biophys Res Commun *48*:391, 1972.

49. Yalow RS, Wu N: Additional studies on the nature of big big gastrin. Gastroenterology *65*:19, 1973.

50. Gregory RA, Tracy HJ: *In* JC Thompson (ed): Gastrointestinal Hormones. A Symposium. Austin and London, University of Texas Press, 1975.

51. Noyes BE et al.: Detection and partial sequence analysis of gastrin mRNA by using an oligodeoxynucleotide probe. Proc Natl Acad Sci USA *76*:4, 1770, 1979.

52. Yoo OJ, Powell CT, Agarwal KL: Molecular cloning and nucleotide sequence of full-length cDNA coding for porcine gastrin. Proc Natl Acad Sci USA *79*:1049, 1982.

53. Boel E et al.: Molecular cloning of human gastrin cDNA: Evidence for evolution of gastrin by gene duplication. Proc Natl Acad Sci USA *80*:2866, 1983.

54. Mevarech M, Noyes B, Agarwal KL: Detection of gastric-specific mRNA using oligodeoxynucleotide probes of defined sequence. J Biol Chem *254*:7472, 1979.

55. Wu V et al.: Regulation of rat antral gastrin and somatostatin gene expression during starvation and after refeeding. Gastroenterology *101*:1552, 1991.

56. Brand SJ, Stone D: Reciprocal regulation of antral gastrin and somatostatin gene expression by omeprazole-induced achlorhydria. J Clin Invest *82*:1059, 1988.

57. Karnik PS, Monahan SJ, Wolfe MM: Inhibition of gastrin gene expression by somatostatin. J Clin Invest *83*:367, 1989.

58. DelValle J, Sugano K, Yamada T: Glycine-

extended processing intermediates of gastrin and cholecystokinin in human plasma. Gastroenterology *97*:1159, 1989.

59. Sugano K, Aponte GW, Yamada T: Identification and characterization of glycine-extended post-translational processing intermediates of progastrin in porcine stomach. J Biol Chem *260*:11724, 1985.

60. Eipper BA et al.: Structure of the precursor to an enzyme mediating COOH-terminal amidation in peptide biosynthesis. Mol Endocrinol *I*:777, 1987.

61. Daugherty DF et al.: Expression and processing of human preprogastrin in murine medullary thyroid carcinoma cells. Am J Physiol *260*:G783, 1991.

62. Marino LR, Takeuchi T, Dickinson CJ, Yamada T: Expression and post-translational processing of gastrin in heterologous endocrine cells. J Biol Chem *266*:6133, 1990.

63. Dickinson CJ, Yamada T: Gastrin-amidating enzyme in the porcine pituitary and antrum. J Biol Chem *266*:334, 1991.

64. DelValle J, Sugano K, Yamada T: Progastrin and its glycine-extended post-translational processing intermediates in human gastrointestinal tissue. Gastroenterology *92*:1908, 1987.

65. Rehfeld JF, Stadil F: Gel filtration studies on immunoreactive gastrin in serum from Zollinger-Ellison patients. Gut *14*:369, 1973.

66. Brand SJ, Wang TC: Gastrin gene expression and regulation in rat islet cell lines. J Biol Chem *263*:16597, 1988.

67. Wang TC, Brand SJ: Islet cell-specific regulatory domain in the gastrin promoter contains adjacent positive and negative DNA elements. J Biol Chem *265*:8908, 1990.

68. Goodley JM, Brand SJ: Regulation of the gastrin promoter by epidermal growth factor and neuropeptides. Proc Natl Acad Sci USA *86*:3036, 1989.

69. Merchant JL, Demediuk B, Brand SJ: A GC-rich element confers epidermal growth factor responsiveness to transcription from the gastrin promoter. Mol Cell Biol *11*:2686, 1991.

70. Wang TC et al.: Gastrin promotes islet cell growth through interactions with transforming growth factor alfa. (Abstract). Regul Pept *40*:275, 1992.

71. Davenport HW: A History of Gastric Secretion and Digestion. Experimental studies to 1975. New York, Oxford University Press, 1992, p. 185.

72. Soll AH et al.: Gastrin receptors on isolated canine parietal cells. J Clin Invest *73*:1434, 1984.

73. Matsumoto M, Park J, Yamada T: Gastrin receptor characterization: Affinity cross-linking of the gastrin receptor on canine gastric parietal cells. Am J Physiol *252*:G143, 1987.

74. Berglindh T, Helander HF, Obrink KJ: Effects of secretagogues on oxygen consumption, aminopyrine accumulation and morphology in isolated gastric glands. Acta Physiol Scand *97*:401, 1976.

75. Chiba T et al.: Carbamoylcholine and gastrin induced inositol phospholipid turnover in canine gastric parietal cells. Am J Physiol *255*:G99, 1988.

76. Chew CS, Brown MR: Release of intracellular Ca^{2+} and elevation of inositol triphosphate by secretagogues in parietal and chief cells isolated from rabbit gastric mucosa. Biochem Biophys Acta *888*:116, 1986.

77. DelValle J, Tsunoda Y, Williams JA, Yamada T: Regulation of $[Ca^{2a}]i$ by secretagogue stimulation of canine gastric parietal cells. Am J Physiol *262*:G240, 1992.

78. Libert F et al.: Selective amplification and cloning of four new members of the G protein-coupled receptor family. Science *244*:569, 1989.

79. Gantz I et al.: Molecular cloning of a gene encoding the histamine H2 receptor. Proc Natl Acad Sci USA *88*:429, 1991.

80. Kopin AS et al.: Expression cloning and characterization of the canine parietal cell gastrin receptor. Proc Natl Acad Sci USA *89*:3605, 1992.

81. Song IL et al.: The human gastrin (cholecystokinin B) receptor gene: Alternative splice donor site in exon 4 generates two variant mRNAs. Proc Natl Acad Sci USA (in press), 1993.

9

History of the Evolution of Ideas in Gastrointestinal Motility

JAMES CHRISTENSEN

THE 19TH CENTURY VIEW

The subject matter of gastrointestinal motility involves a broad range of disciplines. Modern knowledge of the subject therefore awaited advances in a great many basic science topics, including neurosciences, smooth muscle physiology, and gastrointestinal endocrinology. Understanding depended also on the full development of techniques, for methods always limit comprehension. For this reason, the subject flowered rather late in the history of physiology, and then very quickly.

No one knows exactly when the motions of the gut became a matter for serious study. The haruspices, those Greek and Roman diviners whose augury involved the inspection of the viscera of freshly sacrificed animals, must have noticed the entrails moving and may have wondered what meaning those motions might have beyond the magical. And one can imagine that primitive people recognized that eating is somehow related to defecation and surmised that a flow occurred from the mouth to the anus.

But a history requires a more definite starting point. For gastrointestinal motility, Francois Magendie's *Précís Elémentaire de Physiologie* from 1816–17 (1), one of the first textbooks of physiology, can serve that purpose because Magendie had much to say about the matter. And little changed from his time until the 20th century began.

Magendie wrote very early in the history of biology. One of the pioneers in introduc-

ing the rationalism of science (which he called "Baconian induction") into physiology, he wrote his book to report what he had himself observed. Magendie wrote even before the era of histology, when the enteric nervous system remained undiscovered. But his book seems a fair representation of the state of knowledge when the serious study of physiology was just beginning.

He knew that muscles of the lips, cheeks, tongue, and jaws are somatic ("like the muscles of locomotion"), and he recognized that those of the pharynx, palate, and esophagus are different, functioning "without the participation of the will."

He considered swallowing in three phases, the passage of food from mouth to pharynx, its passage through the pharynx, and its movement through the esophagus. He described the motions of the tongue and palate in the first phase of deglutition and of the larynx and hyoid in the second. He knew of the motions of the epiglottis, and denied that it protects the airway from penetration. He gave the third phase, esophageal peristalsis, much less confident and accurate treatment. He considered the esophagus to be no more than an extension of the pharynx, and did not recognize either the cricopharyngeus muscle or its physiologic equivalent, the upper esophageal sphincter. He knew that the behavior of the caudal part of the esophagus differs somewhat from that of the cephalic part. He thought that the bolus is thrust into the esophagus by the pharynx, dilating the esophagus and so exciting fibers of the circular muscle layer above the bolus to contract. This contraction pushes the bolus to a more caudal level, he thought, where distention similarly excites contraction upstream. He seemed here to be anticipating the concept of the peristaltic reflex. Sometimes he saw the bolus ascend the esophagus. He did not know of the lower esophageal sphincter as such. He described it, instead, as a muscular structure, which he believed to be a unique feature of the horse, thinking that it was somehow responsible for the inability of a horse to vomit.

He believed that intragastric pressure rises in direct proportion to gastric filling, and that this "packing" of the stomach requires the presence of unusually strong muscles in the esophagus. He denied the existence of gastric peristalsis. He believed that food remains in the stomach for several hours, and described contractions that press the food from one end of the stomach to the other, in both directions. He claimed that vagotomy does not paralyze the stomach.

He described ring contractions in the small intestine as irregular, involuntary, returning at variable periods, moving sometimes in one direction and sometimes in the other, and occurring simultaneously all along the intestine. He believed that the valvulae conniventes, certain other "aspérities," and the bendings of the canal all retard antegrade flow so that the movement of ingesta is slow and the time of residence in the intestine is long.

Magendie recognized the ileocecal junction as a special region, calling it a "valve" and recognizing its ability to prevent retrograde flow. He described fecal matter as remaining for a long time in the cecum before passing into the colon. He knew that the passage of feces along the colon is very slow and that the contractions of the colonic muscle produce the flow. He recognized the reservoir function of the rectum and the presence of a special muscle structure in the anal canal, which he actually called a "sphincter." He gave the colon itself no place in the expulsion of feces, describing defecation as the result of abdominal and diaphragmatic contractions which compress the rectum to expel its contents through the small opening of the anus.

Much of what Magendie described is related to swallowing and defecation, the two processes that he could observe directly without experimental intervention. He had to study newly killed animals while the gut was still moving to see motions of the esophagus, stomach, and intestine, and the defects of such a crude experimental method show in what he was able to say.

Science relies first of all upon methods. Magendie saw only what he was able to see. One can take his description as the standard of knowledge of the time. Magendie could see very little of gastrointestinal motility, but he tried to interpret what he saw rationally. Magendie used "Baconian induction" to perceive the three essential elements of gastrointestinal motility as separable areas of study. These are *flows,* the *wall motions* that produce these flows, and the *elements in control* of these wall movements.

THE DEVELOPMENT OF METHODS

The Observation of Flows

Aside from Beaumont's famous opportunity in the 1830s in his patient with a gastric fistula (2), no one had any way to examine directly the flow in any part of the gut until more than 50 years later. Beaumont could only make a crude evaluation of gastric flow because his patient's fistula extended into the fundus, and so Beaumont's experiments on flow depended on the measurements of residual volumes collected by aspiration. And gastric emptying was not his major interest. He was more interested in gastric juice and digestion.

The great impetus to the study of flow came with the development of the x-ray tube at the end of the 19th century. Roentgen's development of the concepts and methods for x-ray soon found application in the study of gastrointestinal flow. The pioneers were Bowditch (3) and Cannon, who examined the stomach and intestine by contrast radiography before the turn of the century (4,5). Cannon and others were mainly interested in gastric motility and, indeed, adopted contrast radiography as a new means to study it. They could actually see peristalsis and flow from the stomach. The legacy of Beaumont had created an enormous curiosity about the stomach, and so it was mainly curiosity about gastric flow that drove Cannon and other physiologists, but soon physicians recognized the ability of contrast radiography to demonstrate morphologic lesions in the stomach as well. Hurst (6,7) mainly led this advance in the clinical use of radiography. Not too long afterward, the use of contrast films to observe flow extended to the other organs, including the colon. The biggest problem in the study of flow in the stomach and intestine was the need for rapid changes of film, a need that was fully resolved only when rapid film-changers and cineradiography developed much later.

By 1933, radiographic techniques had revealed so much that an authoritative textbook could be written on the digestive tract from the point of view of the radiologist (8). It contained extensive descriptions of flows in all the organs as well as descriptions of peristaltic wall movements and morphologic abnormalities. Indeed, the descriptions appear quite modern to the contemporary reader.

The limitations of radiographic methods to reveal normal physiology received little notice in the period of the development of methodology. Observations by contrast radiography are hard to quantify, cannot easily be repeated for verification, are usually performed with the subject fasting, and use a remarkably unphysiologic material as the tracer. These problems of radiography to demonstrate motility were overcome only with the development of scintigraphy in the 1980s (9). Scintigraphy made it feasible to do flow studies in routine clinical practice, and it made flow study much more sensitive, but it added little to the fundamental concepts of gastrointestinal flow.

Before the advent of scintigraphy, Hunt had developed a beautifully simple and direct method to advance understanding of gastric emptying, especially of its regulation (10). He used test meals—liquid volumes of variable composition—passed through a nasogastric tube in various volumes and aspirated at variable times afterward to discover the residual volume. He used unanesthetized human subjects, studying the same subjects (including himself) repeatedly because habituation eliminates the inhibition produced by anxiety. Thus, he was able to develop data for the rate of gastric emptying as it is regulated by meal composition, without specific regard to the details of intragastric flows or patterns of wall movements. Hunt's now-classical experiments and concepts remain unsurpassed. They are well summarized in Physiology of the Gastrointestinal Tract (11).

Most discussions of flow in the gut have dealt with bulk flows, the mass translocations of fluid, rather than with microflows. Interest in microflows came about from theoretic considerations of intestinal absorption, in which the presence of an unstirred layer at the luminal surface of the intestine came to be recognized as a limitation to the rate of absorption. Little can be done to study microflows directly, however, because it requires the use of the principles of fluid mechanics, a discipline that is largely as foreign to gastrointestinal physiologists as gastrointestinal physiology is foreign to fluid-mechanicists.

The only efforts to study intestinal flow in any detail beyond bulk flow arose entirely from the initiatives of a fluid mechanicist, Macagno, who was simply curious about flow in a system that seemed unique to him. His extensive experience had focused on flow in rivers and seas. A fluid-mechanical approach to flow in the small intestine by Christensen and Macagno yielded a host of new methods and ideas in the 1970s (12), but the subject languished thereafter. The foundation for a rigorous rheologic study of gastrointestinal microflow was laid then, but it remains to be exploited more fully.

The Observation of Pressures

Magendie knew the general motor function of the gut even if he was not at all clear about the kinds of motions that took place in those regions that he could not see. The radiographers of the early part of this century could estimate rates of transit, and they could see at least the front sides of the peristaltic waves. But they could not easily quantify what they saw, nor could they delineate the sphincters. The concepts of peristalsis and of sphincters existed long before the capacity to demonstrate them more fully became available.

The idea that one could study wall motions by the measurement of pressures in the gut lumen, by kymography (or manometry, as it came to be called later), arose quite early, even before the development of radiographic methods to study flow. It began largely with the use of balloons inflated in the stomach and intestine simply to see what could be discovered, a method used notably by Bayliss and Starling (13), Carlson (14), and Thomas (15), among others. Investigators could record pressure changes in such balloons easily enough, but they had much trouble in interpreting the records. They slowly came to confront the problems of balloon recording, which seem so obvious to us today. The size of the balloon, the degree to which it changes position, the degree to which it stretches the viscus wall, the compressibility of the recording fluid, and the compliance of the system all restrict the reliability of conclusions about the external forces that alter the pressure in such a closed recording system.

The idea of using open-tip catheters rather than balloons to record pressures was explored in the 1920s, but it was most aggressively developed in the 1950s mainly to examine the esophagus. The principal players in this development, which included Code (16) and Ingelfinger, probably sought, at the outset, simply to measure pressures rather than to fully map peristaltic movements. At first, they used air-filled catheters, later changing to water-filled tubes. At some point, they adopted catheters with distal openings placed laterally rather than at the tips of the catheters and observed that, in the esophagus, they could measure the characteristics of peristalsis—velocity and force of contraction—with apparent reproducibility and accuracy. The method was soon improved by Dodds (17) and Hogan and many others. They introduced the continuous perfusion of the catheters with a low-compliance pump (the Arndorfer pump, developed by a colleague of Dodds) and other changes, and the technique soon passed into standard clinical use to describe esophageal motor functions. The technique subsequently has found use in the small intestine, much less so in the stomach and colon. Subsequent experimentation with methods led to developments of much more complex devices in which pressures are measured from miniature pressure transducers mounted on flexible catheters.

These devices, combined with computer-aided analysis of pressure patterns, now promise objective long-term monitoring of motility in all organs. A pressure transducer mounted on a radio signal generator, the "radio-pill," has also found use. Such devices hold the prospect for the demonstration of new motor disorders.

Perfusion manometry and other methods for pressure measurement brought a new importance to the concept of sphincters. Long before the method was developed, physiologists had debated the very existence of sphincters because, aside from the external anal sphincter, the structures could not be directly observed and radiography was scarcely able to show them satisfactorily. Manometry, however, made it possible to define them quite specifically, to describe their dimensions, the timing of their opening and closure, and the force with which they occluded the lumen. Thus, both the upper esophageal sphincter and the esophagogastric sphincter were not clearly described until the mid-1950s. The application of a small balloon, the "Dent sleeve," named for its inventor, Dent, greatly facilitated the study of sphincters. Manometry then became the standard method to describe the function of a sphincter in vivo, and it remains the major clinical and investigative technique to study the sphincters, finding use especially in the esophagus and the anal canal.

The Observations of Wall Movements

Magendie knew what little he did know about the movements of the gut wall from the direct observation of the gut in the opened abdomen, and this remained a major method until after the end of the century, even receiving extensive discussion by Alvarez (18) as late as 1928! After that, the methods to examine flows and hence to infer wall movements (radiography and manometry) captured most of the attention.

The ability to observe wall movements more directly without the artifacts associated with the opening of the abdomen arose in the 1950s with the development of miniature force transducers that could be sewn to the gut wall. Wires from these transducers leading to chronically-implanted cutaneous plugs in experimental animals permitted investigators to record movements (mainly from the stomach and the intestine) over long periods under varying conditions (19,20). Investigators then further developed the use of electrodes implanted in the gut wall to record the electrical events in muscle associated with contractions. Electrodes had been used much earlier, by Alvarez and Mahoney (21), in the 1920s for example, but they were neglected for four decades (22), only to be salvaged for use, especially by Bass, when it was realized that electromyographic tracings greatly supplemented the tracings of wall movements made with chronically-implanted transducers. Now both implanted transducers and implanted electrodes find widespread use in chronic preparations in experimental animals. The obvious problem of providing high resolution is overcome by the use of multiple closely-spaced sensors.

The Observation of the Behavior of Gut Muscle In Vitro

The fact that bits of gut muscle immersed in a physiologic solution keep moving spontaneously led to the study of gut in vitro under various conditions as a means to discover how gut muscle works. Magnus (18), the first to use this method extensively at the beginning of the century, certainly had in mind the goal to understand the nature of the processes responsible for gastrointestinal motility, but that did not long remain the goal of others using the technique. As soon as it was discovered that gut muscle in vitro responds consistently and predictably to autonomic drugs, the use of such muscle preparations in vitro quickly became a standard assay method in the burgeoning field of autonomic pharmacology. The great majority of pharmacologists using preparations of gut muscle in vitro, over the next 50 years, showed little interest in the details of how the tissues were working, only in how they responded to autonomic agonists and antagonists. Differences in responses or in sensitivities between tissues, between guinea pig ileum and rat stomach, for example, certainly perplexed pharmacologists, but not enough that such differences prompted much explorations as to the reasons. Those using muscle preparations in vitro to study motility found themselves looked upon as foolish by others who studied gut motility in whole animals, a dichotomy which, although it never reached print, was apparent in informal discussions among workers in the field in the 1950s and 1960s. Alvarez, a remarkably eclectic investigator in the 1920s (18), wrote approvingly of the study of isolated bowel segments in vitro as a means to advance the understanding of many aspects of motility, but the idea remained so neglected that the approach was touted as a promising new one again in 1971 (23).

NERVES IN THE CONTROL OF GASTROINTESTINAL MOTILITY

The Dogmatic View—Its Origin and Destruction

The idea that nerves regulate gastrointestinal motility can be discerned in the writing of Magendie (1), who noted whether or not cutting the vagi (which he called "the eighth pair") influenced the motions of one organ or another. The idea that the vagus nerves and the sympathetic nerves differ substantially from somatic nerves dates back to the 18th century (24). Winslow introduced the term "sympathetic" to describe the thoracolumbar system in 1732, and as long ago as 1800, Bichat introduced the term *vegetative nervous system* to describe the nerves that contributed to what he conceived of as the organic or vegetative aspects of life, as opposed to the "animal" nerves, which he believed to be involved with animal functions (25). Out of the work of Gaskell, Langley, and others, the modern view of an *autonomic* system with sympathetic and parasympathetic subdivisions emerged around 1900, to persist to this day. The neuroanatomists of the mid-19th century discovered the intramural nerve plexuses and they soon were calling them the *enteric nervous system,* but the term fell out of use for a long time, only to be revived in recent times (25).

This evolution in terminology and anatomic concepts coincided with the evolution of physiologic understanding, so that knowledge of the functions of the enteric nerves matured at the same time that the structure of the enteric nerves became clearer. By about the time of the autonomic neuroanatomy texts of Kuntz (24) and Mitchell (26), anatomy and physiology had so stabilized as to constitute a unified theory that amounted to a virtual dogma, at least with respect to the way in which nerves regulate gastrointestinal motility. A major tenet of this dogma was the "one nerve-one transmitter" rule attributed to Sir Henry Dale, the concept that one type of axon releases one and only one kind of neurohormonal transmitter.

Neurohormonal transmission was not itself a concept that had found immediate acceptance. The idea that nerves form a syncytial union with the tissues they supply prevailed until the end of the 19th century, and the specific idea of neurohormonal transmission was still opposed by stubborn proponents of an electrotonic means of neuromuscular transmission as late as the 1940s. But the Dale hypothesis (not, perhaps, correctly attributed wholly to him) was certainly considered noncontroversial in the 1950s.

The view of nervous control of gut muscle that held from about 1930 for the next three decades proposed that a kind of yin-yang equilibrium prevails, in that two kinds of nerves impinge on gut muscle. The idea was that excitatory (parasympathetic and cholinergic) nerves are constantly opposed by inhibitory (sympathetic and adrenergic) nerves. Contraction occurs, according to this dogma, because of a dominant cholinergic innervation and ceases because of transient sympathetic nerve dominance. Peristaltic contractions, in this view, represent a reflex (the Bayliss-Starling "Law of the Intestine") in which a stimulus at one level excites excitatory (cholinergic) nerves above the stimulus and inhibitory (adrenergic) nerves below it. Sphincters, it was taught, are especially densely innervated and the nerves are reciprocal in effect to those in other regions. That is, cholinergic nerves relax and adrenergic nerves contract sphincters.

When Bayliss and Starling enunciated their "law of the intestine" in 1899, they expanded on an old idea already expressed by Magendie seven decades earlier, but their experiments, carried out in the small intestine, convinced everyone that it is the mechanism for peristalsis and for the con-

trol of sphincters. The rather uncritical acceptance of the implication that the organization of the myenteric plexus everywhere ensures contraction above and inhibition below a point of mechanical or chemical stimulation of the gut at any level undoubtedly delayed further study of motility for a long time. After about 1960, the concept of extrinsic reflexes, in which sensory stimulation of the gut excites responses in the gut through nerve pathways that traverse extrinsic nerve tracts, arose with the demonstration of vago-vagal reflexes inducing gastric accommodation to the volumes of ingesta and of sympathetic pathways through the prevertebral ganglia in colocolonic reflexes. The significance of extrinsic reflexes may have been overstated. Recent studies involving transplanted (and therefore extrinsically denervated) intestine and stomach indicate that their motor function, if not wholly normal, is sufficient to sustain life. This is an example of the principle of redundancy in biology. Several different systems exist side by side to ensure antegrade propulsion in the gastrointestinal tract. The polarity of the intrinsic innervation revealed by the Bayliss-Starling peristaltic reflex provides only one means for polarization.

Although these general ideas prevailed, certainly not everyone accepted them without question. Textbooks as late as the mid-century were vague or elusive about details of the dogma, but they stated one point categorically, that sympathetic axons end by arborizations around smooth muscle cells. This particular aspect of the dogma was shattered when Jacobowitz applied a new fluorescence technique for staining adrenergic nerve fibers to the gut (27). He found that adrenergic fibers are very sparse in the intramural plexuses and that most such fibers (as few as they are) end as arborizations around enteric ganglion cells and around intramural vessels. In fact, there is little or no direct adrenergic innervation of gut smooth muscle itself.

I may have overstated the degree of acceptance of this dogma. Certainly, many experts doubted the validity of such a simple scheme of the neural control of gastrointestinal motility, and so the finding of no direct adrenergic innervation of muscle did not shock everyone. Also, the finding was supported by evidence that came up at about the same time for the existence of another class of inhibitory nerve fibers. This evidence came from studies of muscle strips in vitro.

Magnus, who had first used muscle strips in vitro, was especially concerned with distinguishing myogenic from neurogenic controls (18). His methods did not allow him to do so. What he needed was a nerve-muscle preparation for gut smooth muscle like that which had been so useful in advancing knowledge of somatic muscle physiology. That is, he needed a way to stimulate the nerves without stimulating the smooth muscle at the same time.

Such a preparation came forth in the 1950s from the work of Paton (28,29). Paton, whose field was autonomic physiology and pharmacology, sought a method to investigate the release of acetylcholine from intestinal nerves. Because nerve-muscle preparations with somatic muscle had provided all the evidence on this matter in somatic nerves, it seemed logical to create a similar preparation for gut muscle. He developed a method to place the muscle strip in an electrical field in which, he found, he could obtain selective nerve stimulation at certain frequencies and pulse durations. Paton's technique of electrical field stimulation for the selective excitation of nerves within a smooth muscle mass found further application in the heart (30). But its effect in gastrointestinal motility was much more significant. It led to the discovery of a whole new class of inhibitory nerves, nerves of the greatest importance.

Paton's method, electrical field stimulation of isolated intestinal muscle preparations, did not at first inspire many others to use it, and the procedure languished for a time, perhaps because investigators were not wholly convinced. Only after the purification of the Pacific puffer fish poison, tetrodotoxin, was Paton's method fully accepted. This toxin, purified by toxicologists who sought to discover the method of action of this famous oriental poison (31), was found to block sodium channels but not calcium channels, and so it paralyzed nerves but had no effect on the excitation of contraction in smooth muscle. The poison quickly served to validate Paton's method as a means for selective neural excitation of gut muscle. Further, it provided a simple pharmacologic means to distinguish nerve effects in any preparations of gut muscle in vitro. Any action blocked by tetrodotoxin was, according to this new dogma, neurogenic.

The use of Paton's method and of tetrodotoxin together in many varieties of tissues quickly revealed inhibitory nerves in other organs that are not adrenergic (32). Furthermore, these nonadrenergic inhibitory nerves are not trivial. They seemed to be the major or even the exclusive intrinsic inhibitory nerves in many parts of the gut, in many species. They ultimately came to be called the nonadrenergic noncholinergic (NANC) nerves.

The Search for the NANC Neurohormonal Transmitter

In the early 1960s, everyone who demonstrated NANC nerves wondered what the transmitter might be and sought the possibilities by using the many autonomic receptor antagonists that pharmacologists had made available, mostly through their long interest in the pharmacotherapy of hypertension. Indeed, modern autonomic pharmacology developed almost wholly through the intense effort directed toward the treatment of hypertension in the years after World War II. Gastrointestinal motility seemed not much to occupy the minds of these pharmacologists. It took very little effort to discover, however, that the effect of the NANC nerves could not be blocked by any of the many autonomic receptor antagonists then available. The nature of the inhibitory transmitter remained cryptic.

This all took place in the 1960s. In the same era, chemists began to describe substances other than acetylcholine and catecholamines, which were candidate neurohormonal transmitters. Investigators already knew of a few such substances, like substance P (described by von Euler in the 1930s) and serotonin (described by Erspamer in the 1940s), but most of the new agents, unlike substance P and serotonin, were peptides. Gastrin, secretin, and cholecystokinin, long recognized as gut hormones, were already known to be peptides, and the new agents, as peptides, were first considered to be gut hormones as well. One of the first characterized, vasoactive intestinal peptide (VIP), reflected the work especially of Mutt and Said, who were not gastrointestinal physiologists or neurophysiologists, but when VIP was found in the brain as well as in the gut, it quickly entered the worlds of gastroenterology and neurology (33). The association of VIP with enteric nerves in particular and its potent inhibitory action on gut smooth muscle led to the idea that the NANC nerves act by releasing VIP, and more direct supporting evidence was soon forthcoming, especially in the esophagus (34).

But VIP was not the only early candidate for the NANC neurotransmitter. Burnstock startled the community in 1972 with his proposal that the NANC transmitter is an adenine nucleotide, likely ATP itself (35). He proceeded to develop his ideas at length in a long series of innovative experiments in a variety of tissues. A warm debate soon arose between the advocates of VIP and those of ATP as the NANC neurotransmitter, and it continues to this day.

Meanwhile, the peptide chemists accumulated a long (and still growing) list of other nerve-associated peptides, but none filled the bill so well as VIP and ATP as candidate NANC transmitters. To be fair, one must acknowledge that the list of peptide candidates is so large that its possibilities in gastrointestinal motor physiology are still not adequately explored.

The latest chapter in the story of the search for the NANC transmitter is only a year or two old. Actually, it goes back a little farther, beginning with some old unexplained observations, but the latest candidate transmitter, nitric oxide, did not occur to investigators then as a transmitter. The idea emerged from studies on the endothelial-derived relaxing factor (EDRF), a material whose existence was long suspected from observations made by vascular physiologists. An intense interest in EDRF developed beginning in the 1980s, again largely as part of research in hypertension. By 1987, it was becoming clear that the substance is nitric oxide or something similar (36). Again, in a now-familiar pattern of a raid on another discipline, gastrointestinal motor physiologists seized on nitric oxide and quickly brought forth compelling evidence in its favor as the NANC transmitter

(37-39). The story is not yet over; the hypothesis still requires much clarification. And there is no reason to think that nitric oxide accounts for all NANC transmission in all species.

The Classification of Nerve Cells in the Enteric Plexuses

No one suspected the existence of the enteric nervous system until 1857 and 1862 when the neuroanatomists Meissner and Auerbach first found it, but it was not long before its structural complexity became fully clear. Anatomists then began to relate it to the central nervous system, seeking similarities and interrelationships.

Thus, by the end of the 19th century, it was apparent that the enteric nervous system, like the central nervous system, contained several different kinds of cells, and Dogiel was trying to differentiate them according to their shapes and proposing functions for the different forms. And Langley, not long after, recognized the enteric nervous system as independent and therefore separable, to some degree, from the central nervous system and the parasympathetic and sympathetic systems (25). Langley's classification of the subdivisions of the autonomic nervous system became the standard, and it has withstood 50 years of use. Dogiel's classification of cells on the basis of shape, however, was long debated and remains controversial (40). The central question was always the physiologic relevance of the classifications of cells by structural features, and that question could not be answered by a purely anatomic approach.

Nothing new was possible in the classification of enteric nerve cells for a long time, until the 1970s. Then, the discovery of the nerve-related peptides that began with VIP led to the development of the antibodies necessary for their assay, and that made possible the staining of enteric nerves by immunohistochemistry. This soon led to double-staining techniques, which allowed the discovery of the colocalization of peptides and transmitters in nerves. The discovery of colocalization came as something of a surprise, for Dale's "one nerve-one transmitter" hypothesis had created a mindset against the idea, but that bias was quickly overcome. Soon, almost wholly through the efforts of Furness and Costa (25), it was possible to classify enteric nerve cells according to the immunohistochemically demonstrated peptide and transmitter combinations that they contain, and it is now possible to classify nearly all neurons in the gut wall into the categories defined by these classes.

Electrophysiologists now are also classifying enteric nerve cells on the basis of their evoked and resting behavior as studied with intracellular electrodes (41). This effort, led by Wood, has been remarkably productive. No full correlation between Dogiel's shapes, Furness and Costa's peptide stains, and Wood's electrophysiology has yet been established. Still, the matter has advanced substantially in the past 30 years.

THE ORIGIN OF RHYTHMICITY: "MYOGENIC" FUNCTIONS IN MOTILITY

Myogenic versus Neurogenic

The question of the relative importance of neurogenic and myogenic mechanisms in the motions of the gut must have occurred even to Magendie, because he commented on the functions of the vagi (1). It vexed Magnus as well, and in using his isolated muscle preparations, he attempted to differentiate nerve-regulated functions (18). Out of their studies and those of Alvarez (18), it gradually became clear that the rhythmic contractions that occur in isolated muscle preparations are not neurogenic and hence (by exclusion) must be myogenic. Alvarez, in fact, devoted much of his book in 1922 to a discussion of the subject.

The methods used before the 1960s did not really permit a clear distinction between neurogenic and myogenic functions because they involved variously traumatic treatments of tissues and the use of drugs with actions that were not completely understood. The advent of tetrodotoxin, which selectively abolishes nerve functions, allowed investigators at least to determine what was neurogenic (on the basis of what tetrodotoxin treatment abolished), and the common inference was that what remained was myogenic. The electrical slow waves

of the gut were among the phenomena that remained untouched by tetrodotoxin.

The Electrical Slow Waves of the Gut

Electrophysiology was a fully developed technical discipline in 1939, yet Wiggers could say virtually nothing of the electrical activity of the gut in his textbook (42) of that year: "Numerous attempts have been made to record action potentials from isolated and intact viscera. . . Unfortunately, the arrangement of muscular tissue in these organs is so complex and the electrical variations derived are so complicated that they are for the present difficult to interpret in terms of functional activity." But electrophysiology was the great biologic technology of the time (just as molecular biology is the great technology of ours), and therefore it was not long before ideas and methods were more fully transferred from the heart (where electrophysiology began) to the gut.

As early as 1932, investigators could detect the characteristic electromyogram of the small intestine (43,44) but it remained a seemingly fresh subject when Daniel's thorough review appeared in 1963 (45). The subject advanced rapidly in the 1960s, especially under the guidance of Code and Prosser in America and of Daniel in Canada. The idea of electrical slow waves developed rather slowly, given the ease with which they are detectable and their obvious importance. Thus, it was three decades after the work of Alvarez and Puestow that Code, Daniel, and Prosser took up the subject with their characteristic energy. Investigators focused on the small intestine for a long time, only later extending the method and the concepts to the stomach and colon.

From the beginning, investigators recognized that electrical slow waves govern the rhythmicity of contraction, not merely the fact of contraction. That is, like clocks, the slow waves restrict contractions in time and space, not signaling contractions like the cardiac action potentials, but acting purely as pacemaking signals to which the muscle may or may not respond. Indeed, they were a new sort of phenomenon in having this strictly pacemaker or clock function, and so investigators gave them a variety of names, seeming to feel that existing terminology was somehow inadequate. For some years, "electrical slow waves," "basic electrical rhythm," "pacesetter potentials," and "electrical control activity" competed for usage, to the great confusion of outsiders, and they still do to some extent.

The discovery of the electrical slow waves in the gut satisfactorily unified some old observations. For example, Russian physicians had long toyed with the technology of the electrogastrogram, a device to record the electrical signals of the stomach in analogy with the electrocardiogram. This fascination of the Russians with electrical events in the stomach at a time when they were scarcely thought of in other parts of the world or in other organs reflects the legacy of Pavlov, a legacy which also accounts for the fact that so many of the earliest autonomic neuroanatomists were Russians, or from the Eastern part of Europe. Code, Kelly, Szurszewski, and the others who later did so much to advance understanding of slow waves in the stomach, validated the electrogastrogram, heretofore largely unknown in the West. It has gained renewed currency if not actual vitality. Similarly, the finding of a declining gradient in slow-wave frequency along the small intestine tied in well with the theory of a metabolic gradient along the intestine, which had brought Alvarez to the forefront (18), even into the popular press. The fact that the theory excited some controversy then was partly attributable to the showman personality of Alvarez and his appeals to the press and to the public. His intestinal gradient theory arose again from the ashes on a firm foundation with the discovery of the intestinal slow-wave frequency gradient.

Although the electrical slow waves generated by the stomach and intestine were known long before, they did not attract detailed scrutiny by muscle electrophysiologists until the 1950s and 1960s (46). This was true partly because the early investigators were not, for the most part, themselves highly trained in the electrophysiology of smooth muscle, and partly because the electrophysiology of smooth muscle as studied in vitro did not fully develop as a subject until the 1950s. Bozler in the United States and Bulbring in England especially deserve credit for advancing gut smooth muscle forward as a subject worthy of detailed study in vitro by dedicated electrophysiologists.

Bozler studied the stomach and intestine. Bulbring chose the taenia coli of the guinea pig as her model. It was some time before students of gastrointestinal motility fully realized the significance of the observations of Bozler and Bulbring in their basic electrophysiologic studies. Not until the mid-1960s were their methods and concepts applied to other gut muscles, as prompted in part by curiosity as to the nature of the electrical slow waves.

The Interstitial Cells of Cajal: The Pacemaking System

Many experts now believe the source of the electrical slow waves to be the interstitial cells of Cajal rather than the smooth muscle itself. Although some continue to question this conclusion, at least the prevailing view is negative.

Cajal did not "discover" the interstitial cells that bear his name, but as the mightiest of a group of contemporaneous neuroanatomic giants, he raised them from obscurity at the turn of the century. He viewed these tiny cells as secondary nerve cells forming intermediates in the communication between the axons of enteric nerves and the cells of effector tissues, like smooth muscle and gland cells (47). He thought of them also as forming a terminal syncytium or network of nerve fibers that allowed integrating communication within the substance of the smooth muscle. He described them in the small intestine, pancreas, and salivary glands.

For a long time, neuroanatomists argued about these cells, their function, their distribution, and, indeed, their very existence. Cajal's ideas as to their nature and function were neither disproved nor fully accepted, and they remained cells without a clear function for almost a century. As early as 1925, some investigators had proposed that the cells might be responsible for "myogenic" rhythmic contractions, but on little evidence. Thuneberg revived the idea in 1982 (48), on better evidence, and it has now stimulated the imagination of others who, in fact, have gathered good evidence in its support. And the interstitial cells have subsequently received much attention (49).

It is ironic that the best evidence for the idea that interstitial cells generate the electrical slow waves comes from the colon (of the cat and dog), one of the last places where they were described and the organ where motility is less well understood than in any other structure. The interstitial cells of the mammalian colon were only discovered in 1971, by Stach (50), who found them as a neuroanatomist working on the neglected topic of the innervation of the mammalian colon. He certainly was not looking for pacemakers. The electrical slow waves of the mammalian colon were first described in detail only about the same time, not by design but by accident, the discoverer simply choosing an unexplored tissue in which to demonstrate the use of a new kind of electrode he had devised (51). Thus, with respect to both the electrical pacemaker signals and the cells that probably generate them, the colon was the last organ to come under scrutiny, and it has now become the major one. The small intestine and stomach remain organs in which to test these ideas more fully.

Periodicity in Rhythmic Activity of the Gut

The idea that the pattern or quantity of rhythmic contractions in the gut vary as the animal is fed or fasted goes back a long time. Beaumont, with his limited capacity to see gastric motions in his patient with a fistula to the gastric fundus, concluded that gastric contractions occur only in the fed state, that the stomach becomes quiet after it has emptied itself into the duodenum. Despite casual observations to the contrary, the idea persisted for a long time. But it was not universally held. Carlson (14) cites the writings of an 18th century physiologist, Haller, who believed that hunger represents contractions of the empty stomach, and referred to others who agreed, especially Boldyreff, who had published his observations in 1905 (52). Recording from balloons inflated in the stomach of conscious dogs, Boldyreff saw alternate periods of powerful rhythmic contractions and absolute or relative quiescence over a period of 3 to 4 days of starvation. The periods of contractions lasted for 20 to 30 minutes, the periods of relative quiescence, 1¼ hours or more. Boldyreff noticed that periodic contractions of the intestine accompanied those of the stomach.

Hurst later proposed that these periodic contractions give rise to the sensation of hunger, an idea that Boldyreff had rejected because he saw the contractions become weaker as starvation was prolonged.

Carlson and his colleagues, after further experiments, concluded that hunger is indeed caused by these periodic powerful contractions of the stomach. He described his studies (which involved yet another patient with a gastric fistula) in a monograph in 1916 (14) and the idea of "hunger contractions," of a particular force and regularity that periodically recur in the empty stomach, remained part of standard teaching in gastrointestinal physiology until about the 1940s, when it appears to have died out. Boldyreff's original work and Carlson's observations both have been fully reviewed by Wingate (53).

Although periodicity in gastrointestinal contractions in the fasting animal was established by these studied, the matter soon fell into neglect and was forgotten. The picture of vastly different motility in feeding and fasting did not re-emerge until the work of Ruckebusch (54) in France and of Szurszewski (55) in America. Szurszewski, a gastrointestinal physiologist working in Code's laboratory, viewed himself in the clinical physiology tradition of Boldyreff, Cannon, Carlson, Ivy, and so on. Ruckebusch, in contrast, was a veterinarian who was interested in comparative gastrointestinal physiology. So, whereas Szurszewski and his colleagues confined themselves to man and the dog, Ruckebusch ranged widely across the animal kingdom. Ruckebusch was able to show that periodicity is constant in many herbivores who eat constantly, and that eating interrupts the periodic cycle mostly in carnivores who normally eat meals at wide intervals in time. Ruckebusch's broad interests in comparative animal functions are indicated in the textbook (56) he published not long before his premature death.

Thus, the idea of periodicity of gastrointestinal contractions in fasting arose, apparently from casual observation, very long ago, but it found little use then except by Carlson to explain hunger. Even that idea was forgotten, and motor periodicity in fasting was re-discovered several times, until, finally and firmly re-discovered, the periodic activity of the gut in fasting (newly christened the "migrating motor complex"), has become deeply entrenched in the body of knowledge. It will long remain a subject for study because its importance to the body economy is now well established, and the mechanisms involved remain to be fully determined.

The Concept of Sphincters

The idea of a sphincter originated in ancient times. Indeed, the word had the same meaning to the ancients as it does to us. The anal sphincter, the pupillary sphincters, and the sphincters of various marine invertebrates, all directly and readily visualized, must have provided the prototypes for the concept. Magendie, thus, could speak of the anal sphincter as though it were a familiar structure. He recognized the esophagogastric sphincter only as a strong muscular structure in the horse, which he could feel when he put his fist up into the cardia, not interpreting it as anything related to the anal sphincter. And Magendie apparently considered the anal sphincter to be a fixed constriction, not a tonically contacted muscle whose contraction could transiently disappear and return under control.

Radiographic methods improved the perception of sphincters, but other methods to study them found little use until the 1950s. The advances of the first 50 years can be seen in Wiggers' textbook of 1939 (42). He had somewhat more to say of sphincters in general than Magendie had had a century earlier. Wiggers describes them as thickenings of the circular muscle layer at the cardiac and pyloric ends of the stomach, at the ileocecal junction and at the end of the rectum. He recognized the lower esophageal sphincter closure as a contraction, for he spoke of its "tonicity," but he did not mention its controlled relaxation. He made no mention of the upper esophageal sphincter.

Wiggers knew of the contracted state of the pylorus because, by 1939, it had been thoroughly described by the early radiologists, especially Cannon, and he spoke favorably of Cannon's idea of "acid control" of the pyloric sphincter. Cannon, recognizing that the sphincter must be open to allow the stomach to empty, proposed that antral acidification reflexly relaxes the sphincter, whereas duodenal acidification reflexly

contracts it. But Thomas, Quigley, and others produced evidence against Cannon's idea, and therefore, by Wiggers' time, the pylorus was recognized as a site that is "naturally relaxed," contracting only in coordination with antral peristalsis and during the ensuing bulbar contraction.

Wiggers also spoke of the ileocecal valve as a sphincter whose fluctuations in tonus regulate flow from the small intestine to the colon, a process he called "internal defecation." He believed that this sphincter prevents coloileal reflux and that it regulates antegrade flow. He considered it to be affected by reflexes from both adjacent and distant parts of the gastrointestinal tract.

Wiggers was vague about the anal sphincters. He spoke at one point as though the anal sphincters do not relax, saying, ". . . a mass contraction occurs over the whole colon and, if the tonus of the two sphincters is not great enough to resist the force thus developed, involuntary defecation results." At another point, he acknowledged that distention of the rectum in preparation for defecation diminishes the tonus of the anal sphincter.

It was mainly the advent of radiographic methods that allowed Wiggers to be able to say what was new by then, in comparison to what Magendie knew. Radiographic methods could not readily show the upper esophageal sphincter, nor did they allow measurement of the force of sphincter closure or allow one to distinguish between opening as a passive yielding to a distending force and as a disappearance of contraction force, an active relaxation.

The idea of tonus was well developed by Wigger's time. It had been defined by those who studied gut muscle in vitro, Magnus (18) and those who followed, for they could distinguish readily between rhythmic contractions and the sustained baseline elevations which represented permanent or continuing shortenings of muscle. Thus, when Wiggers spoke of sphincters as showing tonus, he was using what was already a well-developed concept, but not necessarily one that defined sphincters as qualitatively distinct from non-sphincter regions, only quantitatively different.

A qualitative distinction between sphincteric and nonsphincteric muscle became the dogma, proposing the concept of the reciprocal innervation of sphincters, at least of the lower esophageal, pyloric, and ileocecal sphincters. This concept claimed that the sphincters were relaxed by parasympathetic stimulation and contracted by sympathetic stimulation, in reciprocity with the adjacent stomach and intestines. This idea, that sphincters are defined entirely in the nature of the two kinds of innervation, persisted for a long time and continues today.

A challenge to this idea came from Christensen's attempt in 1970 to determine if this reciprocal innervation could be demonstrated through the effects of autonomic drugs (57). The study made use of the lower esophageal sphincter studied in vitro, comparing it with adjacent esophageal wall. The muscle of the sphincter and of the esophageal body responded to all of various excitatory and inhibitory drugs in the same way, differing only in that the sphincter was more sensitive to many than was the adjacent esophageal body. Christensen then compared the same regions by the use of Paton's field stimulation, and it soon became clear that the lower esophageal sphincter is distinguished from the esophageal body mainly by the presence of a high degree of myogenic tone that is resistant to the action of tetrodotoxin (58). A comparatively high degree of myogenic tone soon was shown by others to define other sphincters, namely the pyloric, ileocecal, and internal anal sphincters (59). In all such regions, inhibition results from the actions of the noncholinergic nonadrenergic inhibitory nerves. Therefore the current general definition of a sphincter, a segment possessed of a high degree of myogenic tone which is augmented by cholinergic and perhaps other external excitatory influences (hormones) and which is inhibited by nonadrenergic noncholinergic inhibitory nerves, is only about 20 years old. The studies were made possible by technical advances, improved methods for study of muscle in vitro, the advent of tetrodotoxin, and the use of Paton's method for selective stimulation of nerves by electrical field stimulation. The knowledge that sphincters are defined by the fact that the muscle in these regions is physiologically distinct should prompt studies to determine if the muscle of these regions also is ultrastructurally or chemically distinct. These ideas have only now attracted attention (60,61).

THE EVOLUTION OF CERTAIN ORGAN-SPECIFIC IDEAS IN MOTILITY

The Origin of Peristalsis in the Smooth-Muscle Esophagus

Sixty years after Magendie had described esophageal peristalsis, Kronecker and Meltzer proposed that oropharyngeal contractions squirt liquids to the stomach and that peristalsis conveys only solids. Cannon (62) subsequently fortified this idea when radiographic methods became available.

Meltzer (63) went on to indicate, in 1899, that the programming of the progressive nature of the contraction takes place in the central nervous system and that the brainstem center there could be triggered not only by a swallow but also by oropharyngeal stimulation. The swallowing center received no more notice until Doty (64) took it up in the 1960s. He used classical neuroanatomical methods to localize it precisely in the brainstem.

Meltzer, Doty, and nearly all other experimentalists before 1969 used the dog to study esophageal motor function. The dog resembles most other animals in having an esophagus composed almost entirely of striated muscle. Central programming of peristalsis requires a motor unit organization in which one nerve fiber supplies a certain set of muscle cells. A motor unit organization allows spatial representation of the striated muscle esophagus in the swallowing center so that neurons there can fire in a sequence to produce the spatiotemporal sequence that appears as a peristaltic contraction moving caudad.

In man and other primates, the greater part of the esophagus is smooth muscle. Christensen (65), recognizing that a motor unit organization is unlikely in smooth muscle, and realizing as well that some motor disorders of the esophagus affect only the smooth-muscle segment, proposed that peristalsis in the smooth-muscle segment has a different origin. He set out to find an appropriate experimental animal model for man, to avoid the expense of primates. He soon found that marsupials also have a long smooth-muscle segment in the esophagus, no real surprise in light of the other special anatomic features shared by marsupials and primates. He introduced the American opossum as the appropriate model, and its subsequent use led ultimately to a greater understanding of the process (66).

In the current view, the vagal preganglionic fibers serve as triggers, exciting NANC inhibitory nerves throughout the smooth muscle segment essentially simultaneously. The hyperpolarization these nerves produce in the muscle leads to a rebound depolarization with the accompanying contraction. This contraction follows the hyperpolarization with a latency that progressively increases distally. The opossum esophagus also allowed the in vitro definition of the lower esophageal sphincter; animal investigators could compare one smooth muscle to another. This is not possible in the dog, in which striated muscle extends up to the sphincter region.

Gastric Sieving of Solids and Receptive Relaxation

Magendie recognized that the stomach contracts to shift its contents, and by 1886 Hofmeister and Schütz described gastric peristalsis, but only after the advent of radiography could Cannon really visualize it in vivo. Beaumont had proposed that food entering the stomach follows a pathway along the greater curvature to reach the pylorus. Cannon was able to disprove that idea. He could see the different motor functions of the antrum and fundus and visualized retropulsion of contents in antral contraction. Cannon's views on gastric contractions prevailed for a long time. But the full complexity of gastric flows, including sieving (67), the separation of solids from liquids by the antrum, became clear only after about 1960. Meyer's review contains a full account of this development (68).

Cannon recognized the reservoir function of the stomach, and realized that it expanded with swallowing by the process now called receptive relaxation. But it was not until 50 years later that vagal inhibition of the stomach received careful study, when Harper (69) observed that the electrical stimulation of the central stump of the severed vagus induced gastric relaxation by way of other intact vagus. In the 1960s Jansson (70) and Abrahamson (71) extended the concept of vagally mediated gastric relaxation by demonstrating several reflexes. The excitation of NANC inhibitory nerves mediates these reflexes, for the most part, but Miolan and Roman (72) showed that receptive relaxation also involves the suppression of activity in tonic excitatory fibers to the gastric fundus.

Reverse Peristalsis in the Small Intestine

The idea of reverse peristalsis as a phenomenon underlying vomiting and dyspepsia goes back a long time. Various early writers considered it a well-established pattern of peristalsis in the esophagus, stomach, small intestine, and colon, even though the evidence then existed only from the study of the stomach and colon. Many who studied the small intestine had looked for it in vain. In 1961, Smith and Brizzee (73), investigating vomiting by cineradiography in the cat, observed that apomorphine-induced vomiting produced reverse peristalsis in the small intestine. Weisbrodt and Christensen saw it again in 1972 (74). They used electrodes implanted in the small intestine of the cat. They noted that vomiting was preceded by a complex change. First, the electrical slow waves diminished in amplitude to the point of extinction. Then a prolonged burst of spikes appeared first at the most distal electrode and moved very slowly, 2.8 cm/s, cephalad through the whole segment under study. The animal then vomited. The electrical slow waves returned soon thereafter, running cephalad at first, slowly orienting themselves to the normal cephalo-caudal progression.

Antiperistalsis in the Colon

At the turn of the century, Cannon (5), in studying barium flow at the ileocecal junction, observed antiperistalsis, contractions that arose in the mid-transverse colon and spread toward the cecum, pressing colonic content before them. Soon after, Elliott and Barclay-Smith (75) exposed the colon in situ in a warm bath to watch contractions directly. In the species they examined (guinea pig, cat, rat, ferret, and hedgehog), they saw antiperistaltic contractions in the ascending colon. Barcroft and Steggerda (76) saw them again in 1932. Hurst (77) reported that they were also described by Jacobi in animals in 1890, and by Case in humans in 1913. Christensen (78) began his studies of the electrical slow waves of the cat colon in ignorance of all this previous work. He observed the electrical slow waves in this region to arise commonly at a pacemaking site in the transverse colon and to sweep retrograde to the cecum; contractions accompanied them. He observed also that the pacemaker could migrate from one place to another. The idea of antiperistalsis in the proximal colon still meets resistance, however.

The Effects of the Emotions on Colonic Motility

The idea that the emotions affect colonic motility dates to antiquity, from common first-hand experience. The first objective studies on the matter did not occur until Almy's work of 1947 and later (79). Almy studied normal subjects and patients with the irritable colon syndrome, using manometry to record contractions of the left colon while the subjects were subjected to various kinds of stress. He found that a variety of stresses, such as holding one hand in icewater, painful compression of the skull, insulin-induced hypoglycemia, and overt discussions of anxiety-producing topics all produced colonic spasm or heightened its rhythmic contractions. In contrast, feelings of hopelessness or depression reduced the contractions. Grace, Wolf, and Wolff (80) made similar observations in patients with colostomies.

This evidence found a welcome reception because the idea that some patients suffer an exaggerated colonic response to the emotions already was well established in the concept of the irritable colon syndrome. A host of studies since then have not advanced the matter much further. A major problem is that good methods for long-term monitoring of colonic motility in man remain to be developed.

THE EVOLUTION OF SCIENTIFIC ORGANIZATIONS TO DISSEMINATE KNOWLEDGE IN GASTROINTESTINAL MOTILITY

Until the 1960s, information relevant to motility accrued in separate classes of investigators who belonged to and spoke to separate societies that represented separate academic disciplines. Pharmacologists reported to the American Society of Pharmacology and Experimental Therapeutics (ASPET) and to its publication, the Journal of Pharmacology and Experimental Therapeutics, as well as to a handful of other pharmacologic journals. Physiologists reported to the American Physiological Society (APS) and to its publication, the American Journal of Physiology, as well as to a handful of other physiological journals. Those who studied the behavior of whole organs, mainly clinicians, reported to the American Gastroenterological Association (AGA) and its publication, Gastroenterology, as well as to a handful of clinical journals. Advances in anatomy were confined to anatomic societies and journals, and so on.

One cannot claim an absolute absence of cross-talk among those working in relevant fields, but the separateness of these organizations impeded communication. The ASPET and APS, of course, met jointly once each year as members of the Federated American Societies for Experimental Biology. The structures of the programs, however, did not give gastrointestinal motility a focus sufficient for optimal communication among the different areas within the different societies. The AGA had no designated subsection on motility at its annual meetings, the few papers on motility appearing in a section entitled "miscellaneous" until the late 1960s.

This situation changed slowly in an evolution toward arrangements that enhanced communication among workers in all the varied fields relevant to motility. These changes occurred mainly in two forms, in a gradual restructuring within the AGA annual meeting, and in the evolution of entirely new organizations wholly dedicated to gastrointestinal motility.

The change within the AGA began subtly. About 1963, a group of no more than about 20 persons who studied the esophagus organized a luncheon session at the AGA annual meeting. This group, called The Gullet Club, met mainly to discuss new information about the then-new methodology to record esophageal motility by manometry. Esophageal manometry remained the focus of the investigators for the next 2 to 3 years.

Then, recognizing the limitations of that topic, the group expanded its meeting to take in other subject matter. At the same time, basic scientists began to join the AGA, heretofore a largely clinical organization whose members were mainly academic and practicing clinical gastroenterologists. A deliberate effort was made to expand the size and mission of the Gullet Club, and it quickly became an informal group of one-hundred or more members called the Motility Society. It gained a dedicated evening each year from the AGA and adopted an agenda that included a broad range of topics, focusing on those in which advances were especially rapid.

The development of totally new organizations dedicated to motility began about the same time. The actual beginning came in about 1965, when a group of clinicians, among them Connell, Texter, and VanTrappen, met at Belfast. A second meeting 2 years later was followed by a third, in 1969, at Frascati, near Rome. Here, the International Symposium on Gastrointestinal Motility took on a form that ensured its continuation as the most important central force in organizing all the new ideas coming forth in motility. The Symposium adopted a set of rules that ensured its value down to the present, 20 years later. The rules created a unique kind of organization. The International Symposium was a little like Brigadoon, emerging only in alternate years and flowering only for the 3 to 4 days of its meeting. Between meetings, it existed only as a steering committee, elected at the last meeting. There was no permanent membership. Attendance was invited from members of all relevant scientific disciplines. Hopeful participants were invited to apply for each meeting by submitting an abstract of recent work. The Steering Committee reviewed and accepted abstracts up to the number tolerated by the venue. Attendance was limited to authors and co-authors of accepted abstracts. The maximal attendance, practically, could not exceed about 300. The venue was intentionally kept small, inexpensive, secluded, and far from distractions.

The International Symposium soon resembled an exclusive club, but its rules for attendance ensured a freshness and a constant renewal that could not exist in a larger or more conventional society of fixed membership. Thus, it became a major forum for cross-talk among actively working clinicians, physiologists, and pharmacologists, and, operating under the same rules, it remains so today.

The rules of the International Symposium, by design, slightly favored the participation of European investigators to avoid being outnumbered by Americans. This was accomplished by placing two out of three meetings in Europe. Indeed, American investigators soon came to feel that they were slightly excluded from participation, and so they formed another organization, the American Motility Society, to meet in alternate years, beginning in about 1980. An informal organization at first, it soon became an incorporated society of fixed membership. A parallel European Motility Society was formed at about the same time, having an essentially identical format.

Finally, the fully formed American Motility Society acquired responsibilities for the dedicated programs of the AGA. Thus, the function of the old informal Gullet Club finally evolved into a formal aspect of the operation of the American Motility Society. It was supplanted, finally, by the reorganization of the AGA into sections representing various disciplines, including motility.

These organizations have not been the sole fora for communication among workers in relevant disciplines, but they have become the major ones. They grew up precisely because there was a need for them. Many new ideas have come from their meetings, and their continued growth attests to their usefulness.

REFERENCES

1. Magendie F: An Elementary Compendium of Physiology (Précis Elémentaire de Physiologie) (translated by E. Milligan). 4th Ed. Edinburgh, John Carfrae and Son, 1831.
2. Beaumont W: Experiments and Observations on the Gastric Juice and the Physiology of Digestion. Plattsburg, NY, FP Allan, 1833.
3. Bowditch HP: Movements of the alimentary canal. Science 5:901, 1897.
4. Cannon WB: The movements of the stomach studied by means of the roentgen rays. Am J Physiol 1:359, 1898.

5. Cannon WB: The movements of the intestines studied by means of the roentgen rays. Am J Physiol 6:251, 1902.
6. Hurst AF, Briggs PJ: The diagnosis of gastric and duodenal ulcer with the x-rays. Guy's Hospital Reports 74:278, 1924.
7. Hurst AF, Newton A: The normal movements of the colon in man. J Physiol (Lond.) 47:57, 1913.
8. Barclay AE: The Digestive Tract. A Radiological Study of its Anatomy, Physiology, and Pathology. Cambridge, Cambridge University Press, 1933.
9. Alazraki NP, Fajman WA, Christian PE: Gastrointestinal radionuclide imaging procedures. *In* Yamada T et al. (eds). Textbook of Gastroenterology. Ch. 121. Philadelphia, J.B. Lippincott Co., 1991.
10. Hunt JN: The duodenal regulation of gastric emptying. Gastroenterology 45:149, 1963.
11. Kelly KA: Motility of the stomach and gastroduodenal junction. *In* Johnson LR et al. (eds): Physiology of the Gastrointestinal Tract. 1st Ed., Ch. 12. New York, Raven Press, 1981.
12. Macagno EO, Christensen J: Fluid mechanics of gastrointestinal flow. *In* Johnson LR et al. (eds): Physiology of the Gastrointestinal Tract. 1st Ed., Ch. 10. New York, Raven Press, 1981.
13. Bayliss WM, Starling EH: The movements and innervation of the small intestine. J Physiol (Lond) 24:99, 1899.
14. Carlson AJ: The Control of Hunger in Health and Disease. Chicago, University of Chicago Press, 1916.
15. Wheelon H, Thomas JE: Observations on the motility of the antrum and the relation of the rhythmic activity of the pyloric sphincter to that of the antrum. J Lab Clin Med 6:124, 1920.
16. Code CF et al. (eds): An Atlas of Esophageal Motility in Health and Disease. Springfield, Charles C Thomas, 1958.
17. Dodds WJ, Stef JJ, Hogan WJ: Factors determining pressure measurement accuracy by intraluminal esophageal manometry. Gastroenterology 70:117, 1976.
18. Alvarez WC: The Mechanics of the Digestive Tract. An Introduction to Gastroenterology. 2nd Ed. New York, Paul B. Hoeber, 1928.
19. Farrar JT: Gastrointestinal smooth muscle function. Am J Dig Dis 9:103, 1963.
20. Louckes HS, Quigley JP, Kersey J: Inductograph method of recording muscle activity, especially pyloric sphincter physiology. Am J Physiol 199:301, 1960.
21. Alvarez WC, Mahoney LJ: Action currents in stomach and intestine. Am J Physiol 58:476, 1922.
22. Bass T: In vivo electrical activity of the small bowel. *In* Code CF (ed): Handbook of Physiology. A Critical, Comprehensive Presentation of Physiological Knowledge and Concepts. Section 6: Alimentary Tract, Vol. 4: Motility. Bethesda, American Physiological Society, 1968.
23. Perkins WE: Method for studying electrical and mechanical activity of isolated intestine. J Appl Physiol 30:768, 1971.
24. Kuntz A: The Autonomic Nervous System. Philadelphia, Lea & Febiger, 1953.
25. Furness JB, Costa M: The Enteric Nervous System. Edinburgh, London, Melbourne and New York, Churchill-Livingstone, 1987.
26. Mitchell GAG: Anatomy of the Autonomic Nervous System. Edinburgh, E and S Livingston, Ltd., 1953.
27. Jacobowitz D: Histochemical studies of the autonomic innervation of the gut. J Pharmacol Exper Ther 149:358, 1965.
28. Paton WDM: The action of morphine and related substances on contraction and on acetylcholine output of coaxially stimulated guinea pig ileum. Br J Pharmacol 11:119, 1957.
29. Paton WDM, Vane JR: An analysis of the responses of the isolated stomach to electrical stimulation and to drugs. J Physiol (Lond.) 165:10, 1963.
30. Blinks JR: Field stimulation effecting the graded release of autonomic transmitters in isolated heart muscle. J Pharmacol Exp Therap 151:221, 1966.
31. Kao CY: Tetrodotoxin, saxitoxin and their significance in the study of excitation phenomena. Pharmacol Rev 18:997, 1966.
32. Bennett MR: Rebound excitation of the smooth muscle cells of the guinea pig taenia coli after stimulation of intramural inhibitory nerves. J Physiol (Lond.) 185:124, 1966.
33. Mutt V, Said SI: Structure of the porcine vasoactive intestinal octacosapeptide. Eur J Biochem 42:581, 1974.
34. Christensen J: Motor functions of the pharynx and esophagus. *In* Johnson LR et al. (eds): Physiology of the Gastrointestinal Tract. 2nd Ed. New York, Raven Press, 1987.
35. Burnstock G: Purinergic nerves. Pharmacol Rev 24:509, 1972.
36. Palmer RMJ, Ferrige AG, Moncada S: Nitric oxide release accounts for the biological activity of endothelium-derived relaxing factor. Nature (Lond) 327:524, 1987.
37. Tottrup A, Svane D, Forman A: Nitric oxide mediating NANC inhibition in opossum lower esophageal sphincter. Am J Physiol 260:G904, 1991.
38. Murray J et al.: Nitric oxide: mediator of

nonadrenergic noncholinergic responses of opossum esophageal muscle. Am J Physiol *261*:G401, 1991.

39. Du C, Murray J, Bates JN, Conklin JL: Nitric oxide: Mediator of NANC hyperpolarization of opossum esophageal smooth muscle. Am J Physiol *261*:G1012, 1991.

40. Christensen J: The forms of argyrophilic ganglion cells in the myenteric plexus throughout the gastrointestinal tract of the opossum. J Auton Nerv Syst *24*:251, 1988.

41. Wood JD: Physiology of the Enteric Nervous System. *In* Johnson LR et al. (eds). Physiology of the Gastrointestinal Tract. New York, Raven Press, 1987.

42. Wiggers CJ: Physiology in Health and Disease. 3rd Ed. Philadelphia, Lea and Febiger, 1939.

43. Berkson J, Baldes EJ, Alvarez WC: Electromyographic studies of the gastrointestinal tract. I. The correlation between mechanical movement and changes in electrical potential during rhythmic contraction of the intestine. Am J Physiol *102*:683, 1932.

44. Puestow CB: The activity of isolated intestinal segments. Arch Surg *24*:565, 1932.

45. Daniel EE, Chapman KM: Electrical activity of the gastrointestinal tract as an indication of mechanical activity. Am J Dig Dis *8*:54, 1963.

46. Szurszewski JH: Electrical basis for gastrointestinal motility. *In* Johnson LR et al. (eds): Physiology of the Gastrointestinal Tract. 2nd Ed., Ch. 12. New York, Raven Press, 1987.

47. Cajal SRY: Histologie du système nerveux de l'homme et des vertébrés. Paris, Maloine, 1911.

48. Thuneberg L: The interstitial cells of Cajal: Intestinal pacemaker cells? Adv Embryol Cell Biol *71*:1, 1982.

49. Christensen J: A commentary on the morphological identification of the interstitial cells of Cajal. J Auton Nerv Syst *37*:75, 1992.

50. Stach W: Der Plexus entericus extremus des Dickdarmes und seine Beziehungen zu den interstitiellen Zellen (Cajal). Z. Mikrosk-Anat. Forsch *85*:245, 1972.

51. Christensen J, Caprilli R, Lund GF: Electric slow waves in circular muscle of cat colon. Am J Physiol *217*:771, 1969.

52. Boldyreff WN: Le travail periodique de l'appareil digestif en dehors de la digestion. Arch Sci Biol *11*:1, 1905.

53. Wingate DL: Backwards and forwards with the migrating complex. Dig Dis Sci *26*:641, 1981.

54. Ruckebusch Y, Laplace JP: La motricité intestinale chez le mouton: Phénomènes mécaniques et electriques. CR Soc Biol *161*:2517, 1967.

55. Szurszewski JH: A migrating electric complex of the canine small intestine. Am J Physiol *217*:1757, 1969.

56. Ruckebusch Y: Physiologie Pharmacologie Therapeutique Animales. Paris, Maloine, S.A., 1977.

57. Christensen J: Pharmacological identification of the lower esophageal sphincter. J Clin Invest *49*:681, 1970.

58. Christensen J, Conklin JL, Freeman BW: Physiologic specialization at the esophagogastric junction in three species. Am J Physiol *225*:1265, 1973.

59. Papasova M: Sphincteric function. *In* Wood JD (ed): Handbook of Physiology. A Critical Comprehensive Presentation of Physiological Knowledge and Concepts. Section 6. The Gastrointestinal System. Volume 1; Part 2: Motility and Circulation, Ch. 26. Bethesda, American Physiological Society, 1987.

60. Christensen J, Roberts RL: Differences between esophageal body and lower esophageal sphincter in mitochondria of smooth muscle in opossum. Gastroenterology *85*:650, 1983.

61. Robison BA, Percy WH, Christensen J: Differences in cytochrome C oxidase capacity in smooth muscle of opossum esophagus and lower esophageal sphincter. Gastroenterology *87*:1009, 1984.

62. Cannon WB, Moser A: The movements of the food in the oesophagus. Am J Physiol *1*:435, 1898.

63. Meltzer SJ: On the causes of the orderly progress of the peristaltic movements in the oesophagus. Am J Physiol *2*:261, 1899.

64. Doty RW: Neural organization of deglutition. *In* Code CF (ed): Handbook of Physiology: A Critical, Comprehensive Presentation of Physiological Knowledge and Concepts, Section 6, Vol. IV, Ch. 92. Washington, DC, American Physiological Society, 1861, 1968.

65. Christensen J, Lund GF: Esophageal responses to distension and electrical stimulation. J Clin Invest *48*:408, 1969.

66. Christensen J: The motor functions of the pharynx and esophagus. *In* Johnson LR et al.: Physiology of the Gastrointestinal Tract, 2nd Ed., Ch. 18. New York, Raven Press, 595, 1987.

67. Meyer JH, Thompson JB, Cohen MP, Shadchehr A: Sieving of solid food by the canine stomach and sieving after surgery. Gastroenterology *76*:804, 1979.

68. Meyer JH: Motility of the stomach and gastroduodenal junction. *In* Johnson LR et al. (eds): Physiology of the Gastrointestinal Tract. New York, Raven Press, 1987.

69. Harper AA, Kidd C, Scratcherd T: Vago-

vagal effects on gastric and pancreatic secretion and gastrointestinal motility. J Physiol (Lond) *148*:417, 1959.

70. Jansson G: Extrinsic nervous control of gastric motility. Acta Physiol Scand (Suppl) *326*:1, 1969.

71. Abrahamson H: Studies on the inhibitory nervous control of gastric motility. Acta Physiol Scand (Suppl) *390*:1, 1973.

72. Miolan JP, Roman C: Décharge unitaire des fibres vagales efférentes lors de la rélaxation réceptive d l'estomac du chien. J Physiol (Paris) *68*:693, 1974.

73. Smith CC, Brizzee KR: Cineradiographic analysis of vomiting in the cat. Gastroenterology *40*:654, 1961.

74. Weisbrodt NW, Christensen J: Electrical activity of the cat duodenum in fasting and vomiting. Gastroenterology *63*:1004, 1972.

75. Elliott TR, Barclay-Smith E: Antiperistalsis and the muscular activities of the colon. J Physiol (Lond) *31*:272, 1904.

76. Barcroft J, Steggerda FR: Observations on the proximal portion of exterinized colon. J Physiol (Lond) *76*:460, 1932.

77. Hurst AF: Constipation and allied intestinal disorders. 2nd Ed. London, Oxford University Press, 1921.

78. Christensen J: Motility of the colon. *In* Johnson LR et al. (eds): Physiology of the Gastrointestinal Tract. 2nd Ed., Ch. 21. New York, Raven Press, 665, 1987.

79. Almy TP: Experimental studies on the "irritable colon." Am J Med *10*:60, 1951.

80. Grace WJ, Wolf S, Wolff HG: The Human Colon. An Experimental Study Based on Direct Observation of Four Fistulous Subjects. New York, Paul B. Hoeber, 1951.

10

Progress in Neurogastroenterology

JACKIE D. WOOD

Twentieth-century progress in neurogastroenterology hinged on a conceptual transition from preganglionic/postganglionic to little brain determination of gastrointestinal behavior. The prevailing concept in the first half of the century was classical autonomic organization for neural control. The ganglia within the gut wall were construed as parasympathetic terminal ganglia. Postganglionic parasympathetic neurons with cell bodies in the terminal ganglia released acetylcholine to initiate responses of the musculature or secretory effector systems. This was taught to medical students as the excitatory dimension of gut innervation.

The inhibitory component in the old concept was the sympathetic division of the autonomic nervous system. Postganglionic neurons with cell bodies in abdominal ganglia released norepinephrine to suppress motility and other behaviors. A brake-gas pedal analogy of opposing inhibitory/excitatory input to the muscle or other effectors explained neural control of gut behavior. A balance favoring parasympathetic excitation results in increased activity; balance favoring sympathetic inhibition accounted for suppression of activity.

The groups of neurons in ganglia of the gut were interpreted as relay-distribution centers for signals transmitted from the central nervous system (Fig. 10–1). In this model, all of the decision making and automated control functions were wired into the neural circuitry in the central nervous system. No intelligence was attributed to the nervous system in the gut.

The utmost advance of the century was the enlightened realization that the nervous system of the gut is a minibrain with intelligent circuits. Emergence of the 20th-century heuristic model of the enteric nervous system as a "little brain" (Fig. 10–1) opened the way for basic research and improved understanding of the disordered physiology manifest as disease, including functional disorders in particular.

Functional disorders of the central nervous system, like those of the digestive tract, were designated as such early in the century out of ignorance of the pathophysiologic basis of the disease. Parkinson's disease of the central nervous system was regarded as an idiopathic disorder until the synaptic microcircuits of the basal ganglia and the importance of the neurotransmitter dopamine in the brain were understood. Based on the history of progress in brain research, projection of new understanding of the neural networks of the gut into the 21st century is expected to uncover unrealized explanations for gastrointestinal disorders, as well as rational approaches to therapy.

THE LITTLE BRAIN IN THE GUT

The heuristic model for the enteric nervous system turned out to be the same as for any independent integrative system, whether it be the vertebrate brain or spinal cord or the simple nervous systems of invertebrate animals (Fig. 10–1). Like these systems, the enteric minibrain is synaptically wired for directional flow of information

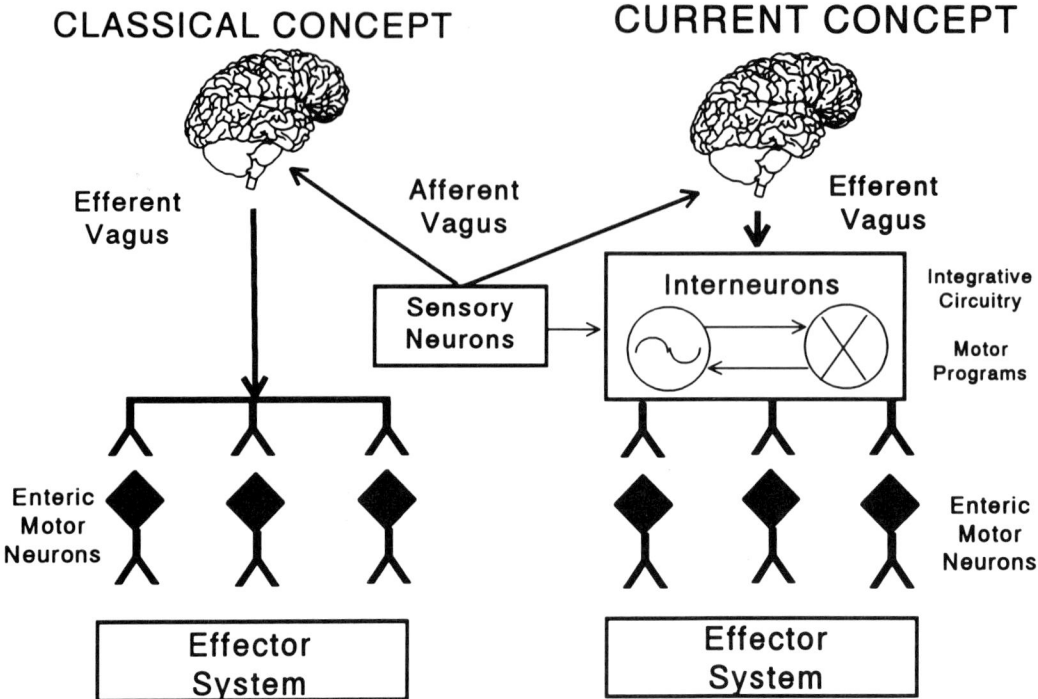

Fig. 10–1. Classical concept, now outmoded, and current concept of relationships between the brain and the digestive tract. The classical concept viewed vagal preganglionic fibers as synapsing directly with enteric motor neurons as illustrated on the left side of the diagram. In the current concept, vagal efferent fibers transmit command signals from the brain to the integrative and motor program circuitry of the enteric nervous system as shown on the right side of the diagram. The integrative and program circuits are assembled from synaptic connections among interneurons and are a component of the enteric minibrain. Sensory neurons and motor neurons also are components of the minibrain.

from sensory neurons to interneurons to motor neurons.

The sensory neurons are specialized for detection of the continuously changing conditions of the digestive milieu and transformation of the information into codes for processing by local area networks. They code information on parameters such as wall tension, acidity, and osmolarity of luminal contents.

Interneurons are synaptically connected into local networks that process the sensory information. Interneuronal networks also hold a library of programs, any of which may be called up for generation of a particular pattern of organized digestive behavior. The interdigestive state of small intestinal behavior and the coordinated secretory and powerful propulsive behavior in response to foreign antigens are examples of programs in the enteric library.

Motor neurons are the links between the

interneuronal networks and the effector systems. They are the final common pathways for output from the nervous system to effectors that include the musculature, secretory epithelium, and blood vasculature. Communication from the interneuronal networks by way of motor neurons directs each effector system to respond with appropriate strength and timing to ensure meaningful coordination with the responses of allied effectors. This is the mechanism by which responses of the musculature, epithelium, and blood vasculature system are organized into a beneficial pattern of behavior at the level of the whole organ.

The Third Division of the Autonomic Nervous System

Johannis Newport Langley, the great British autonomic physiologist of Cambridge's Trinity College, recognized during the first quarter of the century that the ganglia of the gut did more than robotically relay and distribute information from the big brain. He could not reconcile the large disparity between the 2×10^8 neurons in the gut and the few hundred fibers in the vagus nerves other than to suggest that the nervous system of the gut possessed integrative functions independent of the central nervous system (1). This was reinforced by his demonstration of organized propulsion of intraluminal boluses in intestinal segments detached from the body *in vitro* (2). On this basis, he proposed recognition of the gut nervous system as a distinct division of the autonomic nervous system and named it the *enteric nervous system*.

Langley's insightful concept languished for nearly five decades. Nevertheless, now in the last decade of the century, three divisions comprised of parasympathetic, sympathetic, and enteric divisions are accepted by workers the world over as the essence of the autonomic nervous system.

Minibrain Circuits

The prevailing concept of the enteric nervous system, in the waning years of this century, is a minibrain placed in close proximity to the effector systems it controls. Rather than crowding the 2×10^8 neurons required for control of gut functions into the cranial cavity as part of the cephalic brain, and relying on signal transmission over long-unreliable pathways, natural selection placed the integrative microcircuits at the site of the effectors.

The circuits at the effector sites have evolved as an organized array of different kinds of neurons interconnected by chemical synapses. Function in the circuits is determined by generation of action potentials within the boundaries of single neurons and chemical transmission of information at the boundaries of contact between neurons. Action potentials transmit coded information from one region of the neuron to another. Synapses at the boundaries transform the action potential codes to chemical codes. Action potential codes arriving in the presynaptic neuronal terminals are transformed to chemical signals for transmission across the synapse and are then recoded as action potentials in the postsynaptic neurons. Postsynaptic neurons integrate large numbers of synaptic inputs and represent the fundamental component in the computation and processing of neural information. (Progress in understanding details of action potentials and synaptic transmission is described later in the chapter.)

Like the brain and spinal cord, the enteric circuitry processes information and generates patterns of signals that determine the timing and sequence of behavior of muscles and other effector systems. Processing of information in the circuits is a function whereby computation of input signals results in output to the effectors that is a meaningful transform of the input. Like electronic calculators, which receive numbers as input and calculate outputs according to specific equations preprogrammed into the circuits, the neural circuits receive sensory signals and compute outputs that control behavior of the effectors in ways adapted for overall performance of the specialized regions of gut.

Processing of sensory signals is appreciated as one of the major functions of the neural networks of the enteric nervous system. The sensory signals are generated by sensory nerve endings and coded in the form of action potentials. The code may represent the status of an effector system (e.g., tension in a muscle) or may signal a change in a parameter in the environment such as luminal pH. Sensory signals are computed by the neural networks to generate output signals that initiate homeostatic adjustments in the behavior of the effector system.

ENTERIC CIRCUIT FUNCTIONS

Four identifiable functions emerge from the "wiring configurations" (synaptic connectivity) in the enteric neural circuits. These are generalized functions that include: (1) reflexes; (2) pattern generation; (3) coordinated recruitment; and (4) gating. The programs for determination of the variety of intestinal patterns of behavior, described previously, incorporate this group of functions.

Reflexes

Reflex responses of neurally controlled effector systems have several common

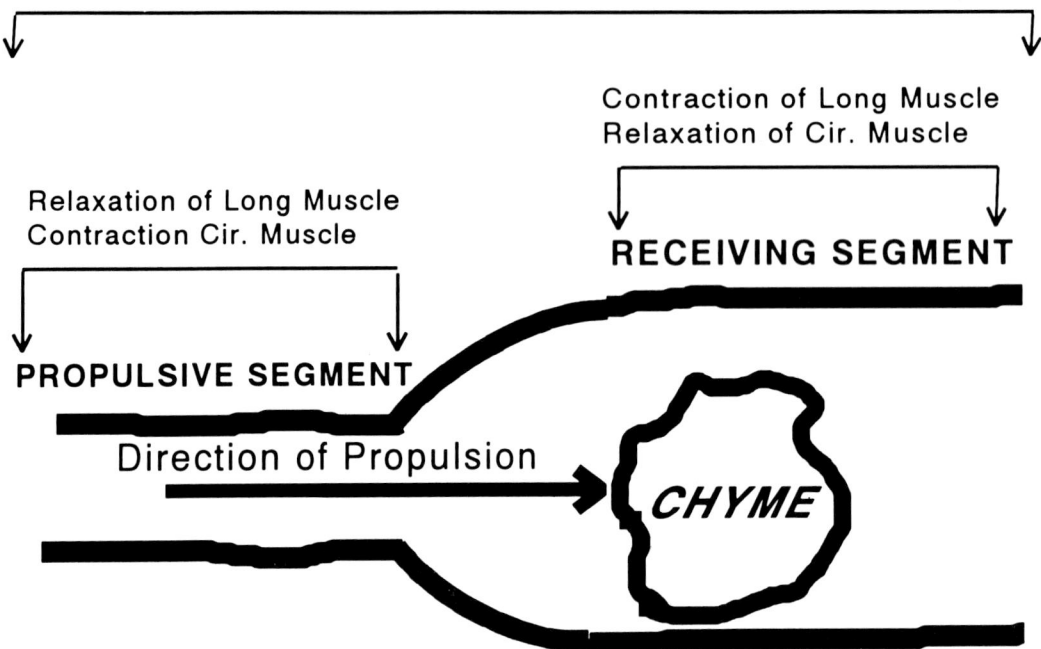

Fig. 10–2.   Peristaltic propulsion is a stereotyped pattern of muscle behavior consisting of a propulsive segment and a receiving segment. The receiving segment is configured by contraction of the longitudinal muscle and inhibition of the circular muscle in that segment. In the propulsive segment, the longitudinal muscle is relaxed and the circular muscle contracts.

characteristics. In the gastrointestinal system and elsewhere in the body, they are a form of effector system behavior that occurs in response to stimulation of sensory neurons. Reflex behavior is stereotyped in the sense that the pattern of effector behavior is reproduced each time the sensory neurons are activated by the preferred stimulus. Reflex behavior is automatic and occurs outside levels of cognitive consciousness. In skeletal muscles, it is a mechanism evolved for speed of response before processing of sensory information to levels of consciousness can occur with the brain. Reflex behavior is generally purposeful in nature (e.g., reflex withdrawal of the hand from a noxious stimulus).

The stereotyped sequence of muscle behavior during peristaltic propulsion (Fig. 10–2) emerges from a reflex pathway. A circuit with fixed connections automatically reproduces the stereotype pattern of behavior each time the circuit is activated. The

minimal circuit for peristaltic propulsion, which is illustrated in Figure 10–3, consists of connections of sensory neurons, interneurons, and motor neurons. It is triggered by sensory inputs or may be activated by command inputs from additional neural circuits. Sensory inputs are derived from distention-sensitive receptors located in the musculature and from mechanical or chemical stimulation of mucosal sensory receptors. Command inputs may be transmitted from the central nervous system or other regions of the enteric nervous system. The output response of the musculature is always the same, consisting of circular contraction and longitudinal relaxation above the point of stimulation and longitudinal contraction and circular relaxation below the point of stimulation.

The peristaltic reflex circuit is a fixed set of connections confined to short segments of intestine. Multiple sets of the same circuit are repeated serially along the intestine.

MINIMAL CIRCUIT FOR PERISTALSIS

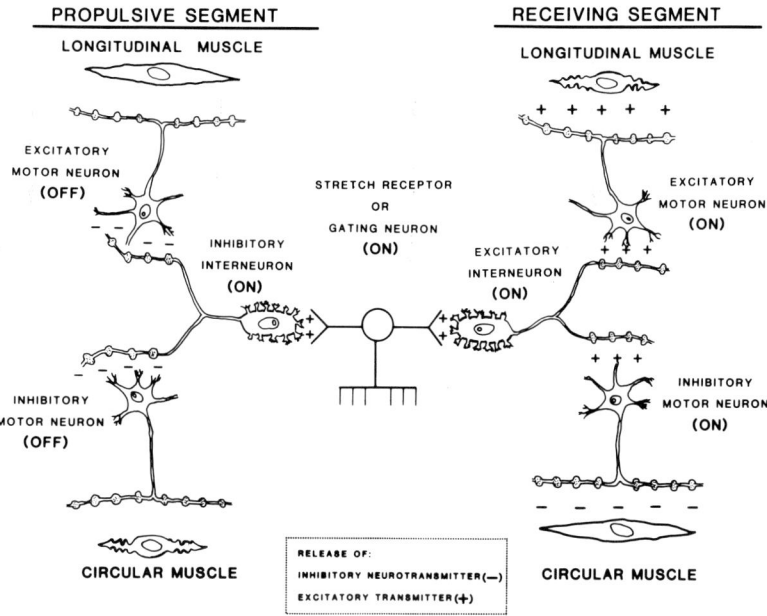

Fig. 10–3. A basic reflex circuit is responsible for the stereotyped behavioral complex of peristaltic propulsion. The basic circuit is organized with synaptic connections among sensory neurons (e.g., mechanoreceptors), interneurons, and motor neurons. Both inhibitory and excitatory motor neurons are required for operation of the circuit. Reproduced with permission from Wood JD: Neurophysiological theory of intestinal motility. Jpn J Smooth Muscle Res *23*:143, 1987.

Repetition of the same basic circuit all along the intestine is revealed by the ability at all levels of the intestine to experimentally evoke the stereotyped behavior characteristic of the peristaltic reflex. Persistence of the reflex in segments cut to a few centimeters in length is evidence that the basic circuit does not occupy an extensive length of intestine when reduced to its basic connections.

The peristaltic reflex circuit is the basic subfunction that underlies all patterns of propulsive motility. Timed sequencing of changes in the contractile state of the musculature in the minimal segment is determined by the permanently connected circuit of Figure 10–3, whereas the repetition rate of the program and the strength of each contractile component of the reflex are adjusted by sensory feedback signals or other modulatory commands to compensate automatically for changes in load and higher functional demands on the whole system.

Blocks of the basic peristaltic reflex circuit are connected in series along the length of the intestine. The strength of muscle responses in a single cycle of the propulsive circuit depends on the intensity of activation of the motor neurons of the circuit and on the number of redundant circuits that are called to activity in parallel. The distance the propulsive complex travels is determined by the number of basic circuits in series that are activated in sequence along the intestine (Fig. 10–4).

The basic circuits are believed to be interconnected by synaptic gates that determine the number of circuits used each time a propulsive event occurs (Fig. 10–4). Propulsive motility is prohibited when all gates are closed. Opening of all gates leads to the strongest muscle responses in a functioning segment and continuous propagation of the propulsive responses throughout long lengths of intestine. (Synaptic mechanisms of gating are discussed subsequently in the chapter.)

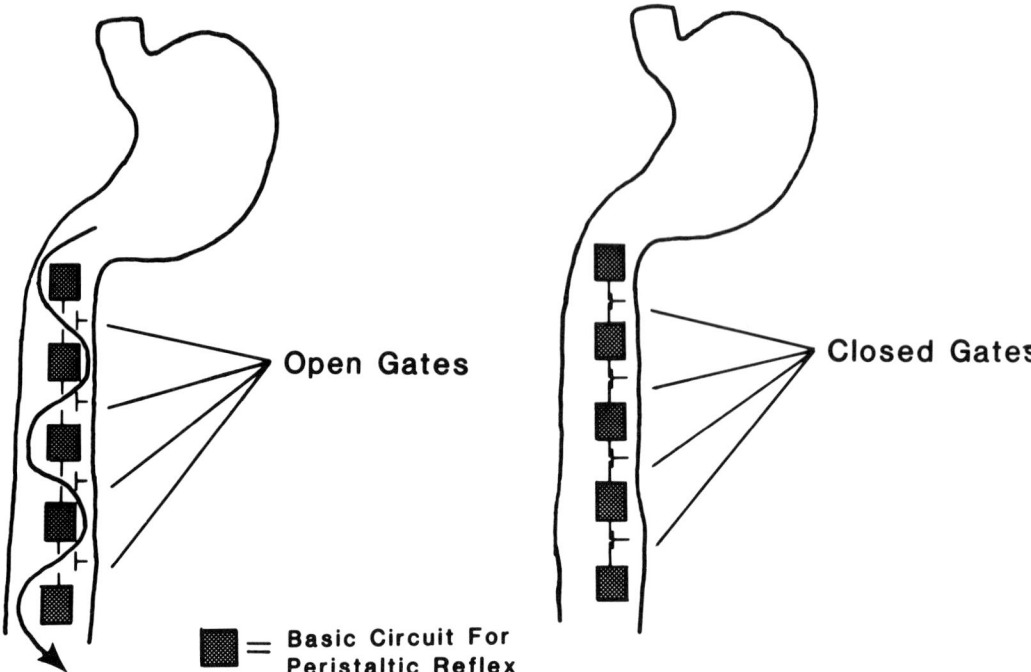

Fig. 10–4. The basic circuit for peristalsis is repeated serially along the intestine. The distance of propagation of peristaltic propulsion is determined by the operation of synaptic gates between the basic blocks of peristaltic circuitry. Opening of the gates between successive blocks of the basic circuit causes extended propagation of the propulsive event. Long-distance propulsion is prevented when all gates are closed. With all gates closed, activation of a single circuit block may result in a motor event that appears like a segmental contraction.

Pattern Generation

Neural pattern generators are neural networks programmed to generate timing and phasing signals for repetitive, rhythmic behaviors of effector systems. Repetitive activation of peristalsis within the activity front of the MMC probably reflects operation of a pattern generator. Short-segment peristalsis, occurring rhythmically at multiple sites along the small intestine during the digestive motility pattern, also appears to be driven by a pattern generator. Likewise, the rhythmic cycles of secretory activity of the colonic mucosa, recently described by Helen Cooke and coworkers at Ohio State University, reflect the output of a pattern generator (4).

Coordinated Recruitment

Populations of motor neurons must be recruited to activity in synchrony to evoke simultaneous responses of the musculature or secretory epithelium in a segment with several square centimeters of surface area. This is a function of enteric "driver circuits."

Driver circuits operate to synchronize motor and secretory events around the circumference of a defined length of intestine. These circuits are believed to provide simultaneous synaptic drive to subpopulations of inhibitory or excitatory motor neurons to the muscle layers during implementation of the propulsive motor programs (Fig. 10–5). They synchronize the discharge of excitatory motor neurons to the colonic crypts to drive the cyclic secretory behavior seen when mucosal mast cells release their mediators in response to antigenic stimulation (3).

The driver networks are "wired" with interneurons identified morphologically as Dogiel Type II and electrophysiologically as AH/Type 2 neurons (see subsequent text). The interneurons are believed to be synaptically connected for feed-forward excitation

FIRST SEGMENT   NEXT SEGMENT

Driver Network   SYNAPTIC   Driver Network
GATE

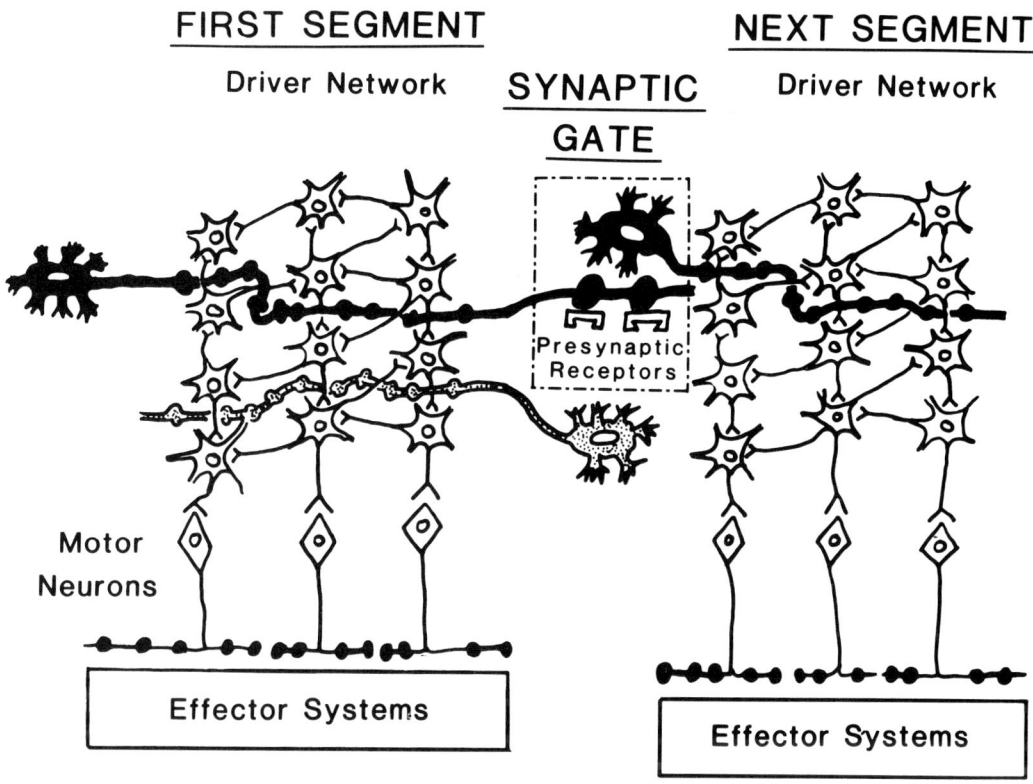

Motor
Neurons

Effector Systems   Effector Systems

Fig. 10–5. Neuronal driver networks use a mechanism of feed-forward excitation to accomplish simultaneous activation of populations of motor neurons within the circumferential and longitudinal boundaries of a segment. The circumference of an intestinal segment is shown. Synaptic gates between driver networks determine the length of intestine over which propulsion occurs. Excitatory interneurons with Dogiel Type I morphology turn on the driver networks. Inhibitory interneurons turn off the driver networks. Synaptic gates between driver networks are closed by activation of presynaptic inhibitory receptors. Closure of the gates prevents activation of the driver network in the next segment, and peristaltic propulsion stops at that segment.

(Fig. 10–5). Feed-forward excitation requires that the neurons in the circuit make recurrent excitatory synaptic connections with each other. This results in a positive feedback mode that accomplishes rapid buildup of excitation within the population of driver neurons. Feed-forward excitation ensures simultaneous activation of the entire network around the circumference of the segment. Simultaneous activation is important for effective application of the forces necessary for propulsion of the luminal contents and for effective secretory responses in the mucosa. Propulsion would be ineffective if, for example, contraction of the circular muscle occurred only partly around the circumference of the propulsive segment or if inhibition were in effect in

only part of the circumference of the receiving segment downstream.

Gating

Gating mechanisms determine the distance of propagation of the peristaltic behavioral complex. Gating, in theory, accounts for ultra-short-distance propagation in the segmentation mode of the digestive pattern. It also can account for extension of the propagation to intermediate distances within the boundaries of the activity front of the MMC and for ultra long-distance propagation associated with power propulsion. Synapses are the gating points that determine when driver circuits connected in series along the intestine are switched on for continued propagation of propulsive motor behavior from segment to segment (Fig. 10–5).

Presynaptic inhibitory mechanisms are implicated in gating the transfer of signals between serially positioned drive networks. Dogiel Type I interneurons (see subsequent text) are candidates for the connecting neurons that transmit signals for coordination of the behavior of driver networks in serial segments (Fig. 10–5). Synaptic connections between the Dogiel I neurons and neurons of the driver network are modeled as gating points for control of the distance of peristaltic propulsion. The presence in the surrounding milieu of neurotransmitters/neuromodulators, which act presynaptically to block the release of transmitter from axons of the Dogiel I connectors, closes the gates for forward transfer of neural signals. When this occurs, propulsion stops because the onward transfer of the signals fails.

The heuristic model of Figure 10–4 shows the basic circuit for the peristaltic behavioral complex as recurrent blocks along the intestine. Synaptic gates connect the blocks of basic circuitry and provide the mechanism for determination of the distance over which the propulsive complex propagates. When the gates are opened, neural signals pass between successive blocks of the basic circuit, resulting in propagation of the peristaltic event over extended distances. Long-distant propulsion is prevented when all gates are closed. With all gates closed, activation of a single block of circuitry may result in motor behavior such as the segmental or mixing contractions of the digestive motility pattern.

MORPHOLOGY OF NEURONS IN THE MINIBRAIN

Development in the 1980s of methods for intraneuronal injection of dyes from recording microelectrodes enabled the identification of morphology in association with electrophysiologic behavior and neurotransmitter content. Gordon Lees in Aberdeen, working at Marischal College in the early 1970s, did this first with a dye that was then new, procion yellow (5). Improvement in intracellular marker dyes, evolving from Lucifer yellow to biocytin and neurobiotin,

greatly facilitated progress in this area in the years that followed (6).

Intracellular marking confirmed most of the earlier histologic impressions of enteric neuronal morphology. These methods revealed the neural networks of the enteric nervous system to be "wired" with neurons belonging to one of four general morphologic categories (Fig. 10–6). Three of these are named Dogiel Types I, II, and III after the 18th century neuroanatomist, A. S. Dogiel. The fourth type, called filamentous neurons, was described recently in the guinea pig by John Furness and associates working at Flinders University in Adelaide.

ENTERIC MOTOR NEURONS

A critical advance toward the minibrain model came in the early 1960s with the discovery of gastrointestinal motor neurons that released neither norepinephrine nor acetylcholine as a neurotransmitter. Some of these were identified as inhibitory neurons that did not release norepinephrine and were therefore divorced from the sympathetic nervous system. The discovery of nonadrenergic inhibitory neurons was followed by findings of excitatory enteric motor neurons that released neurotransmitters other than acetylcholine. Thus, nonadrenergic-noncholinergic (NANC) neurons became the common acronym of escalating usage throughout the latter half of the century.

Inhibitory Motor Neurons

The discovery of nonadrenergic inhibitory neurons was the legacy of Edith Bülbring (1877–1991), "die grosse Dame" of smooth muscle research at Oxford University. She introduced her postdoctoral fellows, Mollie Holman and Geoffrey Burnstock, to the electrophysiology of the guinea-pig taenia coli, and this led to the definitive work on nonadrenergic inhibitory junction potentials (IJPs) in the muscle when they returned to Australia (Monash University and the University of Melbourne, respectively) in 1960–61 (7). Shortly to follow were demonstrations of the NANC inhibitory neurons in other regions by other Bülbring associates, includ-

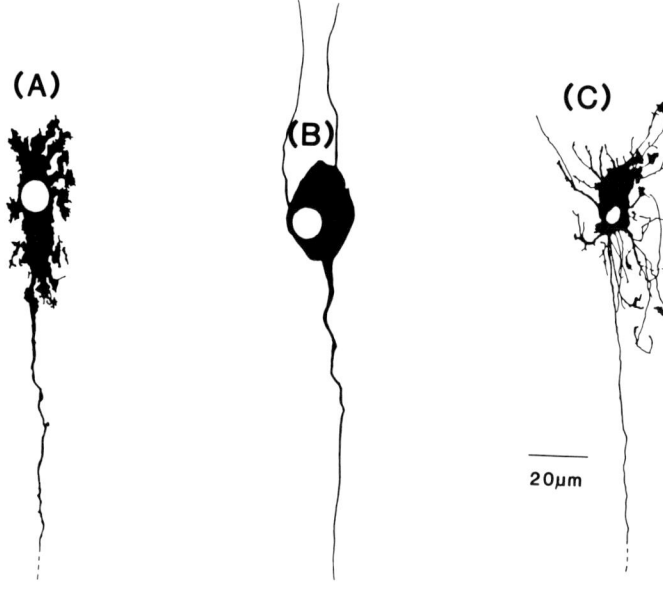

(A)

(B)

(C)

20μm

Fig. 10–6. Dogiel Type I *(A)*, Dogiel Type II *(B)*, and filamentous neurons *(C)* are the general morphologic categories of neurons found in the integrated circuits of the enteric nervous system. Redrawn with permission from Furness JB, Bornstein JC, Trussel DC: Shapes of nerve cells in the myenteric plexus of the guinea-pig small intestine revealed by the intracellular injection of dye. Cell Tissue Res *254*:561, 1988.

ing Antonio Crema at the University of Turin, Italy (8) and Hirosi Kuriyama of Kyushu University, Japan (9).

Work on characterizing the inhibitory actions of the neurons progressed with the input of a variety of students in Burnstock's laboratory including Marcello Costa, Max Bennett, Grahame Campbell, and John Furness (10). The junction potentials were evoked by transmural electrical stimulation of the inhibitory motor neurons. They were hyperpolarizing responses resulting from occupancy of receptors for the inhibitory neurotransmitter on the smooth muscle. The IJPs act to inhibit excitability by hyperpolarizing the membrane potential away from the voltage threshold for discharge of action potentials by the muscle membrane.

After the discovery of IJPs, Burnstock and coworkers, including Grahame Campbell and David Satchell, found the goal of identification of the neurotransmitter released by the inhibitory neurons to be elusive. By 1970, they had evidence that adenosine triphosphate (ATP) was the transmitter and Burnstock's purinergic hypothesis was born to the skepticism of much of the scientific community (11). Others grasped the new investigative opportunity and soon discovered that nonadrenergic inhibitory motor neurons to the circular mus-

cle coat were ubiquitous from the esophagus to the internal anal sphincter.

As work on NANC inhibition escalated around the world, the purinergic hypothesis came under attack and new transmitter candidates emerged. Sammy Said and Viktor Mutt (12), working at the Karolinska Institute in Stockholm, reported a new vasoactive peptide that was to become the next putative inhibitory neurotransmitter. Several principal investigators and their coworkers in the 1970s and 80s, including Harvard University's Raj Goyal, studying the lower esophageal sphincter and the Medical College of Virginia's Gabriel Makhlouf, the intestine, implicated vasoactive intestinal peptide as the transmitter. This marked the beginning of the burgeoning era of peptidergic neurotransmission in the gut. In the 1990s, nitric oxide has become prominent as an inhibitory transmitter candidate that has emerged from the pioneering work of John Gillespie in Glasgow (13–15).

Functional Significance of Inhibition

Progress in understanding neurophysiologic control of the musculature trailed other smooth muscle research and was delayed until a comprehensive picture of the physiology of the smooth muscle emerged (see Chap. 9). The importance of Burnstock's nonadrenergic inhibitory neurons and neural inhibition became apparent, in view of new understanding that the circular muscle layer behaves like a self-excitable syncytium much like cardiac muscle. In the absence of functional innervation, myogenic pacemakers periodically excite the muscle. Once muscle action potentials are triggered by the pacemaker, the excitation and associated contraction spread from muscle fiber to muscle fiber throughout the tissue.

Ongoing activity of the inhibitory motor system to release inhibitory neurotransmitters continuously suppresses excitability of the muscle. In this construct, the circular muscle responds to the ever-running pacemaker only when the inhibition is switched off and spread of muscle action potentials from the pacemaker site is permitted only in sectors of muscle where the inhibitory neurons are not releasing neurotransmitters. The effects of ongoing inhibition are seen when the activity of inhibitory neurons is abruptly blocked by agents, such as tetrodotoxin, which does not affect the muscle directly. Blockade of the neural activity is followed by an increase in action potential discharge in response to the muscle pacemaker and a coincident increase in uncoordinated contractile behavior. Elimination of inhibitory neural activity, or any other circumstance that results in ablation of inhibitory motor neurons, results in the release of uncontrolled chaotic contractile activity.

In the late 1960s, I found evidence that the neural correlate for ongoing inhibition of the circular muscle was the continuous patterned discharge of action potentials that could be recorded in some of the myenteric neurons of dog, guinea pig, cat, and rabbit small intestine (16,17). This neuronal activity results in continuous inhibition of the autogenous activity of the circular muscle. In segments of intestine in vitro, where the neuronal discharge in the myenteric plexus is prevalent, muscle action potentials and associated contractions are absent. I found that contractile responses to electrical stimulation are difficult to evoke in this state. The myogenic slow waves are always present (except in the guinea pig) in this circumstance but are unable to trigger spikes. When the neuronal discharge is blocked,

every cycle of the pacemaker triggers action potentials coupled with large amplitude contractions (18). After neural blockade, electrical stimulation readily evokes sharp phasic contractions of the muscle. Mechanical stimulation also triggers action potentials and large amplitude contractile waves which may propagate for distances of several centimeters in either direction along the segment of intestine (18).

These findings led to the general pathophysiologic rule that any treatment or condition that ablates the inhibitory motor neurons will result in tonic contracture and achalasia of the intestinal circular muscle. Various conditions, with functional ablation of the inhibitory neurons, were found to be associated with conversion from a hypoirritable condition of the circular muscle to a state of hyperirritability. These included (1) local anesthetic drugs (18); (2) long periods of cold storage (18); (3) hypoxic vascular perfusion of an intestinal segment (19); (4) surgical ablation (20); and (5) congenital absence, as in the piebald mouse model for Hirschsprung's disease (21). These states occur because the inhibitory motor innervation is tonically active and blockade or ablation of the motor neurons releases the circular muscle from inhibition permitting myogenic excitation and conduction to proceed unchecked.

The emergent model of the 1970s, in which tonically active inhibitory neurons continuously suppress myogenic activation and conduction of excitation in the circular muscle, included recognition that the patterns of intestinal motor behavior, discussed previously, are dependent on integrated disinhibition of the muscle. In each of the patterns, the interneuronal microcircuits organize the activity of the inhibitory neurons to determine: (1) when a particular pacemaker cycle triggers contractions; (2) the number of muscle fibers activated in parallel and, therefore, the force of the contractile response triggered by a pacemaker cycle; (3) the distance over which action potentials are allowed to spread within the muscular syncytium; and (4) the direction of spread of action potentials and the associated contractions in the syncytium.

In general, the inhibitory motor neurons, outside of the various sphincters, function to continuously suppress the activity of the inherently excitable musculature. Increased activation, within the population of inhibitory motor neurons, sustains circular muscle relaxation within the receiving segment of the peristaltic behavioral complex.

The inhibitory neurons have evolved with the additional functions of mediating vagally induced relaxation of the lower esophageal sphincter and upper stomach during food ingestion and relaxation of tone in other sphincters. Activation of these homologous neurons during swallowing relaxes the lower esophageal sphincter and, during defecation, they are turned on by the local neural networks to relax the internal anal sphincter.

The principal difference in the organization of the inhibitory outflow to the circular muscle of the intestine and the sphincters is tonically active inhibitory motor neurons in the intestine; the inhibitory innervation to the sphincters is normally silent. In the intestine, myogenic contractions occur when ongoing discharge of the inhibitory neurons is suppressed by inhibitory synaptic input from the interneuronal processing circuitry. In the sphincters, myogenic mechanisms maintain contractile tone (i.e., sphincteric muscle is tonically contracted in vivo in the absence of extrinsic nervous input and circulating hormones) and the sphincter relaxes when the normally silent inhibitory neurons are activated by excitatory synaptic input either from interneurons or from signals transmitted by vagal efferent fibers. Relaxation of the internal anal sphincter probably reflects specialized adaptation of the basic peristaltic reflex circuit with the sphincter behaving like a receiving segment at the "end of the line."

Pseudo-obstruction and Hirschsprung's Disease

Michael Shuffler's observations at the University of Washington, Seattle (22) of a loss of enteric neurons in human patients with the diagnosis of pseudo-obstruction suggests that the condition results from absence of neurons and obstructive spasm in the segment with the neuropathology. Consistent with this, Joseph Szurszewski and his coworkers at the Mayo Clinic recently demonstrated that the inhibitory junction potentials were weakened in resected segments from these patients, suggestive of depletion of the inhibitory nerve supply (23).

The inhibitory motor neurons, as well as other circuit components, are missing from the aganglionic segment in Hirschsprung's disease. Consequently, there is no evidence of inhibitory motor function and the segment remains constricted and obstructive in the absence of the peristaltic circuits. In studies of the aganglionic segment of the piebald mouse model, my students and I found that the circular muscle was continuously active in an uncoordinated manner as predicted for loss of inhibition (21,24,25). This explained the chronic constriction and absence of feces in the segment. We could not support the earlier theory that the hypertonic segment was a result of denervation hypersensitivity. In fact, Leonard Johnson of the University of Texas in Houston and I did not find any up-regulation of muscarinic cholinergic receptors on the muscle of the aganglionic segment (26).

Physiologic Ileus

The neurophysiologic explanation for physiologic ileus is ongoing activity of inhibitory motor neurons that results in the continuous release of inhibitory neurotransmitters at the neuromuscular junctions. Quiescence of the circular musculature, in the absence of defined motor patterns, reflects operation of a neural program that holds all gating points within and between peristaltic circuits closed. In this state, the inhibitory neurons are active and responsiveness of the muscle to the myogenic pacemaker is suppressed. This is a normal state persisting, for example, during Phase I of the MMC.

The normal state of motor quiescence becomes pathologic when the gates for propulsive motor patterns are unopenable by functional mechanisms over abnormally long periods of time. In this state, the basic circuits are locked in an inoperable state while unremitting activity of the inhibitory motor neurons suppress myogenic activity. Presence of the inhibitory transmitter prevents the inherent pacemaker system of the muscle from initiating contractions. Blockade of the inhibitory neurons with local anesthetics in animal experiments removes the ongoing inhibition, resulting in continuous contractile activity of the circular muscle layer because of the inherent excitability of the muscle in the absence of inhibition (18).

Excitatory Motor Neurons

The first well-documented evidence of the noncholinergic nature of excitatory transmission to the intestinal musculature was reported by Ambache and coworkers in 1968–70 at Oxford University (27,28). Failure of muscarinic antagonists to block contractile responses to electrical field stimulation and modification of the contractile responses by drugs without cholinergic actions were the early evidence for noncholinergic excitatory transmission.

Recent results with intraneuronal marking techniques, in combination with electrophysiology and immunocytochemical localization of neurotransmitters, indicate that enteric excitatory motor neurons have Dogiel Type I morphology (29). Also, like the inhibitory motor neurons, acetylcholine, acting at nicotinic receptors, is an important mechanism of signal transfer to these neurons.

Transmitters released by excitatory motor neurons to the musculature may trigger contraction by either depolarizing the muscle membrane to the threshold for firing of action potentials or by the direct release of calcium from intracellular stores in the muscle. Transmitters released from excitatory motor neurons to the intestinal crypts (secretomotor neurons) stimulate the secretion of water, mucus, and electrolytes (30–32). Transmitters released from motor neurons to the intestinal vasculature (enteric vasculomotor neurons) dilate the blood vessels and thereby increase mucosal blood flow (33,34).

Acetylcholine and substance P represent the important neurotransmitters released from excitatory motor neurons to the musculature (10,35,36). Vasoactive intestinal peptide and acetylcholine are the significant neurotransmitters presently known to be released from secretomotor neurons at the neuroepithelial junctions (30–32). The watery diarrhea syndrome in humans with tumors that produce high levels of circulating vasoactive intestinal peptide is related to stimulation of secretomotor neurons.

Enteric vasculomotor neurons release acetylcholine and vasoactive intestinal peptide to relax the musculature of submucosal arterioles; substance P constricts the mucosal vessels (30,31). Some of the submucous motor neurons send processes to innervate both the epithelium and vasculature ensuring coordination of function of the two effector systems.

Processes of secretomotor/vasculomotor neurons in the mucosa bind, ingest, and transport cholera toxin. Inside the neurons, the toxin stimulates formation of cyclic AMP which, in turn, enhances the excitability of the neurons, and thereby, the neurogenic drive on secretory behavior (37). This is, undoubtedly, a significant factor in cholera associated diarrhea.

CELLULAR NEUROPHYSIOLOGY OF THE ENTERIC MINIBRAIN

Major advances in enteric neurophysiology developed from application of electrophysiologic methods of recording the electrical and synaptic behavior of single neurons in the enteric nervous system. Investigations of this nature developed into a new subspecialty of gastrointestinal physiology in the latter half of the century. The methods were modified from highly successful approaches that were being applied to the study of neurons in the brain and spinal cord during this period.

The first electrophysiologic study of enteric neurons was reported in 1966 by Syomatu Yokoyama from Fukushima Medical College, Japan (deceased in 1992), working in Klaus Grevan's laboratory in then West Germany (38). He used steel needle microelectrodes to record spike discharge of single neuronal units in the myenteric plexus of the rabbit small intestine.

On the advice of my graduate professor, C. Ladd Prosser, in the Department of Physiology and Biophysics at the University of Illinois, I began single-unit recording from ganglion cells in the cat small intestinal myenteric plexus in 1967, with the first reports appearing in 1969 and 1970 (16,39). Professor Prosser was an authority in comparative neurophysiology, and his tutelage on simple nervous systems of invertebrate animals was invaluable for me later in coalescence of perspectives of an enteric minibrain analogous to these simple systems in control of the behavior of the digestive system.

The work with extracellular recording electrodes was continued by Prosser and Ohkawa, and their papers appeared in 1972 (40–41). Meanwhile, Claus Mayer, from the Physiologisches Institut in Munich, and I continued to use metal extracellular microelectrodes to record from guinea-pig myenteric plexus at the University of Kansas Medical Center in Kansas City (42,43).

During the 1970s, extracellular electrophysiologic studies were done by several groups in the United States, former USSR, and Japan (44–58). Alexander Nozdrachev's group in Leningrad was the first to record from myenteric neurons with the rabbit intestine in situ with blood flow intact (46,47,52). Most of the extracellular work done in the 1970s was on the small or large intestinal myenteric plexus from the guinea pig, cat, or rabbit (see reference 83 for a detailed review of the extracellular work). The primary findings with extracellular electrodes were spontaneous discharge patterns that could account for the ongoing inhibitory drive to the circular muscle, discharge properties of mechanoreceptors and long-lasting trains of spikes that were revealed later by intracellular recording to reflect slow synaptic excitation.

The first studies with intracellular microelectrodes were done almost simultaneously in Australia, Scotland, and the United States. David Hirst, Mollie Holman, and C. Ladd Prosser (59) reported in 1972 on intracellular studies of guinea-pig small-intestinal myenteric neurons done at Monash University in Australia. R. Alan North started intracellular studies of myenteric neurons in Aberdeen, Scotland and continued this work with Shogoro Nishi at Loyola University in Chicago, with the first report appearing in 1973 (60). The work of both groups was done in myenteric neurons in guinea-pig small intestine, which has been the case for most of the others who subsequently applied intracellular methods to study enteric neurons.

Since 1972, the literature on intracellularly determined properties of guinea-pig myenteric and submucous neurons has expanded considerably. Information on the electrical and synaptic behavior of guinea-pig myenteric neurons in specialized regions outside the small intestine is now available for the colon (61), rectum (62,63), gastric corpus (64,65), gastric antrum (66,67), gallbladder (68–70), pancreas (71), and esophagus (72). Reports of similar studies on submucous neurons are available for neurons in the submucous plexus of the small intestine (73,74), cecum (75), and colon (76,77). Fewer reports are available for other species. However, results are available from the cat (72,78), mouse (79), rat (80), and human (81).

Electrical Behavior

Enteric neurons are classified as S/Type 1 or AH/Type 2 on the basis of their electrical behavior recorded with intracellular microelectrodes. Hirst, Holman, and Spence (82) and Nishi and North (60) discovered the two types of neurons simultaneously. The first group used the "S" and "AH" terminology, whereas the latter referred to the cells as Types 1 and 2. It was learned later that the characteristic electrical behavior of the two types is generally related to the Dogiel morphological Types I and II. Dogiel Type I neurons usually have S/Type 1 behavior, whereas AH/Type 2 neurons have Dogiel Type II morphology. Filamentous neurons with a single long process may be one or the other of the two types. (Detailed review of the cellular neurophysiology of enteric neurons appears in reference 83.)

S/Type 1 Electrical Behavior

S/Type 1 neurons are distinguished from AH/Type 2 by the characteristics of the resting membrane potential, the input resistance, and by the way they discharge action potentials. These neurons have lower resting membrane potentials than AH/Type 2 neurons. The smaller membrane potentials are associated with a higher input resistance. S/Type 1 neurons also are more excitable than AH/Type 2 neurons. The elevated excitability is revealed as repetitive discharge of action potentials in response to injection of depolarizing current through the microelectrode (Fig. 10–7). The action potentials are not followed by long-lasting hyperpolarization of the membrane potential as in AH/Type 2 neurons.

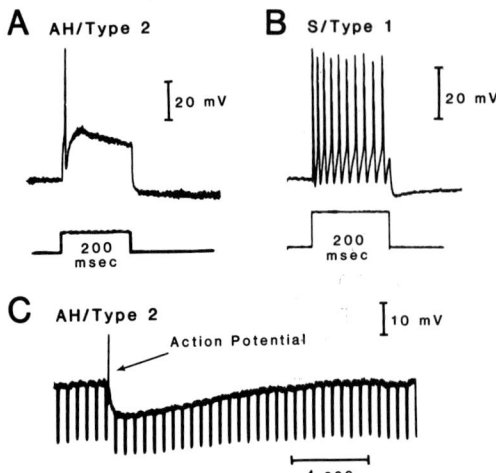

Fig. 10–7. Electrophysiologic behavior of AH/ Type 2 and S/Type 1 enteric neurons. *A.* AH/ Type 2 neuron discharged a single spike at the onset of a prolonged depolarizing current pulse. *B.* S/Type 1 neuron fired repetitively throughout the duration of a prolonged depolarizing current pulse. *C.* The action potential of an AH/Type 2 neuron was followed by a long-lasting hyperpolarizing after-potential. Upper traces in *A* and *B* are the recordings of transmembrane voltage changes; lower traces are records of the depolarizing current pulses injected through the microelectrode into the neuronal cell body. Downward deflections in C are electrotonic potentials produced by injection of repetitive pulses of depolarizing current. Decreased amplitude of the electrotonic potentials during the after-hyperpolarization reflects increased ionic conductance of the cell membrane. Reproduced with permission from Wood JD: Integrated circuits: The basis of gastrointestinal motility programs. *In* Heading RC, Wood JD (eds): Gastrointestinal Dysmotility: Focus on Cisapride. New York, Raven Press, 1992.

AH/Type 2 Electrical Behavior

AH/Type 2 neurons have higher resting membrane potentials associated with lower input resistance than S/Type 1 neurons. The lower input resistance and higher resting potentials reflect more open potassium channels and higher potassium conductance than in S/Type 1 neurons. Excitability of AH/ Type 2 neurons is lower than in S/Type 1 neurons. Injection of depolarizing current in these neurons evokes only one or two action potentials and only at the onset of the current pulse (Fig. 10–7). Repetitive discharge of spikes does not occur in response to current injection when the neuron is in its resting state. Nevertheless, we will see later in the chapter that excitatory neurotransmitters convert AH/Type 2 neurons from the hypo- to hyperexcitability state, with repetitive discharge similar to that seen in S/Type 1 neurons.

Hyperpolarization of several seconds duration follows the action potential in AH/ Type 2 neurons (Fig. 10–7). The after-hyperpolarization is a distinguishing characteristic of AH/Type 2 neurons and the basis for the "AH" designation. It acts to prolong the relative refractory period and results in an automatic mechanism that prevents repetitive spike discharge. The cell bodies of AH/Type 2 neurons are often found in a state of inexcitability. In this condition, they have high resting membrane potentials close to the potassium equilibrium potential and low input resistance indicative of high resting potassium conductance. Injection of depolarizing current does not evoke action potentials in this state; whereas synaptic potentials in response to inputs from other neurons in the circuit may be present. The synaptic potentials do not evoke spikes in this state.

Application of neurotransmitters/neuromodulators often restores excitability to the AH/Type 2 neurons. When this occurs, the cells may discharge action potentials with hyperpolarizing afterpotentials if the concentration of the messenger is low, or they may discharge repetitively like an S/Type 1 neuron if exposed to a higher concentration of the messenger. These neurons are interpreted as interneuronal circuit elements that are not used continuously by the system. When the state of the gut does not require operation of that section of circuitry (e.g., reverse peristalsis), the circuit is inactivated by the low excitability state of its component neurons. The circuit is called to activity by chemical modulators that act to boost the excitability of neurons in the circuit.

Synaptic Behavior

The basic mechanisms for chemically mediated synaptic transmission in the enteric nervous system turned out to be the same as elsewhere in the body. Synaptic transmitters are released by exocytosis from stores localized in vesicles at axonal terminals or transaxonal varicosities. Release is triggered by the arrival of an action potential at the release site. (Details of enteric synaptic transmission are found in reference 83.)

The synaptic events in the circuits of the enteric nervous system were found to be the same as in the brain and spinal cord. Excitatory postsynaptic potentials (EPSPs), inhibitory postsynaptic potentials (IPSPs), and presynaptic inhibition are the principal synaptic events found in the enteric minibrain. Both slow and fast synaptic mechanisms are operational in the gut. Fast synaptic potentials have durations in the millisecond range, whereas slow synaptic potentials last for several seconds or minutes. Fast synaptic potential are usually EPSPs. The slow synaptic events may be either EPSPs or IPSPs.

Fast Excitatory Postsynaptic Potentials

Fast EPSPs were found in the earliest recordings from enteric neurons but only in the S/Type 1 cells by Hirst, Holman, and Spence (82) and Nishi and North (60). They are membrane depolarizations with durations less than 50 ms (Fig. 10–8). Fast EPSPs were subsequently found to occur in S/Type 1 and AH/Type 2 neurons of both myenteric and submucous plexuses in the circuits of all specialized regions of the gastrointestinal tract, gallbladder, and pancreas. They are the sole mechanism of

transmission at the vagal-minibrain interface. Most of the fast EPSPs are mediated by acetylcholine at nicotinic postsynaptic receptors.

Fast EPSPs function in the rapid transfer and transformation of neurally coded information between the elements of the enteric microcircuits. They are the bytes of information in the information processing operations of the circuits. The fast EPSPs in Figure 10–8 recorded from the myenteric plexus of the gastric antrum, corpus, and small intestine reached the threshold for discharge of an action potential, whereas the other EPSPs did not reach threshold. Fast EPSPs do not reach this threshold when the neuronal membranes are hyperpolarized during slow inhibitory postsynaptic potentials. They are most likely to reach spike threshold when the membranes are depolarized during slow excitatory postsynaptic potentials. This fits the definition of neuromodulation, whereby the input-output relations of a neuron to one input are modified by a second synaptic input (84).

Slow Excitatory Postsynaptic Potentials

Enteric slow EPSPs in the late 1970s were unique synaptic events discovered almost simultaneously by R. Alan North and coworkers and by Claus Mayer and me (17,85–87). They are found in both myenteric and submucosal ganglion cells and in both AH/Type 2 and S/Type 1 neurons, but

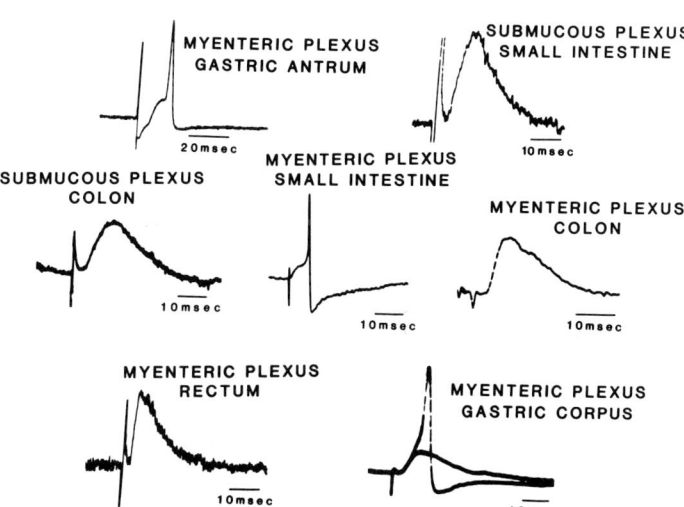

Fig. 10–8. Fast excitatory postsynaptic potentials occur in the millisecond time domain and may evoke action potentials when the depolarization of the membrane exceeds spike threshold. Fast EPSPs are found in the microcircuits of both the myenteric and submucous plexuses and in the various specialized regions of the digestive tract.

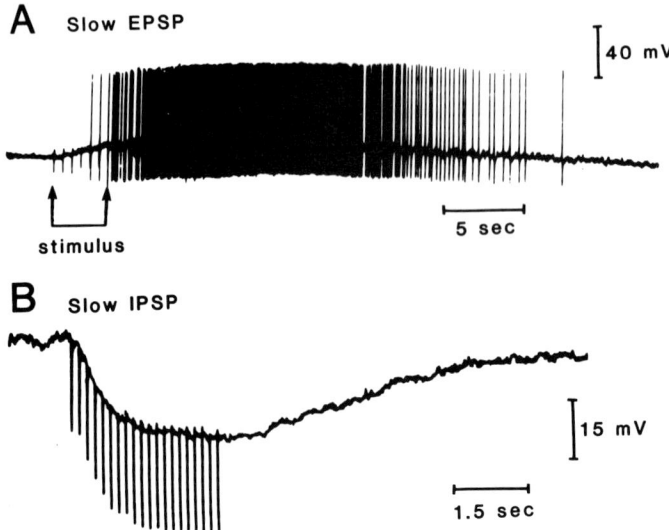

Fig. 10–9. Properties of slow excitatory and inhibitory postsynaptic potentials. *A*. Enhanced excitability during the slow EPSP is reflected by a train of action potentials that continues for several seconds after termination of stimulation of the excitatory axon. *B*. Slow inhibitory postsynaptic potentials are hyperpolarizing potentials. The EPSP and IPSP were recorded in the myenteric plexus of the guinea-pig small intestine.

are most dramatic in AH/Type 2 cells. Neurons with slow EPSPs are found in the small and large intestine and gastric antrum, but not the gastric corpus or gallbladder. They seem to be associated with specialized regions where peristaltic motility is a significant function.

Slowly activating membrane depolarization that is sustained for several seconds to minutes after termination of release of the neurotransmitter from the presynaptic terminal identifies the slow EPSP (Fig. 10–9). Enhanced excitability reflected by a long-lasting train of action potentials during the slow depolarization is the hallmark of the event. Enhanced excitability is apparent experimentally as repetitive spike discharge during depolarizing current pulses. AH/Type 2 neurons, which fire only a single spike at the beginning of a depolarizing current pulse in the inactivated state, fire repetitively in response to depolarizing pulses when the slow EPSP is in effect. When activated by the slow synaptic inputs, the behavior of the AH/Type 2 neurons is much like S/Type 1 neurons.

Postspike hyperpolarization in AH/Type 2 neurons is suppressed during the slow EPSP. Suppression of the after-hyperpolarization is part of the mechanism that permits repetitive spike discharge at increased frequencies during the enhanced state of excitability.

Slow EPSPs provide a mechanism for long-lasting activation or inhibition of gastrointestinal effector systems. The prolonged discharge of spikes during a slow EPSP drives the release of neurotransmitter from the neuron's axon for the duration of the spike discharge. Prolonged inhibition, or excitation at neuronal synapses in the processing circuits and at neuro-effector junctions, is the functional outcome of the slow EPSP. This relates to the functional behavior of the effector systems. Contractile responses of the gut musculature are sluggish events, relative to skeletal muscle, which last for several seconds from start to completion. The trainlike discharge of spikes during slow EPSPs is the neural correlate of long-lasting responses of the muscles in the functioning gastrointestinal tract. Prolonged secretory responses in the intestinal crypts also are related to the sustained discharge during slow EPSPs.

Neuropharmacology of Slow Synaptic Excitation

Several messenger substances found in neurons and endocrine cells of the brain and gut simulate slow synaptic excitation when applied experimentally to enteric neurons. The list, as it presently stands, is as follows:

Histamine	Acetylcholine
Vasoactive	Cholecystokinin
intestinal peptide	Bombesin
Caerulein	Calcitonin gene-
Gastrin-releasing	related peptide
peptide	Corticotropin-
Tachykinins	releasing
(neurokinins)	hormone
Thyrotropin-	Norepinephrine
releasing	Pituitary adenylate
hormone	cyclase
5-Hydroxy-	
tryptamine	
Gamma-	
aminobutyric acid	
Motilin	

Substance P (a tachykinin), 5-hydroxytryptamine, and acetylcholine fulfill criteria for function as neurotransmitters for the slow EPSP. Michael Gershon, of Columbia University, was an advocate for 5-hydroxytryptamine as an enteric neurotransmitter as early as 1967, with subsequent work in his laboratory firmly establishing this biogenic amine as a neurotransmitter (for reviews see 83, 88). Substance P was first proposed by Yoshifumi Katayama of Tokyo Medical-Dental University and R. Alan North, working together at the Massachusetts Institute of Technology, before North's move from Massachusetts to the Oregon Health Sciences Institute in 1986 (85). Claus Mayer and I, working at the Physiologisches Institut in Munich, first described the excitatory action of 5-hydroxytryptamine in 1978 (87).

Neuroimmune Communication

Slow EPSP-like actions of histamine is an example of a paracrine signal to the enteric microcircuits. Histamine is released from mast cells in response to antigenic stimulation. This is an example of neuroimmune communication, whereby the immune system signals the nervous system to change the programming of the effector systems to adapt to perturbations in the lumen (3,89). Enteric neuroimmune communication is a new and rapidly advancing area of investigation likely to expand understanding of irritable conditions in the gastrointestinal tract.

Histamine-containing mast cells in the mucosa behave like sensory receptors endowed with the immune system's ability to detect foreign antigens. Once they are sensitized to an antigen, the mast cells detect the next appearance of the antigen and respond by releasing chemical signals to the nervous system. Histamine is one of the signals. It acts primarily at the H_2 receptor subtype to excite the neurons. We will see further on in this chapter that histamine also has presynaptic inhibitory actions.

The neural response program to foreign antigens appears to be organized with power propulsion in combination with patterns of copious secretion of electrolytes and water in the large intestine. It is integrated behavior designed to eliminate the threatening agent rapidly and effectively from the intestinal lumen. Side effects of operation of the program are diarrhea and lower GI malaise.

Slow Inhibitory Postsynaptic Potentials

Slow IPSPs are characterized by slowly activating hyperpolarization of the membrane potential lasting for several seconds after termination of the release of the neurotransmitter (Fig. 10–9). Slow IPSPs were first reported in small intestinal submucous neurons in 1975 by David Hirst and Hugh McKirdy working at Monash University in Australia (90). Subsequently, Annmarie Surprenant and coworkers contributed significantly to understanding of inhibitory transmission in the submucous plexus (91–92).

Slow IPSPs are found in cell somas of the myenteric and submucous plexuses of the small and large intestine. They are found most frequently in the submucous plexus. The IPSPs are less readily demonstrated in the myenteric plexus because of the simultaneous release of neurotransmitters for slow synaptic excitation in the experimental situation.

Reduced excitability of the somal membrane during the IPSPs decreases the probability of action potential discharge. The probability that the somal membrane will be fired by excitatory synaptic inputs is reduced and is the inverse of the situation with slow EPSPs.

The functional significance of slow synaptic inhibition in the myenteric plexus is termination of the excitatory state of slow synaptic excitation and re-establishment of the low excitability state in the neuronal cell soma. This may be a step in the control of sequentially occurring motor events, such as the conversion from inhibition to excitation in the circular muscle of an intestinal segment during passage of peristaltic propulsion. In the intact animal, there also may be inhibitory modulators of endocrine or paracrine origin that function in particular situations to lock the somal membranes in a low-excitability state.

Neuropharmacology of Slow Synaptic Inhibition

In the years from 1975 to 1992, several putative brain-gut messenger substances were found to mimic slow synaptic inhibition when applied to enteric neurons. The list of substances, which will undoubtedly continue to grow, appears below:

Acetylcholine   Opioid peptides
5-Hydroxytryptamine   Norepinephrine
Neurotensin   Cholecystokinin
Somatostatin   Purine nucleotides
Galanin

Understanding of synaptic inhibition in secretomotor neurons of the submucous plexus of both small and large intestine was a major advance in understanding secretory diarrhea and the mechanism of action of antidiarrheal drugs. The secretomotor neurons were found to have alpha$_2$ adrenoceptors for norepinephrine, delta opioid receptors, and somatostatin receptors. (See references 30–32 for detailed review of neurally evoked secretion.) Activation of any of the inhibitory receptors results in inhibition of firing of the neurons. Enhanced firing of the secretomotor neurons may be a normal functional event or may result from a variety of insults such as inflammation, sensitizing antigens, and bacterial toxins. Inhibition of firing reduces the release of excitatory neurotransmitters at the junction of secretomotor axons with epithelial cells in the crypts. The end result is reduced secre-

tion of water and electrolytes into the intestinal lumen.

The alpha$_2$ inhibitory adrenoceptors on secretomotor neurons are activated by norepinephrine released from postganglionic neurons of the sympathetic division of the autonomic nervous system. No or minimal synthesis of norepinephrine occurs in neurons intrinsic to the enteric nervous system. Neurons with cell bodies in the enteric nervous system also supply inhibitory input to secretomotor neurons. Intrinsic neurons are a source of somatostatin which, when released, inhibits firing of the secretomotor neurons. Intrinsic neurons also are the source of inhibitory opioid peptides such as met-enkephalin, which acts to hyperpolarize secretomotor neurons and reduce the excitatory drive for secretion.

The new understanding of the neuropharmacology of slow synaptic inhibition in the submucous plexus opened the way for explaining the mechanism of action of some antidiarrheal drugs and the constipating action of others. Clonidine, which is an alpha$_2$ agonist and effective antidiarrheal drug, inhibits firing of secretomotor neurons and thereby, reduces neuronal secretory drive to the crypts. Octreotide, the stable somatostatin analog, acts in a similar manner, as does the opioid loperamide. Much of the well-known constipating action of morphine and other narcotic analgesics is undoubtedly related to similar effects of these agents on the secretomotor neurons.

Presynaptic Inhibition

Presynaptic inhibition is the term for mechanisms that suppress release of neurotransmitters from axons. It was first described for the enteric nervous system in 1974 by David Hirst and Hugh McKirdy (93). Presynaptic inhibition is brought about by chemical messengers acting at receptors on the axon. The electrophysiologic studies of the 1970s and 80s uncovered presynaptic inhibition as another significant synaptic event within the enteric microcircuits of the gastric corpus and antrum, as well as the small and large intestine and rectum of the guinea pig (62,65,67,83). It was found to occur at both fast and slow excitatory synapses in the circuits, as well as at neuroeffector junctions.

Presynaptic mechanisms of gating the spread of neural signals utilize presynaptic inhibition to block transmission across synaptic connections within the circuits (see Fig. 10–5). An axon of an enteric interneuron projects only for short distances along the longitudinal direction of the bowel before ending as a synapse with another neuron. The longest projection is, at most, no more than 2 to 3 cm. This suggests that the spread of neuronal signals for propagated behavioral events must cross many synapses for propagation of the event to continue along the intestinal tube. Moreover, each consecutive synapse must transmit unfailingly for propagation to continue. Presynaptic inhibition is an effective mechanism for stopping transmission at synapses. Consequently, activation of presynaptic receptors in the local networks within a given region of intestine brings a propagating event to a halt. Virtually all of the synapses in the neural circuits of the small and large intestine and gastric antrum have presynaptic inhibitory receptors at the release sites for the neurotransmitters. This presents a continuous matrix of sites along the bowel where presynaptic mechanism can gate the distance, as well as the direction of travel of neural signals within the enteric plexuses (94,95).

Neuropharmacology of Presynaptic Inhibition

In the years from 1973 to 92, several putative brain-gut messenger substances were found to activate presynaptic inhibitory receptors. The list of substances appears below:

Norepinephrine	Dopamine
Histamine	5-Hydroxytryptamine
Opioid peptides	Acetylcholine
Neuropeptide Y	Pancreatic polypeptide
Peptide YY	

CONCLUSION

Effective July 25, 1989, U.S. President George H. Bush signed into law a joint resolution of Congress (H. J. Res. 174) declaring January 1, 1990 the start of the decade of the brain. Twentieth-century progress in neurogastroenterology has paved the way for the early 21st century to be the decade of the enteric minibrain in terms of advancement in understanding digestive diseases.

ACKNOWLEDGMENT

Work on neurogastroenterology in my laboratory has been supported by National Institutes of Health research grants RO1 AM26742, RO1 AM16813, RO1 NS17363, RO1 DK37238, RO1 AA07123, RO1 DK39937, and RO1 41825; and a Research Career Development Award. My work in Germany was supported by a fellowship from the Alexander von Humboldt Foundation.

REFERENCES

1. Langley JN: The Autonomic Nervous System, Part I. Cambridge, England, W. Heffer and Sons, 1921.
2. Langley JN, Magnus R: Some observations of movements of the intestine before and after degenerative section of the mesenteric nerves. J Physiol (Lond) *33*:34, 1905.
3. Wood JD: Communication between minibrain in gut and enteric immune system. NIPS *6*:64, 1991.
4. Wang YZ, Cooke HJ: H$_2$ receptors mediate cyclical chloride secretion in guinea pig distal colon. Am J Physiol *258*:G887, 1990.
5. Hodgkiss JP, Lees GM: Correlated electrophysiological and morphological characteristics of myenteric neurones. J Physiol (Lond) *285*:19, 1978.
6. Bornstein JC, Hendriks R, Furness JB, Trussell DC: Ramifications of the axons of AH-neurons injected with the intracellular marker biocytin in the myenteric plexus of the guinea pig small intestine. J Comp Neurol *314*:437, 1991.
7. Burnstock G, Campbell G, Bennett M, Holman ME: Inhibition of the smooth muscle of the taenia coli. Nature (Lond) *200*:581, 1963.
8. Beani L, Bianchi C, Crema A: Vagal noncholinergic inhibition of guinea-pig stomach. J Physiol (Lond) *217*:259, 1971.
9. Kuriyama H, Osa T, Toida N: Nervous factors influencing the membrane activity of intestinal smooth muscle. J Physiol (Lond) *191*:257, 1967.
10. Hoyle CHV, Burnstock G: Neuromuscular transmission in the gastrointestinal tract. *In* Wood JD (ed): Handbook of Physiology,

The Gastrointestinal System, Motility and Circulation, Vol I. Bethesda, Maryland, American Physiological Society, 1989.

11. Burnstock G: Purinergic neurons. Pharmacol Rev *34*:509, 1972.

12. Mutt V, Said SI: Structure of the porcine vasoactive intestinal octacosapeptide. The amino acid sequence. Use of kallikrein in its determination. Eur J Biochem *42*:581, 1974.

13. Gillespie JS: Nonadrenergic non-cholinergic inhibitory control of gastrointestinal motility. *In* Wienbeck M (ed): Motility of the Digestive Tract. New York, Raven Press, 1982.

14. Sanders KM, Ward SM: Nitric oxide as a mediator of nonadrenergic noncholinergic neurotransmission. Am J Physiol *25*:G379, 1992.

15. Grider JR, Murthy KS, Jin J-G, Makhlouf GM: Stimulation of nitric oxide from muscle cells by VIP: Prejunctional enhancement. Am J Physiol *262*:G774, 1992.

16. Wood JD: Electrical activity from single neurons in Auerbach's plexus. Am J Physiol *219*:159, 1970.

17. Wood JD, Mayer CJ: Intracellular study of electrical activity of Auerbach's plexus in guinea-pig small intestine. Pflügers Archiv. *374*:265, 1978.

18. Wood JD: Excitation of intestinal muscle by atropine, tetrodotoxin and xylocaine. Am J Physiol *222*:118, 1972.

19. Hukuhara T, Kotania S, Sato G: Effect of destruction of intramural ganglion cells on colon motility: Possible genesis of congenital megacolon. Jpn J Physiol *11*:635, 1961.

20. Schiller WR, Suriyapa C, Mutchler JHW, Anderson MC: Surgical alteration of intestinal motility. Am J Surg *125*:122, 1973.

21. Wood JD: Electrical activity of the intestine of mice with hereditary megacolon and absence of myenteric ganglion cells. Am J Dig Dis *18*:477, 1973.

22. Schuffler MD, Baird HW, Fleming CR: Intestinal pseudo-obstruction as the presenting manifestation of small cell carcinoma of the lung: A paraneoplastic neuropathy of the gastrointestinal tract. Ann Intern Med *98*:129, 1983.

23. Koch TR, Carney JA, Go VLW, Szurszewski JH: Altered inhibitory innervation of circular smooth muscle in Crohn's colitis. Association with decreased vasoactive intestinal polypeptide levels. Gastroenterology *98*:1437, 1990.

24. Wood JD, Brann LR, Vermillion DL: Electrical and contractile behavior of the large intestinal musculature of the piebald mouse model for Hirschsprung's Disease. Dig Dis Sci *31*:638, 1986.

25. Wood JD, Brann LR: Pharmacological analysis of poststimulus rebound excitation in the large intestine of the piebald mouse model for Hirschsprung's Disease. Dig Dis Sci *31*:744, 1986.

26. Seidel ER, Wood JD, Eikenburg BE, Johnson LR: Muscarinic cholinergic receptors in the piebald mouse model for Hirschsprung's Disease. Gastroenterology *85*:335, 1983.

27. Ambache N, Freeman MA: Atropine-resistant longitudinal muscle spasms due to excitation of non-cholinergic neurons in Auerbach's plexus. J Physiol (Lond) *199*:705, 1968.

28. Ambache N, Verney J, Zar MA: Evidence for the release of two atropine-resistant spasmogens from Auerbach's plexus. J Physiol (Lond) *207*:761, 1970.

29. Brookes SJH, Steele PA, Costa M: Identification and immunohistochemistry of cholinergic and non-cholinergic circular muscle motor neurons in the guinea-pig small intestine. Neuroscience *42*:863, 1991.

30. Cooke HJ: Complexities of nervous control of the intestinal epithelium. Gastroenterology *94*:1087, 1988.

31. Cooke HJ: Neurobiology of the intestinal mucosa. Gastroenterology *90*:1057, 1986.

32. Cooke HJ: Role of the "little brain" in the gut in water and electrolyte homeostasis. FASEB J *3*:127, 1989.

33. Bungardt E et al.: Characterization of muscarinic receptors mediating vasodilation in guinea-pig ileum submucosal arterioles by the use of computer-assisted videomicroscopy. Eur J Pharmacol *213*:53, 1992.

34. Jiang MM, Surprenant A: Re-innervation of submucosal arterioles by myenteric neurones following extrinsic denervation. J Auton Nerv Syst *37*:145, 1992.

35. Daniels EE, Collins SM, Fox JET, Huizinga JD: Pharmacology of drugs acting on gastrointestinal motility. *In* Wood JD (ed): Handbook of Physiology, The Gastrointestinal System, Motility and Circulation Vol I. Bethesda, Maryland, American Physiological Society, 1989.

36. Daniel EE, Collins SM, Fox JET, Huizinga JD: Pharmacology of neuroendocrine peptides. *In* Wood JD (ed): Handbook of Physiology, The Gastrointestinal System, Motility and Circulation Vol I. Bethesda, Maryland, American Physiological Society, 1989.

37. Jiang MM, Kirchgessner A, Gershon MD, Surprenant A: Cholera toxin sensitive neurons in guinea-pig submucosal plexus. Am J Physiol *264*:G86, 1993.

38. Yokoyama S: Aktionspotentiale der ganglienzelle des Auerbachschen plexus in Kaninchendunndarm. Arch Ges Physiol *288*:95, 1966.

39. Wood JD, Prosser CL: Electrical activity from single neurons in Auerbach's plexus of cat intestine. Physiologist *12*:398, 1969.

40. Ohkawa H, Prosser CL: Electrical activity in myenteric and submucous plexuses of the cat small intestine. Am J Physiol *222*:1412, 1972.

41. Ohkawa H, Prosser CL: Functions of neurons in enteric plexuses of cat intestine. Am J Physiol *222*:1420, 1972.

42. Wood JD, Mayer CJ: Patterned discharge of six different neurons within a single enteric ganglion. Pflügers Archiv *338*:247, 1973.

43. Wood JD, Mayer CJ: Properties of mechanosensitive neurons within Auerbach's plexus of the small intestine of the cat. Pflügers Archiv *357*:35, 1975.

44. Dingledine R, Goldstein A: Single neuron studies of opiate action in the guinea-pig myenteric plexus. Life Sci *17*:57, 1975.

45. Ehrenpreis S et al.: Mechanism of morphine block of electrical activity in ganglia of Auerbach's plexus. Eur J Pharmacol *40*:303, 1976.

46. Gnetov AV, Katchalov YP: Use of light director for revealing intramural ganglia and plexus in an intact functioning organ. Sech Physiol J USSR (Engl transl Fiziol Zh SSSR Im Sechenova IM) *61*:794, 1975.

47. Katchalov YP, Gnetov AV: On the microelectrode orientation in regard to the optical axis when studying cells of the intramural nervous apparatus. Sech Physiol J USSR (Engl transl Fiziol Zh SSSR Im Sechenova IM) *61*:791, 1975.

48. North RA, Williams JT: Enkephalin inhibits firing of myenteric neurones. Nature (Lond) *264*:460, 1976.

49. North RA, Williams JT: Extracellular recording from the guinea-pig myenteric plexus and the action of morphine. Eur J Pharmacol *45*:23, 1977.

50. Nozdrachev AD: Functional organization of the myenteral plexus ganglions. Sech Physiol J USSR (Engl transl Fiziol Zh SSSR Im Sechenova IM) *63*:268, 1977.

51. Nozdrachev AD, Kachalov YP, Gnetov AV: Adrenosensitive neurons of the myenteric (Auerbach's) plexus. Bull Exp Biol Med (Engl Transl Bull, Eksp Biol Med) *83*:259, 1977.

52. Nozdrachev AD, Kachalov YP, Gnetov AV: Spontaneous activity of neurons in myenteric plexus of the intestine of intact segments in rabbits. Sech Physiol J USSR (Engl transl Fiziol Zh SSSR Im Sechenova IM) *61*:725, 1975.

53. Nozdrachev AD, Vataev SI: Neuronal electrical activity in the submucosal plexus of the cat small intestine. J Auto Nerv Syst *3*:45, 1981.

54. Sakai KK, Hymson DL, Shapiro R: The mode of action of enkephalins in the guinea-pig myenteric plexus. Neurosci Lett *10*:317, 1978.

55. Sato T, Takayanagi I, Takagi K: Pharmacological properties of electrical activities obtained from neurons in Auerbach's plexus. Jpn J Pharmacol *23*:665, 1973.

56. Sato T, Takayanagi I, Takagi K: Effects of acetylcholine releasing drugs on electrical activities obtained from Auerbach's plexus in the guinea-pig ileum. Jpn J Pharmacol *24*:447, 1974.

57. Yokoyama S, Ozaki T, Kajitsuka T: Excitation conduction in Auerbach's plexus of rabbit small intestine. Am J Physiol *232*:E100, 1977.

58. Yokoyama S, Ozaki T: Polarity of effects of stimulation of Auerbach's plexus on longitudinal muscle. Am J Physiol *235*:E345, 1978.

59. Hirst GDS, Holman ME, Prosser CL, Spence I: Two types of neurones in the myenteric plexus of duodenum in the guinea-pig. J Physiol (Lond) *225*:60P, 1974.

60. Nishi S, North RA: Intracellular recording from the myenteric plexus of the guinea-pig ileum. J Physiol (Lond) *231*:471, 1973.

61. Wade PR, Wood JD: Electrical behavior of myenteric neurons in guinea-pig distal colon. Am J Physiol *254*:G522, 1988.

62. Tamura K, Wood JD: Electrical and synaptic properties of myenteric plexus neurones in the terminal large intestine of the guinea-pig. J Physiol (Lond) *415*:275, 1989.

63. Tamura K: Morphology of electrophysiologically identified myenteric neurons in the guinea-pig rectum. Am J Physiol *262*:G545, 1992.

64. Schemann M, Wood JD: Electrical behavior of myenteric neurones in the gastric corpus of the guinea-pig. J Physiol (Lond) *417*:501, 1989.

65. Schemann M, Wood JD: Synaptic behavior of myenteric neurones in the gastric corpus of the guinea-pig. J Physiol (Lond) *417*:519, 1989.

66. Tack JF, Wood JD: Electrical behaviour of myenteric neurones in the gastric antrum of the guinea-pig. J Physiol (Lond) *447*:49, 1992.

67. Tack JD, Wood JD: Synaptic behavior in the myenteric plexus of the guinea-pig gastric antrum. J Physiol (Lond) *445*:389, 1992.

68. Mawe GM: Intracellular recording from gallbladder neurones of the guinea-pig gallbladder. J Physiol (Lond) *429*:323, 1990.

69. Mawe GM: The role of cholecystokinin in ganglionic transmission in the guinea-pig gallbladder. J Physiol (Lond) *439*:89, 1991.

70. Bauer AJ, Hanani M, Muir TC, Szurszewski

JH: Intracellular recordings from gallbladder ganglia of opossums. Am J Physiol *260*: G299, 1991.

71. Ma RC, Szurszewski JH: 5-hydroxytryptamine (5-HT) evokes fast and slow depolarization in cat intrapancreatic neurons. Gastroenterology *102*:A744, 1992.

72. Janssens W, Tack JF, Janssens J, Vantrappen G: Electrical and synaptic properties of myenteric neurons in the esophageal body of the cat. Gastroenterology *102*:A462, 1992.

73. Surprenant A: Slow excitatory synaptic potentials recorded from neurones of guinea-pig submucous plexus. J Physiol (Lond) *351*: 343, 1984.

74. Surprenant A: The two types of neurones lacking synaptic input in the submucous plexus of guinea-pig small intestine. J Physiol (Lond) *351*:363, 1984.

75. Mihara S: Electrophysiological properties and chemosensitivities of neurons in Meissner's (submucous) plexus of the guinea-pig caecum. J Kurume Med Assoc *41*:1039, 1982.

76. Frieling T, Cooke HJ, Wood JD: Electrophysiological properties of neurons in submucous ganglia of the guinea-pig distal colon. Am J Physiol *260*:G835, 1991.

77. Frieling T, Cooke HJ, Wood JD: Synaptic transmission in submucous ganglia of the guinea-pig distal colon. Am J Physiol *260*: G842, 1991.

78. Wood JD: Intracellular study of effects of morphine on electrical activity of myenteric neurons in cat small intestine. Gastroenterology *79*:1222, 1980.

79. Furukawa K, Taylor GS, Bywater RAR: An intracellular study of myenteric neurons in the mouse colon. J Neurophysiol *55*:1395, 1986.

80. Brookes SJH, Ewart WR, Wingate DL: Intracellular recordings of cells in the myenteric plexus of rat duodenum. Dig Dis Sci *30*:761, 1985.

81. Brookes SJH, Ewart WR, Wingate DL: Intracellular recordings from myenteric neurones in the human colon. J Physiol (Lond) *390*:305, 1987.

82. Hirst GDS, Holman ME, Spence I: Two types of neurons in the myenteric plexus of duodenum in the guinea-pig. J Physiol (Lond) *236*:303, 1974.

83. Wood JD: Electrical and synaptic behavior of enteric neurons. *In* Wood JD (ed): Handbook of Physiology, The Gastrointestinal System, Motility and Circulation, Vol I. Bethesda, Maryland, American Physiological Society, 1989.

84. Wood JD: Neuromodulation in the enteric nervous system. *In* Bloom SR, Polak JM, Lindenlaub E (eds): Systemic Role of Regulatory Peptides. New York, F. K. Schattauer Verlag, 1982.

85. Katayama Y, North RA: Does substance P mediate slow synaptic excitation within the myenteric plexus? Nature (Lond) *274*:387, 1978.

86. Wood JD, Mayer CJ: Intracellular study of tonic-type enteric neurons in guinea-pig small intestine. J Neurophysiol *43*:569, 1979.

87. Wood JD, Mayer CJ: Slow synaptic excitation mediated by serotonin in Auerbach's plexus. Nature (Lond) *276*:836, 1979.

88. Mawe GM, Branchek TA, Gershon MD: Peripheral neural serotonin receptors: Identification and characterization with specific antagonists and agonists. Proc Natl Acad Sci (USA) *83*:9799, 1986.

89. Wood JD: Intestinal neuroimmune interactions. *In* Holle GE, Wood JD (eds): Advances in the Innervation of the Gastrointestinal Tract. Amsterdam, Elsevier, 1992.

90. Hirst GDS, McKirdy HC: Synaptic potentials recorded from neurones of the submucous plexus of guinea-pig small intestine. J Physiol (Lond) *249*:369, 1975.

91. Surprenant A, North RA: Mechanism of synaptic inhibition by noradrenaline acting at alpha 2- adrenoceptors. Proc R Soc (Lond) *234*:85, 1988.

92. North RA, Surprenant A: Inhibitory synaptic potentials resulting from alpha$_2$ adrenoceptor activation in guinea-pig submucous plexus neurones. J Physiol (Lond) *358*:17, 1985.

93. Hirst GDS, McKirdy HC: Presynaptic inhibition at a mammalian peripheral synapse. Nature (Lond) *250*:430, 1974.

94. Furness JB, Bornstein JC, Trussell DC: Shapes of nerve cells in the myenteric plexus of the guinea-pig small intestine revealed by the intracellular injection of dye. Cell Tissue Res *254*:561, 1988.

95. Wood JD: Integrated circuits: The basis of gastrointestinal motility programs. *In* Heading RC, Wood JD (eds): Gastrointestinal Dysmotility: Focus on Cisapride. New York, Raven Press, 1992.

11

The Enteric Flora and Gastrointestinal Disease

ROBERT M. DONALDSON JR.

EARLY CONSIDERATIONS OF THE ENTERIC FLORA

Serious interest in the microbial populations of the intestine began at the end of the 19th century, when the scientific community was increasingly focusing its attention on the bacterial basis of many diseases and on the potency of bacterial toxins. Unquestionably, Elie Metchnikoff was the most influential scientist of that era to emphasize the harm caused by the innumerable microbes normally present in the human colon. Born and educated in Kharkoff (Little Russia), Metchnikoff was a zoologist widely respected as a gifted observer and an astute interpreter. His observations in water fleas led him to discover both the phagocytic functions of human white blood cells and the phenomenon now known as chemotaxis. These discoveries earned him his reputation as "an expert of experts in the science of life" (1), his appointment to the Pasteur Institute in 1888, and the Nobel Prize in Physiology in 1908. It was no wonder, then, that the scientific world paid attention in 1903 when Metchnikoff (2) denounced the colon as a useless organ teeming with bacterial populations which prospered from the remains of undigested food and mucus secretions. He considered the colon the source of many of what he called the "disharmonies" of man, including colorectal cancer, senile dementia, and the process of aging itself. To explain how enteric bacteria could bring about these diverse problems, Metchnikoff affirmed in no uncertain terms the concept of intestinal autointoxication. "Everyone knows," he argued (3), "that a high temperature may be the result of constipation after childbirth or in patients recovering from an operation. This is due to the absorption of substances produced by the microbes of the large intestine. Similar products may be the cause of an attack of acne or of other skin diseases."

Metchnikoff subsequently made it clear in his Harben Lectures of 1906 (4) that the only way to deal with these injurious bacteria was either to remove them by purges or replace them by useful bacteria, among which "the place of honour should be reserved to the lactic bacilli," which produce a "beneficent influence" and which "help to regulate the functions of our intestine and kidneys, rendering valuable service to the entire body." According to this leading Pasteur Institute scientist, lactobacilli were in fact capable of forestalling the ravages of old age.

Metchnikoff's concepts about the colon and its microbial populations exerted a wide influence for several decades. Among his many disciples, however, none was more enthusiastic, wrote more papers, or attracted more attention than Sir W. Arbuthnot Lane. "Willie" Lane, as he was known to his friends, was internationally famous as the leading surgeon of Guy's Hospital, London and as someone who had "performed more colectomies, more often, more perfectly, and more quickly than any other surgeon in the world" (5). Between Metchnikoff's publications of *The Nature of Man* in 1903 and 1938, Lane published nearly 100 papers (6) emphasizing the harmful consequences of chronic constipation and intestinal stasis, disorders which he believed were best treated by partial colectomy and ileocolostomy, the operation which he pioneered.

In *The Nature of Man*, Metchnikoff predicted that one day a surgeon would have the courage to remove the large intestine. When they met in 1904, Lane told the great scientist he had in fact performed many colectomies with salutary results. Both men attributed these good outcomes to a "purification" of the small intestine and its freedom from colonic toxins.

Others quickly grasped the idea of colonic bacterial production of toxins as an important cause of human disease. Intestinal autointoxication, or alimentary toxaemia as it was called in Britain, was of major interest to the Royal Society of Medicine and occupied no fewer than 6 of the Society meetings between March 10 and May 7 of 1913. According to Tanner (6), the meetings were made "notable not only by the fervour with which most of the 60 speakers put forward their views, but also by the fact that none was able precisely to define what he meant by alimentary toxaemia." At the opening meeting, Lane presented a remarkable paper (7) in which he attributed chronic intestinal stasis to improper feeding in early life with subsequent development of peritoneal "bands." These "bands" produced "kinks" in the intestine and consequent stasis of intestinal contents. By facilitating bacterial contamination of the upper intestine, stasis was directly responsible, in Lane's view, for duodenal ulcer, cardiospasm, pancreatitis, cancer of the pancreas, gallstones, and cholangitis. Moreover, he attributed numerous other afflictions to the absorption of toxins produced by colonic bacteria. Lane's list of disorders was remarkably diverse and included degeneration of the heart, arteries, and kidneys, cancer of the breast and colon, goiter, both high and low blood pressure, mental disturbances, tuberculosis, and rheumatoid arthritis.

The cure for these many diseases was, of course, "proper drainage" of the bowel and removal of offending bacteria, a goal best achieved by colectomy. Although completely unsupported by reports of properly followed cases or any other evidence that might be considered acceptable in today's scientific circles, these views nevertheless appealed to many physician-investigators, and for at least two decades, the groundbreaking Royal Society meetings of 1913 spawned a plethora of articles about the causes of, and the medical and surgical treatments for, constipation and intestinal autointoxication. Typical of its literature was a paper in the New England Journal of Medicine in 1931 (8), which extolled in considerable detail the beneficial effects of multiple *small*—as opposed to *large*—enemas in children with "acute intestinal autointoxication" manifested by fever, seizures, and acetonuria.

By the 1930s, the public had enthusiastically embraced these ideas about the harmful effects of constipation and colonic bacteria. "A New Health Society," founded by Sir W. Arbuthnot Lane, effectively popularized the surgeon's ideas throughout Britain. As the popularity of unproven "cures" for constipation and intestinal autointoxication increased during the 1920s and 1930s, serious scientists conducted fewer and fewer inquiries into the biologic or clinical significance of the indigenous enteric flora (9). Instead, scientific investigations from 1930 to 1950 focused on enumerating and identifying gastrointestinal microorganisms (10) and examining their metabolic reactions (11).

THE NATURE AND CONTROL OF ENTERIC MICROBIAL POPULATIONS

Methods

Methodologic advances during the 20th century permitted greater understanding of the enteric flora, although that understanding remains limited because available methodology still is not completely capable of identifying and enumerating microbial populations of the gastrointestinal tract *as they actually exist in the bowel lumen* (12,13). Many methods for culturing both aerobic and anaerobic microorganisms emerged during the latter half of the 19th century, but the limitations of methods for collecting samples forced investigators to confine their studies to human feces and the alimentary canal of experimental animals. As an instructor in surgery at the Johns Hopkins Hospital in 1900, Harvey Cushing (14) described the bacteriology of diseased portions of the human digestive tract which he excised during surgery. Soon thereafter, Hewetson at the University of Birmingham Hospital (15) paid particular attention to anaerobic species and reported the kinds and pathogenicity of bacteria found in surgically removed and therefore diseased digestive tract organs including the stomach, duodenum, jejunum, gallbladder, and biliary ducts.

Examination of the enteric flora of *healthy* subjects became possible only in the early part of the 20th century when many workers developed tubes capable of entering the small intestine (16). The leader in this effort undoubtedly was Max Einhorn (17). Appointed the first head of gastroenterology at the New York Post Graduate Medical School in 1888, Einhorn was an internationally recognized gastroenterologist, known best for inventing many of the specialty's devices and for training many of its future leaders, most notably Henry Bockus (18).

For various reasons (12,13), however, aspiration of intestinal contents proved to be a less than optimal way to collect enteric samples for microbial analysis, even when workers occluded the openings of the tube until they reached the desired site (19), devised special capsules for collecting intestinal contents (20), or resorted to direct needle aspiration of intestinal contents during surgery (21). To date, few studies have compared the efficacy of one collection method over another. Nor have there been any major technologic breakthroughs in the collection of enteric contents for microbial analysis (13), except for the development of nonabsorbable perfusion markers in the 1960s (22), permitting better estimates of concentration changes and completeness of collection.

In contrast, methods for enumerating and identifying enteric microorganisms have continued to advance remarkably during the 20th century. Although Louis Pasteur had demonstrated in 1861 that microorganisms could be cultured both aerobically and anaerobically, practical methods for creating an adequately low redox potential remained unavailable for nearly 100 years. During this interval, available methods were capable of efficiently culturing rapidly growing aerobic

bacteria and some facultative anaerobes, but not obligate anaerobes. Thus, until the middle of the 20th century, most workers continued to believe that species such as Escherichia coli and Streptococcus fecalis dominated the enteric flora. Advances such as Hungate's roll tube technique (23) and gas chromatographic methods for identifying microbial metabolites (24) made it possible to demonstrate, as Table 11–1 shows, that the indigenous organisms of the distal intestine consist almost exclusively of strict anaerobic bacteria, including numerous bacteroides, bifidobacteria, and clostridia species. These and related techniques have considerably improved estimates of both the numbers and diversity of viable intestinal bacteria. For many decades it was apparent that less than one third of fecal organisms counted under the microscope could be cultured, and the number of different bacterial species that could be cultured and identified was relatively small. It was assumed that the majority of fecal bacteria were dead. Subsequent, more rigorous methods for culturing and identifying obligate anaerobes, however, made it clear that up to 90% of microscopically visible bacteria could in fact be cultured and, according to Moore and Holdeman (24), "up to 500 species are present in feces at one time."

Despite these advances, much work remains before investigators can fully realize the goal of characterizing precisely the indigenous flora as it actually exists within the alimentary canal (25). Of particular, but often unrecognized, importance is the inadequacy of traditional "static" culture methods for studying microbial growth in the bowel lumen, where conditions are constantly in flux. Nutrients are continuously being supplied from proximal portions of the gut, while bacteria and their end products are constantly being removed distally. In 1949, Jacques Monod, who subsequently received the Nobel Prize for his work in bacterial genetics, described certain principles of bacterial growth (26) which guided the development of continuous-flow culture systems (27), of which the most widely and longest used was developed by Freter and colleagues (28). Clearly capable of simulating intraluminal microbial interactions more closely than standard culture systems (29,30), continuous-flow techniques con-

Table 11–1
Bacterial Populations of the Human Alimentary Canal*

| | Stomach | Small Bowel | | Large Bowel Cecum/Feces |
		Proximal	Distal	
Intraluminal pH	1.4–3.0	6.5–7.0	7.5	6.8–7.3
Redox potential (mV)	+150	−50	−150	−200
Emptying time (hours)†	0.5–1.0	0.5–1.0	2–4	12–48
Microorganisms‡				
Aerobic genera	0–2	0–4	1–8	8–12
Streptococci	0–2	0–4	2–5	4–9
Staphylococci	0–2	0–2	1–3	3–5
Enterobacteria	0–2	0–3	3–8	5–8
Lactobacilli	0–1	0–4	2–6	6–10
Anaerobic general§	0	0	3–7	8–12
Bacteroides	0	0	0	10–12
Enbacteria	0	0	0	10–12
Fusobacteria	0	0	0	10–12
Bifidobacteria	0	0	0	10–12
Porphyromonas	0	0	0	8–11
Clostridia	0	0	2–4	7–10
Others	0	0	0	6–9

* Data compiled from Simon and Gorbach (13), Moore and Holdemann (24), Wilson (59), and Finegold (89)
† In the fasting state
‡ Log number viable organisms per gram contents
§ More than 20 species can be identified for each anaerobic genus.

tinue to prove particularly valuable for documenting in vitro the ways in which indigenous bacterial populations suppress the growth of bacterial pathogens in vivo.

The Development of Enteric Bacterial Populations

As reviewed by Mackoriack (31), scientists of the 19th century recognized that the fetus is sterile and that the mammalian host derives its indigenous flora entirely from the environment. In his 1899 doctoral thesis at the University of Paris (32), Tissier described the development of the fecal flora in healthy infants and showed that only tiny numbers of enterococci and coliforms are present during the first few hours of life. Once feeding commences, however, bacterial populations increase enormously within a few days. Tissier also observed that breast-fed infants develop a fecal flora that is almost completely dominated by Lactobacillus bifidus, whereas the flora of bottle-fed infants consists of distinctly mixed bacterial populations, including Lactobacillus

acidophilus, coliforms, enterococci, and nonsporulating anaerobes. Tissier attributed the dominance of L. bifidus in breast-fed infants to a "bifidus factor" in breast milk capable of specifically stimulating the growth of L. bifidus. More than 50 years later, investigators amply confirmed Tissier's observations (33–35), and Gyorgy (36) identified "bifidus factor" as a heat-labile polysaccharide.

Two other contributions warrant attention. In 1960, Bishop and Anderson (37) conclusively demonstrated that microbial populations colonize the intestine in an oral-to-anal direction by showing that infants with congenital intestinal atresia consistently yield "colonic type" flora from sites proximal to the bowel obstruction, whereas bowel distal to the site of obstruction is always sterile. In 1977, Long and Swenson (38) compared the fecal flora of newborn infants delivered by Caesarian section with those delivered spontaneously and documented that the earliest enteric microbes were derived from the birth canal.

Dubos and Schaedler (39) showed that

weanling mice, raised in a meticulously clean, but not germ-free, environment could maintain indefinitely the relatively simple, lactobacillus-dominated flora described by Tissier. Under ordinary circumstances, however, this simple flora gradually gives way after weaning to a remarkably complex population consisting of enterococci, coliforms, and lactobacilli but truly dominated by a wide variety of obligate anaerobes. The aerobes initially present generate a redox potential that is sufficiently negative to permit massive growth of diverse obligate anaerobes which ultimately outnumber the aerobes and facultative anaerobes by more than 10,000 to one (Table 11-1).

Surveys conducted by several investigators between 1940 and 1960 (10,35,40) make it abundantly clear that, in contrast to the remarkably similar flora observed in animals of different species before weaning, the bacterial populations harbored by adults vary greatly among species and even from individual to individual within the same species. The results of these surveys strongly suggested that environmental factors were important determinants of the nature of the enteric flora. Nevertheless, as Simon and Gorbach emphasize in their review (13), only drastic environmental changes such as the administration of antibiotics can substantially alter the intestinal bacterial populations of an individual once that individual's "microbial ecosystem" has become firmly established.

The Nature of Enteric Bacterial Populations

Metchnikoff and his contemporaries fully appreciated that the stomach and proximal bowel were only sparsely populated by microorganisms. In fact, Metchnikoff (2) viewed this paucity of bacteria in the "digestive portions" of the gut as evidence that the enteric flora lacked any physiologic importance. As Table 11-1 shows, the pH and redox potential of the gut lumen, as well as each organ's "emptying time," all profoundly influence both the numbers and kinds of microorganisms present in various portions of the alimentary canal. The acid pH of gastric juice largely eliminates the bacteria from the oral cavity as they traverse the stomach, which is usually sterile

or sparsely populated with no more than 100 streptococci, staphylococci, or other aerobes per gram of gastric contents. The pH of the proximal small bowel is more conducive to bacterial growth, and the jejunum is less frequently sterile than the stomach. Nevertheless, the microorganisms in the proximal small bowel remain few in number. Obligate anaerobes are never cultured from the stomach or jejunum, and begin to appear only in the distal small bowel, where an increased number of aerobes and facultative anaerobes and a longer emptying time yield a redox potential that is substantially lower than that of the proximal gut. The enteric flora changes most dramatically across the ileocecal valve. When the cecum is reached, the total number of microorganisms increases by up to a million-fold and the variety of anaerobic species expands enormously. The information conveyed in Table 11-1 remains tentative pending further investigations. Because of continuing methodologic problems (25), for example, the taxonomy of the obligate anaerobes still remains in a state of flux (41).

Factors that Influence and Limit the Enteric Flora

Tissier and other early investigators recognized that diet was an important determinant of fecal flora, a fact that was documented by Dudgeon's systematic surveys as early as 1926 (42). Other investigators soon showed that large quantities of lactose in the diet greatly increase the number of fecal lactobacilli (43), that counts of coliforms and enterococci increase, whereas lactobacilli counts decrease, in response to diets rich in meat proteins (40) or casein (44), and that diets high in butterfat content markedly inhibit growth of E. coli and Proteus vulgaris in the cecum (44). In fact, many other reports published in the period from 1940 to 1965 similarly demonstrated microbial changes in response to distinctly unphysiologic changes in the diets of laboratory animals. Subsequent investigations in adult humans, however, have failed to demonstrate important effects of diet on the enteric flora except when dietary changes are extreme (45,46).

Other environmental changes also must be extreme before they clearly influence the nature of the enteric flora. Thus, animals rigorously maintained in a clean environment, as described previously, consistently demonstrate a characteristic flora (39), whereas preventing coprophagy greatly decreases the number of lactobacilli in cecum or feces (47). Despite these findings, however, stability of the complex microbial populations of the large intestine continues to be their most remarkable feature. Several powerful physiochemical microbial interactions within the bowel lumen appear to bring about the "anticolonizing" and stabilizing effects of the enteric flora (10,12,45).

By the mid-20th century, it was clear that bacterial proliferation rates are such that, unless checked, the growth of the enteric flora would soon overwhelm the host. Smythe (48) calculated, for example, that uninhibited multiplication of two coliform bacilli would produce within 24 hours a bacterial mass possessing the nutritional requirements of a 28-pound child. Thus, much of the 20th century witnessed major investigative efforts to determine the factors that prevent intestinal bacteria from consuming the factors that prevent intestinal bacteria from consuming the host. Zeldow (49) showed that saliva contains potent antibacterial activity against many lactobacilli, streptococci, and staphylococci. Other investigators found that the acid-peptic activity of gastric juice has even more potent antibacterial effects and that achlorydria consistently leads to increased numbers of bacteria in the small bowel (12,45,50).

The striking differences between the flora of the small and large intestine have intrigued many investigators who, since the turn of the century, have intensely examined the microbe-limiting properties of the small intestine (51–53). Although workers have variously attributed antibacterial activity to pancreatic enzymes, lysozyme, bile salts, secretory IgA, and intestinal mucus, these factors do not adequately account for the small numbers of microbes found in the small bowel (12). The studies of Dack and Petran (51) in 1934 and especially of Dixon (52) in 1960 made it abundantly clear that intestinal motility constitutes the major mechanism for limiting the growth of microbial populations within the small bowel lumen and that organisms which enter the duodenum remain viable as they traverse

the length of the small intestine, often held in mucus packets (53). More recently, workers recognized that the interdigestive migratory motor complex is largely responsible for this self-cleansing action of the small intestine (54). Furthermore, whenever small bowel motility is disrupted for any reason, microbial populations soar to numbers usually seen only in the stagnant contents of the colon (55).

As detailed in a previous review (12), investigators also recognized by 1964 that, even within the colon, bacterial growth is limited as a consequence of intermicrobial interactions, which alter luminal pH or redox potential, or which yield either toxic metabolites or antibiotic substances such as colicines or pyocines. The overall result is a powerful "anticolonizing" effect which makes an individual's enteric flora remarkably stable and which protects the host from bacterial pathogens (56). In recent years, sophisticated biochemical and genetic techniques have identified mechanisms of action of enteric antibiotics and have explained why it is that antibiotic-producing bacteria do not destroy themselves (57).

IMPACT OF THE NORMAL ENTERIC FLORA ON THE HEALTHY HOST

Host Resistance and Survival

Pasteur and Metchnikoff held opposing views about the relationship between the animal host and its enteric bacterial populations (31). Pasteur believed that the host derived great benefit from, and in fact could not survive without, these microbes. In contrast, Metchnikoff contended that the host would live a longer, healthier life it it could rid itself of its intestinal bacteria (2,4). Each scientist tried to prove the other wrong by determining how animals fared when raised in a germ-free environment. Attempts to raise germ-free animals were uniformly unsuccessful in that era. Even Madame Metchnikoff's germ-free tadpoles failed to survive, much to her husband's consternation. Pasteur interpreted these results as proof that the host depends vitally on its normal intestinal flora, whereas Metchnikoff believed that only the technical problems created by a germ-free environment prevented animals from surviving.

Within 70 years, it was clear that both scientists had been correct. Metchnikoff was vindicated when it became possible to raise germ-free chicks and mammals and to show that animals with sterile intestines could actually outlive animals reared conventionally (58). Pasteur's view also was upheld, however, because germ-free animals proved to be unusually susceptible to overwhelming, fatal infection by bacterial pathogens that were usually resisted by conventionally reared control animals. As Wilson emphasizes in his recent insightful review (59), we now recognize that this resistance to enteric pathogens results largely from the "anticolonizing" properties of the predominantly anaerobic flora of the normal intestine. Unable to compete with these anaerobes by proliferating within the bowel lumen, bacterial pathogens can infect the host only by developing highly specialized, effective mechanisms for attaching to and penetrating the intestinal mucosa.

Of all the effects of the normal enteric flora on the host, none is more prominent than its impact on the intestine itself. Thus, by the early 1960s, the remarkable effects of the germ-free state on the intestine were understood in considerable detail (12). Many workers found the intestinal wall of the germ-free animal to be thinner and lighter than that of conventionally reared animals. The quantity of reticuloendothelial and lymphatic tissue is greatly diminished, and much fewer leukocytes and macrophages are present in the lamina propria. Because lymphocytic and reticulocytic elements increase rapidly when germ-free animals are monocontaminated with a single indigenous bacterial species, Gordon and coworkers (60) and Sprinz (61) recognized that these changes probably result from the absence of microbial stimulation of the intestinal mucosa, which consequently fails to develop normal antimicrobial immune mechanisms. Sprinz and colleagues (61), working at the Armed Forces Institute of Pathology, further demonstrated that the turnover rate of intestinal epithelial cells was greatly diminished in germ-free guinea pigs. As expected, there was a concomitant increase in villus height and a decrease in crypt depth. In contrast, epithelial cell turnover is greatly increased in celiac sprue and in small intestinal infection, so that crypts expand while villi shorten or disappear altogether. Sprinz (61) thus concluded that the appearance of the intestinal mucosa of conventionally reared animals represented a state of "physiological inflammation" lying between the complete lack of anti-inflammatory immune response that is seen in the germ-free animal and the pathologic inflammatory process characteristic of celiac sprue and other inflammatory disorders.

Investigators of the 1970s and 1980s not only confirmed these observations, but amply demonstrated that the indigenous enteric flora much more dramatically affects the host's intestinal immune system than the latter alters or limits the intestinal flora (59). By the late 1970s, it was clear that animals reared in a germ-free environment possess virtually no antibodies (62). Brown and colleagues at the University of Colorado, on the other hand, showed in the early 1970s that healthy humans developed readily detectable "natural" serum antibodies directed at some of their own enteric microorganisms (63,64). Thus it is now clear that the enteric flora plays a key role in the host's immune resistance, an attribute which is key to survival.

The enteric flora also plays a prominent role in determining the size of the cecum which becomes enormously distended in germ-free rodents but not in other mammals (12,59). The mechanisms responsible for this striking change remain unclear, but cecal size rapidly returns to normal once the bowel is colonized by normal intestinal bacteria or is monocontaminated with E. coli.

Host Nutrition

If the salutary effects of the enteric flora on host resistance and survival supported Pasteur's early views, the flora's impact on host nutrition certainly would be in keeping with Metchnikoff's concepts of the harmful nature of enteric microbes. Because the host and its enteric flora must share the same nutrients, whether ingested by the host or derived from the host's secretions, investigators long suspected that intestinal bacteria might impair the nutritional status of the host. However, solid evidence for this concept developed only with observations of the profound effects of broad spectrum antibiotics on animal nutrition (65,66). In

1950, Stokstad and Jukes (67) showed that the body weight of chicks increased substantially when small quantities of chlortetracycline were added to the diet, a finding that soon led to a massive literature (65,66,68) and a multimillion-dollar investment in antibiotics for animal husbandry. In an astonishing array of experiments, workers added tetracyclines, penicillin, streptomycin, various sulfonamides, and chloramphenicol to animal feed and noted increased growth in chicks, turkey poults, goslings, quail, pheasant, ducks, rats, mice, calves, pigs, dogs, and—to a lesser extent—humans, whereas neomycin, kanamycin, bacitracin, and polymyxin failed to influence growth rates. In his comprehensive 1959 review (65), Luckey delineated the optimal conditions for demonstrating an effect of antibiotics on the growth of domestic animals. The nutritional benefits of antibiotics are most apparent when they are fed from the time of birth, when results are expressed as rates of growth rather than as final weights, when runts or weaker animals in the control and treated groups are compared, when diets of marginal nutritional benefit are used, and when animals are raised in relatively unsanitary quarters. Because of many observations, including the fact that antibiotics had no effect on growth of germ-free animals, it was already apparent by the early 1960s that the growth-promoting effects of antibiotics related primarily to changes in the enteric flora rather than to any direct effect of antibiotics on host tissues or metabolism (69).

Despite a massive research literature, we still do not know precisely how antibiotics alter the enteric flora. As described in early (12,64) as well more recent (59,69) reviews, investigations into the effects of antibiotics on the microbial populations of the bowel frequently are marred by methodologic difficulties and often yield results that are inconsistent, complex, and impossible to interpret. Thus it remains far from clear whether antibiotics improve host nutrition by decreasing the numbers of antagonistic bacteria, by increasing the numbers of beneficial microorganisms, or by diminishing the frequency of subclinical infection.

Most investigators in the 1950s assumed that antibiotics improved nutrition by eliminating those microorganisms capable of successfully competing for and metabolizing dietary nutrients. At the turn of the century, scientists already were well aware of the capability of intestinal microorganisms to metabolize various nutrients. Metchnikoff, for example, commented on the bacterial conversion of meat to indoles and skatoles. During the middle of the 20th century, research focused particularly on microbial breakdown of essential nutrients such as choline (70), folic acid (71), and thiamine (72).

It was equally possible, of course, that antibiotics, by suppressing some bacteria, encouraged overgrowth of other more beneficial microorganisms. It was well established during the 50s that enteric bacteria manufactured many important nutrients including niacin, riboflavin, thiamine, pyridoxine, vitamin B_{12}, folic acid, pantothenic acid, biotin, and vitamin K (73,74).

By the end of the 19th century, it was widely recognized that, in ruminants, essential nutrients are synthesized by bacteria in the gastric rumen, the microorganisms are then destroyed by acid gastric juice, and the released nutrients are absorbed by the small intestine. In nonruminants, on the other hand, microbially synthesized vitamins are manufactured in the colon and therefore are unlikely to be assimilated by the host. Nevertheless, extensive microbial synthesis of vitamins probably accounts for the observation reported in 1927 (75) that rats can remain healthy despite being fed a diet that completely lacks B vitamins. Moreover, the feces of such animals corrects vitamin B deficiency when fed to deficient animals (73). Thus it soon became apparent that ingestion of feces (coprophagy) is crucial for making these vitamins available to the nonruminant host (76). Further support for the nutritional importance of enteric bacteria derived from the fact that folate deficiency in germ-free animals can be readily corrected merely by exposing them to contaminated environs or by monocontamination with E. coli (77).

If the effects of antibiotics on host nutrition resulted merely from eliminating antagonistic bacteria, then growth rates should be substantially increased in germ-free animals. By and large, however, workers have been unable to show that growth is improved in animals raised in germ-free environs, perhaps because of the many problems involved in obtaining proper controls for germ-free experiments and the many ways in which maintaining sterility necessarily restricts and impairs the host. On the other hand, Dubos and Schaedler (39,78–80) conducted a series of experiments in the early 1960s, which convincingly documented the profound effects on host nutrition and resistance from altering the enteric flora. In addition to completing this important work, Rene Dubos distinguished himself as an outstanding investigator at the Rockefeller Institute as the inventor of the Dubos medium for culturing tubercle bacilli, and as the coeditor of a classic medical text, *The Bacterial and Mycotic Infections of Man.* He and Schaedler raised mice in rigorously sanitary, but not germ-free, environs and demonstrated that these "NCS mice" maintained indefinitely a relatively simple enteric flora consisting primarily of lactobacilli and gram-negative anaerobes. Absent from these NCS mice were E. coli, S. fecalis, and the clostridial and proteus species usually found in large numbers in the cecum of conventionally reared mice. Fetal survival and growth rates were substantially greater in NCS mice than in control animals. Mice raised under ordinary laboratory conditions failed to thrive when fed a diet incomplete in protein, whereas NCS mice fed the same diet gained weight. The NCS mice also resisted endotoxin, certain infections, and total body irradiation more successfully than did conventionally reared animals. Dubos and Schaedler's work became particularly important once it was recognized that feeding animals antibiotics engendered transferable antibiotic resistance among enteric bacteria including pathogens (81). Because antibiotics had no effect on the growth of NCS animals (82), it was clear that maintaining a sanitary environment was equally effective and far preferable to the use of antibiotics in animal husbandry.

Intraluminal Metabolism

During the 20th century, investigators became increasingly aware of the broad spectrum of metabolic reactions that microbes carry out in the alimentary canal. Even though it was clear that most of this metabolic activity took place in the colon, given the massive numbers of microorganisms located there, this microbial activity is of great importance to the host and involves a wide variety of endogenous and foreign substrates, including carbohydrates, lipids, steroids, proteins, other nitrogenous substances, and various drugs (11,59,83). Complicating this picture further is the fact that each of the several hundred bacterial species indigenous to the alimentary canal is characterized by its own distinct pattern of metabolic actions. In a landmark publication (11), M. J. Hill and his colleagues have described in considerable detail the development of this vast field of knowledge, but only a few highlights can be mentioned here.

Before the turn of the century, Pasteur recognized that anaerobic bacteria in the gastric rumen or cecum could digest cellulose and other complex polysaccharides that could not be catalyzed by mammalian enzymes (31). Ever since these early observations, bacterial cellulase has fascinated microbiologists, who have long sought a practical means of converting grasses to digestible foodstuffs. In the 1940s, Hungate (27) was investigating the anaerobic breakdown of cellulose when he developed his roll tube technique, which proved to be important for culturing obligate anaerobes. By the late 1970s, it was well recognized that many indigenous enteric species could synthesize the specific enzymes required to hydrolyze cellulose, mucins, pectins, and other complex carbohydrates, which the intestine could neither degrade nor absorb (84,85). When ingested in the diet, these substances transverse the small bowel to reach the colon, where they provide a substantial substrate and nutritional source for colonic microorganisms. Bacterial degradation of these carbohydrates generates as end products acetic, formic, lactic, proprionic, and butyric acids (the volatile fatty acids), as well as methane, hydrogen, carbon dioxide, and water. Levitt (86) took advantage of the microbial generation of hydrogen by using it to measure carbohydrate malabsorption. A decade later, Wrong (87) was able to show that bacterial catabolism of unabsorbed fiber and mucins provides a "colonic salvage mechanism" for the host, because the resulting volatile fatty acids readily diffuse across the colonic mucosa.

Clinicians in the late 1970s noted that

these volatile fatty acids, which are formed in excess when poorly absorbed carbohydrates reach the colon, can cause severe acidosis in patients with resected or bypassed small bowels (85,86). The result can be either metabolic D-lactic acidosis with an altered mental status which resembles alcohol intoxication (88,89) or methylmalonic aciduria which responds to antibiotic therapy and which results from the rare combination of an inherited disorder of propionyl coenzyme A and overproduction of propionic acid by intestinal bacteria (90).

Although these metabolic disorders might be thought of as examples of "intestinal autointoxication," Metchnikoff's century-old ideas come closest to fulfillment in relation to the pathogenesis of hepatic encephalopathy, a malady that undoubtedly results from intestinal bacterial production of ammonia or some other noxious nitrogenous substance (91) and which has been successfully treated by purges and enemas. Although it had been known since the 30s that a urease in colonic bacteria converts urea to ammonia and carbon dioxide, by the 1950s workers also had identified agastric urease. Although apparently an integral part of the gastric mucosa, this urease could be inhibited by antibiotics and was absent from fetal tissue (92). It now seems likely that Helicobacteria pylori may account for this activity because these organisms are rich in urease and adhere closely to gastric antral mucosa (93). By the 1950s, it also was clear to researchers concerned with the pathogenesis of hepatic coma that bacterial metabolism was the major source of intestinal ammonia because portal vein levels of ammonia were distinctly decreased in animals fed antibiotics (94) or raised in a germ-free environment (95). Moreover, work in Wrong's laboratory established in the 1970s that peptides and amino acids, not just urea, served as substrates for the bacterial production of ammonia (96).

Ammonia, although important, is not the only product of enteric bacterial action on nitrogenous substances. It is now clear that these microorganisms also are capable of synthesizing several biologically active amines and a variety of amino acids, including the branched chain amino acids that can result only from microbial metabolism (97). In addition, intestinal bacterial peptidases

inactivate intestinal digestive enzymes (98), whereas other microbial enzymes convert bilirubin to urobilinogen and stercobilin (99), and generate nitrosamines and other mutagenic compounds (83).

Investigators have long recognized the influences of enteric bacteria on the intraluminal metabolism of lipids (100). Not only do bacteria generate substantial quantities of lipid within the bowel lumen (101), the branched chain and hydroxylated fatty acids that these microorganisms tend to synthesize are not found in dietary fats. It was recognized 30 years ago that failure to account for the bacterial production of lipid could result in errors in studies of fat balance (102).

As noted by Talalay in his 1957 review (103), it was only after World War II that investigators began to recognize the important role of the enteric flora in the metabolism of steroids in general and bile salts in particular. New chromatographic methods for analyzing steroids, improved techniques for culturing microorganisms, and evolving germ-free technology all combined to demonstrate that: (1) the liver secretes into bile highly soluble bile salts, which are conjugated with glycine or taurine and which require special mechanisms for absorption by the intestine (104); (2) that intestinal bacterial rapidly hydrolyze these conjugated bile salts to form lipophilic, relatively insoluble bile acids which readily diffuse across the intestinal mucosa (105); (3) that further microbial action converts these deconjugated bile acids to the so-called secondary bile acids, which include deoxycholic acid, lithocholic acid, ketoacids and various other metabolites (106); and (4) that, as a consequence, bile salt turnover is slowed and the bile salt pool is increased in germ-free animals (107). Enteric bacterial actions on other steroidal compounds are extensive but are less important to the host. The extent to which intraluminal bacterial metabolism of estrogens (108) and formation of androgens (109) is important to the host remains unknown at present (59).

The consequences of bacterial metabolism of drugs continue to be of considerable importance to humans (83,110). The major actions of bacteria on drugs include: (1) hydrolysis of sulfasalazine to release its active components, 5-amino salicylic acid; (2) microbial activation of metronidazole; (3) degradation of digoxin to inactive metabolites; (4) increased enterohepatic recycling of chloramphenicol and digoxin as a consequence of bacterial hydrolysis of conjugates of these agents formed in the liver; and (5) inactivation of L-dopa by converting it to dopamine which cannot cross the blood-brain barrier.

THE ROLE OF INDIGENOUS FLORA IN DIGESTIVE DISEASES

Small Bowel Bacterial Overgrowth

According to Ellis and Smith (111), the blind loop syndrome was first recognized in 1890 when White (112) suspected that small bowel strictures might somehow bring about a macrocytic anemia similar to pernicious anemia. It was not until 1924, however, that Seyderhelm and coworkers (113) proved a cause-and-effect relationship by showing that correction of an intestinal stricture cured the associated anemia. During the next 15 years, clinical investigators reported that injections of liver corrected the anemia and its attendant neurologic defects, that diverticula, blind loops, and enteroenterostomies involving the small bowel also caused macrocytic anemia, and that these small bowel lesions also produced steatorrhea. Thus, by 1939, Barker and Hummel were able to document in their classic review (114) all of the salient clinical features of this "blind loop syndrome," so named because it occurred most regularly and obviously after surgical creation of blind loops of small bowel during operations designed to bypass intestinal obstruction. Because each of these lesions was associated with stasis of small bowel contents and consequent bacterial overgrowth, it was not surprising to learn, when broad spectrum antibiotics became available in the 1950s that antibiotic therapy, like surgical correction of intestinal lesions, rapidly corrected steatorrhea and anemia (115). Similarly, once the isolation of pure cobalamin made the necessary measurements possible, there was little difficulty in demonstrating that patients with the syndrome absorbed the vitamin poorly and were vitamin B_{12} deficient (116).

Although an association among small-bowel bacterial overgrowth, vitamin B_{12} deficiency, and steatorrhea was clearly established by 1950, full understanding of the pathogenesis of this syndrome required the development of animal models. In 1950, Aitken, Badenoch, and Spray (117) demonstrates steatorrhea in rats with surgically created blind intestinal pouches. Two years later, Watson and Witts (118) showed that rats with similar lesions called "self-filling diverticula" of small bowel developed weight loss and anemia, whereas control animals with "self-emptying diverticula" remained healthy. Bacteria did not proliferate in self-emptying pouches.

Strauss et al. (119) reported in 1961 that rats with experimental blind loops absorb vitamin B_{12} poorly, and that, as is also true of patients, this malabsorption is corrected by antibiotics but not by an intrinsic factor. By 1962, an extensive series of in vitro and in vivo experiments (120,121) had unequivocally established that vitamin B_{12} malabsorption could be attributed only to direct uptake by bacteria which proliferate within the small bowel lumen and which successfully compete with ileal enterocytes for assimilation of the vitamin. As summarized in Wilson's recent review (59), many investigators subsequently have confirmed these observations without finding evidence of any other explanation for malabsorption of vitamin B_{12}.

Studies in experimental animals also have provided an explanation for steatorrhea in the blind loop syndrome. Studies in blind loop rats reported in 1965 (122) clearly showed that steatorrhea in these animals was caused by fat malabsorption, not increased intraluminal production of lipid by bacteria, and that this malabsorption could not be attributed to impaired digestion of triglycerides, to diminished intestinal mucosal transport of fatty acids, or to decreased re-esterification and export of absorbed fatty acids. It was therefore proposed that bacterial metabolism of bile salts resulted in bile salt deficiency and impaired micellar solubilization of dietary lipids and consequent fat malabsorption (122), a proposal that Kim et al. (123) strongly supported when they reported that feeding conjugated bile salts corrected steatorrhea in dogs with experimental blind loop syndrome. In the clinical syndrome, this proposal was consistent with observations (124) of decreased intrajejunal bile salt concentrations in some patients with bacterial overgrowth.

In subsequent years, investigators identified additional disorders that were conducive to stasis of small intestinal contents and thus resulted in bacterial overgrowth, cobalamin deficiency, and steatorrhea. These included scleroderma involving the small intestine, diabetic enteropathy, intestinal pseudo-obstruction, and afferent loop dysfunction after gastrectomy. Moreover, subsequent work demonstrated that abnormal intraluminal events could not account for all the absorptive disorders observed in the blind loop syndrome and that bacteria proliferating in the small bowel were capable of damaging the mucosal surface. Goldstein (125) reported, but did not document, a patchy small bowel mucosal lesion in patients with bacterial overgrowth. Subsequently, Ament et al. published small bowel mucosal biopsies that documented this lesion (126). It remains unclear whether bacteria damage the mucosal surface by their direct action or by the production of organic acids, hydroxylated fatty acids, unconjugated bile acids, or other noxious agents. Work by Toskes and others in the 1970s, however, established that mucosal surface defects clearly account for the impaired disaccharidase and peptidase activity noted in blind loop rats (127,128). As reviewed by Hill (129), more recent work also has focused on various urinary excretion and breath tests designed to improve the diagnosis of bacterial overgrowth.

Tropical Sprue

During the 1950s, it became increasingly apparent that administration of broad spectrum antibiotics also corrects malabsorption in cases of tropical sprue (130,131), although it remains unclear whether this disease results from a change in indigenous flora or from infection by a pathogen (132). It has been long recognized, however, that the disease often begins as an acute enteritis (133), that its small bowel mucosal lesion is consistent with an infectious process, and that well-documented epidemics have occurred in prison camps and in villages of

South India (134). It also has been clear for many years that tropical sprue differs from the blind loop syndrome in many important respects even though both disorders involve intestinal malabsorption of lipid and cobalamin (13). The intestinal lesion is much more consistent, extensive, and severe in sprue. Antibiotics correct absorptive defects within 7 to 10 days in the blind loop syndrome but require several weeks in tropical sprue. Folate deficiency, a constant feature of tropical sprue, is virtually unheard of in the blind loop syndrome. Finally, it has not been possible to demonstrate in tropical sprue the kind of substantial overgrowth of small bowel bacteria that is a hallmark of the blind loop syndrome. Despite much indirect evidence of an infectious process, numerous attempts during the past several decades have failed to find a microbial agent capable of causing all the clinical features of tropical sprue.

Travelers' Diarrhea

Hippocrates noted 3000 years ago that diarrhea could afflict individuals who traveled to distant lands (135) particularly if such travel involved marked changes in climate. Although reports frequently related the sanitary conditions of a region to the likelihood of developing diarrhea and often incriminated a wide variety of potential pathogens, sound scientific investigations into travelers' diarrhea began when B. H. Kean systematically assessed students traveling to Mexico and Europe in the late 1950s (136) and convincingly used controlled trials to show that broad spectrum antibiotics could effectively prevent the ailment (137). In 1975, Gorbach et al. discovered that enterotoxigenic strains of E. coli could be isolated from the stools of most individuals with travelers' diarrhea (138). It is now clear (139) that at least five strains of E. coli can cause diarrhea. These are known as the enterotoxigenic, enteropathogenic, enteroinvasive, enteroadherent, and enterohemorrhagic strains of E. coli. The latter cause hemorrhagic colitis and the hemolytic-uremic syndrome. Recent studies also have shown the wide variety of agents that can be used to prevent travelers' diarrhea (140,141).

Colorectal Cancer

Both Metchnikoff and Lane attributed cancer of the colon to the large number of bacteria that populate that organ, but only recently have investigators developed evidence to support a relationship between colon bacteria and the development of colorectal cancer. The subject is reviewed in detail by Gorbach and Goldin (83) and is only briefly summarized here. In the late 1960s, Doll (142) and Burkitt (143), two highly respected epidemiologists, described the remarkably low frequency of colon cancer in Asia and Africa compared to its high prevalence in Western countries and suggested that the high-fat, low-fiber intake characteristic of Western-style diets may explain this striking difference. They both noted statistically significant correlations between consumption of animal fats and rates of colon cancer in various countries. Epidemiologic studies in the 1970s confirmed a protective effect of dietary fiber (144–146). How changes in diet might cause colon cancer remains unclear, but experiments with germ-free animals (147) and antibiotics (148) suggest a mediating role for enteric microorganisms.

Several investigators have proposed that dietary fats may serve as the substrate for bacterial enzymes that generate mutagenic compounds. The number of candidate substrates, bacterial enzymes, and mutagenic metabolites continues to grow, but attention has focused particularly on bacterial beta-glucuronidase, nitroreductase, azoreductase (149,150), and production of bile acids by colonic bacteria (151).

Although the concept is provocative, considerable additional evidence is needed to demonstrate that colon cancer results from definable interactions between dietary compounds and the enteric flora. Especially needed are prospective randomized trials to assess the influence of diet on rates of polyp and cancer formation.

Whipple's Disease and Uncultured Bacteria

In 1907, Whipple (152), a pathologist at Johns Hopkins Hospital, who subsequently received the Nobel Prize for other work, described all of the salient features of an intestinal disease characterized by intestinal malabsorption, fever, arthritis, lymphadenopathy, and the infiltration of affected tissues by "foam" cells. These cells are macrophages. Their foamy cytoplasm is packed with particles that stain with periodic acid-Schiff reagent and are composed of bacterial fragments and intact bacteria. Although Whipple himself noted the similarity between this disease and chronic mycobacterial infection, and although investigators have long since established by electron microscopy the presence of a bacillus in the tissues of patients with Whipple's disease, attempts to culture this organism have either been unsuccessful or yielded inconsistent results (153).

As recently reviewed by Tompkins (154), molecular biologic techniques now offer the opportunity to identify, on the basis of their phylogenetically characteristic ribosomal RNA sequences, bacteria that cannot be cultured. Wilson et al. (155) applied this approach to intestinal tissue from one patient with Whipple's disease and amplified a partial 16S rRNA sequence. Relman et al. (156) subsequently reported amplification and identification of complete 16S rRNA sequences obtained both from intestinal mucosa and lymph nodes of patients with Whipple's disease. These sequences were not present in the tissues of appropriate control subjects. As a result of their work, Relman et al. (156) identified actinobacteria as the organism most closely related to the Whipple's bacillus. Investigators now are using this general approach in attempts to identify microbial etiologies of other inflammatory granulomatous disorders such as sarcoidosis (157) and Crohn's disease (158). Given the fact that only 20% of the microorganisms that exist in nature have been cultured (159), the future of these new molecular biologic approaches seems bright indeed.

REFERENCES

1. Mitchell PC: Editor's Introduction to Metchnikoff E: The Nature of Man. Studies in Optimistic Philosophy. New York, G. P. Putnams' Sons, 1903, pp. 1–24.
2. Metchnikoff E: The Nature of Man. Studies in Optimistic Philosophy. New York, G. P. Putnam's Sons, 1903.

3. Ibid, page 73.

4. Metchnikoff E: The New Hygiene. London, William Heneman, 1906.

5. Editorial: Sir Arbuthnot Lane at Guy's Hospital. Brit. J. Surg. *8*:219, 1920.

6. Tanner WE: Sir W. Arbuthnot Lane, His Life and His Work. London, Balliere, Tyndall and Cox, 1946.

7. Lane AW: The consequence and treatment of alimentary toxaemia. Proc Roy Soc Med *vi*(suppl):49, 1912–13.

8. Crawford LP: Treatment of acute intestinal intoxication based upon clinical findings in the colon. N Engl J Med *205*:577, 1931.

9. Rosebury T: Micro-organisms indigenous to man. New York, McGraw-Hill, 1962.

10. Skinner FA, Carr JG (eds): The Normal Microbial Flora of Man. London, Academic Press, 1974.

11. Hill MJ (ed): Microbial Metabolism in the Digestive Tract. Boca Raton, Florida, CRC Press, 1986.

12. Donaldson RM: Normal bacterial populations of the intestine and their relation to intestinal function. N Engl J Med *270*:938, 994, 1050, 1964.

13. Simon GL, Gorbach SL: The human intestinal microflora. Dig Dis Sci *31*(suppl): 147S, 1986.

14. Cushing H: The bacteriology of abdominal organs. Johns Hopkins Hospital Reports *9*: 543, 1900.

15. Hewetson JT: The bacteriology of certain parts of the alimentary canal and of the inflammatory processes arising therefrom. Brit. Med. J. *2*:1457, 1904.

16. Ingelfinger FJ: Tubes. Gastroenterology *74*:310, 1978.

17. Einhorn M: The Duodenal Tube and its Possibilities. Philadelphia, WB Saunders, 1920.

18. Bockus HL: The Einhorn Story. Gastroenterology *74*:949, 1978.

19. Nadel H, Gardner F: Bacteriological assay of small bowel section in tropical sprue. Am J Trop Med Hyg *5*:686, 1956.

20. Shiner M: Capsule for obtaining sterile samples of gastrointestinal fluid. Lancet *i*: 532, 1963.

21. Cregan J, Hayward NJ: Bacterial content of healthy human small intestine. Brit Med J *i*:1356, 1953.

22. Fordtran JS et al.: Permeability characteristics of the human small intestine. J Clin Invest *44*:1435, 1965.

23. Hungate RE: The anaerobic mesophilic cellulytic bacteria. Bacteriol Rev *14*:1, 1950.

24. Moore WEC, Holdeman LV: Identification of anaerobic bacteria. Am J Clin Nutr *25*: 1306, 1975.

25. Moore WEC, Holdeman LV: Special problems associated with the isolation and identification of intestinal bacteria in fecal flora studies. Am J Clin Nutr *27*:1450, 1974.

26. Monod J: The growth of bacterial cultures. Annu Rev Microbiol *3*:371, 1949.

27. Novick A: Growth of bacteria. Annu Rev Microbiol *9*:97, 1955.

28. Freter R et al.: Continuous-flow cultures as *in vitro* models of the ecology of large intestinal flora. Infect Immun *39*:666, 1983.

29. Ransom JP, Finkelstein RA, Ceder RE, Formal SB: Interactions of *Vibrio cholerae, Shigella flexneri,* Enterococci, and Lactobacilli in continuously fed cultures. Proc Soc Exper Biol Med *187*:332, 1961.

30. Freter R: *In vitro* and *in vivo* antagonism of intestinal bacteria against Shigella flexneri. II. Inhibitory mechanisms. J Infect Dis *110*: 38, 1962.

31. Mackowiack PA: The normal microbial flora. N Engl J Med *307*:83, 1982.

32. Tissier, cited by Gyllenberg H and Carlberg G: Dominance of specific intestinal type of *Lactobacillus bifidus* in breast-fed infants. Acta path microbiol Scandinav. *42*:380, 1958.

33. Barbero DJ et al.: Investigations on bacterial flora, pH, and sugar content in intestinal tract of infants. J Pediatr *40*:152, 1952.

34. Gyllenberg H, Carlberg G: Dominance of specific intestinal type of Lactobacillus bifidus in breast-fed infants. Acta Pathol Microbiol Scandinav *42*:380, 1958.

35. Smith HW, Crabb WE: Faecal bacterial flora of animals and man: Its development in young. J Pathol Bacteriol *82*:53, 1961.

36. Gyorgy P: Hitherto unrecognized biochemical difference between human milk and cow's milk. Pediatrics *11*:98, 1933.

37. Bishop RF, Anderson CM: Bacterial flora of stomach and small intestine in children with intestinal obstruction. Arch Dis Child *35*:487, 1960.

38. Long SS, Swenson RM: Development of anaerobic fecal flora in healthy newborn infants. J Pediatr *91*:298, 1977.

39. Dubos RJ, Schaedler RW: Some biological effects of digestive flora. Am J Med Sci *244*: 265, 1962.

40. Porter JR, Rettger LF: Influence of diet on distribution of bacteria in stomach, small intestine and cecum of white rat. J Infect Dis *66*:104, 1940.

41. Finegold SM: Anaerobic gram-negative rods. *In* Gorbach SL, Bartlett JG, Blacklow NR (eds): Infectious Diseases. Philadelphia, WB Saunders, 1992.

42. Dudgeon LS: Study of intestinal flora under normal and abnormal conditions. J Hyg *25*: 119, 1926.

43. Wilbur RD et al.: Intestinal flora of pig as influenced by diet and age. J Nutrition *71*: 168, 1960.

44. Bergeim O, Hanszen AH, Pincussen L, Weiss E: Relation of volatile fatty acids and hydrogen sulphide to intestinal flora. J Infect Dis *69*:155, 1941.

45. Simon GL, Gorbach SL: Intestinal flora in health and disease. Gastroenterology *86*: 174, 1984.

46. Finegold SM, Attebery AR, Sutter VL: Effect of diet on human fecal flora. Comparison of American and Japanese diets. Am J Clin Nutr *27*:1456, 1974.

47. Gustafsson BE, Fitzgerald RJ: Alteration in intestinal microbial flora of rats with tail cups to prevent coprophagy. Proc Soc Exper Biol Med *104*:319, 1960.

48. Smyth PM: Changes in intestinal bacterial flora and role of infection in kwashiorkor. Lancet *ii*:724, 1958.

49. Zeldow BJ: Studies on antibacterial action of human saliva. II. Observations on mode of action of Lactobacillus bactericidin. J Dent Research *40*:446, 1961.

50. Wirts CW, Goldstein F: Studies of mechanism of postgastrectomy steatorrhea. Ann Intern Med *58*:25, 1963.

51. Dack GM, Petran E: Bacterial activities in different levels of intestine and in isolated segments of large and small bowel in monkeys and in dogs. J Infect Dis *54*:204, 1934.

52. Dixon JMS: Fate of bacteria in small intestine. J Pathol Bacteriol *79*:131, 1960.

53. Florey HW: Observations on functions of mucus and early stages of bacterial invastion of intestinal mucosa. J Pathol Bacteriol *37*:283, 1933.

54. Code CF, Marlet JA: The interdigestive myoelectric complex of the stomach and small bowel of dogs. J Physiol (Lond.) *246*: 387, 1975.

55. Donaldson RM: Small bowel bacterial overgrowth. Adv Intern Med *16*:191, 1970.

56. Halbert SP: Antagonism of coliform bacteria against Shigellae. J Immunol *58*:153, 1948.

57. Kundliff E: How antibiotic-producing organisms avoid suicide. Annu Rev Microbiol *43*:207, 1989.

58. Gordon HA, Pesti L: The gnotobiotic animal as a tool in the study of host-microbial relationships. Bacteriol Rev *35*:390, 1971.

59. Wilson KH: The gastrointestinal microflora. *In* Yamada T et al. (eds): Textbook of Gastroenterology. New York, Lippincott, 1991.

60. Gordon HA: Germ-free animal: Its use in study of "physiologic" effects of normal microbial flora on animal host. Am J Digest Dis *5*:841, 1960.

61. Sprinz H: Morphological response of intestinal mucosa to enteric bacteria and its implication for sprue and Asiatic cholera. Fed Proc *21*:57, 1962.

62. Hashimoto K, Handa H, Umehara K, Sasaki S: Germfree mice reared on an "antigenfree" diet. Lab Anim Sci *28*:38, 1978.

63. Brown WR, Lee EM: Radioimmunologic measurements of naturally occurring antibodies. I. Human serum antibodies reactive with *Escherichia coli* in gastrointestinal and immunologic disorders. J Lab Clin Med *82*: 125, 1973.

64. Brown WR, Lee EM: Radioimmunologic measurements of naturally occurring antibodies. II. Human serum antibodies reactive with *Bacteriodes fragilis* and *Enterococcus* in gastroenterological and immunological disorders. Gastroenterology *66*:1145, 1974.

65. Luckey D: Antibiotics in nutrition. *In* Goldberg HS (ed): Antibiotics, Their Chemistry and Non-medical Uses. Princeton, NJ, Van Nostrand, 1959.

66. Jukes TH: Antibiotics in Nutrition (Antibiotics Monographs No. 4), New York, Medical Encyclopedia, 1955.

67. Stokstad ELR, Jukes T: Further observations on "animal protein factor." Proc Soc Exper Biol Med *73*:523, 1950.

68. Stokstad ELR: Antibiotics in animal nutrition. Physiol Rev *34*:25, 1954.

69. Finegold SM, Sutter VL, Matheson GE: Normal indigenous intestinal flora. *In* Hentges DJ (ed): Human Intestinal Microflora in Health and Disease. New York, Academic Press, 1983.

70. de la Huerga J et al.: Effects of antimicrobial agents upon choline degradation in intestinal tract. J Clin Invest *33*:1117, 1953.

71. Wood RC, Hitchings JH: Studies of uptake and degradation of folic acid, citrovorum factor, aminopterin, and pyramethamine by bacteria. J Biol Chem *234*:2381, 1959.

72. Fujita A et al.: Studies of thiaminase. I. Activation of thiamine breakdown by organic bases. J Biol Chem *196*:289, 1952.

73. Kon SJ, Porter KWG: Intestinal synthesis of vitamins in ruminant. Vitam Horm *12*: 53, 1954.

74. Mickelson O: Intestinal synthesis of vitamins in nonruminant. Vitam Horm *14*:1, 1956.

75. Fridericia LS et al.: Reflection, transmissible change in intestinal content, enabling rats to grow and thrive without vitamin B in food. J Hyg *27*:70, 1927.

76. Barnes RH: Nutritional implications of coprophagy. Nutrition Rev *28*:289, 1962.

77. Daft FS et al.: Role of coprophagy in utili-

zation of B vitamins synthesized by intestinal bacteria. Fed Proc 22:129, 1963.

78. Dubos RJ, Schaedler RW: Effect of intestinal flora on growth rate of mice and on their susceptibility to experimental infections. J Exper Med 111:407, 1960.

79. Dubos RJ, Schaedler RW: Effect of bacterial endotoxins on water intake and body weight of mice. J Exper Med 113:921, 1961.

80. Schaedler RW, Dubos RJ: Fecal flora of various strains of mice: Its bearing on their susceptibility to endotoxin. J Exper Med 115:1149, 1962.

81. Spika JS et al.: Chloramphenicol-resistant *Salmonella newport* traced through hamburger to dairy farms. N Engl J Med 316:565, 1987.

82. Dubos RJ, Schaedler RJ, Costello RL: Effects of antibacterial drugs on weight of mice. J Exper Med 117:245, 1963.

83. Gorbach SL, Goldin BR: The intestinal microflora and the colon cancer connection. Rev Infect Dis 15 (suppl 2):s252, 1990.

84. Salyars AA, Vercellotti JR, West SEH, Wilkins TD: Fermentation of mucins and plant polysaccharides by *Bacteroides* from the human colon. Appl Environ Microbiol 33:319, 1977.

85. Hill MJ: Metabolism of carbohydrates and glycosides. *In* Hill MJ (ed): Microbial Metabolism in the Digestive Tract. Boca Raton, Florida, CRC Press, 1986.

86. Levitt MD: Production and excretion of hydrogen in man. N Engl J Med 281:122, 1969.

87. Wrong OM, Edmonds CJ, Chadwick VS: Short chain organic acids. *In* The Large Intestine: Its Role in Mammalian Nutrition and Homeostasis. New York, John Wiley and Sons, 1981.

88. Oh MS et al.: D-lactic acidosis in a man with the short bowel syndrome. N Engl J Med 301:249, 1979.

89. Stolberg L et al.: D-lactic acidosis due to abnormal gut flora. N Engl J Med 306:1344, 1982.

90. Bain MD et al.: Contribution of gut bacterial metabolism to human metabolic disease. Lancet 140:1078, 1988.

91. Chalmers TC: Pathogenesis and treatment of hepatic failure. N Engl J Med 263:23 and 77, 1960.

92. Kornberg HL, Davies RE: Gastric urease. Physiol Rev 35:169, 1955.

93. Marshall BJ: Campylobacter pyloridis and gastritis. J Infect Dis 153:650, 1986.

94. Silen W, Harper HA, Mawdsley DL, Weirich WL: Effect of antibacterial agents within intestine. Proc Soc Exper Biol Med 88:138, 1955.

95. Warren KS, Newton WL: Portal and peripheral blood ammonia concentrations in germ-free and conventional guinea pigs. Am J Physiol 197:517, 1959.

96. Vincent AJ et al.: Generation of ammonia from non-urea sources in a faecal incubation system. Clin Sci Mol Med 51:313, 1976.

97. Vincent AJ: Metabolism of ammonia, urea, and amino acids, and their significance in liver disease. *In* Hill MJ (ed): Microbial Metabolism in the Digestive Tract. Boca Raton, Florida, CRC Press, 1986.

98. Borgstrom B et al.: Trypsin, invertase, and amylase content of feces of germfree rats. Proc Soc Exper Biol Med 102:154, 159.

99. Gustafsson BE, Lanke LS: Bilirubin and urobilins in germfree, ex-germfree, and conventional rats. J Exper Med 112:975, 1960.

100. Asselineau F, Lederer E: Chemistry and metabolism of bacterial lipides. *In* Bloch K (ed): Lipid Metabolism. New York, Wiley, 1960.

101. Webb JPW, James AT, Kellogg TD: Influence of diet on quality of faecal fat on patients with and without steatorrhea. Gut 4:37, 1963.

102. Jover A, Gordon RS Jr: Procedure for quantitative analysis of feces with special reference to fecal fatty acids. J Lab Clin Med 59:878, 1962.

103. Talalay P: Enzymatic mechanism in steroid metabolism. Physiol Rev 37:362, 1957.

104. Dietschy JM: Mechanisms for the intestinal absorption of bile acids. J Lipid Res 9:297, 1968.

105. Norman A, Sjovall J: On transformation and enterohepatic circulation of cholic acid in rat. J Biol Chem 233:872, 1958.

106. Portman OW, Shah S, Antonis A, Jorgensen B: Alteration of bile salts by bacteria. Proc Soc Exper Biol Med 109:599, 1962.

107. Gustafsson BE, Norman A, Sjovall J: Influence of *E. coli* infection on turnover and metabolism of cholic acid in germ-free rats. Arch Biochem 91:93, 1960.

108. Jarvenpaa P, Kosunen T, Fotsis T, Adlerkreutz H: In vitro metabolism of estrogens by isolated intestinal micro-organisms and by human fecal microflora. J Steroid Biochem 13:345, 1980.

109. Bokkenheuser VD et al.: Biosynthesis of androgen from cortisol by a species of *Clostridium* recovered from human fecal flora. J Infect Dis 149:489, 1984.

110. Boxenbaum HG, Bejersky I, Jack ML, Kaplan SA: Influence of gut microflora on bioavailability. Drug Metab Rev 9:259, 1979.

111. Ellis H, Smith HD: The blind-loop syndrome. Monogr Surg Sci 4:193, 1967.

112. White WH: On the pathology and prognosis of pernicious anemia. Guy's Hosp Rep *47*: 149, 1890.

113. Seyderhelm R, Lehman W, Michels P: Experimentelle intestinale perniziose Aneamie beim hund. Klin Wchnschr *2*:1439, 1924.

114. Barker WH, Hummel LE: Macrocytic anemia in association with intestinal strictures and anastomoses. Bull Johns Hopkins Hosp *46*:215, 1939.

115. Donaldson RM: Intestinal bacteria and malabsorption. Ann Intern Med *64*:948, 1966.

116. Halsted JA, Lewis PM, Gasster M: Absorption of radioactive vitamin B12 in the syndrome of megaloblastic anemia associated with intestinal stricture or anastomosis. Am J Med *20*:42, 1956.

117. Aitken MA, Badenoch J, Spray GH: Fat excretion in rats with intestinal cul-de-sacs. Brit J Exper Path *32*:355, 1950.

118. Watson GM, Witts LJ: Intestinal macrocytic anemia. Br Med J *1*:13, 1952.

119. Strauss EW, Donaldson RM, Gardner FH: Relationship between intestinal bacteria and absorption of vitamin B_{12} in rats with diverticula of small bowel. Lancet *2*:736, 1961.

120. Donaldson RM: Malabsorption of Co^{60-} labeled cyano-cobalamin in rats with intestinal diverticula. 1. Evaluation of possible mechanisms. Gastroenterology *43*:271, 1962.

121. Donaldson RM, Corrigan H, Natsios G: Malabsorption of Co^{60-} labeled cyanocobalamin in rats with intestinal diverticula. II. Studies on contents of diverticula. Gastroenterology *43*:262, 1962.

122. Donaldson RM: Studies on the pathogenesis of steatorrhea in the blind loop syndrome. J Clin Invest *44*:1815, 1965.

123. Kim YS et al.: The role of altered bile salt metabolism in the steatorrhea of experimental blind loop syndrome. J Clin Invest *45*:956, 1966.

124. Tabaqchali S, Booth CC: Jejunal bacteriology and bile salt metabolism in patients with intestinal malabsorption. Lancet *2*:12, 1965.

125. Goldstein F: Mechanisms of malabsorption and malnutrition in the blind loop syndrome. Gastroenterology *61*:784, 1971.

126. Ament MD, Shimoda SS, Saunders DP, Rubin CE: Pathogenesis of steatorrhea in three cases of small intestinal stasis syndrome. Gastroenterology *63*:728, 1972.

127. Toskes PP, Donaldson RM: The blind loop syndrome. *In* Sleisenger MH, Fordtran JS (eds): Gastrointestinal Disease: Pathophysiology, Diagnosis, Management. 4th Edition. Philadelphia, WB Saunders Co., 1989.

128. Toskes PP et al.: Small intestinal mucosal injury in the experimental blind loop syndrome. Gastroenterology *68*:1173, 1975.

129. Hill MJ: Bacterial metabolism and the diagnosis of small bowel and gastric overgrowth. *In* Hill MJ (ed): Microbial Metabolism in the Digestive Tract, Boca Raton, Florida, CRC Press, 1986.

130. French JM, Gaddie R, Smith NM: Tropical sprue: Study of 7 cases and their response to combined chemotherapy. Quart J Med *25*:333, 1956.

131. Sheehy T, Perez-Santiago E: Antibiotic therapy in tropical sprue. Gastroenterology *41*:208, 1961.

132. Cook GC: Aetiology and pathogenesis of post infective tropical malabsorption (tropical sprue). Lancet *i*:721, 1984.

133. Gardner FH: Tropical sprue. N Engl J Med *258*:791 and 835, 1958.

134. Mathan VI, Baker SJ: An epidemic of tropical sprue in southern India. Ann Trop Med Parasitol *64*:439, 1970.

135. Gorbach SL: Travelers' diarrhea. *In* Gorbach SL, Bartlett JG, Blacklow NR (eds): Infectious Diseases. Philadelphia, WB Saunders Co., 1992.

136. Kean BH, Waters SR: The diarrhea of travelers. N Engl J Med *216*:71, 1959.

137. Kean BH, Schaffner W, Brennan RW, Waters SR: The diarrhea of travelers. V. Prophylaxis with phthalylsulfathiazole and neomycin sulphate. JAMA *180*:367, 1962.

138. Gorbach SL et al.: Travelers' diarrhea and toxigenic *Escherichia coli*. N Engl J Med *292*:933, 1975.

139. Levine MM: *Escherichia coli* that cause diarrhea: Enterotoxigenic, enteropathogenic, enteroinvasive, enterohemorrhagic, and enteroadherent. J Infect Dis *155*:3777, 1987.

140. Dupont HL et al.: Prevention of travelers' diarrhea by the tablet formulation of bismuth subsalicylate. JAMA *257*:1347, 1987.

141. Johnson PK et al.: Lack of emergence of resistant fecal flora during successful prophylaxis of travelers' diarrhea with norflaxicin. Antimicrob Agents Chemother *30*:671, 1986.

142. Doll R: The geographical distribution of cancer. Brit J Cancer *23*:1, 1969.

143. Burkitt DP: Epidemiology of cancer of the colon and rectum. Cancer *28*:3, 1971.

144. Burkitt DP: Colonic-rectal cancer: Fiber and other dietary factors. Am J Clin Nutr *31*(10 suppl.):58, 1978.

145. Modan B et al.: Low-fiber intake as an etiologic factor in cancer of the colon. J Natl Cancer Inst *55*:15, 1975.

146. Dales LG et al.: A case-control study of

relationships of diet and other traits to colorectal cancer in American blacks. Am J Epidemiol *109*:132, 1979.

147. Reddy BS, Watanabe K: Effect of intestinal microflora on 3,2'-dimethyl-4-aminobiphenyl-induced carcinogenesis in F344 rats. J Natl Cancer Inst *61*:1269, 1986.

148. Goldin BR, Gorbach SH: Effect of antibiotics on incidence of rat intestinal tumors induced by 1,2 dimethylhydrazine dihydrochloride. J Natl Cancer Inst *67*:877, 1981.

149. Goldin BR, Gorbach SL: The relationship between diet and rat fecal bacterial enzymes implicated in colon cancer. J Natl Cancer Inst *57*:371, 1976.

150. Goldin BR et al.: Influence of diet and age on fecal bacterial enzymes. Am J Clin Nutr *31*(10 suppl.)S136, 1978.

151. Hill MJ et al.: Bacteria and etiology of cancer of large bowel. Lancet *i*:95, 1971.

152. Whipple GH: A hitherto undescribed disease characterized anatomically by deposits of fats and fatty acids in the intestinal and mesenteric lymphatic tissues. Bull Johns Hopkins Hosp *18*:382, 1907.

153. Dobbins WO III: Whipple's Disease. Springfield, Illinois, Charles C Thomas, 1987.

154. Tompkins LS: Use of molecular methods in infectious diseases. N Engl J Med *327*:1290, 1992.

155. Wilson KH, Blitchington R, Frothingham R, Wilson JAP: Phylogeny of the Whipple's-disease-associated bacterium. Lancet *338*:474, 1991.

156. Relman DA et al.: Identification of the uncultured bacillus of Whipple's disease. N Engl J Med *327*:293, 1992.

157. Saboor SA, Johnson NM, McFadden J: Detection of mycobacterial DNA in sarcoidosis and tuberculosis with polymerase chain reaction. Lancet *339*:1012, 1992.

158. Moss MT et al.: Specific detection of Mycobacterium paratuberculosis by DNA hybridization with a fragment of the insertion element IS900. Gut *32*:395, 1991.

159. Olsen GJ et al.: Microbial ecology and evolution: A ribosomal RNA approach. Annu Rev Microbiol *40*:337, 1986.

Colon and Rectum

12

Intestinal Gas

MICHAEL D. LEVITT

Medical interest in intestinal gas dates back nearly to the beginning of recorded history, as evidenced by a treatise by Hippocrates entitled "The Winds" (1). Over the ensuing centuries, this topic has been a source of fascination for the layman and has been discussed by such lay literary greats as Geoffrey Chaucer, Benjamin Franklin, and Mark Twain. However, the first major investigational paper concerning gas (a comprehensive analysis of human flatus) did not appear until 1862 (2), and this report was followed by a relatively fallow 100-year period during which gas received only limited scientific attention. The development and application of gas chromatography in the mid-1960s marks the beginning of the modern history of investigation in the field of intestinal gas. Thus, the fertile period has been very brief, with most major advances occurring in the past 30 years. I was fortunate to have had this "golden age" of gas coincide with my career in gastroenterology, and this chapter will largely consist of a review of the scientific advances in intestinal gas as seen through my eyes as both a spectator and an active participant.

The first rigorous scientific paper concerning intestinal gas appeared in 1862, when Emil Ruge in Vienna published his finding that human flatus contained large quantities of CO_2, H_2, swamp gas (CH_4), and unidentified gases (2). Very little O_2 or H_2S was observed. His collection device consisted of a rubber nipple (that fit into the rectum) attached to a glass tube that led through a hole in a chair to a water displacement system. Interestingly, Ruge discussed

the difficulty he encountered with plugging of the tube, a problem that still bedevils attempts to obtain long-term collections of flatus. Cumbersome and time-consuming analytic techniques were required: CO_2 was measured by the volume that disappeared when the flatus was passed through a base, and H_2 and CH_4 were determined by complicated combustion techniques. Although subsequent technologic advances have markedly simplified the analysis of flatus, the many studies of this topic published over the past 150 years (3–6) have served mostly to confirm Ruge's initial observations as well as demonstrating that his unidentified gas largely consists of N_2. Of particular interest was his observation that flatus H_2 increased in some subjects when they ingested a diet high in milk, a finding confirmed about 115 years later, when the breath H_2 test was used to identify lactase deficiency (7).

With several striking exceptions, the period between 1862 and 1965 was a "dark age" for gas research. There are several possible explanations for this dearth of investigation. Before 1960, the methodology required for the analysis of gas was complicated, time-consuming, and insensitive. In addition, intestinal gas was probably considered by many to be a more appropriate topic for scatologic humor than serious scientific investigation. Lastly, gas research can be initially disconcerting to the investigator accustomed to handling liquids such as blood and urine because gas is invisible, difficult to collect, store, and dilute without leakage and contamination; and difficult to quantitate because the volume varies with temperature and pressure.

One important piece of research was carried out in the 1930s in the laboratory of Dr. Owen Wangensteen, the legendary Chief of Surgery at the University of Minnesota from 1930 to 1967. Wangensteen's training program was unique in that the surgical fellows were required to obtain a Ph.D., usually in physiology. As a result, his large program generated an enormous quantity of research and an inordinate number of chiefs of surgical sections. Wangensteen's group (8–10) reported that gaseous distension played an important role in the mortality of experimental small bowel obstruction in dogs, and the prevention of air swallowing by esophageal ligation eliminated this accumulation of bowel gas. Although these studies provided the basis for use of gastric suction in the treatment of bowel obstruction, they also led to the incorrect conclusion that virtually all the gas in the gut was swallowed air, a concept that was widely held for the subsequent 30 years.

By far the most extensive study ever published concerning the volume and composition of human flatus appeared in 1949. By means of a rectal tube and a siphon leading to a water trap, Kirk (3) obtained over 70 five-hour collections of flatus. His data indicated that subjects on standard and high-cabbage diets, respectively, passed an average of 1.55 and 2.34 mL of gas per minute. These 5-hour values extrapolate to flatus volumes of about 2000 and 3000 mL per day. Although these volumes are frequently cited as the daily output of flatus, it is almost certainly incorrect to extrapolate the daily output from 5-hour collections, given the temporal variations in passage of flatus.

Although most excretory products are readily collected, it is surprisingly difficult to obtain long-term, quantitative collections of flatus, free from atmospheric contamination. The investigator using the rectal tube rapidly learns that this instrument is uncomfortable, has a tendency to plug rapidly with fecal material, and frequently provides contaminated samples, as evidenced by the presence of appreciable O_2. Attempts to use a colostomy stomal patch over the anus also have not been fully satisfactory. Thus, the intestinal gas field is plagued by a lack of information on such seemingly mundane questions as how much flatus is excreted per day by healthy subjects, and whether patients complaining of flatulence actually excrete excessive gas.

Recently, Christl and coworkers (11) in Cambridge, England, described the use of an elegant technique in which subjects were housed in a small airtight room. The airflow through the room was controlled at a rate of 100 L/minute and the excretion rate of H_2 and CH_4 was determined from the difference between the concentrations of these gases in the air entering and leaving the room. This technique made possible the first long-term measurements of the excretion rate of H_2 and CH_4 under relatively physiologic conditions. Unfortunately, the excretion of N_2 and CO_2 in flatus cannot be assessed with this technique, and the world still awaits a method that will make possible long-term measurements of total flatus excretion.

In the 1930s, Dr. Walter Alvarez proved that not all important scientific advances require complicated measurements. Alvarez noted that patients complaining of excessive "gas" as the cause of their abdominal distension could reduce their abdominal girth on command, whereas subjects with a true increase in abdominal contents, such as those with ascites, could not (1). This led him to conclude that the origin of abdominal distension was not usually excessive "gas" but rather an unconscious lowering of the diaphragm and relaxation of abdominal muscles. He then performed studies on himself in which he attempted to predict, based on his sense of distension, how much intestinal gas would be present on his abdominal roentgenogram. He found little or no correlation between his sense of distension and the volume of his bowel gas. These observations were confirmed 30 years later when quantitative measurements of the volume of intestinal gas showed that subjects complaining of bloating and distension caused by a self-perceived increase in "gas" had perfectly normal volumes of intestinal gas (12).

The renaissance of intestinal gas research was triggered in the early 1960s by the lowly jelly bean. Doris Calloway (Fig. 12–1), a Ph.D. nutritionist working at the Armed Forces Food and Container Institute, was presented with the complaint that black jelly

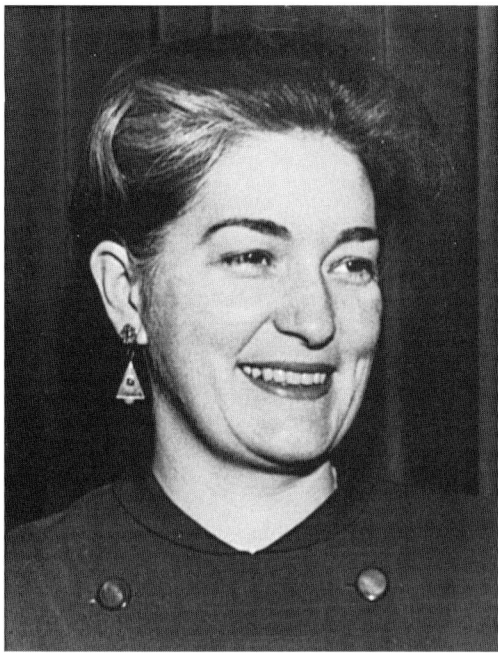

Fig. 12–1. Doris Calloway in 1966.

beans seemed to be particularly flatogenic for pilots flying at high altitude. Although the putative gaseousness of black jelly beans was never resolved, this question prompted Dr. Calloway and her coworkers to look into the possibility that newly developed chromatography techniques might provide a useful means of analyzing intestinal gases. They fabricated their first gas chromatograph, and shortly thereafter these instruments became commercially available. Using sensitive gas chromatographic techniques, Calloway and coworkers carried out a series of innovative studies, the most important of which showed that the intestinal gases, H_2 and CH_4, could be detected on the breath and that breath H_2 concentration varied with the diet (Fig. 12–2) (13). At approximately the same time (1965–66), Frederick Steggerda, a Ph.D. physiologist at the University of Illinois, carried out studies of flatus using gas chromatography and showed that the ingestion of baked beans markedly increased both the concentration and the rate of rectal passage of CO_2 and H_2 (14).

The increased interest in intestinal gas research that has characterized the last 30 years largely reflects the development of gas chromatographic techniques in the early 1960s. In contrast to the hours of analytic time required for the chemical analysis of a gas sample, gas chromatography requires only minutes to determine accurately the composition of an unprepared gas sample. Of particular importance is the exquisite sensitivity of this technique, which can accurately measure concentrations of a part per million or less, thus making it possible to measure the concentration of intestinal gases in expired air.

I had the good fortune to begin my gastrointestinal fellowship training with the legendary Dr. Franz Ingelfinger at Boston University in 1965, the dawn of the golden age of gas. By chance, I came to the fellowship with an interest in this topic. During my medical residency, I concocted and tested the idea that the gas content of blood in the stomach could be used to determine the source of upper gastrointestinal bleeding. The idea was that a gas ([131] xenon in my studies) would be infused into the colon of an upper gastrointestinal bleeder. The gas should be absorbed into portal blood and carried to the lungs, where it would be efficiently cleared in expired air. Thus, blood obtained from the stomachs of patients with bleeding esophageal varices (portal blood) would have a high concentration of the test gas as opposed to the low concentration present from bleeding caused by a peptic ulcer or gastritis (systemic blood).

Ingelfinger was not impressed with my Rube Goldberg scheme to diagnose the source of blood loss. However, he did have a long-standing interest in intestinal gas, and it was alleged that for many years he had tried, without success, to induce his fellows to study gas. Among Ingelfinger's many talents were his prescience with regard to potentially productive research topics, coupled with an extraordinary ability to stimulate his fellows to perform this research, a stimulation that usually took the form of negative reinforcement. According to Ingelfinger, "gas" was the perfect topic for someone with my limited research talents because nothing was known about this topic; hence, if I were lucky enough to stumble across some observation, I would have at least one publishable finding to show for my fellowship. He backed up this over-

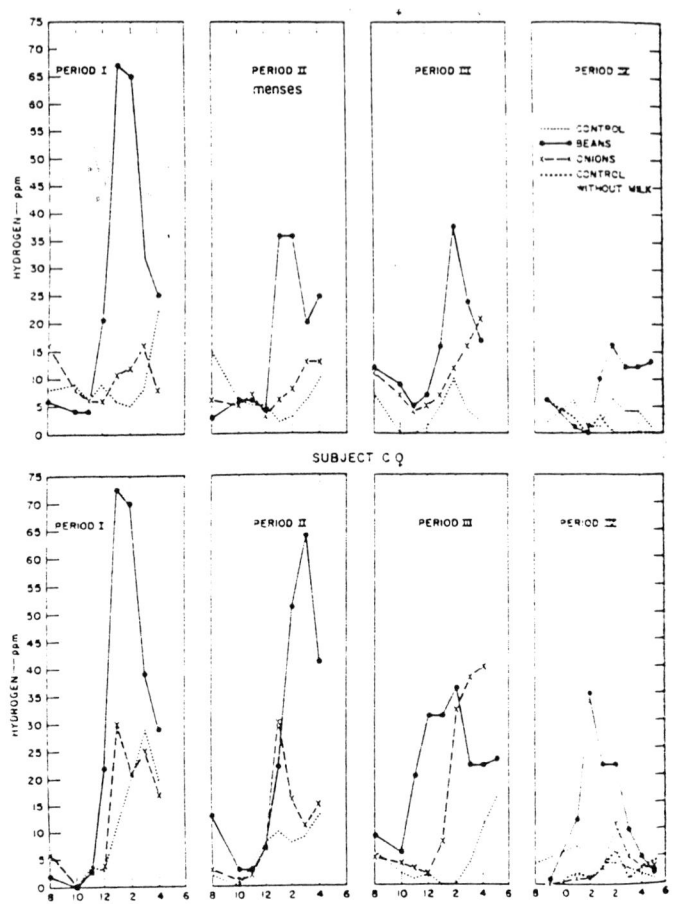

Fig. 12–2. The influence of ingestion of beans and onions on breath H_2 concentration. Reproduced with permission from Calloway DH: Respiratory hydrogen and methane as affected by consumption of gas-forming foods. Gastroenterology *51*:383, 1966.

whelming confidence in my abilities with the offer to send me to the laboratory of Dr. Calloway, who had moved from the military to the University of California at Berkeley. Dr. Calloway very kindly showed me her laboratory and equipment, and I returned to Boston and bought a gas chromatograph.

Ingelfinger was not one to spend money frivolously on trips and equipment for his fellows, and I was made acutely aware that I had better produce something worthwhile. About the only research technique with which I was familiar was the constant perfusion method developed by John Fordtran (a recent graduate of Ingelfinger's program) to study absorption from liquid infusates in the human intestine. I slightly altered Fordtran's technique to make possible measurement of the site and rate of H_2 and CH_4 production in the human intestine. The subject swallowed a triple-lumen, mercuryweighted polyvinyl tube, which was allowed to pass until the distal orifice was in the terminal ileum. By means of an orifice located in the proximal jejunum, the intestine was constantly and rapidly perfused with nitrogen containing a nonabsorbable marker gas, sulfur hexafluoride. Gas was found to be rapidly propelled through the gut, and within 30 minutes of starting the infusion, nitrogen was exiting from the rectum at a rate approximating the jejunal infusion rate. After establishment of a steady state, gas samples were collected from the proximal and distal ileum and rectum and analyzed for H_2, CH_4, and sulfur hexafluoride. The latter gas provided a means of measuring the rate of movement of gas past a collecting site, analogous to the use of polyethylene glycol in perfusion studies with liq-

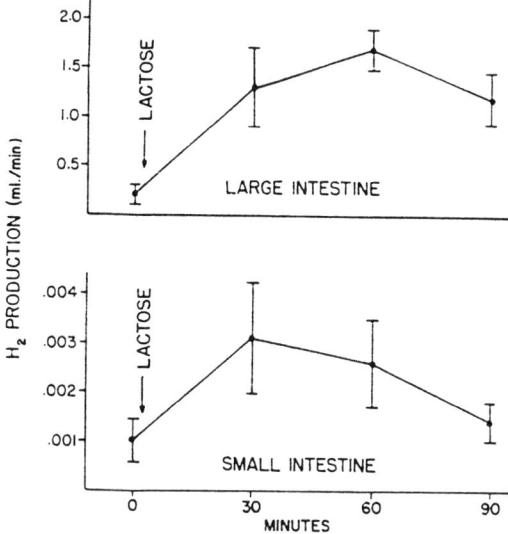

Fig. 12-3. Measurements of H_2 production in the small bowel and colon before and after instillation of two g of lactose into the proximal and distal ileum and colon. Reproduced with permission from Levitt MD: Production and excretion of hydrogen gas in man. N Engl J Med *281*:122, 1969.

uids. We found that H_2 and CH_4 were produced only in the colon (15). Of particular interest was the finding that an infusion of a small amount of lactose into the small bowel and colon caused an enormous increase in the colonic production of H_2 (but not CH_4), whereas small bowel H_2 production remained negligible (Fig. 12-3). It was concluded that nearly all H_2 production resulted from fermentation of malabsorbed carbohydrate by the colonic bacteria. In addition, H_2 excretion on the breath was found to correlate closely with the rate of H_2 production in the colon, with a mean of 14% of the colonic production appearing on the breath. Thus, breath H_2 excretion could be used as a simple, noninvasive marker of colonic H_2 production. Ingelfinger and I submitted this work to the Journal of Clinical Investigation, from which it rebounded with probably the shortest rejection message ever produced by this august journal, which I reproduce in toto:

"The paper contains very little that is new compared to its length. The experimental design and techniques seem adequate to support the conclusions drawn by the paper, which seems rather consistent but not very novel."

By the time of this rejection, Ingelfinger had become editor of the New England Journal of Medicine. He removed his name from authorship and suggested submission to the New England Journal, where, no doubt with his assistance, it was rapidly accepted for publication (15).

The observation that gas infused into the upper jejunum was rapidly propelled through the gut suggested that useful information could be obtained from a jejunal infusion of a gas not present in the gut (such as argon) that would "wash" out the native bowel gases. If all gas washed out at the rectum were quantitatively collected and analyzed for the bowel gases, one should be able to determine directly the volume and composition of the intestinal gas. Before this study, two groups had attempted to measure the volume of gas in the gut using the body plethysmograph and had reported values of about 2000 mL (16) and 200 mL (17). Our washout studies demonstrated that normal subjects had less than 200 mL of gas in their small and large bowels (12) and that subjects complaining of bloating and distension had normal volumes of bowel gas (18). Analysis of the relative proportions of bowel gases provided the first and only data concerning the composition of the entire intestinal gas pool (as opposed to the composition of flatus). Although N_2 was usually the predominant bowel gas, in some subjects the bacterially produced gases, H_2, CO_2, and CH_4, were predominant. The discrepancy between our findings in healthy human subjects and the observation of Wangensteen and coworkers that virtually all intestinal gas in dogs was swallowed air (10) probably reflects differences in experimental design. In the dog studies, the esophagus was ligated and no food entered the gastrointestinal tract; hence, no substrate was available in the intestine for bacterial gas production.

The results of studies of H_2 production and excretion suggested that measurements of breath H_2 excretion might have clinical utility as a simple, noninvasive, qualitative test for carbohydrate malabsorption; i.e., an increase in breath H_2 excretion after ingestion of a carbohydrate should indicate that the carbohydrate was malabsorbed and delivered to the colonic bacteria. The accuracy of this test was confirmed by comparing the breath H_2 excretion rate to the blood glucose rise that followed ingestion of 50 g of lactose by lactose-tolerant and intolerant subjects (7). However, the widespread use of this technique awaited the publication of two additional studies in prominent journals. First, Newcomer and coworkers (19) at the Mayo Clinic fed subjects lactose and compared the results of breath H_2 excretion rate and blood glucose measurements to the "gold standard" measurements of lactase activity in small bowel biopsies. Their observation that H_2 excretion perfectly distinguished lactase-deficient from lactase-persistent subjects (Fig. 12–4) provided instant credibility for the H_2 breath test. Second, the technique I used relied on measurement

of total breath H_2 excretion, a measurement requiring analysis of a timed collection of expired air. Metz and coworkers (20) in Toronto reasoned that subjects at rest have a relatively constant alveolar ventilation; thus, the irritatingly simple determination of alveolar H_2 concentration could be substituted for my more complicated measurement of H_2 excretion rate. Most recently, simple alveolar breath samplers and relatively inexpensive gas chromatographs dedicated to H_2 analysis have become commercially available, making breath H_2 analysis a routine office procedure.

Gastroenterologic investigators around the world apparently were eagerly awaiting the development of the H_2 breath test to assess carbohydrate absorption in light of its subsequent application in hundreds of studies over the past 20 years. In my opinion, the widespread appeal of this test is largely attributable to its simplicity and noninvasive nature, rather than the clinical value of the information provided.

As initially employed, breath H_2 testing only yielded qualitative information concerning carbohydrate malabsorption in that near-complete absorption was distinguished from very appreciable malabsorption. However, in many situations it was of interest to quantitate carbohydrate malabsorption, and we wondered if the amount of H_2 excreted on the breath correlated with the amount of carbohydrate not absorbed. To determine if this were the case, it obviously was necessary to compare breath H_2 measurements with some independent "gold standard" measurement of carbohydrate malabsorption. The only accepted direct means of quantitating such malabsorption was, and still is, aspiration from the perfused terminal ileum, a complicated, time-consuming, uncomfortable, and expensive technique when carried out in paid volunteers. However, it was known that some carbohydrates such as the synthetic disaccharide, lactulose, are totally nonabsorbable in the small bowel, but readily fermented by the colonic bacteria. Thus, as a shortcut, healthy volunteers were fed varying doses of lactulose, and their breath H_2 response was monitored. John Bond (my lowly fellow at that time and now the distinguished past president of the ASGE) found that a subject's breath H_2 excretion in-

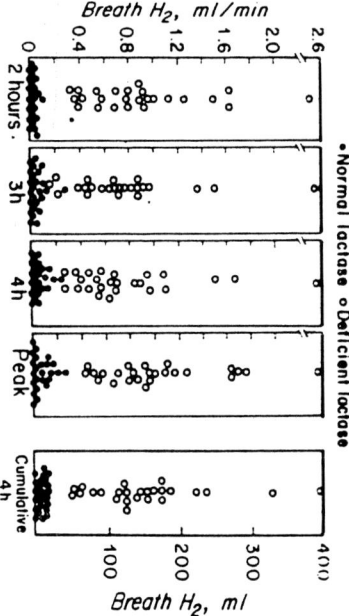

Fig. 12–4. Breath H_2 excretion of lactase deficient and lactase persistent ("normal lactase") subjects after ingestion of 50 g of lactose. Note that an H_2 excretion rate of about 0.2 mL/min at 2 hours provided perfect separation between the two groups of subjects. Reproduced with permission from Newcomer AD, McGill DB, Thomas PJ, Hofman AF: Prospective comparison of indirect methods for detecting lactose deficiency. N Engl J Med *293*:1232, 1975.

creased linearly with increasing dosage of lactulose, indicating that breath H_2 excretion could serve as a semiquantitative, as well as qualitative, indicator of malabsorption (21). Although far from perfect, the lack of other quantitative measures of carbohydrate malabsorption led to the widespread use of H_2 measurements for this purpose.

Breath H_2 measurements also have been used as a measure of small bowel transit time. The time elapsing between ingestion of a nonabsorbable carbohydrate and a rise in breath H_2 excretion serves as a reasonably accurate indicator of the time required for the head of a carbohydrate load to traverse the small bowel (22). Over 40 papers have been published using this technique. Once again, the widespread use of this method is largely attributable to its simplicity and the lack of other available techniques, rather than the clinical utility of measurements of small bowel transit time.

Initially, I presumed that the rate of H_2 excretion was determined simply by the amount of carbohydrate delivered to the colonic bacteria and the number of these bacteria that are able to carry out H_2-releasing fermentation reactions. However, various subsequent studies, many published in the Journal of Clinical Investigation, have demonstrated the inaccuracy of this simplistic scenario. First, Perman and coworkers showed that fecal H_2 production was inhibited by acid pH and postulated that this mechanism explained the reduced breath H_2 excretion observed with chronic ingestion of lactulose (23). French workers next demonstrated that the fecal bacteria adapt to chronic carbohydrate malabsorption with the induction of reactions that shunt carbohydrate away from H_2-producing reactions (24). Most importantly, it has been shown that colonic bacteria consume, as well as produce, H_2. I first became aware of this phenomenon while carrying out experiments designed to study the rate of absorption of gases from segments of rat intestine isolated between ligatures. The rats were housed in a closed chamber, and the absorption rate of the gases was determined from their excretion rate into the chamber. When a mixture of H_2 and He was instilled into the ceca of fasting rats, virtually all the He was absorbed and excreted, whereas only about 10% of the instilled H_2 was recovered

in the chamber, the remainder having disappeared irreversibly in the rat. Infusion of these two gases into the small bowel of the conventional rat or into the cecum of germ-free rats demonstrated nearly complete recovery of both gases. Thus, it was concluded that colonic bacteria can consume H_2, and that all vivo studies of intact humans or animals or in vitro studies with fecal homogenates had assessed net, rather than absolute, H_2 production (25).

Recently, Dr. Alessandra Strocchi, an Italian fellow working in my laboratory, showed that H_2 consumption is proportional to the H_2 tension in the fecal homogenate and that consumption could be totally inhibited if H_2 tension were maintained at a very low level (26). Comparison of H_2 release from human fecal homogenates incubated at very low versus physiologic H_2 tension suggested that the vast majority of H_2 produced in feces is consumed, with only a small fraction becoming available for excretion. The major nonbacterial factor influencing H_2 tension in fecal material is the extent to which the material is stirred, good mixing releases H_2 from the feces, thus reducing the H_2 tension and consumption. The efficiency of H_2 consumption also is influenced by the bacteria present in the feces. Methanogens are particularly efficient H_2 consumers, utilizing four moles of H_2 to produce one mole of CH_4 (26). Only about 40% of the population have a methanogenic flora (27), and these bacteria are localized almost entirely to the left colon (28).

These observations indicate that H_2 excretion is determined by the complex interaction of a variety of factors in addition to the simple availability of carbohydrate and the numbers of H_2-producing bacteria. A subject with poor luminal stirring and an efficient H_2 consuming flora may excrete very little H_2 despite appreciable carbohydrate malabsorption. Excretion of H_2 following malabsorption of slowly fermented carbohydrates may be minimal because these carbohydrates will make their way to the left colon where the presence of methanogens and poor stirring in the more solidified feces dramatically enhances H_2 consumption. This hypothesis is supported by observations showing that malabsorption of slowly fermented, resistant starch in bananas and cold potatoes results in far less H_2 than does an equivalent malabsorption of the rapidly fermented sugar, lactulose (29).

No doubt future studies will be directed toward determining whether flatulent patients have enhanced absolute H_2 production and/or defective H_2 consumption. The development of means to enhance the efficiency of H_2-consuming bacteria would be a far more acceptable form of therapy for the flatulent patient than is a diet low in nonabsorbable carbohydrates, the only available therapy at the present time.

Two other gases, CH_4 and CO_2, are produced in large quantity by the intestinal bacteria. Carbon dioxide production in the gut has received limited attention, probably because such studies require collections directly from the intestinal tract. (Breath measurements cannot distinguish between the relatively small amounts of CO_2 liberated in the gut and production by the subject's cellular metabolism.) Outside of the many measurements of CO_2 in flatus, the only important research study involving intestinal CO_2 was carried out by Rune (30) in Denmark, who demonstrated the importance of the interaction of acid and duodenal bicarbonate in the generation of CO_2. He showed that, during periods of high acid secretion, duodenal contents had a PCO_2 of approximately 500 torr. Because the partial pressure of pure CO_2 would be about 760 torr, it is apparent that the bulk (about 5/7) of the gas in the duodenum was CO_2. Although this CO_2 is absorbed rapidly, the possibility remains to be investigated that accumulation of this CO_2 in a loop of gut could play a role in the discomfort of conditions such as nonulcer dyspepsia.

Methane, like H_2, is produced solely by the colonic bacteria, and measurements of breath CH_4 provide a simple means of assessing the in situ function of the methanogens. Although the feces of all subjects contain appreciable numbers of H_2-producing bacteria, a study of the breath CH_4 concentration of 170 healthy individuals showed that only about one third of the population had a sufficient number of functioning methanogens to raise their breath CH_4 above the background atmospheric level of about 1.5 ppm (27). Using a rebreathing system, we were able to sensitively measure CH_4 excretion, and found that healthy individuals differed by over one millionfold in their rate of breath CH_4 excretion. Such enormous individual differences have never been observed for metabolites derived from the host's cellular metabolism, but may exist for bacterial products because of the great variability in numbers and types of bacteria that can inhabit the human colon.

The studies of breath CH_4 provided a clear-cut demonstration of how the colonic bacteria can influence both the environment of the entire body (as well as the colonic lumen) when they produce an absorbable metabolite, such as CH_4. Attempts to link a CH_4-producing flora to some disease state is an obvious avenue of research that thus far has not been very rewarding. Initial observations suggested an unusually high prevalence of CH_4 production in patients with colonic carcinoma (30), but subsequent studies failed to support this relationship (31). Despite these initial failures, the possibility remains that study of CH_4 or some other volatile bacterial metabolites excreted in expired air will provided useful information on disease processes related to colonic bacterial metabolism. The simplicity of this technique is illustrated by our ability, in a few days, to measure the breath CH_4 concentration of 170 individuals, whereas it would have required months to carry out bacterial studies of feces passed by such a large number of subjects.

No discussion of gas research would be complete without some mention of work performed to identify the odoriferous components of flatus. None of the quantitatively important gases has an odor; thus this property must be attributed to gases present in only trace concentrations. Identification of odors is a difficult area of research and only a few studies of human feces have been reported. Extremely sensitive methodology is required because the human nose can detect one part in one billion of a noxious gas. In addition, there is a very inexact relation between the chemical structure of a compound and its smell; thus, the only detector that can determine if an isolated compound is the source of a specific, noxious odor is the human nose (often referred to as an "experienced human sniffer" in research publications). The only serious study of fecal odors to date suggested that sulfur-containing gases, methanethiol and dimethyl sulfide, were responsible for the unpleasant odor of human feces (32).

Our understanding of the physiology of intestinal gas has improved somewhat during the past 30 years. However, compared to most areas of intestinal physiology, gas has received a minimum of attention and much remains to be learned. In particular, there is no effective therapy for gaseousness. Thus, Ingelfinger's suggestion to a novice investigator 27 years ago still seems like good advice for today's young scientist: study gas because so little is known about this topic that almost any observation is likely to be new and publishable.

REFERENCES

1. Alvarez WC, *cited in*. An Introduction to Gastro-Enterology, 4th Ed. New York, Hoeber, 1948.
2. Ruge E: Beitrag zur kennuness der darmgase. Sitzber Kaiserlicken Akad *44*:739, 1861.
3. Askevold F: Investigations on the influence of diet on the quantity and composition of intestinal gas in humans. Scand J Clin Lab Invest *8*:87, 1956.
4. Beazell JM, Ivy AC: The quantity of colonic flatus excreted by the "normal" individual. Am J Digest Dis *8*:128, 1941.
5. Steggerda FR, Dimmick JF: Effect of bean diets on concentration of carbon dioxide in flatus. Am J Clin Nutr *19*:120, 1966.
6. Tomlin J, Lowis C, Read NW: Investigation of normal flatus production in healthy volunteers. Gut *32*:665, 1991.
7. Levitt MD, Donaldson RM: Use of respiratory hydrogen (H_2) excretion to detect carbohydrate malabsorption. J Lab Clin Med *75*:937, 1970.
8. Paine JR, Carlson HA, Wangensteen OH: The postoperative control of distension, nausea, and vomiting. JAMA *100*:1910, 1933.
9. Hibbard JS, Wangensteen OH: Character of the gaseous distension in mechanical obstruction of the small intestine. Proc Soc Exp Biol Med *31*:1063, 1934.
10. Hibbard JS: Gaseous distention associated with mechanical obstruction of the small intestine. Arch Surg *33*:146, 1936.
11. Christl SU, Murgatroyd PR, Gibson GR, Cummings JH: Quantitative measurement of hydrogen and methane from fermentation using a whole body calorimeter. Gastroenterology *98*:A164, 1990.
12. Levitt MD: Volume and composition of human intestinal gas determined by means of an intestinal washout technique. N Engl J Med *284*:1394, 1956.
13. Calloway DH: Respiratory hydrogen and methane as affected by consumption of gas-forming foods. Gastreonterology *51*:383, 1966.
14. Steggerda FR: Gastrointestinal gas following food consumption. Ann NY Acad Sci *150*:57, 1968.
15. Levitt MD: Production and excretion of hydrogen gas in man. N Engl J Med *281*:122, 1969.
16. Blair HA, Dern RJ, Bates PL: The measurement of volume of gas in the digestive tract. Am J Physiol *149*:688, 1947.
17. Bedell GN, Marshall R, DuBois AB, Harris JH: Measurement of the volume of gas in the gastrointestinal tract. J Clin Invest *35*:336, 1956.
18. Lasser RB, Bond JH, Levitt MD: The role of intestinal gas in functional abdominal pain. N Engl J Med *293*:524, 1975.
19. Newcomer AD, McGill DB, Thomas PJ, Hofmann AF: Prospective comparison of indirect methods for detecting lactase deficiency. N Engl J Med *293*:1232, 1975.
20. Metz G et al.: Breath hydrogen as a diagnostic method for hypolactasia. Lancet *i*:1155, 1975.
21. Bond JH, Levitt MD: Use of pulmonary hydrogen (H_2) measurements to quantitate carbohydrate malabsorption: Study of partially gastrectomized patients. J Clin Invest *51*:1219, 1972.
22. Bond J, Levitt MD: Use of breath hydrogen (H_2) to quantitate small bowel transit time following partial gastrectomy. J Lab Clin Med *90*:30, 1977.
23. Perman JA, Modler S, Olson AC: Role of pH in production of hydrogen from carbohydrates by colonic bacterial flora. J Clin Invest *67*:643, 1981.
24. Florent C et al.: Influence of chronic lactulose ingestion on the colonic metabolism of lactulose in man (an *in vivo* study). J Clin Invest *75*:608, 1985.
25. Levitt MD, Berggren T, Hastings J, Bond JH: Hydrogen (H_2) catabolism in the colon of the rat. J Lab Clin Med *84*:163, 1974.
26. Strocchi A, Levitt MD: Factors affecting hydrogen production and consumption by human fecal flora: The critical role of hydrogen tension and methanogenesis. J Clin Invest *89*:1304, 1992.
27. Bond JH, Engel RR, Levitt MD: Factors influencing pulmonary methane excretion in man. J Exp Med *133*:572, 1971.

28. Flourie B: Comparative study of hydrogen and methane production in the human colon using caecal and faecal homogenates. Gut *31*:684, 1990.

29. Cummings JH, Englyst HN: Breath hydrogen (H₂) may not be a reliable way of quantitating starch fermentation. Gastroenterology *98*:A166, 1990 (Abstract).

30. Haines A et al.: Breath methane in patients with cancer of the large bowel. Lancet *i*:481, 1977.

31. Karlin D et al.: Breath methane excretion in patients with unresected colorectal cancer. J Natl Cancer Inst *69*:573, 1982.

32. Moore JG, Jessop LD, Osborne DN: A gaschromatographic and mass spectrometric analysis of the odor of human feces. Gastroenterology *93*:1321, 1987.

13

Irritable Bowel Syndrome

MARVIN M. SCHUSTER

Progress in our understanding of the irritable bowel syndrome (IBS) over the past century is reviewed in six categories which emphasize how the changes in focus of attention at different stages have shaped research and knowledge of this disorder.

DESCRIPTIVE ERA

At a time when observational powers were strengthened and finely honed by the lack of more modern diagnostic technology, clinical descriptions of diseases and syndromes were based on the historical reporting of symptoms and careful observations of signs, and this information was then used as a basis for rational speculation on etiology, a predominantly inductive process. It is interesting that one of the earliest accounts of IBS in the English literature (1) omits the description of symptoms other than to state that they manifest themselves "by various anomalous and distressing symptoms" and that "they are sufficiently characteristic to admit of clinical isolation, and to justify our classification of such cases under the designation of mucous disease of the colon" (1). Attention was focused on mucus as the characteristic sign of the disorder, and much time and energy were expended on descriptions of mucus. Clark (1) commented that the disorder is a "frequent occurrence and seems incidental to advanced civilization." He attributed the cause to overeating, overdrinking, and excess of "sexual or other emotional excitement, sedentary life, damp or hot atmo-

sphere, and the abuse of purgatives, but above all aloes." He furthermore postulated a pathogenesis based on local capillary congestion and "highly excitable condition of nervous centers." He hypothesized that the "fermentation" of the mucus induced fermentation of bowel contents, producing gases that poisoned the blood. He proposed a therapeutic program consisting predominantly of dietary exclusions, daily exercise, avoidance of emotional excitement, and bowel regulation. An earlier description of IBS by Howship (2) postulated an etiology based on "a spasmodic stricture in the sigmoid flexure of the colon."

IBS was first described in the American literature in 1871 by Mendes daCosta, who also focused on the mucus in the stools which represented the most readily observable sign of the disorder he called "membranous enteritis." He made the enigmatic observation that the disorder "is not very common; yet it is not very uncommon" (3).

In 1905, White (4) presented 60 cases in an address delivered before the Devon and Exeter Medical Society and published in the Lancet. He apparently was not aware of previous publications because he lamented the fact that, although the disorder was "not rare and many cases have been published in France, Germany and America, no series of cases has been recorded in this country (England)." He recognized the limitations of the term "membranous colitis" as well as the disadvantages of other labels such as mucus colic, glary enteritis, glutinous diarrhea, tubular diarrhea, mucus affection of the intestine, and intestinal croup. Like his predecessors, he focused on the observable mucus and therefore suggested membranous colitis as the appropriate term, emphasizing that the disease was limited to the colon. He was wise enough to caution that this term was acceptable only provided "we do not bind ourselves to the proposition that there is inflammation of the colon." He suspected a neurotic etiology because of "its greater frequency among the middle and upper classes and among women," and occurring most commonly between the ages of 20 and 30 and only infrequently after age 45. He also recognized the benign nature of the disorder, stating that "membranous colitis of itself hardly, if ever, kills." He commented that he or a colleague inspected the bowel movements in nearly all instances and noted hard masses of varying shapes with constipation predominating in almost all patients but occasionally alternating with liquid feces.

White noted that "all writers are so agreed that membranous colitis occurs, as Nothnagel says, in nervous neurasthenic, hypochondriacal, hysterical individuals that there is no need to go into this in detail." These biases have been transmitted through generations of students to the present day. Apparently, however, the irritable bowel syndrome was not separated from what is recognized today as inflammatory bowel disease because three stages of mucus disease were described; first, the expulsion of mucus; second, tubular casts of the gut; and third, the evacuation of shreds of "lymph" mixed with blood and pus.

William Osler (5) also focused on the mucus of IBS as the sign, which provided its name "mucous colitis," and he described patients manifesting "hysterical, hyperchondriacal and neurasthenic personalities." Later authors also viewed the disorder as a nervous response to stress (6). The concept of hypovagotonia evolved in an attempt to explain the visceral manifestations of stress or personality disorder (7).

Chaudhary and Truelove (8) refined the definition and provided more thorough epidemiologic and demographic evidence of the disorder; they also defined two types of IBS: spastic colon consisting of painful constipation, diarrhea, or alternation of the two, and the other, painless diarrhea. The concept of a painless form of the disorder persisted for another two decades.

Epidemiological Advances

As with many other aspects of IBS, advances in knowledge of epidemiologic features have occurred predominantly over the past several decades. Many refinements have appeared since Clark described the condition as "common" (Lancet) and DaCosta described it as not very common and yet "not very uncommon" (3). Mendeloff was the first to recognize its surprisingly high prevalence as both a primary and secondary diagnosis in hospitalized populations (9). This was unanticipated, particularly because irritable bowel syndrome is treated predominantly on an ambulatory basis. The recorded prevalence also represents a minimal estimate because this disorder is not reportable, and many individuals with IBS do not seek medical attention.

Attention to the socioeconomic effects of the disorder developed only recently with the recognition that it ranks close to the common cold as a leading cause of absenteeism from work due to illness (10). Several well-designed epidemiologic studies have demonstrated in community samples that 15 to 20% of the general population have symptoms satisfying the criteria for irritable bowel syndrome, but these individuals have never consulted a physician for these symptoms (11,12).

REFINEMENTS IN THE DEFINITION: APPLICATION OF STATISTICAL METHODS

A major obstacle to improved understanding of irritable bowel syndrome until recent times has been the lack of appropriate diagnostic criteria. The first modern scientific attempt to establish diagnostic criteria was in 1978 (13). The authors administered a questionnaire to patients with IBS and compared their response to those of patients with organic diseases attending a GI clinic. Four symptoms were found to occur statistically more frequently in IBS patients than among individuals with organic gastrointestinal disorders and two additional symptoms showed a strong trend toward significance. These findings have been reproduced by others (14,15), and subsequently became the basis for the diagnostic criteria established by an International Working Team in Rome (16), which used a system similar to the DSM III system for psychiatric diagnosis, requiring certain major features and a specified number of minor features from a list of possible symptoms. Unfortunately, the original wording of these criteria permitted the diagnosis of IBS in the absence of pain. This definition, therefore, was refined in a subsequent publication of the working team, which incorporated abdominal pain as a necessary part of the diagnosis (17). The inclusion of pain was in agreement with a simpler definition formulated from an earlier meeting in Droitwich, England (18). Until then, painless diarrhea had been accepted as a form of irritable bowel syndrome (7). Because of their simplicity, the Droitwich criteria tend to be used more commonly in the clinical setting, whereas the Rome criteria, because they are more restrictive, are more suitable for research purposes.

Another area of interest has been the investigation of abnormal motor responses in areas of the gastrointestinal tract other than the colon in patients with IBS. A second Rome working team, avoiding direct confrontation with this issue, identified subgroups of functional gastrointestinal disorders ranging in location from the esophagus to the anal sphincters. Under this schema, irritable bowel syndrome was one of five functional bowel disorders (19).

PSYCHOLOGIC THEORIES AND CORRELATIONS

The concept that emotions influence the body dates to antiquity. Plato said, "for this is the great error of our day, that physicians separate the psyche from the soma." These concepts eventually evolved into the belief that the irritable bowel syndrome was a psychosomatic disorder. Engel proposed a biopsychosocial model that incorporated biologic, psychologic, and social factors into an integrated whole with complex interactions between these components resulting in a dynamic continuum. These concepts empha-

sized illness as opposed to disease and persons as opposed to organs (20).

Freudian psychoanalysis stressed the role of symbolism as an expression of unconscious drives that could be expressed in somatic fashion. Franz Alexander, who used psychoanalytic theory to account for psychosomatic disorders, sought to explain organ specificity in terms of vulnerability to a specific emotional conflict (21). He postulated that the gastrointestinal tract was particularly vulnerable to dependency conflicts, whereas the cardiovascular system was more vulnerable to rage. Alexander characterized a number of disorders, including ulcerative colitis, duodenal ulcer, asthma, rheumatoid arthritis, essential hypertension, neurodermatitis, and thyrotoxicity as psychosomatic but, interestingly, irritable bowel syndrome was not included. Similarly, the general psychiatric literature concentrated heavily on peptic ulcer disease and ulcerative colitis and paid little attention to irritable bowel syndrome. Peptic ulcer disease was thought to result from unresolved dependency-independency conflicts. As a precipitating factor in ulcerative colitis, Engel emphasized the loss (real or imagined) of a key figure occurring in a "personality type" that was predisposed to develop that disorder (22,23).

An investigation of peptic ulcer, assumed at that time to be classically psychosomatic, prompted the conclusion that peptic ulcers resulted from a genetic susceptibility in conjunction with a personality profile that created vulnerability (24). This study, involving army recruits, demonstrated that psychologic testing could identify gastric hypersecretors and predict development of ulcers under periods of stress.

The Russian physiologist I.T. Kurtsin, working with Bikov, took issue with the French physiologist, Bichat, who divided all bodily activity into animal functions (interacting with the external environment) and vegetative functions (interacting with internal organs). Like Pavlov, he did not accept Langley's theory that the vegetative nervous system was independent of the central nervous system.

Almy and co-workers (25–28), using pressure recordings, demonstrated that stressful interviews could induce either spasm or inhibition of colonic contractions, even when the topic under discussion in each instance was the same. What differed was not the stimulus but the patient's reaction to it (the induced effect). When the patient's reaction was that of anger and hostility, colonic motility was augmented. When the effect was depression, colonic contractions were inhibited. The question was raised as to whether the alternating constipation and diarrhea seen in irritable bowel syndrome might be explained by the affective state of the patient. It was noted that these responses were not specific to patients with irritable bowel syndrome, but represented an exaggeration of responses that also occurred in normal individuals. Wolf also reported that colonic motility was responsive to emotional stimulation and that hypomotility was induced during states of emotional dejection, whereas hypermotility was associated with anger and resentment (29). These findings were based on observations in individuals obtained by balloon kymography, barium enema x-rays, and direct observations of colonic mucus fistulas. He, too, postulated that the alternating constipation and diarrhea of irritable colon syndrome might be induced in this manner by altered emotions.

Although there are few objective studies of the effects of stress in IBS, there are many comments on the importance of stress. Mendeloff reported on historical recollections of the existence of stress before the onset of the syndrome (30). However, approximately 50% of people without bowel disorders also report bowel symptoms during stressful periods (11). Other studies have demonstrated that patients with irritable bowel syndrome tend to exhibit "somatizing" behavior (a tendency to develop somatic symptoms when stressed psychologically) (12,31). Patients with IBS also were found to seek medical attention for non-IBS related problems more often than the general population (32) and to have sought nontraditional medical approaches such as acupuncture more often (33). Studies uniformly report a greater anxiety, neuroticism, and closer relationship of illness to psychosocial stresses in IBS patients than in ulcerative colitis patients (34–36).

It has become apparent that patients with IBS who seek medical attention differ psychologically from those with IBS who do not seek medical attention. The 15% of the general population who qualify for the diagnosis of IBS but have not consulted physicians score within the normal range on psychologic tests, whereas IBS patients who seek medical attention score high on the scale of neuroticism and psychologic distress (12). Furthermore, it was shown that patients with IBS were not simply neurotic complainers who were supersensitive to any type of pain, because IBS patients could tolerate the cold pressor test with immersion of the hand in iced water longer than could normal subjects (12). This observation suggested that IBS patients were not simply overresponsive to all types of pain, but rather were sensitive specifically to intestinal pain. Whether this is because the intestines of these patients are hyperresponsive to stimuli such as eating or intraluminal distension, or whether this response is a perceptual phenomenon is presently under investigation. The finding of an abnormal colonic myoelectric frequency in patients with IBS also suggests a target organ abnormality (37).

Numerous studies have demonstrated an increase in psychologic distress and neuroticism among patients with irritable bowel syndrome (30,38). However, more recent investigations have demonstrated a pronounced difference in this regard between patients with irritable bowel syndrome who seek medical attention, and the 15% of the general population who have the symptoms of irritable bowel syndrome but who do not (11). Psychologic distress and neuroticism appear more important in determining medical attention-seeking behavior than in determining the underlying illness.

Recent psychologic attention has turned to factors present in the backgrounds of patients who present for medical attention with symptoms of functional gastrointestinal disorders. For example, more than 50% of women who presented with functional gastrointestinal disorders had a history of sexual or physical abuse. The significance of this observation also is being evaluated.

THE ERA OF PHYSIOLOGIC STUDIES

For decades, the colon was the focus of attention in physiologic investigations in

IBS, but recently abnormalities have been demonstrated in other areas of the tubular gut (39). Most studies of the colon have not demonstrated abnormalities in the resting motility of the colon, but have shown abnormal motor activity following stimulation by meals (40), hormones (41), stress (25), and intraluminal distention (42). These findings emphasize the presence of disordered motility in the irritable bowel syndrome and the fact that this disorder is precipitated by numerous stimuli. Although stress is recognized as an important factor, it is not the only one supporting the concept that irritable bowel syndrome is not purely a psychosomatic disorder (43). The abnormal response is usually that of excessive contractions in the colon. By contrast, abnormal baseline contractions have been demonstrated in the small bowel in patients with IBS (44), whereas stress seems to inhibit small bowel contractions (45,46). Some reports find a correlation between spastic colonic contractions and abdominal pain (47).

In attempting to elucidate the mechanism of altered bowel habits in the irritable bowel syndrome, Connell (48) demonstrated a paradoxic motility in patients with constipation and diarrhea. Although it appears logical that diarrhea would be associated with increased motility and constipation with decreased motility, the opposite actually is true; hence the paradox. The reason for this response is that when the normal haustral contractions of the colon are exaggerated, as they are in spastic constipation, the transit of stool in a caudad direction is delayed. Inhibition of these contractions, which results in effacement of haustra, lessening impeding contractions characterizes diarrheal states. Waller (49) also found increased motility in constipation-predominant IBS as compared to diarrhea-predominant IBS. Other observers, however, failed to confirm decreased motility in diarrhea-predominant IBS (25,50), but, in fact, observed increased motility in pain-associated diarrhea, perhaps because the earlier studies included patients with painless diarrhea as well as painful diarrhea. It is now inappropriate to combine all patients with IBS into a single category. A preferable classification might be diarrhea-predominant or constipation-predominant groups.

Continuing investigations also have underscored the importance of other types of motility in explaining the occurrence of constipation and diarrhea, including high-amplitude progressive contractions (HAPCs) that sweep down the colon six to eight times a day (51). These contractions cluster around meals and bowel movements and are markedly suppressed in constipation-predominant IBS patients. Obviously, at least two (and probably more) mechanisms can explain the altered bowel habits of irritable bowel syndrome.

The finding of an abnormal baseline myoelectric activity in the smooth muscle of the colon is important in two respects. First, it indicates that there may be an inherent (congenital or acquired) abnormality in the target organ; and second, it may provide a clue as to abnormalities that predispose to disordered motility in irritable bowel syndrome (37,40,52).

ALTERED PAIN PERCEPTION

The altered bowel habits of the irritable bowel syndrome may consist of diarrhea or constipation or a combination of the two; but, by definition, pain is common to all patients with the irritable bowel syndrome (18,53). Numerous studies have shown patients with irritable bowel syndrome to be more sensitive than controls to colonic distention (42,54).

The fact that the site of pain in patients with irritable bowel syndrome varied from individual to individual and could be located anywhere in the abdomen was long held as corroborative evidence that the irritable bowel syndrome is "functional" and not physiologic or organic. However, it was demonstrated that the pain induced by balloon distention in a specific part of the colon could be referred to almost any site of the abdomen so that even the site of physiologic pain was not necessarily at the trigger site (55). This finding might also explain why distention of the rectum or rectosigmoid (the most common site in experimental situations) often does not reproduce the patient's complaint of pain, even though it almost invariably induces spastic contractions in patients with irritable bowel syndrome. Much of today's research revolves around studies of perception and mechanisms of altered perception.

CONCEPTS OF TREATMENT

Because early concepts focused on mucus as the critical underlying pathology, it is not surprising that the treatment prescribed by Clark included the removal of accumulated mucus and the prevention of subsequent excessive secretion. The editor of Lancet (1) said that "Dr. Clark has at last, after many suggestive failures (and what honestly recorded failures are not eminently successful and useful?)" arrived at the conviction that the most successful scheme of treatment involved removing the mucus by internal use of alkalies with gentle laxatives. Preventive measures included: (1) solid diet, excluding hard substances such as vegetables and fruits; (2) abstinence from tea, coffee, beer, and all hot liquids; (3) gradual increase of daily exercise; (4) avoidance of emotional excitement and hot and damp atmospheres; (5) astringents and tonics; (6) bowel regulation; (7) counterirritation to the abdomen; and (8) in obstinate cases, the introduction of astringent solutions into the bowel per rectum.

W. Hale White (4) emphasized that "by far the most important part of treatment is to keep the large bowel empty." He used castor oil for this purpose. He recognized that "there is, however, no doubt that lavage is more effectual when carried out at Pombiers than when used in this country. If, therefore, treatment by simple aperient fails that patient should be sent to Pombiers." For more severe cases, he advocated "allowing all the feces to escape by a right sided colostomy." He reported that some cases respond to high-frequency electrical currents. We also are told that treatment should be directed to the underlying nervous conditions by "appropriate means," but it is not easy to such means, and even if they are found, "attention to them might unduly attract our energies from the one thing needful—viz. to keep the large bowel empty."

In a paper entitled "Mucous Colitis: Observations in 500 cases," presented in May 1929, J. Friedenwald and associates accepted the theory that, because "mucus colitis has its origin in an imbalance of the vegetative nervous system and is therefore a purely functional affection, the method of treatment becomes evident. Inasmuch as the disease is observed in psychoneurotics, careful analysis into the patient's emotions and mental state must be undertaken. Reeducation is essential." He added, "the constitutional factor must also be taken into consideration. The exhaustion of the nervous system, which is the cause of the physical and mental fatigue, still further depresses the already weakened constitutional defect." He therefore advocated avoidance of overwork and stressed the importance of rest and diversion. Although he appreciated the significant role of diet, Friedenwald recognized that "authorities have not been in accord regarding the character of the diet to be prescribed." Some authorities at the time advocated large portions of indigestible residue with an excess of fat and recommended that this change be brought about suddenly and not gradually. Others advocated bland diets with small residue. Friedenwald favored an initially bland diet with gradual increase in roughage. He suggested avoiding colonic irrigations with medicated solutions, but indicated that olive oil enemas retained in the bowel overnight were soothing. He stated that drugs play "a very unimportant role in the treatment of mucus colitis." Atropine and belladonna were recommended for overcoming spasm and bromides to provide sedation.

Dietary recommendations for the irritable bowel syndrome have varied from time to time, as with diverticulosis, being influenced by both empiric observations and prevailing theories. In the time of Walter Alvarez, the "smooth diet" (the Alvarez diet) was advocated. It was felt that roughage would irritate the sensitive lining and produce more mucus and perhaps more spasm. The British surgeon, Dennis Burkitt, working in Africa, observed that both diverticulosis and irritable bowel syndrome were uncommon among African natives, and he correlated this situation with a high-fiber African diet in contrast to the Western low-fiber diet. This observation has led to numerous studies of the effects of fiber in both the irritable bowel and diverticular disease of the colon, with mixed results. One of the major problems concerns the very high placebo response characterizing the irritable bowel syndrome, and complicates evaluation of the efficacy of fiber. This has been true also in the use of drugs. However, some reports indicate a beneficial effect of fiber on constipation but not on pain. At present, high-fiber diets and hydrophilic bulking agents are commonly prescribed.

Attempts to implicate food allergies or intolerance generally have been disappointing except that food intolerances have been observed in some patients who manifest predominantly diarrhea (56).

Because of the demonstrated colonic spasms in the irritable bowel syndrome and the contribution of spasm to the pain, antispasmodics have been widely used in treatment. But the only study in this country that demonstrated efficacy involved a 6-week trial using a dose double the amount normally prescribed, and one that resulted in a high incidence of anticholinergic side effects (57).

Antispasmodics generally are prescribed for symptomatic relief of pain. Sedatives and tranquilizers are avoided, but tricyclic antidepressants have achieved fairly general acceptance, both for their analgesic effect and because they have been found empirically helpful in small single doses during the evening. Relaxation tapes also have been found useful.

Investigation of the possible role of neuropeptides in the irritable bowel syndrome has increased, including the possible development of competitive ligands, which might prove beneficial by binding at receptor sites. 5 HT3 antagonists (such as Cisapride) are undergoing clinical trial, and 5 HT4 agonists are being developed for future study.

Treatment, in addition to pharmacotherapy, has included for the first time controlled trials of psychotherapy, hypnotherapy, and behavioral therapy. Brief periods of psychotherapy over a 3-month period produced improvement in gastrointestinal and psychologic symptoms (58). Some of the studies of psychologic therapy suggest improvement of gastrointestinal symptoms of IBS without change in psychologic status; others do not. The beneficial effect of tranquilizers, particularly benzodiazepines, is not impressive. Biofeedback therapy apparently has succeeded in reducing colonic spasm (59), but was no more successful than

relaxation training in alleviating symptoms (41). Hypnotherapy produced significant reductions in abdominal pain, distention, and altered bowel habits when compared to controls (60).

CONCLUSION

The history of IBS begins with the descriptive era that followed initial recognition of this disorder during the 19th century. At that time, the focus of attention was on its most recognizable feature, the mucus that gave the disorder its initial name, "mucous colitis." As the science of epidemiology developed, demographic information concerning IBS became more available, altering concepts of its definition. The application of newly developed statistical methods permitted further refinement of the definition and the development of a more homogenous patient population.

Theories of etiology ranged from initial concepts that inflammation produced spasm and overproduction of mucus to psychologic theories that evolved through successive stages as psychiatry and psychology developed new insights and new etiologic hypotheses.

Physiologic investigation, often combined with studies of the effect of provocative stimuli, especially stress and psychosocial factors, has increased during recent decades. Modern research has revealed potentially significant insights into the role of intestinal neurotransmitters recently demonstrated to coexist in both the central nervous system and the gut. These observations indicate complex brain-gut interactions and represent the most important new areas of research into the nature of the irritable bowel syndrome.

In the years ahead, it will be important to determine whether the altered physiologic events that are being increasingly recognized play a causative role or simply represent a response to various precipitating factors. Nevertheless, pathophysiologic insights provide a rational basis for developing effective therapy. Improved understanding of the neurologic and neurohumoral mechanisms regulating gut activity will provide increased opportunities for fruitful research.

REFERENCES

1. Editorial: Clinical illustrations of mucous disease of the colon. From Notes of Various Cases under the Care of Dr. Andrew Clark. Lancet *ii*:614, 1859.
2. Howship J: Practical Remarks on the Discrimination and Successful Treatment of Spasmodic Stricture in the Colon. London, Burgess and Hill, 1930.
3. DaCosta JM: Membranous enteritis. Am J Med Sci *62*:321, October 1871.
4. White WH. A study of 60 cases of membranous colitis. Lancet *ii*:1229, 1905.
5. Osler W: The Principles and Practice of Medicine. Appleton, New York, 1892.
6. Bockus HL, Bank J, Wilkinson SA: Neurogenic mucous colitis. Am J Med Sci *176*:813, 1928.
7. Barker L: Management of the spastic colon and mucous colopathy, especially in hypovagotonic persons. Amer J Med Sci *178*:606, 1928.
8. Chaudhary NA, Truelove SC: Irritable colon syndrome. J Med *31*:307, 1962.
9. Mendeloff AI: Epidemiology of irritable bowel syndrome. Practical Gastroenterology *3*:12, 1979.
10. Almy TP: Digestive disease as a national problem. II. A White paper by the American Gastroenterological Association *53*:821, 1967.
11. Drossman DA, Sandler RS, McKee BC, Lovitz AJ: Bowel patterns among subjects not seeking health care. Gastroenterology *82*:529, 1982.
12. Whitehead WE et al.: Symptoms of psychologic distress associated with irritable bowel syndrome: Comparison of community of medical clinic sample. Gastroenterology *95*: 709 1988.
13. Manning AP, Thompson WG, Heaton KW, Morris AF: Toward positive diagnosis of irritable bowel. Br Med J *2*:653, 1978.
14. Talley NJ et al.: Diagnostic value of the Manning criteria in irritable bowel syndrome. Gut *311*:71, 1990.
15. Whitehead WE et al.: Existence of irritable bowel syndrome supported by factor analysis of symptoms in two community samples. Gastroenterology *98*:336, 1990.
16. Thompson WG et al.: Irritable bowel syndrome: Guidelines for the diagnosis. Gastroenterol Internat *1*:92, 1989.
17. Thompson WG et al.: Functional bowel disease and functional abdominal pain. Gastroenterol Internat *5*(2):75, 1992.
18. Reed NW (ed): Irritable Bowel Syndrome. London, Grune and Stratton, 1985.
19. Drossman DA et al.: Identification of subgroups of functional gastrointestinal disorders. Gastroenterol Internat *3*:159, 1990.
20. Engel GL: The need for a new medical model: A challenge for biomedicine. Science *196*:129, 1977.
21. Alexander F: Psychosomatic Medicine, Its Principles and Applications. New York, Norton, 1950.
22. Engel GL: Studies of ulcerative colitis. III. The nature of the psychologic processes. Am J Med *19*:231, 1955.
23. Engel GL: Studies of ulcerative colitis. V. Psychological aspects and their implication for treatment. Am J Dig Dis *3*:315, 1958.
24. Weiner H, Thaler M, Resier MF, Mirsky IA: Etiology of duodenal ulcer. I. Psychosomatic Medicine *9*:1, 1957.
25. Almy TP, Abbot FKJ, Hinkle LE: Alteration in colonic function of distress. Gastroenterology *15*:95, 1950.
26. Almy TP, Tulin M. Alterations in colonic function in man under stress: experimental production of changes simulating the "irritable colon." Gastroenterology 8:616, 1947.
27. Almy TP, Kern F, Tulin M: Alterations in colonic function under stress. II. Experimental production of sigmoid spasm in healthy persons. Gastroenterology *12*:425, 1949.
28. Almy TP, Hinkle LE, Berle B, Kern F: Alterations in colonic function under stress. III. Experimental production of sigmoid spasm in patients with spastic constipation. Gastroenterology *12*:437, 1949.
29. Grace WJ, Wolf S, Wolff HG: The role of the colon in bodily economy and common colonic disorders in the human colon: An experimental study based on direct observations of 4 fistulous subjects. New York, P.B. Hoeber, Inc. 1951.
30. Mendeloff AI, Monk M, Siegel CI, Lillienfeld A. Illness experience in life stresses in patients with irritable colon and with ulcerative colitis. N Engl J Med *282*:14, 1970.
31. Whitehead WE, Enck P: Psychopathology in patients with irritable bowel syndrome. *In* Singer MC, Doebell H (eds): Nerves and the Gastrointestinal Tract. Falk Symposium, Lancaster, United Kingdom, Kluwer Academic Publishers, 1989.
32. Fielding JF: Surgery and the irritable bowel syndrome: The singer as well as the song. Ir Med J *76*:33, 1983.
33. Smart HL, Mayberry JF, Atkinson M: Alternative medicine. Consultations and remedies in patients with irritable bowel syndrome. Gut *27*:826, 1986.
34. Esler MD, Goulston KJ: Levels of anxiety in colonic disorders. N Engl J Med *288*:16, 1974.

35. Fava GA, Pavan L: Large bowel disorders. I. Illness configuration and life events. Psychopathol Psychosomat 27:93, 1976.

36. Mendeloff AI: The epidemiology of idiopathic inflammatory bowel disease. *In* Kirsner JB, Shorter RG (eds): Inflammatory Bowel Disease. Philadelphia, Lea & Febiger, pp. 3–19, 1975.

37. Snape WJ, Carlson GM, Matarazzo SA, Cohen S: Evidence that abnormal myoelectrical activity produces colonic motor dysfunction in irritable bowel syndrome. Gastroenterology 72:383, 1977.

38. Liss JL, Alpers DH, Woodruff RA: The irritable colon syndrome and psychiatric illness. Dis Nerv Sys 34:151, 1973.

39. Kumar D, Wingate DL: Irritable bowel syndrome: A paroxysmal motor disorder. Lancet *ii*:973, 1985.

40. Snape WJ, Carlson GM, Cohen S: Colonic myoelectric activity in irritable bowel syndrome. Gastroenterology 70:326, 1978.

41. Harvey RF, Read AE: Effect of cholecystokinin on colonic motility and symptoms in patients with irritable bowel syndrome. Gut 13:837, 1972.

42. Whitehead WE et al.: Tolerance for rectosigmoid distension in irritable bowel syndrome. Gastroenterology 98:1187, 1990.

43. Whitehead WE, Schuster MM (eds): Gastrointestinal Disorders: Behavioral and Physiological Basis for Treatment. New York, Academic Press, 1985.

44. Kellow JE, Phillips SF: Altered small bowel motility as correlated with symptoms in irritable bowel syndrome. Gastroenterology 92:1885, 1987.

45. Kumar D, Wingate DL: The irritable bowel syndrome: A paroxysmal motor disorder. Lancet *ii*:973, 1985.

46. Kellow JE, Gill RC, Wingate GL: Prolonged ambulant recordings of small bowel motility demonstrate abnormalities in the irritable bowel syndrome. Gastroenterology 98:1208, 1990.

47. Holdstock DJ, Misiewicz JJ, Waller SL: Observations of mechanisms of abdominal pain. Gut *10*:19, 1969.

48. Connell AM: The motility of the pelvic colon. II. Paradoxical motility in diarrhea and constipation. Gut 3:342, 1962.

49. Waller SL: The irritable bowel syndrome: Clinical and pathophysiological features. Rondiconti D Gastroenterologia 3:809, 1971.

50. Whitehead WE, Engel BT, Schuster MM: Irritable bowel syndrome: Physiological and psychological differences between diarrhea-predominant and constipation-predominant patients. Dig Dis Sci 25:404, 1980.

51. Crowell MD et al.: Method for prolonged ambulatory monitoring of high-amplitude propagated contractions from colon. Am J Physiol 24:G263, 1991.

52. Taylor I, Darby C, Hammond P, Basu P: Is there myoelectric abnormality in irritable colon syndrome? Gut 19:391, 1978.

53. Schuster MM: Irritable bowel syndrome. *In* Sleisenger M, Fordtran J (eds): Gastrointestinal Disease, Fifth edition. Philadelphia, WB Saunders Co, 1992.

54. Ritchie J: Mechanisms of pain in irritable bowel syndrome. Gut *14*:125, 1973.

55. Swarbrick ET et al.: Site of pain from the irritable bowel. Lancet *ii*:443, 1980.

56. Nanda R, James R, Smith H: Food intolerance in irritable bowel syndrome. Gut *30*:1099, 1989.

57. Page JG, Dirnberger GM: Treatment of irritable bowel syndrome with Bentyl (dicyclomene hydrochloride) J Clin Gastroenterol 3:153, 1981.

58. Svedlund J, Sjodin I, Otosson JO, Dotevall G: Psychotherapy in irritable bowel syndrome: A controlled outcome study. Acta Psychiatr Scand 67: (Suppl) *306*:1, 1983.

59. Bueno F, Cerulli M, Schuster MM: Operant condition of colonic motility in irritable bowel syndrome. Gastroenterology 70:867, 1976.

60. Whorwell PJ, Prior A, Colgan SM: Hypnotherapy in severe irritable bowel syndrome, further experience. Gut 28:423, 1987.

14

Historical Antecedents of Inflammatory Bowel Disease Concepts*

JOSEPH B. KIRSNER

The idiopathic inflammatory bowel diseases (IBDs), ulcerative colitis and Crohn's disease, are "old" rather than "new" diseases. B. Morson's review (1) of Matthew Baillie's 1793 *Morbid Anatomy of Some of the Most Important Parts of the Human Body* "strongly suggests that patients were dying from ulcerative colitis during the latter part of the 18th century." The first "impact" description of "ulcerative colitis" by Samuel Wilks of London in 1859 (2) concerned a 42-year-old woman who died after several months of diarrhea and fever. Autopsy demonstrated a transmural ulcerative inflammation of the colon and terminal ileum, originally designated as "simple ulcerative colitis," but a century later identified as Crohn's disease (3). The 1875 case report of Wilks and Moxon (4) of extensive ulceration and inflammation of the entire colon in a young woman who had succumbed to severe bloody diarrhea also was labeled "simple ulcerative colitis." By 1907, 317 patients had been admitted to seven London hospitals with an inflammatory and ulcerative disease of the colon (5). Nearly half of the patients died from perforation of the colon and peritonitis, hemorrhage, and complications including "nephritis," "infective endocarditis," sep-

sis, hepatic abscess, fatty liver, and pulmonary embolism.

ULCERATIVE COLITIS

When the 20th century began, similar instances were being reported in Europe and in the United States. In 1902, R. F. Weir (6) performed an appendicostomy in a patient to facilitate colonic irrigation with a 5% solution of methylene blue alternating with a 1:5000 solution of silver nitrate or of bismuth, presumably to eliminate an "infection." J. P Lockhart-Mummery of London (7) in 1907 diagnosed carcinoma of the colon in 7 of 36 patients with ulcerative colitis and recommended use of the recently developed electrically illuminated proctosigmoidoscope. Reports of ulcerative colitis from France, Germany, Italy, and England also increased during the early years of the 20th century and ulcerative colitis was a major subject of the 1913 Paris Congress of Medicine.

During the second quarter of the 20th century, A. F. Hurst of London (8), implicating an organism "related to B. dysenteriae," recommended as treatment daily irrigations of the colon with dilute solutions of silver nitrate or tannic acid, and the intravenous administration of a "polyvalent antidysenteric serum."

During the 1930s through the 1950s, etiologic speculation, including food and pollen allergy, deficiency of an "intestinal protec-

* Based in part on Kirsner, Joseph B.: The Historical Basis of Etiopathogenetic Concepts in Inflammatory Bowel Disease in *Bockus Gastroenterology*, with permission of the editors, J. E. Berk, R. G. Farmer, W. M. Haubrich, and F. Schaffner. Philadelphia, W. B. Saunders Co., 1993.

tive substance," various aerobic and anaerobic intestinal bacteria, and a psychiatric disorder (e.g., an "ulcerative colitis personality"). Patients underwent extensive psychiatric scrutiny and prolonged psychotherapy without sustained benefit. Treatment improved following the availability of sulfanilamide in 1938, penicillin in the 1940s, ACTH and adrenal steroids in 1950, and their derivative compounds. In 1951, Kirsner et al. (9) documented the complete clinical and radiologic reversibility of ulcerative colitis in a group of patients who had responded promptly and consistently to therapy.

Pathology

Pathologic descriptions of ulcerative colitis, almost from the beginning, emphasized the diffuse, predominantly mucosal/submucosal involvement, typically beginning in the rectum and rectosigmoid, limited to the left colon in some patients but in others advancing to involve the entire colon. In 1933, Buie and Bargen (10) of the Mayo Clinic implicated vascular "thrombotic phenomena" as the pathologic basis for ulcerative colitis, and in 1937 Bargen designated the disease as "thrombo-ulcerative colitis." In 1954, S. Warren and S. Sommers (11) classified 10% of their 1949 series as "colitis gravis" with 'inflammatory necrosis of arteries, veins, or both, leading to vascular occlusions and infarction of a part or all of the adjacent colon."

A review of 120 surgically treated patients and 60 autopsied cases by S. Warren and S. C. Sommers of Boston (12) in 1949 re-emphasized the mucosal involvement. None of the prevailing etiologic hypotheses seemed acceptable. However, the presence of a "damaging substance" in the fecal stream was acknowledged as a possibility, as had been suggested by P. Manson-Bahr in 1943, and even earlier by B. Dawson (13) in the 1909 London Symposium. Experiments in our laboratory during the 1950s included the repeated instillation of fecal discharges from patients with severe active ulcerative colitis into self-retaining ileocolonic pouches constructed in dogs, with negative results. The direct intramucosal injection of ulcerative colitis fecal filtrates also failed to induce inflammation of the rectum in monkeys. R. T. Stoughton (14) in

1953 isolated a substance (possibly proteolytic enzyme), not pancreatic trypsin, probably originating in the gut microflora (possibly bacterial endotoxin), from fecal filtrates of patients with ulcerative colitis, capable of digesting epidermal cells even after the skin has been fixed in formalin. However, the "acantholysis" was noted also with fecal extracts from individuals without colonic disease.

Morson (15) later provided a comprehensive overview of the pathology,

"In active ulcerative colitis, the mucous membrane shows diffuse infiltration with chronic inflammatory cells, mainly lymphocytic and plasma cells but also eosinophiles. There is also a variable degree of vascular congestion and intra-mucosal hemorrhage. The epithelium shows goblet cell depletion and reactive hyperplasia, and some of the tubules contain an accumulation of polymorphonuclear leukocytes, so called crypt abscesses. With remission the first change is restoration of the goblet cell population, accompanied by a reduction in the amount of inflammation and the disappearance of crypt abscesses. The mucous membrane can return entirely to normal but if there have been repeated attacks of severe colitis, atrophy will develop as judged by a reduction in the number of epithelial tubules per unit area, loss of their parallelism and failure of the bases of the crypts to reach right down to the mucularis mucosae. Although none of these features are specific for ulcerative colitis, together they create a characteristic histologic picture."

The etiologic concepts of the 1950s (16) and 1960s, which included infection, allergy, "nonspecific damage" to colonic epithelium, "vascular disease," and a locally "injurious agent" in the fecal stream, generated little research activity at that time.

"Natural" and Experimental Colitis

By the 1950s, questions arose as to the possibility of naturally occurring animal counterparts of the disease that were known to veterinarians. Numerous inflammatory diseases of the colon had been identified in animals (dogs, cats, horses, cattle, sheep, swine, rodents), presumably caused by bacteria or viruses (17). However, despite morphologic similarities, none truly duplicated human IBD (chronicity, recurrences, extra-intestinal complications). Only the colitis observed in captive cottontop tamarins (saguinus oedipus) resembled human ulcerative colitis in its clinical and histologic features, responded to sulfasalazine and was complicated by colonic carcinoma. The absence of colitis among the wild cottontop tamarins of the Colombian rain forest suggested an environmental (possibly infection, "cold stress") cause for the captive tamarin colitis.

Many attempts were made during the 1920s through 1960 (17,18) to reproduce ulcerative colitis in animals (rabbits, guinea pigs, hamsters, dogs, mice, rats), including nutritional deficiencies (vitamin A, pantothenic acid, pyridoxine, folic acid), the local application of Shiga and staphylococcal toxins to colonic explants in dogs, the vasoconstriction induced by adrenalin hydrochloride injected intraperitoneally in dogs, the intraperitoneal infusion of lipopolysaccharide, the intravenous injection of staphylococcus toxin in rabbits, and the administration of the enzymes collagenase and lysozyme intrarectally and intraarterially. The small and large intestine were readily damaged by these manipulations, but the lesions healed rapidly. In 1969, ulcerations in the right colon were produced in guinea pigs and rabbits given orally a 5% aqueous solution of carrageenan, a sulfated polysaccharide of high molecular weight extracted from red seaweed (chondrus crispus, euchema spinosum) (19). The reaction was enhanced immunologically by a component of the outer cell wall of Bacterioides vulgatus, inhibited by the addition of metronidazole, and was not reproducible in germ-free animals. Although the inflammatory reaction mimicked ulcerative colitis (mucus depletion, diffuse inflammation and pseudopolyps), granulomas also developed. Later, topically (colonic) applied compounds (4 to 10% acetic acid, trinitrobenzene sulfonic acid in 50% alcohol), orally administered drugs (indomethecin, mitomycin-c), and inhibition of fatty acid oxidation (20) induced colonic injury, but none reproduced human ulcerative colitis.

CROHN'S DISEASE

Inflammatory bowel disease consistent with Crohn's disease was described 300 years ago (21,22). Similar cases were reported during the early part of the 19th century (23–26). The "ulcerative colitis" described by Samuel Wilks in 1859 in the celebrated case of Isabella Bankes, as already noted, was reclassified later as Crohn's disease of the colon. "The intestines lay in a coil adherent by a thin layer of lymph indicative of recent inflammation. The ileum was inflamed for three feet from the ileocecal valve, though otherwise the small intestine looked normal. The large intestine was ulcerated from end to end with ulcers of varying size, mostly isolated though some had run together. . . . inflammation was most marked at the proximal colon and the cecum appeared to be sloughing, causing the peritonitis."

In 1889, Samuel Fenwick of London (27) observed, in a 27-year-old woman with a history of diarrhea and weight loss that "many of the coils of intestine were adherent and a communication existed between the cecum and a portion of the small intestine adherent to it. Whilst the sigmoid flexure was adherent to the rectum and a communication also existed between them, the lower end of the ileum was much dilated and hypertrophied and the ileocecal valve was contracted to the size of a swan's quill."

Early in the 20th century, case reports from France, Germany, and Great Britain documented the increasing frequency of this disease and the similar presenting feature: mass lesion of the abdomen, superficially resembling a tumor; arbitrarily assumed to be "malignant" and, at a time of limited abdominal surgery, arbitrarily dismissed as "untreatable." R. Shapiro (28) in a 1939 review identified many instances of apparent Crohn's disease masquerading as abdominal "tumors" among the 413 cases he collected from the literature.

The 1913 paper by T. Kennedy Dalziel, (Fig. 14–1) a Glasgow surgeon (29), including 13 patients is noteworthy for its classic findings. The first patient, a physician, had experienced since 1901 bouts of cramping abdominal pain and diarrhea progressing to intestinal obstruction and death. At autopsy, the entire small intestine was chronically inflamed and the mesenteric lymph nodes were enlarged. Dalziel distinguished the process from tuberculosis and related his "chronic intestitial ileitis" to Johne's

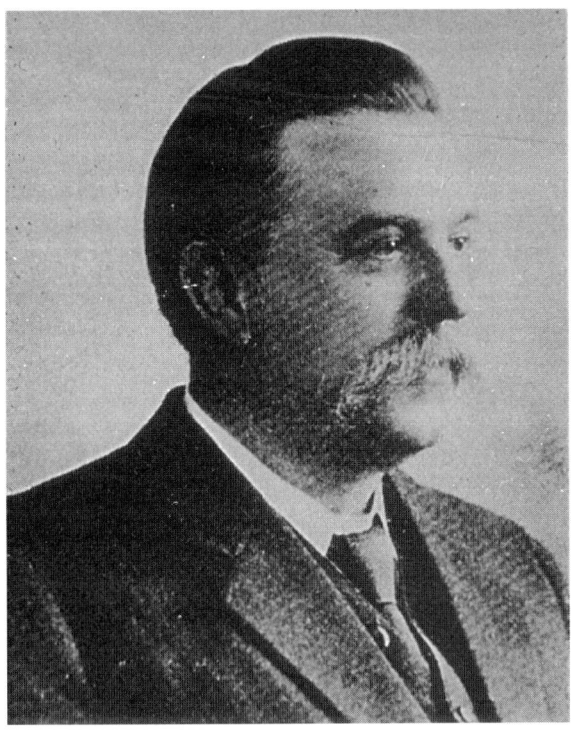

Fig. 14–1.   Sir T. Kennedy Dalzeil.

mycobacterial intestinal disease of cattle, but, of course, could not provide microbiologic documentation.

By 1920, American physicians were reporting instances of "nonspecific" hyperplastic and granulomatous lesions of the intestinal tract, previously identified as "hyperplastic intestinal tuberculosis" (30). The clinical and pathologic features were remarkably similar: relatively young patients, children, teenagers, and young adults, often operated upon for "appendicitis," symptoms of fever, abdominal cramps, diarrhea, and weight loss; the disease appeared to involve mostly the terminal ileum or ileocecal area. In the United States, England, and Sweden (Malmo), Crohn's disease was more common among Jewish people regardless of native birth, immigrant history, or orthodoxy; they were Ashkenazi rather than Sephardic Jews. However, the Jewish predominance was not observed in other countries (e.g., Denmark, Norway).

Immediately preceding the pivotal paper by Crohn, Ginzburg, and Oppenheimer (31) in 1932, F. J. Nuboer of Holland (32) and M. Golob of New York (33) (1932) reported strongly suggestive instances of a similar disease. In 1934, A. S. Bissell of the University of Chicago (34) described two male patients, ages 28 and 39, with ileocecal masses requiring resecton, but the report aroused little attention. Harold Edwards of London (35) in 1936 characterized the resected bowel from a 23-year-old woman as having the "consistency of a hose pipe;. . . . it was well to remember that Crohn's disease was a rather fatal condition." In the 1936 series of Koster et al. (36), 13 patients had had a preoperative diagnosis of appendicitis.

Etiologic speculation focused upon bacteria, viruses, protozoa (e.g., Entameba histolytica), "achylia gastrica," foreign bodies, abdominal trauma, impaired vascular and lymphatic circulation, and intestinal allergy. The concept of an underlying endolymphangitis with lymphatic obstruction provided the rationale for the 1936 experiments of Reichert and Mathes (37), who injected fine sand and a sclerosing solution of 26% bismuth oxychloride with and without Escherichia coli into the cannulated mesenteric lymphatics of dogs. Edema of the ileocecal area developed, but mucosal ulceration and granulomas were not demonstrated. Chess (38) in 1950 fed dogs silica and talc; and Kalima et al. (39) in 1976 injected formalin solution into the mesenteric lymphatics. Endolymphangitis developed with edematous thickening of the distal small bowel and ileocecal area. Histologic examination demonstrated occasional foreign body giant cells and inflammation, but regional enteritis was not reproduced. Van Patter and Bargen et al. (40) suggested that "the causative agent may be found in the fecal stream and ... appears initially in the proximal part of the small intestine. . . . Tubercles and lymphoid hyperplasia develop when the etiologic agent gains entrance into the interstitial space of the intestinal wall. The further course of the agent appears to be by way of the lymphatic vessels where it causes focal intralymphatic endothelial hyperplasia, lymphatic obstruction, and dilatation, lymphoid hyperplasia and lymphatic endothelial proliferation."

Mt. Sinai, New York 1932 Paper

The New York Mt. Sinai experience began with E. Moschowitz and A. O. Wilensky (41), who in 1923 described four patients with "nonspecific" granulomas of the intestine. In the first patient, an acute appendicitis was followed by a mass formation (granuloma of the bowel), then bowel obstruction, and subsequently a peritonitis. Microscopically, the intestinal mass was characterized by numerous giant cells. The second patient also had an attack suggestive of acute appendicitis and then developed an inflammatory mass in the ascending colon. A similar sequence of events occurred in the third, fourth, and fifth patients. Leon Ginzburg (Fig. 14–2), associated with the surgeon A. A. Berg, who had operated on all these patients, and Gordon Oppenheimer, then resident in surgical pathology, collected a series of 12 patients dating back to 1920, characterized by an hypertrophic and ulcerative stenosis of the distal two or three feet of the terminal ileum, "ending rather abruptly at the ileocecal valve." Amebiasis, syphilis, and actinomycosis apparently were eliminated. Intestinal tuberculosis was excluded by negative results after guinea pig intraperitoneal injection and by the absence of acid-fast bacilli histologically. In 1930 Burrill Crohn had under his care two young patients with a similar process. Crohn's first case was a 16-year-old boy with diarrhea, fever, a mass in the right lower abdominal quadrant, and pain, requiring ileocecal resection. The patient's sister also required an operation for regional ileitis several years later. The two groups united at the suggestion of Dr. Paul Klemperer, Chairman of the Department of Pathology, providing the 14 cases published in the 1932 JAMA article as "terminal ileitis." J. A. Bargen, anticipating the more extensive involvement of the small intestine, suggested the term "regional enteritis."

More 20th Century Reports

In 1934, Brown, Bargen, and Weber (42), describing involvement of the entire ileum

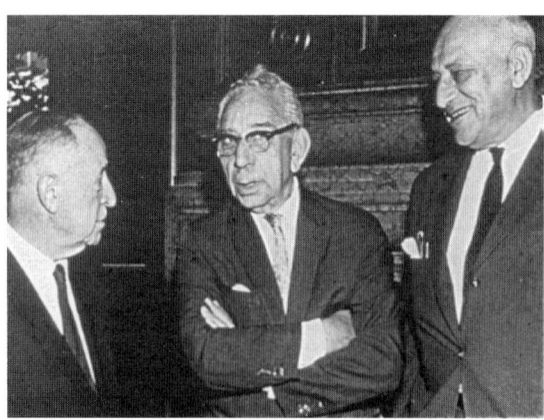

Fig. 14–2. Left to right: L. Ginzburg, B. Crohn, G. Oppenheimer.

and jejunum, re-emphasized the term "regional enteritis." In 1936, Crohn and B. D. Rosenak (43) described nine instances of combined ileitis and colitis and considered the colitis a form of ulcerative colitis. I. Snapper, A. Pompen, and J. Groen (44) (1936) implicated intestinal stagnation proximal to the ileocecal valve and noted the psychogenic concomitants and the apparent Jewish predilection.

Crohn's disease by now was global in its distribution. Fone (45) of Melbourne, Australia, observed that 40 of 41 patients already had had at least one additional operation! Other reports described the radiographic features of regional jejunitis (1937), involvement of the stomach in association with the terminal ileum and sigmoid (1939), and fistula formation (46).

Crohn's Disease of the Colon

Despite early European and American reports of colonic involvement by Crohn's-like inflammatory lesions, the papers of Dalziel in 1913 and Moschowitz and Wilensky in 1923, describing "non-specific granulomatous lesions" in both the small and large intestine, descriptions of a right-sided colitis in 1930 by Bargen and Weber and by Crohn and Berg of New York, the concept of a "Crohn's colitis" for unaccountable circumstances was not completely accepted in America during the 1940s and 1950s. Ginzburg and Oppenheimer's 1932 paper (47) on "Nonspecific Granulomata of the Intestines, Inflammatory Tumors and Strictures of the Bowel" was the first American reference to "Crohn's colitis." Charles Wells of Liverpool (48) in 1952 recognized "segmental colitis" as a variant of Crohn's disease. W. T. Cooke in 1955 and working with B. Brooke in 1959 conclusively identified "right-sided colitis" as Crohn's disease. But not until the reports of H. E. Lockhart-Mummery and B. C. Morson (49) in 1959 and 1960 was Crohn's colitis finally accepted as a distinct entity in the U.S.

Pathology of Crohn's Disease

In 1938, Coffey (50) emphasized the subacute or chronic, granulomatous inflammatory process, the tendency to stenosis of the bowel, the fistula formation, and the lack of evidence of a tuberculous process. In 1939,

G. Hadfield of England (51) was impressed by the thickening of the wall of the ileum, fistulas from the bowel to the abdominal wall and to the bladder, the superficial ulcerations, the giant-cell systems in the submucosa and in the regional lymph nodes, and the obstructive lymphedema of the submucosa. Hadfield implicated Boeck's sarcoidosis, but this was refuted by Crohn and Yarnis (52). The significance of the granuloma in Crohn's disease has remained unclear throughout, and it is possibly a response to the etiologic agent (e.g., antigen) (53).

In 1943, Tallroth (54), impressed with the many eosinophils in histologic sections, termed the disease "ileitis allergica," a "local anaphylactic reaction in the nature of an Arthus phenomenon." The 1948 study of 120 cases by S. Warren and S. C. Sommers of Boston (55) emphasized the cicatrizing nature of the tissue reaction: "A progressive sclerosing granulomatous lymphangitis, probably as a reaction to an irritative lipid substance." Interestingly, Coffey's 1938 study of Crohn's disease had included the finding of lipid particles, possibly residual food constituents, in multinucleated giant cells.

H. Rappaport et al. (56) in 1951 studied 100 cases at the U.S. Armed Forces Institute of Pathology, including 85 bowel resections and 15 autopsies. In 72 instances, sections from mesenteric lymph nodes and 35 appendices were available for study. The "tubercle-like granuloma observed in about half of the group, differed from foreign body granulomas and from the sarcoid lesion. Lymphedema and lymphangiectases were common."

In 1954, Warren and Sommers (57) suggested that, while "nonspecific ulcerative colitis is probably a disease of the whole body, with its most striking manifestation in the colon, the histopathology of regional ileitis would suggest a reaction to irritative lipid substances. It appears possibly to represent a by-product of some biochemical abnormality of lipid absorption in the intestine." B. C. Morson (58) (Fig. 14–3) for many years had noted foci of vasculitis (arteritis) in surgically resected and in biopsy tissue of Crohn's disease and "I often wondered about the importance of this lesion." Interest has developed recently in the possi-

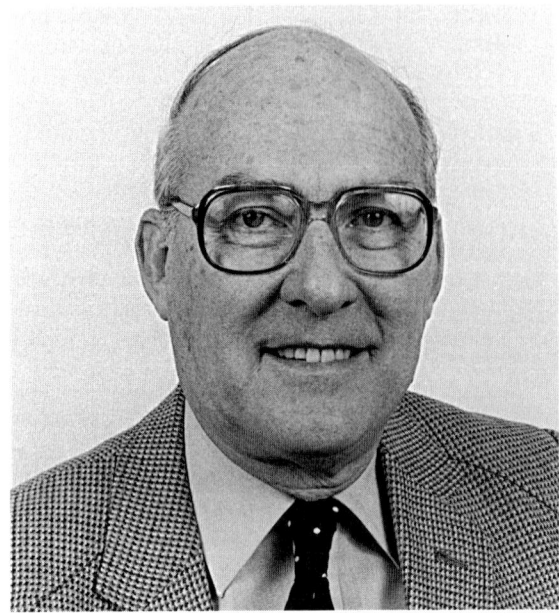

Fig. 14–3. Basil Morson.

bility of a focal "granulomatous" mesenteric vasculitis involving mucosal and submucosal vessels. Morson emphasized the gross features of thickened adherent mesentery, thickened loops of distal small bowel, enteric fistulas, one or several areas of narrowing, aphthous ulcers, and linear serpiginous ulcers, a cobblestone appearance to the mucosa, and the asymmetric distribution of the disease. Distinctive histologic findings include focal lesions, transmural inflammation, dilated submucosal lymphatics, prominent lymphoid aggregates, knife-like fissuring ulcerations, granulomas, hypertrophy of the muscular layer, and neural hyperplasia.

The earliest lesion of Crohn's disease is apparently the tiny slit-like ulcer, located precisely over the M cell in the epithelium overlying a lymphoid follicle in Peyer's patches (59). This lesion, the granulomas, the focal distribution of Crohn's disease, the lymphatic dilatation, and the lymphoid prominence seem to reflect the pathogenesis of the disease.

Eponym of Crohn's Disease

Reports of "granulomatous inflammation" of the small bowel in Great Britain in the 1930s occasionally referred to the condition as Crohn's disease. R. F. Barbour and A. B. Stokes (60) wrote in 1936, "To this localized condition the name of regional enteritis was given, although in America it also became known as Crohn's disease." A. F. Hurst in 1937 also referred to the condition as Crohn's disease. In the United States, B. C. Cushway (61) of Chicago in a 1934 case report used the title "Chronic Cicatrizing Enteritis, Regional Ileitis (Crohn)." The term Crohn's disease probably was first used as a synonym by F. I. Harris (62) (1933) in the article "Chronic cicatrizing enteritis of the ileum: Regional Ileitis (Crohn)." To some American observers, this entity might well have been called "CGO disease" to reflect the contributions of not only Crohn, but also Ginzburg and Oppenheimer, who provided 12 of the 14 cases in the 1932 report. The term Crohn-Dalziel disease will appeal to many, in recognition of Dalziel's significant 1913 description of this condition. Whatever the "labeling" circumstances, the entity today carries the eponym Crohn's disease as the most convenient designation, now sanctioned by worldwide usage, for a unique inflammatory process involving any part of the gastrointestinal tract, characterized by chronicity, recurrences, and numerous complications. G. Armitage and M. Wilson (63) in 1939 concluded that the term "cicatrizing enteritis though a fair term is far from euphonious." "The name Crohn's disease has been adhered to in most cases at this hospital (Leeds). It avoids confusion, makes no pretense of pathological exactitude, conveys an exact meaning, is easily remembered by students, and pays a well deserved tribute."

On the matter of eponyms, the comment of Thomas Lewis (64) in 1944 is relevant: "Diagnosis is a system of more or less accurate guessing, in which the end point achieved is a name. These names applied to disease come to assume the importance of specific entities . . . whereas they are, for the most part, no more than insecure and therefore temporary conceptions." Presumably, the Crohn's designation will yield to the etiology of the disease once it is discovered!

EPIDEMIOLOGY OF IBD

Although John Snow (65) had published his "epidemiologic classic," *On the Pathology and Mode of Communication of Cholera,* in 1849 and W. Budd (66) had documented the water-borne distribution of typhoid fever, an epidemiologic approach to the study of inflammatory bowel disease conceptually and practically was not feasible until the 1950s. E. I. Spriggs of London (67), in a 1934 analysis of 35 patients, had estimated the rate as "5 in a thousand." A. G. Melrose in 1956 (68) collected information on 1425 patients with chronic idiopathic ulcerative colitis for the years 1946 to 1950 and proposed an overall incidence of 10.9% per 10,000 general admissions. The rate of 6.9% for the five Scottish towns in contrast to 15.5% for the London hospitals was early recognition of the urban:rural IBD incidence differential.

Houghton and Naish in 1958 (69) identified 170 patients with ulcerative colitis and 32 with ileitis from the records of the three main hospitals in Bristol, England for the years 1953, 1954, and 1955. The estimated annual incidence figures of 0.85 per 1000 for ulcerative colitis and 0.14 per 1000 for regional ileitis were similar to those of E. I. Spriggs (1934) and A. G. Melrose (1956). H.

J. Ustvedt (70) in 1958, reviewing hospital admission rates on all patients discharged from Norwegian hospitals during the 10 year period from 1945 to 1955 noted a mean annual rate of 1.2 per 100,000 population.

Acheson in 1960 (71) reviewed the data for all 2320 male veterans discharged from the 174 hospitals of the U.S. Veterans Administration with diagnoses of regional ileitis, ulcerative colitis, or enteritis not specified as ulcerative, and observed a fourfold increase of Jewish patients, over a sample of all discharges, regardless of geographic origin of birth within the USA. Acheson also noted a 20-fold increase in the incidence of ankylosing spondylitis among the 2320 U.S. veterans with IBD (72). J. G. Evans and E. D. Acheson (73), in a 1965 study in Oxford, England for the 1951 to 1960 period, confirmed the rising incidence of ulcerative colitis and demonstrated a bimodal age incidence pattern.

In perhaps the first population study of IBD, Iversen, Bonnevie, Riis, and Anthonisen (74) in a 1968 survey of ulcerative colitis in Copenhagen county (Denmark) for the period from 1961 to 1966, reviewed 310 patients (excluding proctitis). The prevalence rate was 44.1 per 100,000 inhabitants. Considering only the 231 patients in whom ulcerative colitis was diagnosed for the first time (1961 to 1966), the incidence of the disease averaged 7.3 per 100,000 per year, contrasting with 1.6 per 100,000 found by Lindenberg and Aagard (1964) (75) during the years 1940 to 1951 excluding proctitis. The prevalence of diagnosed cases was 109 per 100,000. A population study of two counties in central Sweden for the period from 1956 to 1967 (76) revealed a mean incidence of 2.5 per 100,000 for the first 6 years of the 12-year span and 5.0 during the second 6-year period.

Epidemiologic studies by Mendeloff et al. (77–80) in the well-defined Baltimore area during the 1960s documented higher hospital incidence and prevalence rates for both ulcerative colitis and regional enteritis for whites than non-whites, for Jews than non-Jews, and the rising incidence of ulcerative colitis during the first half of the 20th century, exceeding Crohn's disease in a proportion of 4 to 5:1. Mendeloff characterized the IBD population as follows: (1) males and females nearly equally affected; (2) patients more commonly western than oriental; much more often of northern European origin; (3) more often urban than rural; (4) more often Caucasian than black; (5) the diseases more common among Jews living in Europe and North America than among non-Jews, but not as common among Israelis; and (6) IBD more common in families than expected.

According to Kyle (81), Crohn's disease was "most common in northwest Europe and in the north-east part of North America. . . . Caucasians living in the southern hemisphere were less liable to develop Crohn's disease."

Reviewing the period between 1960 to 1979 in the Baltimore area, B. M. Calkins and A. I. Mendeloff (82) noted an increase in the age-adjusted rate for Crohn's disease over ulcerative colitis for whites of both sexes and for nonwhite women from the first to the second analysis. Mendeloff confirmed the "striking" bimodality of the age-specific incidence of both Crohn's disease and ulcerative colitis reported by Acheson; the first mode during the third decade and the second mode (for men) from ages 55 to 60.

Subsequent regional epidemiologic surveys (83) documented the worldwide distribution of IBD and, with several geographic exceptions (northeast Scotland, Israel, Iceland), the initially increased and now stabilized incidence of ulcerative colitis, the still-rising incidence of Crohn's disease, appearing also in formerly "lagging" countries (Brazil, South Korea), and the unexpectedly high incidence of inflammatory bowel disease (especially Crohn's disease) in such areas as the North Tees Health District of England.

SMOKING AND IBD

The relationship between ulcerative colitis and non-smoking (84), especially the occurrence of ulcerative colitis among former smokers, was first reported by S. M. Samuelsson (85) in a 1976 thesis (University of Upsala, Sweden). In response to my inquiry as to the origin of his interest in IBD and tobacco, Professor John Rhodes of Cardiff, Wales (86), relates the following: "Between 1980 and '81 I had working with me a research registrar, Dr. Tony Harries, who has recently been appointed to a Chair of Tropical Medicine in Blantyre, Malawi. Dr. Harries was doing his research into nutritional problems in Crohn's disease and was particularly assessing the value of anthropometric measurements, relating them to other nutritional parameters. The mid-arm circumference was one of the simple measurements and assessment involved taking into account several variables—age, sex, dominant arm, and smoking status. The rule of thumb we had at the time was that smokers on average were 10% lighter in weight than non-smokers and it was, therefore, important to take this factor into consideration when making comparisons with controls.

"The group of patients with Crohn's disease under study were to be compared with controls (taken from a normal population attending an Orthopedic Clinic) but we also wanted to include a patient group and what better group than ulcerative colitis. At first we had 100 patients with colitis, taken at random and the results which related to smoking status were 'irritating.' This was because hardly any of them were smokers, which made it difficult to get meaningful statistics from the comparison. After musing over the figures however, we wondered whether it might just be a possibility that patients with colitis were largely non-smokers. This prompted us to carry out a larger survey of both patients with colitis and Crohn's disease with matched controls. Unfortunately, the original matching with controls was between colitis and normal controls. The patients with Crohn's disease did not have any tight matching with controls and results looked similar to the control population at that time (only subsequently did the story develop showing that those with Crohn's tended to be smokers compared with the general population). Because the finding of 'non-smoking' status with UC was new we determined to do no further work on it for a time—but would await data from other groups to see whether or not they confirmed our observations.

"I often relate the story because it is curious and fascinating. The observation was made during the course of a piece of research where we allowed ourselves the liberty of looking at data and rather than discarding useless statistics, raised another possibility to account for them. Out of interest we have worked in the last three years on this problem and are close to resolving the mechanisms involved."

Harries, Baird, and Rhodes of Cardiff, Wales, reported in the 1982 mail questionnaire a hitherto underemphasized infrequency of cigarette smoking in patients with ulcerative colitis and an excess of cigarette smoking in Crohn's disease or controls: 8% of the ulcerative colitis series were current cigarette smokers compared with 42% of the group with Crohn's disease and 44% of controls. Of the ulcerative colitis group, 48% had never smoked compared with 30% for Crohn's disease and 36% for controls. This finding was rapidly confirmed by Bures et al. of Czechoslovakia in a study of 50 patients with ulcerative colitis and 31 with Crohn's disease. In the same year, De Castella described a young woman whose ulcerative colitis began when she stopped smoking cigarettes, subsided on resumption of smoking, and returned when she again discontinued the use of tobacco. Roberts and Diggle described the case of a woman with severe ulcerative colitis who recovered after 3 years of symptoms when she began to smoke cigarettes. After 7 "smoking" years of well-being, she stopped smoking, with prompt return of the ulcerative colitis. Nicotine chewing gum containing 40 mg of nicotine subsequently maintained remission of the disease.

The negative association between ulcerative colitis and cigarette smoking was reaffirmed by observers from many geographic areas. Also, the risk of ulcerative colitis was greater among ex-smokers than in those who had never smoked. The tobacco connection is not exclusive to inflammatory bowel disease. A similar negative relationship has been observed in patients with Parkinson's disease (87).

PSYCHOGENIC RELATIONSHIPS IN IBD

The relationship of mind and body has interested mankind from earliest times (88,89). Scientific awareness of the physiologic responses of the body to emotional stress probably originated with the classic observations of C. Darwin (1872) (90), and of I. P. Pavlov (91) and W. B. Cannon (early 1900s) (92).

Psychogenic factors were "formally" implicated in ulcerative colitis by the reports by Murray (1930) (93) and Sullivan (1932) (94). Murray studied 12 patients with ulcerative colitis. In each, he observed a chronologic relationship between an emotional disturbance and the onset of bowel symptoms. Traits of fearfulness, emotional immaturity, and instability were common. None of the seven men in the series had been married or had ever been away from his mother. The five women each had emotional disturbances involving their marriage or home life. Sullivan's second series of 15 patients featured prolonged emotional tension involving marital and fiscal difficulties. Five men were described as having a "mother complex." In 11 patients, diarrhea had begun within 48 hours of an emotional upset.

Psychiatric precepts during the 1930s, 1940s, and 1950s emphasized an "ulcerative colitis personality," characterized by immaturity of the patient, sensitivity, indecisiveness, overdependence, and inhibited interpersonal relationships. Decisive emotional events included the loss of a loved one, feelings of social rejection, and maternal dominance. Many of the early clinical reports implicating emotional difficulties in ulcerative colitis originated in subjective clinical impressions, and retrospective reviews of past hospital records and lacked "control" groups of patients. Later observations (1940s, 1950s) came from controlled clinical scrutiny and direct physiologic studies (95,96). The experiments of T. P. Almy and M. Tulin (97) and of W. J. Grace, S. Wolf, and H. Wolff (95) documented the significant physiologic effects of emotional stress on the normal colonic mucosa (hyperemia, vascular engorgement, increased secretion of mucus, and augmented colonic motor activity). Such responses were intensified and more prolonged in the ulcerative colitis colon. Grace, Wolf, and Wolff (1951) (95) further described the "hyperdynamic response and the diarrhea of disturbed colonic function as consisting of hyperemia, contraction of longitudinal muscles with shortening of the colon and increased rhythmic contractile activity of circular muscles in the caecum, ascending and transverse loops, while the descending and sigmoid colon'' . . . assumed a rigid tubular shape due to longitudinal muscle activity . . . This emptying reaction of the colon was evoked by words or events with special meaning to the individual eliciting reactions of anger, resentment, guilt, humiliation, and anxiety. A similar colonic response could be initiated or augmented by parasympathomimetic agents. Wener and Polonsky (98), observing a transverse colostomy in a patient with ulcerative colitis, described a ''sympathetic and parasympathetic response'' characterized by pronounced hyperemia and edema of the colon, increasing the vulnerability of the ''friable mucous membrane'' to trauma. To evaluate the possible role of parasympathetic hyperactivity, Moeller and Kirsner in 1954 (99) injected dogs repeatedly over long periods of time with parasympathomimetic drugs (methacholine, neostigmine) and noted only transient superficial ulcerations in the colon mucosa.

In 1955, G. Engel (100), reviewing the nature of ''the somatic process'' and the adequacy of psychosomatic hypotheses in ulcerative colitis, stated: ''It is clear that none of the psychosomatic hypotheses so far advanced has fulfilled the requirements both of correctly identifying the somatic processes and of indicating how psychic processes are related to the somatic. . . . . . these data suggest that . . . the bowel appears to be responding to local areas of surface irritation rather than as part of an integrated excretory act.''

Clinical opinions varied widely as to the presence and the significance of emotional disturbances manifested by patients with ulcerative colitis. Nevertheless, psychotherapy, supportive, conventional and psychoanalytical, was encouraged by many physicians, and though prolonged and demanding, was an important part of the medical treatment of patients with ulcerative colitis during the 1940s and 50s. In 1954 Grace, Pinsky, and Wolff (101) reported lower operability rates, fewer serious complications, and lower mortality rates in a series of 34 patients with ulcerative colitis treated by therapy emphasizing the alleviation of stress compared to a matched group of 34 patients in whom treatment consisted mainly of diet and medication.

Contrary results were reported by others (102–104). In a series of 70 patients with severe ulcerative colitis treated on the Psychiatric Service at Mt. Sinai Hospital, New York, by psychoanalytically oriented psychotherapy for an average period of 3 months, '' no specific value was observed in preventing surgical intervention on severe recurrences.'' Even more persuasive was the ''psychological improvement'' of the ulcerative colitis patient after successful surgical therapy (ileostomy; ileostomy and colectomy) (105). Feldman et al. (106), in a study including two control groups of individuals, found no evidence of a psychogenic causation in 34 patients with ulcerative colitis.

In 1970, Kirsner (107) stated: ''The continuing unsettled role of psychogenic influences in the pathogenesis of ulcerative colitis reflects the prolonged preoccupation with earlier anecdotal psychiatric approaches and with subjective attempts to establish an exclusive or primary psychogenic etiology. Emotional disturbances are common in patients with ulcerative colitis; and they undoubtedly contribute to the exacerbation, chronicity, and the severity of ulcerative colitis. However, they are not specific for ulcerative colitis and they reflect in part, secondary emotional responses of the chronically ill patient.''

A. Karush et al. (108) in 1977 summarized the views of many psychiatrists: ''We do not claim that ulcerative colitis is 'caused' by unusual reactions of the mind alone, we claim only that these reactions almost always play a vital role in the interaction of the four etiological determinants, genetic endowment, constitutional vulnerability, intrapsychic processes, and the external environment. The intrapsychological processes may, for example, predispose to the actual development of the disease; in many cases, however, they may be secondary reactions to the symptoms and to the disability caused by the disease . . . They may also reflect a combination of causal ingredients, which seems to be the usual situation in chronic ulcerative colitis . . . As do other humanist physicians, the psychiatrist who works with somatic illness tries to view the patient as a whole and to see his illness as an outcome of many operant pathogenic factors.''

Crohn's Disease

B. B. Crohn was never persuaded of an etiologic role for emotional disturbances in Crohn's disease, and opinions as to the importance of psychiatric disturbances in Crohn's disease varied even more than in ulcerative colitis. Blackburn in 1939 had found a majority of 24 patients "abnormally introspective," Bockus in 1945 described patients with regional enteritis as "emotionally immature, sensitive, and rather excitable people." Grace (109) and others were impressed with the relationship between stress and the onset or relapse of Crohn's disease. On the other hand, Kraft and Ardali (110) regarded the psychologic difficulties as nonspecific consequences of chronic, recurrent, and frustrating illness. Crockett (111) in 1952, in a study of 16 patients, had concluded: "Routine psychiatric examination does not give substantial support for the suggestion that emotional stress is a major aetiological factor in Crohn's disease." The conflicting views perhaps reflect insufficient distinction between "mental illness" versus "emotional disturbances" and differing physician attitudes toward the physiologic alterations induced by "everyday" emotional disturbances.

Lysozyme

A concept allied to psychogenic hypothesis in the 1950s involved the bacteriolytic and mucolytic enzyme lysozyme present in nasal secretions, saliva, and tears, originally discovered by A. B. Fleming (112) in 1922. K. Meyer et al. (113) (1948) and Grace et al. (1949) reported increases in the level of lysozyme in the blood and in the feces of patients with active ulcerative colitis and regional enteritis during periods of emotional stress, diminishing when the stress subsided. Lysozyme allegedly destroyed the protective mucus lining the surface of the colon, rendering the colon more vulnerable to invading pathogenic bacteria and other cytolytic substances (114).

Interest in the role of lysozyme as a pathophysiologic expression of emotional stress subsided after the observation of large nonspecific increases in fecal lysozyme in the dog following electrocautery of the rectal mucosa (115), the failure of large quantities of crystalline lysozyme to damage ileocolonic pouches in dogs, the absence of a lysozyme substrate in the colon and rectum of normal individuals and patients with ulcerative colitis, and the demonstrated inability of lysozyme to digest or dissolve human mucus (116).

MICROBIAL ASPECTS

Ulcerative Colitis

Possible bacterial causes of ulcerative colitis attracted attention during the latter years of the 19th century and early in the 20th century, a time when many bacterial causes of intestinal disease were being identified. In 1906, S. Flexner and J. E. Sweet had observed small hemorrhages, ulcerations, and a fibrinous exudate in the colon of rabbits injected intravenously with Shiga and Flexner dysentery bacilli or their toxins. In 1907, H. de R. Morgan had produced diarrhea in rats and rabbits fed a gram-negative bacillus isolated from the feces of infants suffering with "summer diarrhea." Many other bacteria were implicated on little or no evidence, including Bacillus coli (1909), streptococci (1911), and B. Coli communis (1913). None of these organisms fulfilled Koch's postulates. Yet, bacterial possibilities influenced the treatment of ulcerative colitis for many years. A. F. Hurst (117) administered a "polyvalent anti-dysenteric serum" intravenously, and J. Leusden (118) advocated an autologous vaccine of fecal bacteria. Typhoid vaccine (119) and autogenous vaccines (120) of dysentery and other organisms were administered with questionable benefit.

Focal infection (e.g., dental infection, "chronic cholecystitis") was a commonly emphasized cause of disease in the United States during the 1920s that resulted in "wholesale" removal of teeth and gallbladders with questionable benefit. The apparent precipitation of ulcerative colitis in several patients following the extraction of infected teeth (or tonsils) increased interest in the possibility of oral (dental bacteria) as a cause of ulcerative colitis. In 1924, J. A. Bargen (121) (Fig. 14–4) reported the development of bloody diarrhea in rabbits injected intravenously with bacterial cultures prepared from the feces of patients with ul-

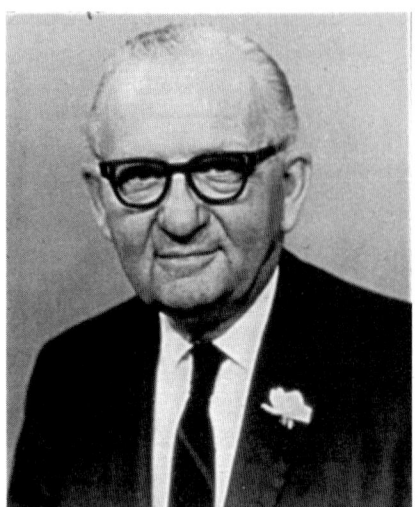

Fig. 14–4.   J. A. Bargen.

cerative colitis (presumably containing diplostreptococci). Autopsy demonstrated petechial to massive submucosal hemorrhages and superficial ulcers in the rabbit rectum, progressing proximally to involve much of the colon, "resembling human ulcerative colitis." Diplostreptococci were cultured from the ulcers. Bargen and Logan (122) in 1925 reported positive cultures from the rectal ulcerations in 80% of 68 ulcerative colitis patients. Colonic lesions developed in 45 of 139 rabbits injected intravenously with 5 to 15 mL of the broth containing diplostreptococci. Cook (123), working with Rosenow in 1931, injected rabbits with the diplostreptococci cultured from the abscessed teeth of patients with active ulcerative colitis. Sixty percent of 60 injected rabbits developed a "diffuse hemorrhagic infiltration" of the colon. Cook also inoculated artificial cavities created in the teeth of 15 dogs with a diplostreptococcus isolated from the teeth of patients with ulcerative colitis. Diarrhea developed in seven animals and colonic ulcerations were observed proctoscopically for as long as 8 to 16 months after the dental inoculation. Bargen implicated the fecal diplostreptococci and subsequently treated patients with an autologous vaccine including diplostreptococci. Others dismissed the "Bargen diplostreptococcus" as "simply a form of the normal enterococci present in all stools and often found in normal people." Subsequent studies by M.

Paulson (124) of Baltimore and by Mones and Sanjuan (125) failed to confirm the 1924 and 1925 experiments of Bargen and the diplostreptococcus concept soon lost scientific credibility.

Many other bacteria were implicated during the 1920s and 1930s and similarly dismissed for lack of decisive evidence: the anaerobe spherophorus necrophorus (126) (1930s), bacillus Morgagni, pseudomonas aeruginosa, hemolytic and non-hemolytic Escherichia coli, parasites (Entareka histolytica), and viruses (e.g., lymphopathia venereum). Felsen (127) in 1936 reviewed 583 cases of acute bacillary dysentery and suggested a "common pathogenesis," i.e. bacillary dysentery, for acute and chronic distal ileitis and chronic ulcerative colitis, but Penner in 1936 found the evidence inconclusive. Following the 1933–34 Chicago epidemic of amebic dysentery, E. histolytica was implicated as a cause. I later treated several patients who had had a confirmed amebic dysentery in 1933 and 1934, and then presented in the 1940s as a "typical ulcerative colitis;" a sequence of events consistent with a "sensitization" of the bowel induced by the earlier amebic infection, perhaps "priming" the colon's mucosal immune system for the later development of ulcerative colitis.

Viruses also have been implicated in the etiology of ulcerative colitis. However, serologic evidence of excessive exposure to known viruses (influenza, mumps, measles, herpes, Cocksackie A, B, Echo, E-B, adenovirus in ulcerative colitis and Crohn's disease was never obtained. The occasional increased titers of cytomegalovirus have been in malnourished, secondarily immunodeficient patients. The clinical and proctoscopic similarity of the ulcerative colitis caused by the lymphopathia venereum (chlamydia) to ulcerative colitis (128) led to studies of a possible etiologic relationship in the 1940s, with negative results (129,130).

Crohn's Disease

A microbial cause always seemed more likely in Crohn's disease than in ulcerative colitis (131). In 1913, Dalziel compared regional ileitis to Johne's mycobacterial disease of cattle. In the 1932 New York series, tuberculosis was excluded by negative cultures, and by animal inoculations, syphilis was excluded serologically and actinomycosis by the differing histology. In 1938, Pumphrey of the Mayo Clinic (132) carefully investigated the bacterial etiology in 13 cases with negative results. In 1943, Rodaniche, Kirsner, and Palmer, because of the clinical and proctoscopic resemblance of Crohn's disease to lymphopathia venereum (lymphoid prominence, cicatrizing tendency), studied four patients with this disease. Frei skin tests with mouse and human antigens were negative, and the serum was negative for neutralizing antibodies against the virus.

Because of the histologic resemblance of the Crohn's disease granulomatous lesion to Boeck's sarcoidosis, this possibility received early consideration, but no supporting evidence could be elicited. The many bacteria implicated in Crohn's disease over the years included, in addition to the tubercle bacillus, mycobacteria (Kansasii [1978], paratuberculosis) (133) anaerobic organisms (including Eubacteria strains Me_{46}, Me_{47}, B. vulgatus, peptostreptococcus, aerobacter aerogenes, coprococcus, bifidobacteria), and more recently, Campylobacter fetus ssp. jejuni, Yersinia enterocolitica, Chlamydia trachomatis); none achieved etiologic status. Serologic evidence of exposure to Epstein-Barr, Echo A,B adenovirus, as in ulcerative colitis, and to rotavirus and Norwalk virus, also was negative.

Microbial possibilities in Crohn's disease also have included a slowly growing pleomorphic mycobacterial variant (Mycobacterium linda) (134), the possible role of bacterial components (lipopolysaccharides, peptidoglycans, oligopeptides) (135), metabolic products (toxins, necrosins), "normal" intestinal bacteria, and viral protein elements (virions, prions). The injection of sterile nonviable bacterial (Group A streptococci) cell wall fragments into the cecal wall and ileal mesentery induced a "classic granulomatous inflammation" attributed to the peptidoglycan-polysaccharide complex. Another bacterial cell wall constituent, A,E diaminopimelic acid, demonstrated in rectal biopsy tissue from patients with ulcerative colitis in 1965 (136), has not been studied.

Specific infections of the terminal ileum and colon in animals have been associated with tissue changes partially resembling Crohn's disease, including an enterocolitis in cocker spaniels (1954), mycobacterial paratuberculosis infection of the terminal ileum in cattle (Johne's disease) (1913), a terminal ileitis in swine, and a granulomatous colitis of boxer dogs (137). However, none of the animal diseases duplicated Crohn's disease.

IMMUNE MECHANISMS

In 1801, Edward Jenner (138) observed that "infection can alter the body in a manner that will cause its tissues to react with increased intensity to subsequent contact with the infective agent." More than 100 years elapsed before the important role of the gastrointestinal tract in the immune homeostasis of the body was demonstrated (139). In 1919, Besredka (140) showed that oral "immunization of rabbits provided protection against otherwise fatal Shiga bacillus infection." Subsequent studies established "the efficacy of oral immunization in the prevention of dysentery." In 1922, Davies (141) documented the presence of fecal antibody in the stools of patients with bacillary dysentery before serum antibody appeared. Subsequent observations by Heremans (1960) (142), and Tomasi et al. (1965) (143), among others, identified the IgA class of immunoglobulins and their role in the emerging field of mucosal immunity of the gastrointestinal tract.

In 1938, I. Gray and M. Walzer (144), studying hypersensitivity reactions in mucous membranes, demonstrated an allergic reaction in the passively sensitized rectal mucosa of human subjects and the rhesus monkey. After sensitization of the rectal mucosa with human serum containing atopic reagins, a local inflammatory reaction was induced within 10 to 15 minutes by feeding the specific protein, characterized by pronounced edema, erythema, and hypersecretion of mucus. This observation was extended to the mucosa of the ileum and the colon in man (1940), documenting the immune responsiveness of the gastrointestinal mucosa (145,146).

The major concept of an altered gut mucosal immune system in the pathogenesis of inflammatory bowel disease (147) also developed in the context of early interest in hypersensitivity (allergy) of mucous membranes of the gastrointestinal tract to foods, pollens, and other allergens (148,149). However, general acceptance of gastrointestinal allergy as a common cause of disease in the adult was hampered by the subjectivity of the diagnosis and the lack of objective evidence. A. F. R. Andresen and A. H. Rowe, comparing the ulcerative colitis reaction to an eczema-like allergic response, postulated an allergic basis for both chronic ulcerative colitis and regional enteritis, implicating pollens as well as foods (milk, eggs, wheat, potato, coffee, tea, and chocolate). Rider and Moeller (150) injected extracts of wheat, eggs, and milk directly into the rectal mucosa of patients with ulcerative colitis, but the "nonspecific" hyperreactivity of the ulcerative colitis mucosa negated the importance of the mucosal reactions. Thus, although allergy to foods occurs in a few unusually atopic adult patients (for example, allergy to fish in an individual whose serum contained a reagin that could be passively transferred to the skin of a normal person), because of the subjectivity of the clinical observations (151), food allergy was abandoned in the 1950s as the cause of "nonspecific" ulcerative colitis or Crohn's disease.

Immune mechanisms in the late 1940s were implicated in various diseases of unknown cause (e.g. rheumatoid arthritis). A series of clinical events during the 1930s and 1940s suggested to me their involvement also in ulcerative colitis (152). These events included the abrupt onset of severe ulcerative colitis in a young woman who, with many others, had developed acute food poisoning at a family picnic in New York state. Everyone recovered within 24 to 48 hours except for the patient, who died after several years of severe ulcerative colitis. Other events were the occasional association of ulcerative colitis with other immune diseases (e.g., autoimmune hemolytic anemia, systemic lupus erythematosus, Hashimoto's thyroiditis); the ulcerative colitis developing years later in individuals who had experienced an acute amebic dysentery (1933–1934), the familial occurrences of inflammatory bowel disease, and the beneficial therapeutic effects of ACTH and the adrenal corticosteroids.

James Gear (153) increased interest in immunologic mechanisms in 1955: "Many important diseases of man may result from the action of autoantibodies developed against tissues made autoantigenic by some alteration to the tissue cells. Such an alteration may be caused by infections, drugs and other chemicals, and by physical agents, including x-rays, heat, and cold." Although the concept of ulcerative colitis and Crohn's disease as "immune-mediated" diseases imparted a sense of conceptual progress in the 1950s, just what "immune-mediated" connoted was not clear (154). The immunologic resources and responses of the gastrointestinal tract, despite the earlier observations of Besredka, Davies, Gray, and Walzer, had not been fully appreciated, and uncertainty persisted as to an immunologic role for the gastrointestinal tract in these diseases. In 1956 and 1957, Kirsner and Elchlepp, using the 1920 J. Auer (155) principle of local autosensitization to foreign protein, as demonstrated in the rabbit ear exposed to dilute xylol, produced immune complexes to crystalline egg albumin in rabbits, as documented later immunologically (156). The complexes were localized to the distal bowel via the rectal instillation of a non-inflammatory, very dilute solution of formalin. An ulcerative colitis promptly developed in precisely the areas of the rectum demonstrated immunologically to contain the immune complexes and nowhere else. Repeated "Auer-Kirsner" reactions in the colon produced chronic ulcerative inflammation of the bowel. The Auer-Kirsner phenomenon was reproduced in 1962 by Callahan, Goldman, and Vial (157) in colon-sensitized inbred mice. The Auer-Kirsner colitis with modifications today is utilized as an experimental model of human ulcerative colitis. Kirsner and Goldgraber in 1958 and 1959 also demonstrated the positive response of the rabbit colon to the Arthus and the Shwartzman reactions, re-confirming the immunologic responsiveness of the bowel. Elsewhere, colon "auto-antibodies" were produced by the injection of colon tissue and bacteria. Delayed hypersensitivity to 2,4 dinitrochlorobenzene in guinea pigs and miniature swine produced inflammation and ulceration of the colon. The same tissue reaction could be induced by the application of DNCB in orobase to the colon and was intensified by prior skin sensitization to DNCB.

Studies by Kirsner and Bregman (158), by O. Broberger and P. Perlmann of Stockholm (159) during the 1950s, and by Bernier et al. of Paris (160) had demonstrated heterogeneous hemagglutinating and precipitating "antibodies" reacting with antigens of human colon mucosa in the sera of children and adult patients with ulcerative colitis. These early observations were followed by comprehensive studies of the immunology of the gastrointestinal tract, especially ulcerative colitis. Kirsner and Palmer (161) wrote in 1954: ". . . Perhaps future studies should include the concept of vulnerability of the host, a person more susceptible to ulcerative colitis because of tissue hyper-reactivity, biological as well as psychogenic in origin." This hypothesis was validated scientifically in the next decade.

Wright and Truelove (162) (Fig. 14-5) in 1965 had raised the question of early wean-ing with loss of the usual defenses of the infant gut conferred by human breast milk, including secretory IgA as a risk factor in the development of ulcerative colitis. Shorter (1972) (163), in recognition of the infant's permeable intestine and immature intestinal defenses permitting the entry of bacteria (enterobacteriacae) and other antigens, suggested the very early "priming" of the gut-associated mucosal immune system as "preparing" the bowel for the later development of an inflammatory bowel disease, a sequence of events similar to that implied earlier in patients with food poisoning and amebic dysentery.

By now (1960s), the immunology of the gastrointestinal tract and the possible role of immune mechanisms in ulcerative colitis and Crohn's disease had become the most active area of IBD research. Early interest focused upon "autoimmunity," the possible identity of intestinal antigens, the search for anticolon antibodies, abnormal serum

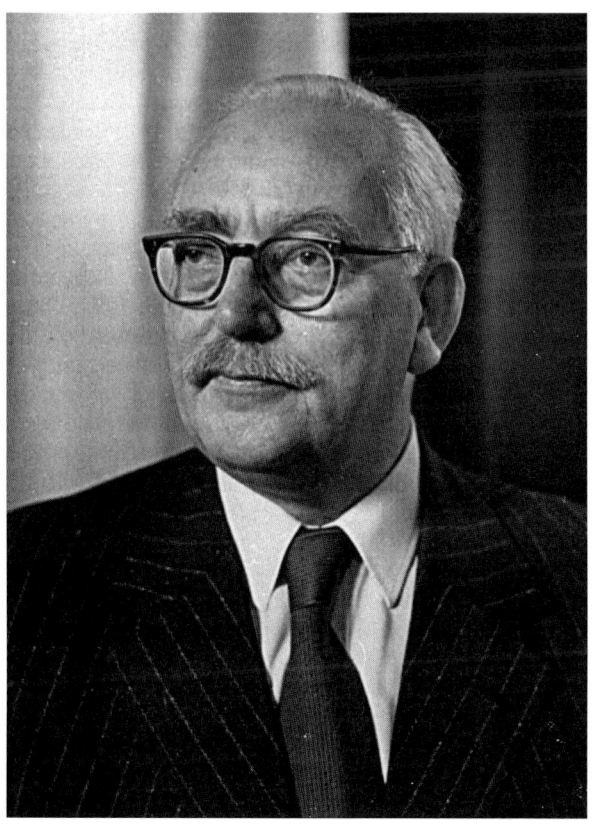

Fig. 14–5. Sidney Truelove.

immunoglobulins as a reflection of an immune process (164), and experimental attempts to produce an immune colitis. The methodology was crude; the "antigens" and "antibodies" were inadequately characterized, and their relationship to IBD was never established. F. C. Shean et al. (165) produced hemorrhagic colitis in the dog by the intravenous injection of rabbits with anti-dog-colon serum. However, attempts to induce chronic colitis by long-term exposure to autologous colon were unsuccessful. J. J. Bernier et al. of Paris (166) in 1963 induced bloody diarrhea in guinea pigs injected with large quantities of an anti-guinea-pig-colon serum.

These observations notwithstanding, there was no evidence of an immunologic abnormality preceding the onset of IBD or in healthy members of IBD families. Nor was there convincing evidence for an autoimmune pathogenesis. Most, if not all, the immunologic phenomena in IBD, appearing and disappearing with the activity and the quiescence of ulcerative colitis or Crohn's disease, represented secondary events, reflections of a chronically activated gut mucosal immune system. These events are generally independent of the type, severity, and duration of the disease.

Immunologic studies after approximately 40 years (1950s through 1990s) have advanced from early limited interest in a possibly abnormal systemic immunity and the experimental induction of an immunologic ulcerative colitis to more fundamental studies of the immunophysiology of the gut, the gut-associated mucosal immune system, antigen-access M and dendritic cells in the intestinal epithelium, possible autoimmune reactions, and T cell antigen receptors (167–169). Interest also is developing in the identification of the several antigen(s) recognized by the serum neutrophil cytoplasmic antibodies found in ulcerative colitis and sclerosing cholangitis. The present view is that some imbalance in the gut mucosal immune system plays a significant role in the pathogenesis of ulcerative colitis; that in Crohn's disease immunologic mechanisms are involved but secondary to an intestinal inflammatory reaction induced by intestinal microorganisms and their metabolites.

M CELL

Two additionally important components of the immune response in IBD involve the intestinal (antigen access) M cell and the role of lymphokines/cytokines. The M (membranous) cell is a specialized epithelial cell characterized by luminal surface microfolds rather than microvilli overlying the gut-associated (also bronchi-associated) lymphoid tissues, distributed in the intestine among the absorptive cells (also present in the colon and the appendix), which transport bacterial, viral, or food antigens from the intestinal lumen to the extracellular space, allowing access to lymphocytes, macrophages, and plasma cells. The M cell of the intestinal epithelium was identified in 1922 when K. Kumagai (170) demonstrated the uptake of ink, carmine dye, powdered erythrocytes, and living or dead mycobacteria from the intestinal lumen into the rabbit appendix and/or Peyer's patches, by means of specialized cells in the intestinal epithelium. In 1965, J. F. Schmedtje (171), studying the epithelium of the rabbit appendix, designated such cells overlying lymphoid follicles as "lympho-epithelial cells." R. L. Owen and A. L. Jones (1974) (172) coined the term M cells. Their status in inflammatory bowel disease, especially as to permeability and antigen access, is under investigation.

INFLAMMATION, LYMPHOKINES, CYTOKINES

Cytokines are proteins produced by "producer" cells responding to various inducing stimuli by influencing the behavior of particular target cells by means of specific surface receptors. Cytokines participate in the regulation of the immune response and help orchestrate the complex process of inflammation. Lymphokines is the arbitrary term applied to cytokines produced by or acting upon cells of the immune system. The interrelationship of the immune response in IBD with the inflammatory process and the regulatory role of the lymphocytes/cytokines produced by immunologic effector cells and lamina propria cells are important in understanding the nature of IBD. Interest in the biology of inflammation and its involvement in immune reactions dates back nearly 100 years to the observations on cellular immunity (i.e., phagocytosis) by Elie Metchnikoff in 1882 (173), on humoral immunity by Paul Ehrlich (1908) (174), and in the 1930s and 1940s to the biochemical studies of inflammation by Valy Menkin (175).

"McCord and Fridovich (176) in 1969 were the first to discover the enzyme superoxide dismutase (SOD) and proposed that the superoxide anion free radical is produced in mammalian systems. Up to that time, no one actually believed that reactive free radicals could be produced in living systems." "Bernard Babior (177) apparently was the first to demonstrate that activated polymorphonuclear cells produce large quantities of the superoxide anion radical. The importance of PMN-derived free radicals as important antibacterial agents later was confirmed using PMNs from patients with chronic granulomatous disease."

The first demonstration that reactive oxygen metabolites could play a major role in intestinal pathophysiology was reported by Neil Granger and colleagues (178), who demonstrated that postischemic microvascular injury in the small bowel could be attenuated by the intravenous administration of superoxide dismutase.

The review by M. B. Grisham and D. N. Granger (179) was one of the first on the possibility that immunologically activated phagocytic leukocytes (e.g., PMNs, eosinophils, and macrophages) could be important contributors to the mucosal injury observed during active colonic and intestinal inflammation. They also demonstrated the inhibitory effect of five amino salicylic acid on free oxygen radicals with subsequent healing of the intestinal lesions.

In 1975, Gould of England (180) found increased levels of the cyclooxygenase-derived prostaglandins (PGE₂) in the stools of patients with ulcerative colitis. Sharon, Ligumsky, Rachmilewitz, and Zor (181) extended these observations in 1978 and also noted elevated levels of prostaglandins of the cyclooxygenase pathway in the colonic mucosa, the serum, and the stools of patients with ulcerative colitis. Subsequently, Sharon and Stenson demonstrated a 50-fold increase in the leukotriene LTB4 and mono HETEs in the colonic mucosa of ulcerative

colitis, and postulated a proinflammatory role for LTB4 in both ulcerative colitis and Crohn's disease.

Interest in lymphokines/cytokines dates to the 1972 discovery of a factor produced by macrophages stimulating T cell responses to antigens, later designated as interleukin-1 (IL-1) (perhaps known earlier in the 1940s as endogenous pyrogen) (182) and to the discovery of interleukin-2 (IL-2) by Paetkau et al. (183) and by Chem and di Sabato (184) in 1976. Investigation of the role of cytokines, including nitric oxide, in the tissue reaction of ulcerative colitis and of Crohn's disease and in the nature of the inflammatory reaction (e.g., role of vascular adhesion molecules) is in its early stages (185).

GENETIC ASPECTS OF INFLAMMATORY BOWEL DISEASE—EARLY OBSERVATIONS

The first published instances of familial IBD from the 1909 London symposium on ulcerative colitis: (a) brother and sister, (b) father and sibling, and (c) father and sister of a third patient were labeled as "coincidences," and this view prevailed for more than 50 years. Reports of "familial" inflammatory bowel disease appeared in the 1960s and subsequently increased, clinically indicating a genetic relationship in IBD (186–189).

Ulcerative Colitis

In 1936, Moltke (190) described 5 families with ulcerative colitis (mother and daughter, 2; brother and sister, 2; and father and daughter, 1). Sloan, Bargen, and Gage (1950) (191) noted 26 positive family histories among 2000 patients; Kirsner and Palmer (1954) reported 6 family occurrences; and Banks, Korelitz, and Zetzel (1957), 9 families among 244 patients. Schlesinger and Platt (1958) obtained a family history of ulcerative colitis in 17% of 60 children with ulcerative colitis; fourfold higher than the usual ethnic distribution of the hospital population. The 1963 Chicago study included multiple family occurrences in 66 of 1084 patients with ulcerative colitis. An unusual sequence involved two brothers, who developed ulcerative colitis and succumbed to carcinoma of the colon within 15 years after onset of the disease (192).

Crohn's Disease

Crohn (193), referring in 1934 to the regional ileitis in a brother and sister, stated: "The occurrence may be purely accidental or it may have significance as to a congenital predisposition or a transmissible causative agent. . ." Early familial instances of regional enteritis subsequently were reported by many observers (194–196). In the family reported by Kuspira et al. (197), six members were affected, spanning three generations.

Crohn and Yarnis in 1958 (198) wrote: "Ulcerative colitis . . . rarely occurs in more than one member of a family . . . on the other hand, regional ileitis or enteritis occurs in multiple instances in intimately blood-related members of a family sufficiently often to warrant attention." They recorded 12 instances of familial involvement including three family groups: (1) young woman, brother, and half-brother with ileitis and father with ulcerative colitis; (2) ileitis, segmental colitis, and ulcerative colitis in three adult siblings; and (3) a child and her two blood-related aunts all having ileitis, confirmed at operation.

FAMILIAL PATTERNS

Familial distributions of IBD involved first-degree relatives (parent, child, or siblings) more often than second-degree or third-degree relatives (aunts, uncles, nieces, and nephews) in accord with a polygenic inheritance. In the 1963 Chicago study for ulcerative colitis, 50 of the 89 family members were brothers and sisters and cousins, approximately the same generation as that of the probands, and 11 were grandparents. For regional enteritis, 15 of 22 family members included brothers, sisters, and first cousins.

De Matteis (1963) (199) summarized 5 reports on ulcerative colitis comprising 20 parent-child combinations; mother and child were involved in 16 and father and child in 4. Among 32 reports on Crohn's disease involving 72 familial instances, mother and child were affected in 7 instances and father and child in 3, involving father and son in one instance, excluding a role for sex-linked genes.

The occurrence of IBD in three or more members of the same family, a possibility estimated as one in 12 billion, strongly supported a genetic relationship. Early three-member family reports included Spriggs (1934): ulcerative colitis in two brothers and a sister; Moltke (1936): brother, sister, and maternal aunt; Brown and Schieffley (1939) (94): two sisters and one brother; Houghton and Naish (1958) (69): (1) ulcerative colitis in three members of one family, (2) mother and three daughters with ulcerative colitis and a nephew with regional enteritis; Jackman and Bargen (1942) (200): (1) mother, son, and mother's brother; (2) mother and two daughters with ulcerative colitis and nephew with regional enteritis; and Bacon (1958): twin brothers and a sister. In the 1963 Chicago study, triple or more familial occurrences of inflammatory bowel disease included: (1) mother, brother, and sister with ulcerative colitis; (2) two sisters and a grandfather with ulcerative colitis; (2) three sisters with ulcerative colitis; and (3) three sisters and one brother with ulcerative colitis.

Thayer's (1972) (201) unusual family included a 21-year-old man with ulcerative colitis from the age of 8 who developed a carcinoma of the descending colon. A maternal aunt developed ulcerative colitis at the same time. One year after the death of the index patient, his brother, 2 years younger, developed ulcerative colitis and required colectomy and ileostomy. Within a year after this operation the boy's father developed ulcerative colitis and, after 5 years of medical treatment, also underwent a colectomy and ileostomy. The eight members of the Morris family (1965) represented three generations, all with ulcerative colitis, four males and four females, a distribution compatible with the influence of an autosomal dominant gene.

The seven affected members of the Ashkenazi Jewish family studied by Sherlock et al. (1963) included five with regional enteritis and two with ulcerative colitis. The index patient was a woman of 48 with regional enteritis of 25 years' duration. Regional enteritis was present in a sister aged 47, brothers aged 53 and 55, and a male first cousin aged 62. Ulcerative colitis was present in a married sister aged 46 and a nephew aged 16. Seven IBD-uninvolved relatives of the family had varying degrees of deafness.

INTERMINGLING OF DISEASES—TWINS— GENETIC ASSOCIATIONS

Ulcerative colitis was more likely to occur than Crohn's disease among the families of probands with ulcerative colitis and the same relationship held for probands with Crohn's disease, but the disease incidence was mixed in approximately 25% of families suggesting an etiologic relationship. The association of ulcerative colitis and Crohn's disease with genetically mediated conditions, such as for ulcerative colitis: ankylosing spondylitis and Turner's syndrome; and for Crohn's disease: psoriasis and the Hermansky-Pudlak syndrome added to the evidence.

The survey of monozygotic twins demonstrated moderate concordance for ulcerative colitis and strong concordance for Crohn's disease, powerful evidence for a genetic influence in inflammatory bowel disease. Discordance was more common for ulcerative colitis than for Crohn's disease.

The series of Binder et al. (1966) (202) included eight families with additional affected members (5 to 30%); whereas the control group had one family (0 to 73%). In the 1971 Chicago study (189), a positive family history for IBD was documented in 113 of 646 personally examined patients, 17.5%. As further validation, 150 of the 646 patients were selected at random and were matched by age, sex, race, religion, and social status with 150 apparently healthy individuals from the community. A positive family history was noted in 11% of the patients and in 4% of the controls.

HLA GENES

Because the major histocompatibility complex controls a spectrum of genes involved in immune regulation, associations between HLA genes (particularly Class II gene products) and disease susceptibility

have been actively investigated in IBD. However, extensive surveys, other than revealing ethnically related differences, have not demonstrated a dominant or specific HLA distribution in IBD, with the exception of HLA B_{27} in patients with ulcerative colitis and ankylosing spondylitis, an association between HLA-DR2 phenotype and ulcerative colitis, between DR1, DWQ_w5 or $B44C^2w5$ phenotypes with Crohn's disease, and HLA-DQB-1 genotype with Crohn's disease in children.

In summary, the genetic mechanism implicated in the individual vulnerability to IBD is not known. The genetic abnormality probably involves the combined interaction of several genes and the polygenic or multifactorial type of inheritance, interacting with environmental influences to precipitate inflammatory bowel disease in susceptible individuals.

OVERVIEW

The chronologic events described for ulcerative colitis and for Crohn's disease reveal "old" rather than "new" diseases, at least several centuries old. The changing epidemiologic patterns; the steady increases during the 19th century, especially in northern Europe and England, extending to the United States in the early 20th century; the prominence of ulcerative colitis during the first half and of Crohn's disease during the second half of this century; their frequency in the industrialized countries contrasted with their infrequency in under developed countries; their appearance in previously lagging, increasingly industrialized areas (e.g., Japan, Brazil), are all consistent with environmental causes (bacteria, mycobacteria, viruses, dietary substances, food additives, industrial, atmospheric, and water pollutants, chemicals, "stress," etc.) not exclusive to any particular geographic area or to any ethnic group.

The remarkable integrity of the gastrointestinal epithelium, exposed continuously to large numbers of aerobic and anaerobic bacteria and viruses, their constituents and metabolic products, endotoxins, and the many other elements of the gut microflora under healthy circumstances, is incompletely understood. The small intestine and the large intestine are readily damaged experimentally by a wide variety of injurious agents. However, no true analogues of IBD have as yet been found to occur naturally, and none have been induced experimentally.

Therapeutic responses in inflammatory bowel disease have been unrevealing as to etiology. Suppression of the proinflammatory molecules by sulfasalazine, the mesalamines (5ASA), steroids, and antileukotrienes also benefits experimental bowel injury. Antibiotics do not cure and occasionally exacerbate IBD. The clinical response of Crohn's disease to "immunosuppresssants" requires continued medication, and the precise mechanisms involved are incompletely understood.

The two diseases share comparable epidemiologic and demographic features except for the infrequency of smokers among patients with ulcerative colitis and their excess among patients with Crohn's disease. Familial occurrences are more common in Crohn's disease. Clinically, skip lesions and the ileal, perianal, and perineal involvements of Crohn's colitis contrast with the diffuse inflammation of the colon in ulcerative colitis, beginning in the rectum to affect exclusively the entire colon, although instances of a Crohn's type of proctitis have been observed. Involvement of the upper gastrointestinal tract and perianal abscess and fistula formation are typical of Crohn's disease. Sclerosing cholangitis is more often associated with ulcerative colitis. Histologically, mucosal-submucosal involvement of ulcerative colitis contrasts with the transmural Crohn's disease, and the prominent lymphoid aggregates, dilated submucosal lymphatics, and granulomas distributed throughout the bowel wall of Crohn's disease are not seen in ulcerative colitis. The recurrence of Crohn's disease of the small bowel after intestinal resection and anastomosis, the continued inflammation and ulceration, and the intestinal recurrences after total proctocolectomy and ileostomy are in contrast to the cure of ulcerative colitis following total colectomy and ileostomy or ileoanal anastomosis. Both diseases are associated with increased rates of surgery and mortality and in both the risk of intestinal cancer is increased. Nevertheless, the majority of patients, with strong family and physician support, can live reasonably "normal" lives despite their chronic recurrent disease, perhaps more so in ulcerative colitis than Crohn's disease (203).

The individual identities of ulcerative colitis and Crohn's disease are supported by the following. The increased titers of serum antineutrophil antibodies to an antigen (204) (possibly cytoplasmic granules) differ from the antigen recognized by the antineutrophil antibodies in vasculitis, in patients with ulcerative colitis and their first-degree relatives and the antibodies against goblet cells (205), not exclusive to ulcerative colitis but more frequent in ulcerative colitis than in Crohn's disease. The colon tissue levels of angiotensin I and II are increased in Crohn's disease (206). Antibodies to a trypsin-sensitive antigen in pancreatic juice are present in Crohn's disease but not in ulcerative colitis (206). The IgA antibodies to a soluble antigen of the yeast Saccharomyces cerevisae are increased, and the expression of CD25 (interleukin 2 receptor) on T cells and macrophages differs (on T cells in Crohn's disease and on macrophages in ulcerative colitis). Antiendothelial cell antibodies are found in both Crohn's disease (207,208) and in ulcerative colitis, correlating with circulating van Willebrand factor, a serologic indicator of vascular injury. The recent demonstration of increased interleukin-2 messenger RNA in the intestinal mucosal lesions of Crohn's disease and not in ulcerative colitis adds to the evidence that the pathogenesis is different in Crohn's disease and ulcerative colitis (209).

In contrast to earlier hypotheses, etiologic concepts in 1994 revolve around immunologic mechanisms in ulcerative colitis and microbially related events for Crohn's disease (bacteria, enteroviruses, bacterial metabolites), but coupled with genetic and environmental factors, possibly including an acquired or genetically mediated gut mucosal immune vulnerability to environmental agents.

Present evidence suggests that ulcerative colitis and Crohn's disease are genetically and clinically heterogeneous diseases with overlapping morphologic features and multifactorial origins. Collagenous colitis and lymphocytic colitis probably relate pathogenetically to ulcerative colitis. Ulcerative colitis and Crohn's disease probably result from the conjunction of multiple etiologic factors (genetic endowment, host gut defenses, abnormalities of colonic epithelial cells, prior antigenic (bacterial) experience of the intestinal mucosal immune system, and various nonspecific triggering events. Predisposing circumstances include an abnormal intestinal epithelium, increased intestinal permeability (M cell) to bacteria, viruses, and other antigens, and perhaps an immunoregulatory defect (hyperreactivity of intestinal lamina propria T_h cells), genetically determined or acquired. Precipitating agents include antibiotics altering the gut microflora, bacterial metabolites (endotoxin, peptidoglycan-PS), and "stress" expressed by way of the interacting central and enteric nervous systems. The IBD reaction perhaps initiated and sustained by the incorporation of bacterial and other (possibly lipid) elements into bowel wall involves a series of coordinated proinflammatory events mediated by lymphokines, cytokines, and leukotrienes of the lipoxygenase pathway, insufficiently balanced by protective cyclo-oxygenase products (e.g., prostaglandin E_2), with important contributions by activated macrophages and inflammatory cells (polymorphonuclear cells, lymphocytes, eosinophils, mast cells, and Paneth cells).

Thus, ulcerative colitis and Crohn's disease are not only distinctive but also definitive, albeit distantly related, diseases; environmental and genetic factors are important in their pathogenesis; and climate and industrializaton are important contributing circumstances.

The study of ulcerative colitis and Crohn's disease today involves numerous scientific disciplines: genetic, geographic, and sociocultural epidemiology, molecular microbiology, immunology, molecular genetics, biochemistry, the biology of the intestinal epithelium in health and in disease, and gastrointestinal neuroendocrinology, reflecting the broadening scope of IBD concepts in 1994. The challenge for the future will be to utilize the newer scientific advances in cellular and molecular biology in the more coordinated interdisciplinary investigation towards the ultimate conquest of two of the most challenging diseases in all of medicine.

REFERENCES

Ulcerative Colitis

1. Morson BC: Current concepts of colitis. The 1970 Lettsomian Lectures, Trans Med Soc London *86*:159, 1970.
2. Wilks S: Morbid appearances in the intestine of Miss Bankes. London Medical Gazette *2*:264, 1859.
3. Fielding JF: "Inflammatory" bowel disease. Br Med J *290*:47, 1985.
4. Wilks S, Moxon W: Lectures on Pathological Anatomy. 2nd ed. Philadelphia, Lindsay and Blakiston, 1875.
5. Cameron HC, Rippman CH: Statistics of ulcerative colitis from London hospitals. Proc R Soc Med *2*:100, 1909.
6. Weir RF: A new use for the useless appendix in surgical treatment of obstinate colitis. Med Rec *62*:201, 1902.
7. Lockhart-Mummery JP: The causes of colitis: With special reference to its surgical treatment, with an account of 36 cases. Lancet *i*:1638, 1907.
8. Hurst AF: Ulcerative colitis. Guy's Hosp Rep *71*:26, 1921.
9. Kirsner JB, Palmer WL, Klotz AP: Reversibility in ulcerative colitis. Radiology *57*:1, 1951.
10. Buie LA, Bargen JA: Chronic ulcerative colitis—A disease of systemic origin. JAMA *101*:1462, 1933.
11. Warren S, Sommers SC: Pathology of regional ileitis and ulcerative colitis. JAMA *154*:189, 1954.
12. Warren S, Sommers SC: Pathogenesis of ulcerative colitis. Am J Pathol *25*:657, 1949.
13. Dawson B: Discussion of ulcerative colitis. Proc R Soc Med *2*:94, 1909.
14. Stoughton RB: Enzymatic cytolysis of epithelium by filtrates of feces from patients with ulcerative colitis. Science *116*:37, 1952.
15. Morson BC: Pathology of ulcerative colitis. *In* Kirsner JB, Shorter RG (eds): Inflammatory Bowel Disease. Philadelphia, Lea & Febiger, 1975.
16. Kirsner JB, Palmer WL: Ulcerative colitis (considerations of its etiology and treatment). JAMA *155*:341, 1954.
17. Cave DR, Kirsner JB: Animal models of inflammatory bowel disease. Ztschr. f. Gastroenterologie *17*(Suppl):125, 1979.
18. Strober W: Animal models of inflammatory bowel disease. Am J Dig Dis *30*(Suppl):3S, 1985.
19. Marcus R, Watt J: Seaweeds and ulcerative colitis in laboratory animals. Lancet *ii*:489, 1969.

20. Roediger WEW, Nance J: Metabolic induction of experimental ulcerative colitis by inhibition of fatty acid oxidation. Br J Exp Pathol 67:773, 1986.

Crohn's Disease

21. Fabry W: Ex scirrho et ulcere cancioso in intestino cocco exorta iliaca passio. *In* Opera, Observatio LXI, Centuriae I. Frankfort:31. J.L. Dufour, 1682: 49 cited by Fielding, J.F. Crohn's disease and Dalziel's syndrome. J Clin Gastroent 10:279, 1988.
22. Morgagni GB: The seats and causes of disease investigated by anatomy. *In* Johnson, Payne (eds): Five Books Containing a Great Variety of Dissections with Remarks (Translated from the Latin of John Baptist Morgagni by Benjamin Alexander.) In Three Volumes. London, A. Millar and T. Cadell, 1769.
23. Combe C, Saunders H: A singular case of stricture and thickening of ileum. Med Trans Roy Coll Phys Lond 4:16, 1813.
24. Abercrombie J: Pathological and Practical Researches of the Stomach, the Intestinal Tract, and Other Viscera. Edinburgh, Waugh and Innes, 1828.
25. Colles A: Practical observations upon certain diseases of intestines, colon and rectum. Dublin Hosp Reports 5:131, 1830.
26. Bristowe JS: Ulceration, stricture, perforation of the small intestines. Trans Path Soc Lond 4:152, 1853.
27. Fenwick S: Clinical Lectures on Some Obscure Diseases of the Abdomen. London, Churchill, 1889.
28. Shapiro R: Regional ileitis—a summary of the literature. Am J Med Sci 198:269, 1939.
29. Dalziel TK: Chronic interstitial enteritis. Br Med J (Clin Res) 2:1068, 1913.
30. Coffen TH: Nonspecific granuloma of the intestine causing intestinal obstruction. JAMA 35:1303, 1925.
31. Crohn BB, Ginzburg L, Oppenheimer GD: Regional ileitis: A pathologic and clinical entity. JAMA 99:1323, 1932.
32. Nuboer FJ: Chronische phlegmone van het ileum. Med J Geneesk 76:2989, 1932 Cited by Weterman, I: Course and Long Term Prognosis of Crohn's Disease. Delft, Holland, W. D. Meinema BV, 1976.
33. Golob M: Infectious granuloma of the intestines. Med J Rec 135:390, 1932.
34. Bissell AD: Localized chronic ulcerative ileitis. Ann Surg 99:957, 1934.
35. Edwards H: Specimen of Crohn's disease. Med Soc Trans 59:87, 1936.
36. Koster H, Kasman LP, Sheinfeld W: Regional ileitis. Arch Surg 32:789, 1936.

37. Reichert FL, Mathes ME: Experimental lymphoderma of the intestinal tract and its relation to regional cicatrizing enteritis. Ann Surg 104:601, 1936.
38. Chess SD et al.: Production of chronic enteritis and other systemic lesions by ingestion of finely divided foreign materials. Surgery 27:221, 1950.
39. Kalima TV, Saloniemi H, Rahko T: Experimental regional enteritis in pigs. Scand J Gastroenterol 11:353, 1976.
40. Van Patter WN et al.: Regional enteritis. Gastroenterology 26:347, 1954.
41. Moschowitz E, Wilensky AO: Nonspecific granulomata of the intestine. Am J Med Sci 166:48, 1923.
42. Brown PW, Bargen JA, Weber HM: Inflammatory lesions of the small intestine (regional enteritis). Am J Dig Dis Nutr 1: 426, 1934.
43. Crohn BB, Rosenak BD: A combined form of ileitis and colitis. JAMA 106:1, 1936.
44. Snapper I, Pompen AWM, Groen J: Ileite regionale. Ann Med Intern (Paris) 29:5, 1936.
45. Fone DJ: Regional enteritis (Crohn's disease). Med J Austr 1:865, 1966.
46. Hurst AF: Regional ileitis—Three cases with fistula formation. Guy's Hosp. Rep 89: 54, 1939.
47. Ginzburg L, Oppenheimer GB: Nonspecific granulomata of the intestines, inflammatory tumors and strictures of the bowel. Ann Surg 1046, 1933.
48. Wells C: Ulcerative colitis and Crohn's disease. Ann Roy Coll Surg Engl 11:105, 1952.
49a. Lockhart-Mummery HE, Morson BC: Crohn's disease (regional enteritis) of the large intestine and its distinction from ulcerative colitis. Gut 1:87, 1960.
49b. Morson BC, Lockhart-Mummery HE: Crohn's disease of the colon. Gastroenterologia 92:168, 1959.
50. Coffey RJ: Pathologic manifestations of regional enteritis. Mayo Clin Proc 13:541, 1938.
51. Hadfield G: The primary histological lesion of regional ileitis. Lancet ii:773, 1939.
52. Crohn BB, Yarnis H: Regional Ileitis. 2nd Ed. New York, Grune and Stratton, 1958.
53. Chambers TJ, Morson BC: The granuloma in Crohn's disease. Gut 20:269, 1979.
54. Tallroth A: Regional enteritis with special reference to its etiology and pathogenesis. Acta Chir Scand 88:407, 1943.
55. Warren S, Sommers SC: Cicatrizing enteritis (regional ileitis) as a pathologic entity: Analysis of 120 cases. Am J Pathol 24:475, 1948.
56. Rappaport H, Burgoyne FH, Smetana HF:

The pathology of regional enteritis. Milit Surg *109*:463, 1951.

57. Warren S, Sommers SC: Pathology of regional ileitis and ulcerative colitis. JAMA *154*:189, 1954.

58. Morson BC: Personal communication, 1991.

59. Rickert RR, Cantor HW: The "early" ulcerative lesion of Crohn's disease corrective light and scanning electron microscopic studies. J Clin Gastroenterol *2*:11, 1980.

60. Barbour RF, Stokes AB: Chronic cicatrizing enteritis. Lancet *i*:299, 1936.

61. Cushway BC: Chronic cicatrizing enteritis—Regional ileitis (Crohn). Illinois Med J *66*:525, 1934.

62. Harris F, Bell G, Brunn H: Chronic cicatrizing enteritis: regional ileitis (Crohn). Surg Gynecol Obstet *57*:637, 1933.

63. Armitage G, Wilson M: Crohn's disease—A survey of the literature and a report on 34 cases. Br J Surg *38*:182, 1950.

64. Lewis T: Reflections upon reform in medical education. I. Present state and needs. Lancet *i*:619, 1944.

Epidemiology

65. Snow J: On the mode of communication of cholera. Lond Med Gaz *9*:745, 923, 1849. 2nd edition 1855. Reprinted in Frost WH (ed): Snow on Cholera. New York, The Commonwealth Fund, 1936.

66. Budd W: Typhoid fever, its nature, mode of spreading and prevention. London, Longmans Green, 1873. Reprint, New York, Grady Press, 1931.

67. Spriggs EI: Chronic ulceration of the colon. Quart J Med *27*:549, 1934.

68. Melrose AG: The geographic incidence of chronic ulcerative colitis in Britain. Gastroenterology *29*:1055, 1955.

69. Houghton EAW, Naish JM: Familial ulcerative colitis and ileitis. Gastroenterologia *89*:65, 1958.

70. Ustvedt HJ: Ulcerative colitis: A study of all cases discharged from Norwegian hospitals in the ten year period 1945–55. *In* Pemberton J, Willard H (eds): Recent Studies in Epidemiology. London, Oxford Press, 1958.

71. Acheson ED: The distribution of ulcerative colitis and regional enteritis in United States veterans with particular reference to the Jewish religion. Gut *1*:291, 1960.

72. Acheson ED, Nefzger MD: Ulcerative colitis in the United States Army in 1944—Epidemiology: Comparisons between patients and controls. Gastroenterology *44*:7, 1963.

73. Evans JG, Acheson ED: An epidemiological study of ulcerative colitis and regional enteritis in the Oxford area. Gut *6*:311, 1965.

74. Iversen I, Bonnevie O, Anthonison P, Riis P: An epidemiological model of ulcerative colitis. Scand J Gastroenterol *3*:432, 593, 1968.

75. Lindenberg J, Aagard P: Colitis ulcerosa in Denmark. Ugeskr Larg *126*:781, 1963.

76. Norlan BJ, Krause U, Bergman L: An epidemiological study of Crohn's disease. Scand J Gastroenterol *5*:385, 1970.

77. Monk M et al.: An epidemiologic study of ulcerative colitis and regional enteritis among adults in Baltimore. I. Hospital incidence and prevalence 1960–1963. Gastroenterology *53*:198, 1967.

78. Monk M, Mendeloff AI, Siegel CE, Lilienfeld A: An epidemiological study of ulcerative colitis and regional enteritis among adults in Baltimore. II. Social and demographic factors. Gastroenterology *56*:847, 1969.

79. Mendeloff AI: The epidemiology of idiopathic inflammatory bowel disease. *In* Kirsner JB, Shorter RG (eds): Inflammatory Bowel Disease. Philadelphia, Lea & Febiger, 1975.

80. Garland CF et al.: Incidence rates of ulcerative colitis and Crohn's disease in fifteen areas of the United States. Gastroenterology *81*:1115, 1981.

81. Kyle J: Crohn's Disease. New York, Appleton-Century-Crofts, 1972.

82. Calkins BM, Lilienfeld AM, Garland CF, Mendeloff AI: Trends in incidence rates of ulcerative colitis and Crohn's disease. Digest Dis Sci *19*:913, 1984.

83. Whelan G: Epidemiology of inflammatory bowel disease. Med Clin North Am *74*:1, 1990.

84. Osborne MJ, Stansby GP: Cigarette smoking and its relationship to inflammatory bowel disease. A review. J R Soc Med *85*:214, 1992.

85. Samuelsson SM: Ulceros colit och proktit. Thesis, University of Upsala 182, 1976.

86. Rhodes JM: Personal communication, Oct. 14, 1991.

87. Kessler H, Diamond KI: Epidemiological studies of Parkinson's disease. I. Smoking and Parkinson's disease. Am J Epidemiol *94*:16, 1971.

Psychogenic

88. Palmer WL: The patient, the physician, and the gut—A consideration of mind and matter. Dallas Med J *52*:500, 1966.

89. Wolf S: Studying the person in the patient. The Pharos 38, Spring 1990.

90. Darwin C: Expression of emotion in men and animals. London, John Murry, 1872.
91. Pavlov I: Conditioned Reflexes (Trans GV Anrep). New York, Oxford, 1927.
92. Cannon WB: Bodily Changes in Pain, Hunger, Fear and Rage. 2nd Ed. New York, Appleton, 1929.
93. Murray CD: Psychogenic factors in the etiology of ulcerative colitis. Am J Dig Dis *180*:239, 1930.
94. Sullivan AJ: Psychogenic factors and ulcerative colitis. Am J Dig Dis 2:651, 1935.
95. Grace WJ, Wolf S, Wolff HG: The Human Colon. New York, P. B. Hoeber, Inc., 1951.
96. Lium R: Observations on the etiology of ulcerative colitis. IV. The rectometrogram and the rectal reactions of eight normal subjects and one patient with ulcerative colitis before and after spinal anethesia. A preliminary report. Am J Med Sci *197*:841, 1939.
97a. Almy TP, Tulin M: Alterations in colonic function in man under stress. I. Experimental production of changes simulating the irritable colon. Gastroenterology 8:616, 1947.
97b. Almy TP, Kern F, Tulin M: Alterations in colonic function in man under stress. II. Experimental production of sigmoid spasm in healthy persons. Gastroenterology *12*: 425, 1949.
98. Wener J, Polonsky A: The reaction of the human colon to naturally occurring and experimentally induced emotional states: Observations through a transverse colostomy in a patient with ulcerative colitis. Gastroenterology *15*:84, 1950.
99. Moeller HC, Kirsner JB: The effect of drug-induced hypermobility tract on the gastrointestinal tract of dogs. Gastroenterology *26*:303, 1954.
100. Engel GL: Studies of ulcerative colitis. II. The nature of the somatic processes and the adequacy of psychosomatic hypotheses. Am J Med *16*:416, 1954.
101. Grace WJ, Pinsky RH, Wolff H: Treatment of ulcerative colitis. Gastroenterology 26: 462, 1954.
102. McKegney FP, Gordon RD, Levine SM: A psychosomatic comparison of patients with ulcerative colitis and Crohn's disease. Psychosom Med *32*:153, 1970.
103. Alpers DH: Psychiatric illness and inflammatory bowel disease. *In* Rachmilewitz D (ed): Inflammatory Bowel Diseases. The Hague, Martinus Nijhoff Publishers, 1982.
104. Aronowitz R, Spiro HM: The rise and fall of the psychosomatic hyothesis in ulcerative colitis. J Clin Gastroent *10*:298, 1988.
105. White BV: Effect of ileostomy and colectomy on personality adjustment of patients with ulcerative colitis. N Engl J Med *244*: 537, 1951.
106. Feldman F, Cantor D, Soll S, Bachrach W: Psychiatric study of a connective series of 34 patients with ulcerative colitis. Br Med J 2:16, 1967.
107. Kirsner JB: Ulcerative colitis—1970—Recent developments. Scand J Gastroenterol 6(Suppl 6):63, 1970.
108. Karush A, Daniels GE, Flood C, O'Connor JF: Psychotherapy in Chronic Ulcerative Colitis. Philadelphia, WB Saunders Co., 1977.
109. Grace WJ: Life stress and regional enteritis. Gastroenterology 23:542, 1953.
110. Kraft IA, Ardali C: Psychiatric study of children with diagnosis of regional ileitis. South Med J *57*:599, 1964.
111. Crockett RW: Psychiatric findings in Crohn's disease. Lancet *i*:946, 1952.
112. Fleming A: On a remarkable bacteriolytic element found in tissues and secretions. Proc R Soc Lond 93:306, 1922.
113. Meyer K et al.: Lysozyme activity in ulcerative alimentary disease. Am J Med 5:496, 1948.
114. Prudden F, Meyer K: Lysozyme (mucolytic enzyme) activity in chronic ulcerative colitis, with a preliminary report on antilysozyme therapy. *In* Postgraduate Gastroenterology. Philadelphia, WB Saunders, 1950.
115. Moeller HC, Klotz AP, Kirsner JB: Lack of effect of crystaline lysozyme in the isolated intestinal pouch of the dog. Gastroenterology 20:604, 1952.
116. Glass GBJ, Pugh BL, Grace WJ, Wolf S: Observations on the treatment of human gastric and colonic mucus with lysozyme. J Clin Invest 29:12, 1950.

Microbiology

117. Hurst AF: Ulcerative colitis. Guy's Hosp Rep 85:317, 1935.
118. Leusden JT: Observations on colitis ulceration with a contribution to the knowledge of the pathogenetic effects of colon bacilli. Nederlandisch Tijdschr v Geneesk 2:2890, 1921.
119. Lups S: Vaccine therapy in ulcerative colitis. Am J Dig Dis Nutr 2:65, 1935.
120. Maratka Z, Wagner F: The treatment of nonspecific ulcerative colitis by autogenous vaccine—Correlated bacteriological and immunological studies. Gastroenterology *113*:34, 1948.
121. Bargen JA: Experimental studies on the etiology of chronic ulcerative colitis (preliminary reports). JAMA *83*:332, 1924.

122. Bargen JA, Logan AH: The etiology of chronic ulcerative colitis. Experimental studies with suggestions for a more rational form of treatment. Arch Intern Med *36*:818, 1925.

123. Cook TJ: Focal infection of the teeth and elective localization in the experimental production of ulcerative colitis. J Am Dent Assoc *18*:2290, 1931.

124. Paulson M: Chronic ulcerative colitis with reference to a bacterial etiology. Exper Stud Arch Intern Med *41*:75, 1928.

125. Mones PG, Sanjuan PD: Colitis ulcerosa graves non amibianas: Etiologia, diagnostico and tratamiento medico. Barcelona, Salvat Editores S.A., 1935, p. 49.

126. Dack GM, Heinz TE, Dragstedt LR: Ulcerative colitis. Study of bacteria in the isolated colons of three patients by culture and by inoculation of monkeys. Arch Surg *31*:225, 1935.

127. Felsen J: The relationship of bacillary dysentery to distal ileitis, chronic ulcerative colitis and nonspecific intestinal granuloma. Ann Intern Med *10*:645, 1936.

128. Paulson M: Intracutaneous responses, comparable to positive Frei reactions, with colonic exudate from chronic ulcerative colitis cases with positive Frei tests. Am J Dig Dis *3*:667, 1936.

129. Rodaniche EC, Kirsner JB, Palmer WL: Lymphogranuloma venereum in relation to ulcerative colitis. JAMA *115*:515, 1940.

130. Victor R, Kirsner JB, Palmer WL: Failure to induce ulcerative colitis experimentally with filtrates of feces and rectal mucosa. Gastroenterology *14*:398, 1950.

131. Neilsen K: Regional enteritis in domestic animals. *In* Engel A, Larson T (eds): Regional Enteritis (Crohn's Disease). Stockholm, Nordiska Bokhandelns Forlag, 1971.

132. Pumphrey RE: Studies on the etiology of regional ileitis. Proc Staff Meet Mayo Clin *13*:539, 1938.

133. Burnham WR, Lennard Jones JE, Stanford JL, Bird G: Mycobacteria as a possible cause of Crohn's disease. Lancet *ii*:693, 1978.

134. Chiodini RJ et al.: Characteristics of an unclassified mycobacterium species isolated from patients with Crohn's disease. J Clin Microbiol *20*:966, 1984.

135. Sartor RB et al.: Granulomatous enterocolitis induced in rats by purified bacterial cell wall fragments. Gastroenterology *89*:587, 1985.

136. Bregman E, Kirsner JB: Amino acids of colon and rectum. Possible involvement of diaminopimelic acid of intestinal bacteria in antigenicity of ulcerative colitis colon. Proc Soc Exp Biol Med *118*:727, 1965.

137. Van Kruiningen HG: Granulomatous colitis of Boxer dogs: Comparative aspects. Gastroenterology *53*:114, 1967.

Immune Mechanisms

138. Jenner E: An inquiry into the causes and effects of the variolae vaccinae. A disease discovered in some of the counties of England, particularly Gloucestershire, and known by the name of the cow pox. Lancet, 3rd Edition, D. N. Shury, London, p 13, 1801.

139. Bienenstock J: The physiology of the local immune response. *In* Asquith P (ed): Immunology of the Gastrointestinal Tract. London, Churchill Livingstone 1979.

140. Besredka A: La vaccination contre les etats typhoides par la voie buccale. Ann Inst Pasteur *33*:882, 1919.

141. Davies A: An investigation into the serological properties of dysentery stools. Lancet *ii*:1009, 1922.

142. Heremans JF: Les globulines sériques du système gamma, leur nature et leur pathologie. Arcia, Brussels, 1960.

143. Tomasi TB, Tan EM, Solomon A, Prendergast RA: Characteristics of an immune system common to certain external secretions. J Exp Med *121*:101, 1965.

144. Gray I, Walzer M: Studies in mucous membrane hypersensitiveness. III. The allergic reaction of the passively sensitized rectal mucous membrane. Am J Dig Dis Nutr *4*:707, 1938.

145. Gray I, Harten M, Walzer M: Studies in mucous membrane hypersensitiveness: Allergic reactions in passively sensitized mucous membrane of ileum and colon in humans. Ann Intern Med *13*:2050, 1940.

146. Walzer M, Gray I, Straus HW, Livingston S: Studies in experimental hypersensitiveness in the Rhesus monkey: Allergic reaction in passively locally sensitized abdominal organs. J Immunology *34*:91, 1938.

147. Kirsner JB: Inflammatory bowel disease—Overview of etiology and pathogenesis. *In* Berk JE (ed): Bockus Gastroenterology. Philadelphia, WB Saunders Co., 1985.

148. Andresen AFR: Ulcerative colitis—An allergic phenomenon. Am J Dig Dis Nutr *9*:91, 1942.

149. Rowe AH: Chronic ulcerative colitis: Allergy in its etiology. Ann Intern Med *17*:83, 1942.

150. Rider JA, Moeller HC: Food hypersensitivity in ulcerative colitis. Further experience with an intramucosal test. Am J Gastroenterol *37*:497, 1962.

151. Bleumink E: Food allergy and the gastroin-

testinal tract. *In* Asquith P (ed): Immunology of the Gastrointestinal Tract. London, Churchill Livingstone, 1979.

152. Kirsner JB, Goldgraber MB: Hypersensitivity, autoimmunity and the digestive tract. Gastroenterology *38*:536, 1960.

153. Gear J: Autoantibodies and the hyper-reactive state in the pathogenesis of disease. Acta Med Scand *152*(Suppl 306):39, 1955.

154. Kraft SC, Kirsner JB: Immunological apparatus of the gut and inflammatory bowel disease. Gastroenterology *60*:922, 1971.

155. Auer J: Local autoinoculation of the sensitized organism with foreign protein as a cause of abnormal reactions. J Exp Med *32*: 427, 1920.

156. Kirsner JB, Elchlepp J: The production of an experimental colitis in rabbits. Trans Assoc Am Phys *70*:102, 1957.

157. Callahan WS, Goldman RG, Vial AB: The Auer phenomenon in colon-sensitized mice. J Surg Res *3*:395, 1963.

158. Bregman E, Kirsner JB: Colon "antibodies" in ulcerative colitis (Abstract). J Lab Clin Med *56*:785, 1960.

159. Broberger O, Perlmann P: Autoantibodies in human ulcerative colitis. J Exp Med *110*: 657, 1959.

160. Bernier JJ, Lambling A, Cornelis W: Sur la presence d'anticorps anti-colon dams le serum de malades atteints de colite ulcereusa. Bull Miem Soc Méd Hopitaux Paris *28–29*:1129, 1960.

161. Kirsner JB, Palmer WL: Ulcerative colitis—Considerations of its etiology and treatment. JAMA *155*:341, 1954.

162. Wright R, Truelove SG: Early weaning in ulcerative colitis. Br Med J *2*:138, 1965.

163. Shorter RG, Huizenga KA, Spencer RJ: A working hypothesis for the etiology and pathogenesis of nonspecific inflammatory bowel disease. Dig Dis Sci *17*:1024, 1972.

164. Brandtzaeg P, Baklien K, Fausa O, Hael PS: Immunohistochemical characterization of local immunoglobulin formation in ulcerative colitis. Gastroenterology *66*:1123, 1974.

165. Shean FC, Barker WF, Fonkalsrud EW: Studies in active and passive antibody induced colitis in the dog. Am J Surg *107*:337, 1964.

166. Bernier JJ, Lambling A, Terris G, Cornelis W: Autosensitization in hemorrhagic rectocolitis (ulcerative colitis) and experimental colitis induced by hetero- and auto-antibodies. Arch Mal App Dig *51*:1161, 1962.

167. Elson CO: The immunology of inflammatory bowel disease. *In* Kirsner JB, Shorter RG (eds): Inflammatory Bowel Disease. Philadelphia, Lea & Febiger, 1988.

168. Kirsner JB, Shorter RG: Recent developments in "nonspecific" inflammatory bowel disease. N Engl J Med *306*:775 and 837, 1982.

169. MacDermott RP, Elson CE: Preface to mucosal immunology. I. Basic principles. Gastroenterol Clin North Am *20*:397, 1991.

170. Kumagai K: Uber den resorptions vorgang der corpuscularen bestandteile im darm. Berichte Gesamte Physiol Exp Pharmacol *17*:414, 1923.

171. Schmedtje JF: Some histochemical characteristics of lymphoepithelial cells of the rabbit appendix. Anat Rec *151*:412, 1965.

172. Owen RL, Jones AL: Epithelial cell specialization within human Peyer's patches. An ultrastructural study of intestinal lymphoid follicles. Gastroenterology *66*: 189, 1974.

173. Metchnikoff E: Untersuchungen uber die intracellularle verdauung bei wirbellosen thieren. Arbeit Zool Inst Univ Wien *5*:141, 1883. See also O. Metchnikoff! Life of Elie Metchnikoff. New York, Houghton Mifflin Co., 1921.

174. Ehrlich P: Experimental researches on specific therapy on immunity with special reference to the relationship between distribution and action of antigens. *In* Vol. 3. Himmelwert F (ed): Collected Papers. New York, Pergamon Press, 1960 (originally published 1908).

175. Menkin V: Studies on inflammation; measure of permeability of capillaries in inflamed area. J Exper Med *51*:285, 1930.

176a.McCord JM, Fridovich I: Superoxide dismutase. An enzymic function for erythrocuprein (hemocuprein). J Biol Chem *244*: 6049, 1969.

176b.Fridovich I: The biology of oxygen radicals. Science *201*:875, 1978.

177. Babior BM, Kipnes RS, Curnutte JT: Biological defense mechanisms, the production by leukocytes of superoxide—A potential bactericidal agent. J Clin Invest *52*: 741, 1973.

178. Granger DN, Rutili G, McCord JM: Superoxide radicals in feline intestinal ischemia. Gastroenterology *81*:22, 1981.

179. Grisham MB, Granger DN: Neutrophil mediated mucosal injury—Role of reactive oxygen metabolites. Dig Dis Sci *33*:6S, 1988.

180. Gould SR: Prostaglandins, ulcerative colitis, and sulphasalazine. Lancet *ii*:988, 1975.

181. Sharon P, Ligumsky, Rachmilewitz D, Zor U: Role of prostaglandins in ulcerative colitis—Enhanced production during active disease and inhibition by sulfasalazine. Gastroenterology *75*:638, 1978.

182. Atkins E: Pathogenesis of fever. Physiol Rev *40*:580, 1960.

183. Paetkau V, Mills G, Gerhart S, Monticone V: Proliferation of murine thymic lymphocytes in vitro is mediated by the concanavalin-a-induced release of a lymphokine (costimulator). J Immunology *117*:1320, 1976.

184. Chem DM, di Sabato G: Further studies on the thymocyte stimulating factor. Cell Immunol *24*:211, 1976.

185. Dinarello CA: Interleukin-1 and Interleukin-1 antagonism. Blood *77*:1627, 1991.

Genetic Aspects

186. Kirsner JB: Genetic aspects of inflammatory bowel disease. Clin Gastroenterol *2*: 557, 1973.

187. Sherlock P, Bell BM, Steinberg H, Almy TP: Familial occurrence of regional enteritis and ulcerative colitis. Gastroenterology *45*:413, 1963.

188. Kirsner JB, Spencer JA: Family occurrences of ulcerative colitis, regional enteritis, and ileocolitis. Ann Intern Med *59*:133, 1963.

189. Singer HC, Anderson JGD, Frischer H, Kirsner JB: Familial aspects of inflammatory bowel disease. Gastroenterology *61*: 423, 1971.

190. Moltke O: Familial occurrence of non-specific ulcerative colitis. Acta Med Scand *78*(Suppl 72):426, 1936.

191. Sloan WP, Bargen JA, Gage RP: Life histories of patients with ulcerative colitis: A review of 2000 cases. Gastroenterology *16*: 25, 1950.

192. Gassaniga AB, Gassaniga DA: Carcinoma of the colon following chronic ulcerative colitis. Report of two unusual cases in brothers. Dis Colon Rectum *5*:437, 1962.

193. Crohn BB: The broadening concept of regional ileitis. Am J Dig Dis *1*:97, 1934.

194. Brown PW, Schieffley CH: Chronic regional enteritis occurring in three siblings. Am J Dig Dis Nutr *6*:257, 1939.

195. Cornes JS, Stecher M: Primary Crohn's disease of the colon and rectum. Gut *2*:189, 1961.

196. Armitage G, Wilson M: Crohn's disease: Survey of literature and report of 34 cases. Br J Surg *38*:182, 1950.

197. Kuspira J, Bhambhani R, Singh SM, Links H: Familial occurrences of Crohn's disease. Hum Hered *22*:239, 1972.

198. Crohn BB, Yarnis H: Regional Ileitis—2nd Edition, New York, Grune and Stratton, 1958.

199. de Matteis V: L'aspetto familiare della malattia di Crohn. Annali Italiani di Chirurgia *39*:936, 1963.

200. Jackman RJ, Bargen JA: Familial occurrence of chronic ulcerative colitis (thrombo ulcerative colitis). Am J Dig Dis Nutr *9*:147, 1942.

201. Thayer WR Jr: Personal communication, 1972.

202. Binder V et al.: A genetic study of ulcerative colitis. Scand J Gastroenterol *1*:49, 1966.

Overview

203. Farmer RG, Easley KA, Farmer JM: Quality of life assessment by patients with inflammatory bowel disease. Cleveland Clin J Med *59*:35, 1992.

204. Targan S, Sexon A, Landa SC: Serum antineutrophil cytoplasmic autoantibodies to distinguish ulcerative colitis from Crohn's disease patients. Gastroenterology *96* (Suppl):A505, 1989.

205. Seibold F, Weber P, Jenss H, Wiedmann KH: Antibodies to a trypsin sensitive pancreatic antigen in chronic inflammatory bowel disease: Specific markers for a subgroup of patients with Crohn's disease. Gut *32*:1192, 1991.

206. Jaszewski R et al.: Increased colonic mucosal angiotension I and II concentrations in Crohn's colitis. Gastroenterology *98*: 1543, 1990.

207. Sawyer AM, Pottinger BE, Wakefield AJ: Serum antiendothelial cell antibodies are present in Crohn's disease but not ulcerative colitis. Gut *31*:A1169, 1990.

208. Stevens TRJ, Harley SL, Blake DR, Rampton DS: Anti-endothelial cell antibody-positive ulcerative colitis serum promotes the adherence of neutrophils to vascular endothelial cells (Abstract). Gut *33*(Suppl):S63, 1992.

209. Mullin GE et al.: Increased interleukin-2 messenger RNA in the intestinal mucosal lesions of Crohn's disease but not ulcerative colitis. Gastroenterology *102*:1620, 1992.

15

Acute Appendicitis

NORTON J. GREENBERGER

INTRODUCTION

Acute appendicitis is a relatively common cause of abdominal pain in all age groups and the most frequent cause of *severe* acute abdominal pain in children and teenagers that results in urgent evaluation by a physician. Appendicitis in its classic form is easily diagnosed, but in the very young and the elderly it often is atypical and presents a diagnostic problem. This occurs in spite of the fact that acute appendicitis should always be considered in the differential diagnosis of "acute abdomen," which is better termed severe acute abdominal pain.

This chapter reviews the following features of acute appendicitis:

- Historical background with special reference to the contributions of Fitz and Osler
- Incidence and epidemiology with emphasis on changes that have occurred during the past 20 years
- Pathophysiology and pathogenesis
- Clinical manifestations
- Ultrasonography in the diagnosis of acute appendicitis
- Appendicitis in the elderly
- Differential diagnosis
- Treatment

HISTORICAL BACKGROUND

Fernel's chapter on causes and signs of diseases of the intestines from his book *Universa Medicina* (1,2), published in 1581, is believed by many to be the first description of acute appendicitis. Subsequent reports by Heister (1755) (1,3), Mestivier (1759) (1,4) and Parkinson (1812) (1,5) described instances of acute appendicitis with perforation and/or peritonitis. In 1824, Lauyer-Villermay (6) reported two cases of appendicitis and Melier in 1827 (7) reported four additional cases and first described an appendiceal abscess.

The classic description of appendicitis was the paper by Fitz (1,8) read at the first meeting of the Association of American Physicians in 1886 and subsequently published in the forerunner of the New England Journal of Medicine (8). The paper is remarkably prescient. Ralph Major's summary of this paper (1) also is a classic and is reproduced here with minor editing.

"A historical statement was made of the origin of the terms typhlitis, perityphlitis, and perityphlitic abscess. The want of exact agreement as to what was understood by these terms was emphasized. Attention was called to the importance of bearing in mind that in the vast majority of cases, the primary disease was an inflammation of the caecal appendix. The term appendicitis was preferred to typhlitis, as avoiding the possibility of a misunderstanding, and as localizing the disease in its usual place of origin.

The paper was based upon an analysis of two hundred and fifty-seven cases of unquestionable perforating ulcer of the appendix, and of two hundred and nine cases diagnosed as typhlitis, perityphlitis, and perityphlitic abscess. In the latter series, the diagnosis was clinical, not anatomical.

The important features in the etiology of

appendicitis were considered, also the limitations as to sex and age. It was found that the disease occurred most frequently among previously healthy youths and young adults, especially males; that a faecal concretion or foreign body was present as a local cause in more than three-fifths of the cases. Attacks of indigestion and acts of violence, especially when indirect, were exciting causes in one-fifth of the cases. The action of these causes was favored by a constipated habit, or by congenital or acquired irregularities in the position and attachment of the appendix. The first characteristic symptom of a perforating appendicitis was found to be a sudden, severe, abdominal pain. This occurred in eighty-four percent of the cases, and usually in the right iliac fossa, where tenderness could always be found, even when the pain was referred to some other locality. The pain was attributed to the actual perforation or detachment of fresh adhesions. Fever was the next characteristic symptom and occurred in the course of twenty-four hours. Finally came the swelling which made its appearance in the course of three days. The chief source of danger from the appendicular peritonitis arose from its becoming generalized. Such a result followed most frequently between the second and fourth days. More than two-thirds of the patients died during the first eight days and two-thirds of these between the fourth and eight days, inclusive.

The question of a differential diagnosis was then discussed. The termination in resolution was referred to. It was considered to take place in about one-third of the cases as approximately determined from the recorded cases of typhlitis and perityphlitis. Even resolution might be undesirable since the number of cases of recurrent disease is considerable, and might have been prevented by appropriate treatment. The reader recommended at the outset, the opium treatment with rest and a liquid diet, the food being given in small quantities, frequently repeated. If it became evident that general peritonitis was imminent at the end of twenty-four hours after the sudden intense pain, the appendix should be exposed and removed. Usually the symptoms were not so urgent that the appearance of the swelling could not be awaited. Although Willard Parker advised that the abscess might be opened as early as the fifth day, the practice has been to operate at a later date. Forty-seven percent of the cases were operated upon in the second week and twenty-six percent after the third week. More favorable

results in the future were to follow the earliest possible opening of the swelling. This in most instances was at the outset, a sac formed by a circumscribed peritonitis. It was usually present on the third day of the disease, dating from the pain, its first characteristic symptom. Negative results from a diagnostic puncture did not contraindicate the operation."

Thus, Fitz's major contribution was the definition of acute appendicitis and the suggestion that early appendectomy was essential to cure. Senn (9) was the first surgeon to correctly diagnose acute appendicitis before rupture, to perform an urgent appendectomy, have the patient recover, and to report his experience.

Osler's description of appendicitis also is a major contribution, and selected portions are cited directly. One cannot help but marvel at the clarity of this description, published in 1912 (10).

"Inflammation of the vermiform appendix is the most important of acute intestinal disorders. Formerly the "iliac phlegmon" was thought to be due to disease of the caecum—typhlitis—or of the peritoneum covering it—perityphlitis; but we now know that with rare exceptions the caecum itself is not affected, and even the condition formerly described as stercoral typhlitis is in whole question on a rational basis.

Etiology.—The exciting causes of appendicitis are not always evident. An infection is the essential factor. The lumen of the appendix forms a sort of test-tube, in which the faeces lodge and are with difficulty discharged, so that the mucosa is liable to injury from retention of the secretions or from the presence of inspissated faeces or occasionally foreign bodies. In some instances the appendicitis is a local expression of a general infection. The causes of the undoubted increase of the disease are not known; some have attributed it to the prevalence of influenza. By others the poison of rheumatic fever is believed to be a cause, and just as it may excite tonsillitis, so it may cause inflammation of the lymphatic tissues of the appendix. It is remarkable, too, that there may be two or three cases of appendicitis at the same time in one family. The acute catarrhal form may be associated with pneumonia or typhoid fever or any of the acute infections. Direct injury, as in straining and heavy lifting, is an occasional exciting cause.

The bacteriology of the disease is most varied. The Bacillus coli is present in a large number of cases, and the pyogenic organisms, particularly the Streptococcus pyogenes. The disease may be produced experimentally in rabbits by the intravenous injection of pneumococci and other oganisms; Poynton and Paine have caused it with the organism isolated from rheumatic cases.

Faecal Concretions.—The lumen of the appendix may contain a mould of faeces, which can readily be squeezed out. Even while soft, the contents of the tube may be moulded in two or three sections with rounded ends. Concretions—enteroliths, coproliths—are also common. Of 700 cases of foreign bodies there were 45 percent of faecal concretions (J. F. Mitchell). The enteroliths often resemble date stones in shape. The importance of these concretions is shown by the great frequency with which they are found in all acute inflammations of the appendix.

Foreign Bodies.—Of 1,400 cases of appendicitis collected by J. F. Mitchell these were present in 7 percent; in 28 cases pins were found. It is well to bear in mind that some of the concretions bear a very striking resemblance to cherry and date stones.

Symptoms.—In a large proportion of all cases of acute appendicitis the following symptoms are present: (a) Sudden pain in the abdomen, usually referred to the right iliac fossa; (b) fever, often of moderate grade; (c) gastrointestinal disturbance–nausea, vomiting, and frequently constipation; (d) tenderness or pain on pressure in the appendix region.

Pain.—A sudden, violent pain in the abdomen is, according to Fitz, the most constant, first, decided symptom of perforating inflammation of the appendix, and occurred in 84 percent of the cases analyzed by him. In fully half of the cases it is localized in the right iliac fossa, but it may be central, diffuse, but usually in the right half of the abdomen. Even in the cases in which the pain is at first not in the appendix region it is usually felt here within thirty-six or forty-eight hours. It may extend toward the perineum or testicle. It is sometimes very sharp and colic-like, and cases have been mistaken for nephritic or for biliary colic. Some patients speak of it as a sharp, intense pain-serous-membrane pain; others as a dull ache-connective tissue pain. While a very valuable symptom, pain is at the same time one of the most misleading. Some of the forms of recurring pain in the appendix region Talamon has called appendicular colic.

The condition is believed to be due to partial occlusion of the lumen, leading to violent and irregular peristaltic action of the circular and longitudinal muscles in the expulsion of the mucus.

Fever.—Fever is always present in the early stage, even in the mildest forms, and is a most important feature. J. B. Murphy states that he would not operate on a case in which he was confident that no fever had been present in the first thirty-six hours of the disease. An initial chill is very rare. The fever may be moderate, from 100° to 102°; sometimes in children as the very outset the thermometer may register above 103.5°. When a localized abscess has formed, and in some very virulent cases of general peritonitis, the temperature may be normal, but at this stage there are other symptoms which indicate the gravity of the situation. The pulse is quickened in proportion to the fever.

Gastrointestinal Disturbance.—The tongue is usually furred and moist, seldom dry. Nausea and vomiting are symptoms which may be absent, but which are commonly present in the acute perforative cases. The vomiting rarely persists beyond the second day in favorable cases.

Local Signs.—Inspection of the abdomen is at first negative; there is no distention, and the iliac fossae look alike. On palpation there are usually from the outset two important signs—namely, great tension of the right rectus muscle, and tenderness or actual pain on deep pressure. The muscular rigidity may be so great that a satisfactory examination cannot be made without an anaesthetic. McBurney has called attention to the value of a localized point of tenderness on deep pressure, which is situated at the intersection of a line drawn from the navel to the anterior-superior spine of the ilium, with a second, vertically placed, corresponding to the outer edge of the right rectus muscle. Firm, deep, continuous pressure with one finger at this spot causes pain, often of the most exquisite character. In addition to the tenderness, rigidity, and actual pain on deep pressure, there is to be felt, in a majority of the cases, an induration or swelling. In some cases this is a boggy, ill-defined mass in the situation of the caecum; more commonly the swelling is circumscribed and definite, situated in the iliac fossa, two or three fingers' breadth above Poupart's ligament. Some have been able to feel and roll beneath the fingers the thickened appendix. The later the case comes under observation the greater the probability of the existence of a well-marked tumor mass. It is not to be forgotten that there may be neither tumor mass nor induration to be felt in some of the most intensely virulent cases of perforative appendicitis. The pain may be mistaken for that of hip joint disease.''

INCIDENCE AND EPIDEMIOLOGY: CHANGES DURING THE PAST 50 YEARS

Relevant data on the incidence and epidemiology of acute appendicitis are summarized in Table 15–1. The maximum inci-

dence of acute appendicitis occurs in the second and third decades of life, with approximately two thirds of the cases occurring during this time interval. The disease is much less frequent before the age of 10 and after the age of 50. Although males generally have predominated, in two recent reports, females predominate by a ratio of almost 2:1 (11,12). The absolute incidence of the disease has decreased by about 40% between 1940 and 1960 but since then has remained relatively stable. The incidence of appendicitis is now about 10 per 100,000 population, and the overall risk of developing appendicitis has fallen to approximately

Table 15–1
Appendicitis: Review of Two Large Series

	Osler (10)	University of California (11)	Kaiser, Los Angeles (12)	
Number of cases	1223	1000	1013	
Period reviewed		1963–1977	1976–1978	
Females:Males (%)		64:36	66:34	
Age distribution				
<10	5.6	9.1%		
11–20	19.5	31.9%		
21–30	21*	35.5%		
31–40		8.2%		
41–50		5.4%		
>50		9.9%		
Normal appendix		20.7%	14.7%	
Men		12%		
Women		34%		
PID/gynecologic problem		32%		
Perforated appendix				
Overall		27.3%	18.9%	
<10 years		38.7%	<15 years	41%
11–30 years		19.1%		
31–50 years		26.3%	>35 years	36%
>50 years		64.6%		
Symptoms				
Pain				
Periumbilical		10%		
RLQ		75%		
Diffuse		7%		
Anorexia		92%		
Nausea		78%		
Vomiting		64%		
Previous similar episodes				
1		9%		
>2		4%		
Appendolith		1.4%		

* Ages 21–25 only

7%. The comparable figures at the turn of the century were 15 in 100,000, with the risk of developing appendicitis about 15% during a lifetime. In a recent study from Los Angeles, appendectomies accounted for approximately 1.4% of hospital admissions and about 11.5% of general surgical operations during a 2-year period (12). For reasons that are unclear, the overall incidence of appendicitis is much lower in underdeveloped countries, especially parts of Africa, and in lower socioeconomic groups. Since 1960, the clinical pattern of appendicitis has been changing. Patients under 10 years of age and over 50 years of age are arriving at hospitals at later stages of appendicitis, and this has been associated with a significant increase in the incidence of perforation (Table 15-1). The overall incidence of perforation in two large series was 27.3% and 18.9% respectively. Although the current overall mortality risk of appendicitis is less than 1%, the proportion of fatal cases is six times as great in perforated appendicitis as in those operated on in an earlier stage (12).

PATHOPHYSIOLOGY

Two theories have been prominent regarding the initiation of acute appendicitis. The primary pathogenetic mechanism in acute appendicitis has been luminal obstruction, which in turn results in infection, the bacteria involved being those of the fecal flora normally occupying the lumen of the appendix. Obstruction has been noted in approximately 30 to 40% of cases and, when present, is most commonly caused by a fecalith. The second theory postulates that ulceration of the mucosa is the initial event and that the subsequent inflammatory reaction results in obstruction of the tiny appendiceal lumen. The unifying hypothesis would hold that obstruction can either precede or follow the onset of the disease. Once obstruction occurs, mucus accumulates in the appendiceal lumen and fecal bacteria multiply and invade the appendiceal wall. Venous engorgement and subsequent arterial compromise result from high intraluminal pressures. The most common bacteria in the appendix include Bacteroides fragilis, Escherichia coli, Klebsiella enterobacter, Streptococcus faecalis, and anaerobic streptococci. If perforation occurs and the process evolves slowly, contiguous organs such as the terminal ileum, cecum, and omentum may wall off the appendiceal area so that a localized abscess develops.

CLINICAL MANIFESTATIONS

The clinical manifestations of appendicitis are summarized in Table 15-2 (13). The history and sequence of development of symptoms are among the most important diagnostic features of appendicitis. Abdominal pain is almost invariably the initial symptom. It is frequently poorly localized to the epigastrium and periumbilical area, reaches a peak of intensity at approximately 4 to 6 hours and then may subside. It reappears in the right lower quadrant as a progressively severe steady pain aggravated by motion or cough. The shift from diffuse abdominal pain to the right lower quadrant occurs in 50 to 60% of patients. Anorexia, nausea, and vomiting also are common symptoms (Tables 15-1 and 15-2), and one of these symptoms is present in 90% of cases. In another 25% of the cases, pain begins in and is confined to the right lower quadrant. If the symptoms of right lower quadrant pain have been present for a longer period of time, i.e., 2 weeks, and especially if accompanied by weight loss greater than 10 pounds, anemia, or occult blood in the stool, the diagnosis is more likely to be Crohn's disease rather than appendicitis. However, it should be recalled that Crohn's disease does involve the appendix in 5 to 10% of cases, and patients can present with acute onset of symptoms that clearly simulate acute appendicitis.

The physical findings also are summarized in Table 15-2. Low-grade fever ranging from 99 to 101° is common. A fever above 100°F (38.3°C) should raise the question of perforation. Physical findings may vary according to the location of the appendix and with time after the onset of the illness. The physical signs to search for include local tenderness, rebound tenderness, muscle guarding, and muscle rigidity. With gentle palpation of the abdomen, one can usually detect the presence of tenderness which, as noted previously is most often localized to the right lower quadrant at or near

Table 15–2
Acute Appendicitis*

I. History and physical examination
    A. Abdominal pain—almost invariably the initial symptom
        1. Frequently poorly localized to epigastrium and periumbilical area
        2. Reaches peak of intensity in 4 to 6 hours, then may subside
        3. Reappears in RLQ as progressively severe steady pain aggravated by motion or cough
    B. Anorexia, nausea, vomiting (one of these symptoms present in 90% cases)
        1. Presence of hunger distinctly unusual
    C. Abdominal tenderness found in locations corresponding to location of appendix (abdomen, flank, pelvis)
        1. RLQ tenderness (especially at McBurney's point)
        2. Percussion, rebound tenderness, referred rebound tenderness, jar tenderness—signs of peritoneal irritation
    D. Low-grade fever (99–101°) common
    E. If chronic symptoms, weight loss > 10 lbs or anemia—consider Crohn's disease
II. Laboratory studies
    A. Modest leukocytosis (12,000 to 16,000 WBC/mm^3)
    B. Appendolithiasis seen on plain film of the abdomen (1.5% of cases)
    C. Ultrasound examination showing a thickened appendix (positive in 65 to 70% of cases)
III. Diagnosis of appendicitis in the elderly
    A. Diagnosis often is overlooked because symptoms and signs mild and diagnosis is not considered
    B. Pain often is minimal or even absent
    C. Shift of pain to RLQ occurs in only 20%
    D. Temperature may be elevated only slightly
    E. Abdominal tenderness may be deceptively mild
    F. Can present with a painless mass (appendiceal mass)
IV. Differential diagnosis
    A. Most common conditions discovered at operation when acute appendicitis is erroneously diagnosed
        1. Mesenteric lymphadenitis (? viral, Yersinia)
        2. Acute pelvic inflammatory disease
        3. Mittelschmerz (rupture of an ovarian follicle)
        4. Twisted ovarian cyst
        5. Regional enteritis
        6. Ruptured ectopic pregnancy
    B. Other disorders presenting diagnostic difficulties
        1. Cholecystitis, pancreatitis, diverticulitis, ureteral calculus, Meckel's diverticulitis, perforated ulcer

* With permission from Greenberger NJ, Hinthorn DR: History Taking and Physical Examination: Essentials and Clinical Correlates. St. Louis, CV Mosby Co., 1992, p. 247.

McBurney's point. The diagnosis of acute appendicitis cannot be established unless tenderness is elicited. It should be emphasized, however, that abdominal tenderness could be absent if a retrocecal or pelvic appendix is present, in which circumstance the cardinal physical finding could well be tenderness in the flank or on rectal and pelvic examination. If the appendix has ruptured, physical signs change. Diffuse tenderness may supervene and rebound tenderness and muscle rigidity become more obvious. A mass may develop if localized perforation has occurred. Therefore, rectal and pelvic examinations are essential in every patient with the abrupt onset of severe abdominal pain and in every patient suspected of having appendicitis. In addition, it should be done to exclude diseases of the pelvic organs. A few patients with acute appendicitis may complain of increased tenderness as the tip of the examining finger in the rectum gently palpates the right side.

Laboratory studies are not necessary to establish a diagnosis of appendicitis, but usually are obtained to provide supporting information. Modest leukocytosis with white blood cell counts ranging from 12,000 to 16,000 WBC/mm^3 is characteristic, and a white blood cell count greater than 20,000 cells per microliter should raise the question of perforation. In many patients, even if the leukocyte count is normal, there will be a shift to the left in the differential white blood cell count. Thus, only 5% of patients with appendicitis have both a normal differential and a normal total leukocyte count. The presence of anemia or blood in the stool should suggest another diagnosis, i.e., regional enteritis or carcinoma of the cecum. Urinalysis should be obtained to exclude genitourinary conditions that may simulate acute appendicitis. Plain films of the abdomen are rarely of value except when a fecalith is observed in the right lower quadrant. In a recent series (Table 15-1), fecalith was noted in only 1.4% of the patients.

ULTRASONOGRAPHY IN THE DIAGNOSIS OF ACUTE APPENDICITIS

The overall accuracy of the preoperative clinical diagnosis of acute appendicitis ranges from 70 to 78%. This is because the typical clinical signs and symptoms are nonspecific and, before high-resolution sonography, no noninvasive imaging technique was available to enable direct visualization of the inflamed vermiform appendix. Schwerk et al. (14) carried out a prospective study of the routine use of high-resolution sonography in 523 patients with suspected acute appendicitis. Criteria for ultrasound diagnosis included visualization of a noncompressible aperistaltic appendix with a target-like appearance in transverse view and a diameter of at least 7 mm. In 115 of 130 patients with proven appendicitis, the inflamed appendix or appendiceal abscess was visualized, yielding a sensitivity of 88.5%. Ultrasonically visible appendices had a mean diameter of 11.4 mm. The overall accuracy of sonography was 95.7% and specificity was 98%. The predictive value of a positive test was 94.5% and of a negative test, 96.3%. In 24 (89%) of the 27 patients with appendiceal rupture the correct

diagnosis was made with ultrasound. In the other 3 (11%), the diagnosis was missed. The authors concluded that high-resolution, real-time sonography is a sensitive, specific imaging technique for diagnosing acute appendicitis and its complications. Routine use of ultrasonography significantly improved the diagnostic accuracy in patients with suspected appendicitis and reduced the negative laparotomy rate from 22.9 to 13.2%.

Several additional studies attest to the validity and utility of sonography in the diagnosis of acute appendicitis (15,16). Larson et al. (15) examined 206 patients with suspected appendicitis with sonography over a 6-month period in 3 community teaching hospitals. Of 41 patients in whom the surgeons judged the clinical findings severe enough to warrant immediate surgery (group A), 34 (83%) had appendicitis, and sonography had a sensitivity of 76%, a specificity of 71%, and an accuracy of 76%. Of 165 patients in whom the surgeons judged the clinical findings severe enough to warrant hospitalization for observation but not immediate surgery (group B), 51 (32%) had appendicitis at subsequent surgery. Sonography had a sensitivity of 96%, a specificity of 94%, and an accuracy of 95%. Of 49 surgeons surveyed, the mean testing threshold (i.e., the probability of appendicitis below which they would send the patient home without further tests or observation) was 0.11, and the mean treatment threshold (i.e., the probability of appendicitis above which they would operate immediately) was 0.82. The post-test probability of appendicitis with findings indicating appendicitis present on sonography was 0.93 in group A and 0.88 in group B, and with findings absent on sonography it was 0.62 in group A and 0.02 in group B. Larson et al. conclude that in group A patients the use of sonography remains controversial in the diagnosis of appendicitis, but in group B patients it is both valid and useful.

Fa and Cronan (16) reassessed 70 ultrasonographic examinations and retrospectively re-analyzed these studies using the most recently published criterion, which requires a maximal appendiceal diameter of more than 6 mm. Ultrasonography was shown to be 80.0% sensitive, 95.0% specific, and 92.9% accurate in diagnosing appendicitis, with a positive predictive value of 72.7% and a negative predictive value of 96.6%. Ultrasonographic examination provided additional findings, predominantly gynecologic or obstetric, in 52% of the women, leading to an alternative diagnosis in one third of these patients who complained of abdominal pain. Ultrasonographic study provided additional findings in 12% of the men, leading to alternative diagnoses in 12%. Ultrasonographic results directly influenced clinical management in 18% of the patients.

These studies indicate that appendiceal ultrasonographic examination is a reliable ancillary technique in diagnosing or excluding appendicitis. It is indicated in patients with an atypical or equivocal presentation; those with a firm clinical diagnosis do *not* require ancillary diagnostic aids and should proceed immediately to surgical intervention. The predominant role of ultrasonography in evaluating appendicitis is not as an independent diagnostic determinant. Rather, it is most useful as a means of improving decision making when considered in combination with a thorough history and physical examination in patients who represent diagnostic dilemmas.

APPENDICITIS IN THE ELDERLY AND IN PREGNANCY

The diagnosis of appendicitis in the elderly may be particularly difficult. This diagnosis often is overlooked because symptoms and signs are mild and the diagnosis is not considered. Accordingly, pain is often minimal and may even be absent. The shift of pain to the right lower quadrant occurs in only 20% of patients. The temperature may be elevated only slightly and abdominal tenderness may be deceptively mild. Patients can present with a painless right lower quadrant mass, which may reflect an appendiceal abscess. Finally, it should be noted that appendicitis occurs about once in every 1000 pregnancies and is the most common extrauterine condition requiring an abdominal operation.

DIFFERENTIAL DIAGNOSIS

More than 40 disorders can cause acute abdominal pain and discussing them is be-

yond the scope of this presentation. Accuracy in establishing a diagnosis of acute appendicitis is about 75 to 80% for experienced clinicians. A normal appendix was removed 20.7% and 14.7% of the time in two series each including 1000 patients with acute appendicitis (Table 15-1). The diagnosis is more likely to be erroneous in women than in men (Table 15-1). The most common conditions discovered at operation when acute appendicitis is erroneously diagnosed include mesenteric lymphadenitis, adult pelvic inflammatory disease, mittelschmerz, twisted ovarian cysts, regional enteritis, and ruptured ectopic pregnancy. The "negative" appendectomy rate in young women ranges from 35 to 45%. This has led to the increased use of ultrasound in young women with abrupt onset of severe abdominal pain (see previous text). In doubtful cases, 4 to 6 hours of careful observation is usually more beneficial than harmful. However, further delay can be associated with perforation and its attended increased morbidity and mortality. In appendicitis without perforation, the mortality rate is in the order of 0.1%. With perforated appendicitis, the mortality rate is approximately 3%, and this increases dramatically in the elderly to a 15% mortality rate.

TREATMENT

The treatment for acute appendicitis is surgical removal of the appendix. Because mortality and morbidity correlate with perforations and perforation correlates with duration, early diagnosis and appendectomy are essential. In most series, the removal of a normal appendix has occurred in 15 to 20% of cases (Table 15-1). It is reasonable to assume that virtually all such operations were carried out to avoid the catastrophe of unoperated-upon acute appendicitis. Patients with obvious acute appendicitis for whom no surgeon or surgical facilities are available can be treated with antibiotics and intravenous fluids. The usual regimen includes an aminoglycoside such as gentamicin, an antibiotic such as clindamycin for anaerobes, and ampicillin. It must be emphasized that such treatment is only temporizing and does not obviate the need for appendectomy to be carried out.

Laparoscopic Appendectomy

The successful introduction of laparoscopic cholecystectomy triggered a series of attempts to replace standard operative procedures with endoscopic techniques. Several reports attest to the efficacy of laparoscopic appendectomy. A representative study is that of Pier et al. (17). For a 4½-year period, this group of surgeons operated on 997 patients who presented with typical signs and symptoms of appendicitis. Conventional appendectomy was performed on 64 patients. The remaining 933 patients underwent attempted laparoscopic appendectomy. The procedure was converted to an open procedure in 18 cases (2%) because of extensive adhesions, extreme obesity, bleeding, abnormal vermix position, abscess, or perforation. Most of these cases occurred early during the days when the procedure was being mastered. The results obtained show that laparoscopic appendectomy is feasible, rapid, and as safe as open surgery. Few wound infections, minimal pain, and rapid postoperative mobilization are the main arguments in favor of laparoscopic appendectomy. The most important potential benefit, a low incidence of long-term complications such as adhesive intestinal obstruction, remains to be confirmed by prolonged follow-up of these patients. Importantly, the rate of complications in this particular series interoperatively was 0.2% and postoperatively 0.8%. A randomized, prospective trial of laparoscopic versus traditional open appendectomy will be of interest, and such studies are in progress.

REFERENCES

1. Major RH: Appendicitis in Classic Descriptions of Disease. 7th printing. Springfield, Charles C Thomas, 1947.
2. Fernel J: Universa Medicina. De partium morbis et symptomis. Liber VI, Frankfort, Wechelus, 1581, p. 592. Cited in reference #1.
3. Heister L: Medical, Chirurgical, and Anatomical Cases and Observations by Laurence Heister. Translated by George Wirgman, and printed in London by J. Reeves 1755. Cited in reference #1.
4. Mestivier M: An unusual tumor of the appendix (trans). J Med Chir Pharm, Paris, 1759, x, 441, 1759. Cited in Reference #1.
5. Parkinson J. Case of Diseased Appendix Vermiformis. Med Chir Tr, London, 1812, III, p. 57. Cited in Reference #1.
6. Louyer-Villermay JB: Observations pour servir à l'histoire de inflammations de l'appendice du caecum. Arch Gen Med Paris 5:246, 1824.
7. Melier F: Mémoire sur des tumeurs phlegmoneuses occupant la fosse de l'appendice cécal. J Gen Med Chir Pharm 100:317, 1827.
8. Fitz RH: Perforating inflammation of the vermiform appendix, with special reference to its early diagnosis and treatment. Boston Med Surg J 115:13, 1886.
9. Senn N: A plea in favor of early laparotomy for catarrhal and ulcerative appendicitis, with report of two cases. JAMA 12:630, 1889.
10. Osler W: Appendicitis. In The Principles and Practice of Medicine. 10th Edition. 1912. New York and London, D. Appleton Co., 1912, p. 531.
11. Lewis FR et al.: Appendicitis: A critical review of diagnosis and treatment in 1,000 Cases. Arch Surg 110:675, 1975.
12. Silberman VA: Appendectomy in a large metropolitan hospital. Retrospective analysis of 1,013 cases. Am J Surg 142:615, 1981.
13. Greenberger NJ, Hinthorn DR: History Taking and Physical Examination: Essentials and Clinical Correlates. St. Louis, CV Mosby Co., 1992, p. 247.
14. Schwerk WB, Wichtrup B, Rothmund M, Rüschoff J: (Philipps-Univ of Marburg, West Germany): Ultrasonography in the diagnosis of acute appendicitis: A prospective study. Gastroenterology 97:630, 1989.
15. Larson JM et al.: The validity and utility of sonography in the diagnosis of appendicitis in the community setting. AJR 153:687, 1989.
16. Fa EM, Cronan JJ: Compression ultrasonography as an aid in the differential diagnosis of appendicitis. Surg Gynecol Obstet 169:290, 1989.
17. Pier A et al.: Laparoscopic appendectomy. World J Surg 17:29, 1993.

16

Diverticular Disease

JAMES L. ACHORD

Throughout the 19th and into the 20th century, diverticular disease of the colon was unknown to the practicing physician. Descriptions of diverticula did not regularly appear in textbooks of medicine until about 1920 (1). Even then, emphasis was chiefly on the complications of the diverticula: peritonitis, abscesses, or fistula. Opinions as to the etiology of intestinal diverticula were confined to possible anatomic explanations, but their epidemiology, demography, or pathogenesis was unknown. Not until radiology of the colon was fully developed, well into the 20th century, was their frequency appreciated.

Current information indicates that diverticula of the colon are present in more than 20% of adults in the U.S. and in 33% of those over 50 years of age (2). About 50% of individuals in their 80s have diverticula (3,4). Interestingly, the frequency of diverticula in Sweden is only 5.2% and, in Norway, 15.8% (5). Thus, diverticulosis coli has been called a disease of western civilization (6). With better understanding and especially the introduction of antibiotics, treatment has improved dramatically. However, it is not yet certain that these advances have had a significant impact on prevention of the problem or the frequency of its complications.

HISTORY

Although many authors cite Sommering's translation of Baillie's *Morbid Anatomy* (1794) as the first anatomic description of diverticula of the colon, Telling and Gruner reviewed the original and found that polyps, not diverticula, were described (7). Voigtel (1804) reported descriptions earlier than 1794 by Schrock, Roilan, Gunz, Morgagni, and Haller (8).

Diverticula of the gut were considered medical curiosities until just before the turn of the century, when the German physician Graser (1898) demonstrated that they were not uncommon (7,9). Most published reports in the first 15 years of the 20th century consisted of one to three cases, and not all of these were valid examples of colon diverticula. The first comprehensive review by Telling and Gruner (7) in 1917, included 324 cases and over 200 references. Of the 85 case histories in which age was given and excluding two children, ages 6 and 7 years, the average age of patients was 52.5 years. In early published reports, the disease was identified by its complications, including peritonitis, colonic obstruction, peridiverticular abscesses, and fistulas; death was common.

DIAGNOSIS

A history of radiology by Ronald L. Eisenberg (10) includes comprehensive discussions of the development of gastrointestinal radiology, critical to the increased awareness of diverticula of the gastrointestinal tract. The following synopsis is derived from this outstanding contribution.

In 1895, Roentgen discovered the nature of x-rays, for which he received the first

Nobel prize in physics in 1901. Roentgen clearly understood the potential medical application of his discovery, and the first human radiograph was that of the left hand of his wife. Just one year later, Enrico Salvioni developed the principle of fluoroscopy. Thomas Edison developed the first practical, through dangerous, fluoroscope ("Vitascope"), also in 1902. By the early 1900s, commercial production of fluoroscopes was flourishing and the instruments became widely available, to those without medical training as well as to physicians. However, the dangers soon became apparent and the use of fluoroscopy diminished. By early 1887, Walter B. Cannon was using bismuth subnitrate to study the swallowing mechanism of experimental animals. Bismuth subnitrate is reduced to its toxic nitrite form by hydrochloric acid and soon proved too dangerous for clinical use. Bachem and Gunther (1910) already had found that barium sulfate was inert, inexpensive, and satisfactory (11); it became the preferred medium.

Early attempts to visualize the colon in humans involved the ingestion of large amounts of bismuth salts. Review of the few published pictures makes it obvious why this was a poor method of examining the colon. Schule (1904) performed the first colon examination, using a radiopaque solution as an enema (12); Case published a demonstration of multiple colon diverticula 10 years later (13). DeQuervain published early x-ray studies of the gut in 1914 (14). The procedure was refined by Haenisch (1874–1952), using barium sulfate, to more or less its present technique. Fischer (1923) introduced the "double-contrast" (air contrast) technique (15). By the middle 1930s, present methods of barium enemas were well established and readily available to clinicians. Improved recording films by Kodak and others in the 1970s and the application of ultrasonography and computed scanning advanced the diagnostic approach.

CHANGES IN CONCEPTS OF ETIOLOGY

Diverticulosis

Until well into the 20th century, little or no etiologic distinction was made between diverticula in the colon and those that occur elsewhere in the gut, although their anatomic differences were recognized (7). For colonic diverticula, that the outpouching occurs along the course of blood vessels penetrating the muscularis of the colon was recognized by Klebs (1868) (16) and confirmed later by many observers (17,18). Klebs (16) implicated traction on the bowel by the mesentery, as did Fisher in 1900, as the cause (19), while Hansemann in 1896 (20) favored pulsion as the mechanism. Early experiments in filling human colons at autopsy (21) or the living colons of anesthetized animals (9) with water to the point of rupture did little to clarify the problem. No conclusive data were available for either pulsion or traction, and the controversy persisted. By 1917, anatomic observations had provided no support for mesenteric traction as a significant factor. The most commonly held opinions then were that diverticula were caused by pulsion, the result of a presumably weakened colonic musculature, or both (7). The intraluminal force was considered to be excessive gas and fecal stasis, explaining the predominant location in the sigmoid. Weakness of the wall of the colon caused by the natural process of aging was regarded as the explanation for the greater frequency of diverticula in the older age groups. By 1930, the view was firmly established that diverticula of the colon were the result of pulsion and that the outpouching occurred at the weakest point in the wall, defined by penetrating blood vessels. Intraluminal propulsive forces were considered to result from abdominal straining during defecation and exaggerated by constipation (7,9). Despite data indicating that less than half of the patients with colonic diverticula actually had constipation (19,22–24), this concept has persisted (25–27).

Disorders of colonic muscle size and arrangement were recognized when the disorder was first described. In 1910, Keith described circular, concertina-like folds in some patients with diverticula of the colon that ". . . so deeply invade the lumen as seriously to obstruct the forward movement of the faeces" (28). This situation he attributed to tonic contractions of the taenia coli in the segment of the gut containing diverticula. In 1963, Morson (29) described the muscular hypertrophy present in numerous patients, many of whom had diverticulosis. Arfwidsson suggested that patients with such muscular changes but no diverticula were, in fact, "pre-diverticular" (30). Morson's findings later were confirmed by Fleischner (31), who used the terms "simple massed diverticulosis" and "spastic sigmoid or myochosis" to explain symptoms of diverticulitis without other evidence of inflammation. He related this apparent work hypertrophy to an abnormality of muscular contractions as a late consequence of the irritable bowel syndrome (32). Horner previously had suggested a relationship between "spastic colon" and diverticulosis (24). Although similar motor abnormalities of the colon were demonstrated in both irritable bowel syndrome and symptomatic diverticulosis (4,33), individual variations (34) did not consistently support a relationship. For example, one study followed 77 patients with irritable bowel syndrome for a mean period of 6 years (but up to 14 years in some patients) and failed to demonstrate the development of diverticula (35). In another study, patients in Scandinavia with the irritable bowel syndrome were reported to develop diverticula twice as frequently as matched controls from the general population (36). Although diverticulosis and irritable bowel syndrome share similar symptoms, the relationship between the two remains uncertain (37), perhaps because of inability to precisely define the irritable bowel syndrome.

In the mid-1960s, Painter and Truelove published a series of careful cineradiographic observations and simultaneous pressure measurements in the human sigmoid colon. They were able to demonstrate that the colon becomes segmented, creating closed compartments (38–41). When muscle contraction occurred within the segments, pressures increase as high as 90 mm Hg, with simultaneous distention of diverticula. Painter and colleagues suggested that the process of segmentation and the development of diverticula were more likely in the relatively narrow sigmoid colon of patients on low-residue diets (41). Wells found that West African natives, who eat a very bulky and high-fiber diet, have very large colons and no diverticula (42). Urbanization of South African blacks, including changes in their traditional diet, results in the appearance of diverticular disease (43). Similar changes have been observed in Japanese immigrants to Hawaii (44). Interestingly, Carson and Hoelzel demonstrated the development of diverticula in rats fed a low-residue (low-fiber) diet (45), but this experiment has never been confirmed (46).

Almy pointed out that Laplace's law, which states that the tension in the wall of a hollow cylinder is proportional to its radius multiplied by the pressure within the cylinder ($T = P \times R$), can explain why diverticula are more likely to form in the relatively narrow sigmoid (because $P = T/R$) (47). Theoretically, bulk produced by high-fiber diets reduces the pulsion pressure within the lumen by increasing the radius and presumably also reduces the segmentation described by Painter. Diverticulosis, therefore, has been described as a chronic fiber deficiency disease characteristic of populations eating highly refined, low-fiber diets (48,49). Since segmentation has not been documented to occur in the right colon, the formation of diverticula in this area requires another explanation.

The concept of colon diverticula formation thus has moved from one of pulsion by intraluminal gases, constipation, and straining at defecation to the formulation that intraluminal pressure is generated by contraction of colonic musculature. Further, compartmentalization of the colon into closed segments allows very large amplitude inner pressures to develop that tend to force the mucosa through weaknesses in the musculature; the most prominent located immediately adjacent to the penetrating nutrient vessels of the colonic wall. The most susceptible length of colon is the narrowest, the sigmoid. Epidemiologic data indicate that the population groups with wider sigmoid colons are those who ingest a diet high in undigestible fiber. Diverticulosis is rare in these people unless they move, at an early age, to cultures emphasizing highly refined, low-fiber diets. The relationship, if any, between colon diverticulosis and gastrointestinal motility disorders, as in the irritable bowel syndrome, remains unclear. From the available data, the variably increasing weakness of the wall of the colon with age (33,50,51) seems to explain, in part at least, the increasing frequency with aging in susceptible populations.

Diverticulitis

At the beginning of the 20th century, patients were discovered to have diverticula when they presented to the physician with a complication, such as an intra-abdominal abscess or enteric fistula. With the development of diagnostic radiology, the presence of diverticulosis could be discovered before complications occurred and the clinical signs and symptoms of diverticulitis were confirmed. When acute diverticulitis was suspected, cautious single contrast enemas were the only recourse and continue to be used today (52) to confirm the diagnosis. In this circumstance, colonoscopy usually is omitted to avoid the risk of unsealing a localized perforation. In recent years, abdominal computed tomography (CT) has been helpful in difficult cases, not only for diagnosis (53,54) but also for percutaneous drainage of pericolic abscesses (55–57), although concern has been expressed that the diagnostic advantages of CT do not justify the increased expense (58).

Thus, the early knowledge of diverticulosis consisted almost entirely of observations on the complications initiating clinical attention; namely, abscess, perforation, and obstruction. Because no applicable data were specifically concerned with the etiology of these complications (and there still are none), conclusions were limited to experiences with analogous blind structures with narrow orifices and the observation of fecaliths within diverticula (59). It was assumed that obstruction of the orifice of the sac caused stasis and fecalith formation, leading to the subsequent inflammatory process or diverticulitis. In addition, fecaliths were assumed to cause pressure necrosis and erosion of the mucosa of the diverticular sac. Although this sequence of events seems logical, little evidence exists that erosion by fecaliths initiates the infection or the "microperforation" commonly assumed to trigger a diverticulitis (59–61). In 1965 (62) and again in 1975 (3), the inflammatory process was found to begin in the peridiverticular tissue, not in the mucosa of the sac as might be predicted if fecalith erosion were implicated. Further, no microscopic evidence of inflammation is found in almost half of the resected specimens from symptomatic patients (29,32) and no correlation was found between relevant symptoms and pathologic evidence of inflammation at autopsy in unrelated deaths (1,63). Nevertheless, in the absence of alternative explanations of the factor(s) that initiates the local infection, fecaliths continue to be implicated (60,61,64).

CHANGES IN TREATMENT

Diverticulosis

Until about 25 years ago, it was common practice to restrict the diet in patients who were discovered to have diverticulosis, with or without symptoms. Since no data existed before the mid-1960s to suggest that diverticulosis actually could be prevented, this prescription was directed at prevention of complications. Because obstruction of the narrow neck of diverticula appeared to be the cause of diverticulitis, a low-fiber ("non-irritating") diet devoid of particulate matter such as corn, grape skins, and seeds (65,66) was recommended. Until at least the decade of the 1960s, this diet was commonly prescribed in asymptomatic diverticulosis (25,65). No satisfactory investigations were published that demonstrated the effectiveness of a bland, "low-residue" intake, but it had the strong support of centuries of empiric dietary manipulation in many illnesses. By 1960, multiple observations had documented the relative infrequency of complications of incidentally discovered diverticula (24,67) regardless of diet and most physicians no longer insisted on a low residue intake in asymptomatic individuals with diverticulosis.

The observations of Painter (38–41), Burkitt (6), and others led to abandoning low-fiber diets in favor of high-fiber intake in an attempt to influence the development of colonic diverticula. "Fiber deficiency" also has been incriminated in the etiology of colon cancer (68,69). Because a high-fiber intake, at least theoretically, mitigates against segmentation of the colon, it would be expected not only to reduce the frequency of diverticula but to reduce symptoms in those with diverticula. Although high-fiber intake has been associated with decreased abdominal pain in symptomatic patients (60), no prospective study has yet demonstrated a reduction in the risk of developing either diverticulosis or diverticulitis (46). Nevertheless, clinical experience and circumstantial evidence have established the high-fiber diet as the most appropriate diet for colonic diverticulosis in addition to its other benefits (48,49,68–71).

Diverticulitis

Before the antibiotic era, the treatment of painful diverticula and complications of diverticulosis was surgical. Mayo described diverting colostomy and resection in 1907 (56). Because of persistently high mortality rates largely related to infection, Smithwick (1942) advised a multistage procedure (72) that became the conventional approach (59); that is, an operation to drain the abscess and provide a diverting colostomy; a second procedure to resect the diseased segment, and a third to close the colostomy and re-establish bowel continuity. From 1950 to 1970 or so, an aggressive or even prophylactic one-stage surgical resection to avoid complications was advocated by many surgeons (73–77). However, experience with incidentally discovered diverticula did not support prophylactic therapy (24,67). On the other hand, about 70 to 80% of patients treated for acute diverticulitis with antibiotics and no surgical procedure had no further symptoms or did not require hospital admissions for their disease (78,79). By 1970, antibiotics had had a significant impact in reducing morbidity and mortality. Further, the ability to percutaneously drain abscesses (57) made resection and reanastomosis as a single-stage procedure the therapy of choice in complicated acute diverticulitis. Currently, textbooks of both gastroenterology and surgery advise medical treatment for the first episode and surgery only for unresolved or recurrent episodes of acute diverticulitis, using a one-stage primary resection in most instances (60,61,63).

SUMMARY

Medicine has advanced from a position of recognizing diverticulosis of the colon only in the presence of a complication to its recognition as a common disease. Clinical information gradually is being accumulated to provide a more rational therapeutic approach. Preventive methods have yet to be fully established. Although the accumulated data are compatible with the hypothesis that colonic diverticulosis is a problem of aging in association with a biologically inappropriate diet, many questions remain that are difficult to resolve without further investigation and the long-term observation of large numbers of patients.

REFERENCES

1. Parks TG: Postmortem studies of the colon with special references to diverticular disease. Proc R Soc Med *61*:932, 1968.
2. Smith CC, Christensen WR: The incidence of colonic diverticulosis. AJR *82*:996, 1959.
3. Morson BC: Pathology of diverticular disease of the colon. Clin Gastroenterol *4*:37, 1975.
4. Hughes LE: Post mortem survey of diverticular disease of the colon. Part II. The muscular abnormality in the sigmoid colon. Gut *10*:344, 1969.
5. Kohler R: The incidence of colonic diverticulosis in Finland and Sweden. Acta Chir Scand *126*:148, 1963.
6. Painter NS, Burkitt DP: Diverticular disease of the colon: A deficiency disease of Western civilization. Br Med J *2*:450, 1971.
7. Telling WHM, Gruner OC: Acquired diverticula, diverticulitis, and peridiverticulitis of the large intestine. Br J Surg *4*:468, 1917.
8. Voigtel FG: Handbuch der pathologischen anatomie, Vol 2, page 575, 1804. Quoted by Telling and Gruner (7), Fisher (19) and Slack (17).
9. Beer E: Some pathological and clinical aspects of acquired (false) diverticula of the intestine. Am J Med Sci *128*:135, 1904.
10. Eisenberg RL: Radiology. An Illustrated History. Chicago, Mosby Year Book, 1992.
11. Bachem C, Gunther H: Barium sulfate as a shadow-forming contrast agent in roentgenologic examinations. Zietschr fur Rontenkunde, *12*:369, 1910. Quoted by Eisenberg (10), p. 264.
12. Schule A: Intubation and radiography of the large intestine. Arch Verdauungskr *10*:111, 1904. Quoted by Eisenberg (10), p. 278.
13. Case JT: The roentgen demonstration of multiple diverticula of the colon. AJR *2*:654, 1914.
14. DeQuervain F: Zur diagnose der erworbenen dick arm divertikel und der sigmoiditis

diverticularis. Deutsche ztschr F Chir *128*: 67, 1914. Quoted by Rege, RV and Nohrwold: Diverticular disease. Curr Probl Surg *26*:133, 1989.

15. Fischer AW: A new roentgenologic method for examination of the large intestine. A combination of the contrast material enema and insufflation with air. Klin Wschr *2*:1595, 1923. Quoted by Eisenberg (10), p. 280.

16. Klebs E: Die Veranderurgen der gan zen darmwand. Handbuch Pathologischen. Path Anatomie, 1867, p. 271. Quoted by Telling and Gruner (7), Beer (9), and Fisher (19).

17. Slack WW: Diverticula of the colon and their relation to the muscle layers and blood vessels. Gastroenterology *39*:708, 1960.

18. Noer RJ: Hemorrhage as a complication of diverticulitis. Ann Surg *141*:674, 1955.

19. Fisher MH: False diverticula of the intestine. J Exp Med *5*:333, 1900.

20. Hansemann D: Ueber die Emtgstehorg falscher Darmdivertikel. Virch Arch, 1846. Quoted by Telling and Gruner (7), Beer (9).

21. Quoted by Beer (9).

22. Spriggs EI, Marxer OA: Intestinal diverticula. Quart J Med *19*:1, 1927.

23. Willard JH, Bockus HL: Clinical and therapeutic status of cases of colonic diverticulosis seen in office practice. Am J Dig Dis *3*: 580, 1936.

24. Horner JL: Natural history of diverticulosis of the colon. Am J Dig Dis *3*:343, 1958.

25. Palmer ED: Clinical Gastroenterology. New York, Paul B. Hoeber, Inc., Harper & Brothers, 1957.

26. Mendeloff AI: Diseases of the colon and rectum. *In* Wintrobe M et al. (eds): Harrison's Principles of Internal Medicine, Sixth Edition, New York, McGraw-Hill, 1970, p. 1500.

27. Spiro HM: Clinical Gastroenterology. Toronto, The Macmillan Co., 1970, pp. 550.

28. Keith A: Diverticula of the alimentary tract of congenital or of obscure origin. Br Med J *1*:376, 1910.

29. Morson B: The muscle abnormalities in diverticular disease of the colon. Br J Radiol *36*:385, 1963.

30. Arfwidsson S: Pathogenesis of multiple diverticula of the sigmoid colon in diverticular disease. Acta Chir Scand *130*(Suppl):342, 1965.

31. Fleischner FG, Ming S, Henken EM: Revised concepts on diverticular disease of the colon. I. Diverticulosis: Emphasis on tissue derangement and its relation to the irritable colon syndrome. Radiology *83*:859, 1964.

32. Fleischner FG: Diverticular disease of the colon. New observations and revised concepts. Gastroenterology *60*:316, 1971.

33. Eastwood MA, Watters DAK, Smith AN: Diverticular disease—is it a motility disorder? Clin Gastroenterol *11*:545, 1982.

34. Eastwood MA, Brydon WG, Smith AN, Pritchard J: Colonic function in patients with diverticular disease. Lancet *i*:1181, 1978.

35. Holmes KM, Salter RH: Irritable bowel syndrome—a safe diagnosis? Br Med J *285*: 1533, 1982.

36. Havia T, Manner R: The irritable colon syndrome. Acta Chir Scand *137*:569, 1971.

37. Connell AM: Applied physiology of the colon: Factors relevant to diverticular disease. Clin Gastroenterol *4*:23, 1975.

38. Painter NS, Truelove SC: The intraluminal pressure patterns in diverticulosis of the colon. 1. Resting patterns of pressure. Gut *5*:201, 1964.

39. Painter NS, Truelove SC: The intraluminal pressure patterns in diverticulosis of the colon. 2. The effect of morphine. Gut *5*:207, 1964.

40. Painter NS, Truelove SC: The intraluminal pressure patterns in diverticulosis of the colon. 3. The effect of prostigmine. Gut *5*: 365, 1964.

41. Painter NS, Truelove SC, Ardran GM, Tuckey M: Segmentation and the localization of intraluminal pressures in the human colon, with special reference to the pathogenesis of colonic diverticula. Gastroenterology *49*:169, 1965.

42. Wells C: Diverticula of the colon. Br J Radiol *22*:449, 1949.

43. Segal I, Solomon A, Hunt JA: Emergence of diverticular disease in the urban South African black. Gastroenterology *72*:215, 1977.

44. Stemmermann GN, Yatani R: Diverticulosis and polyps of the large intestine: A necropsy study of Hawaii Japanese. Cancer *31*:1260, 1973.

45. Carlson AJ, Hoelzel F: Relation of diet to diverticulosis of the colon in rats. Gastroenterology *12*:108, 1949.

46. Almy TP, Howell DA: Diverticular disease of the colon. N Engl J Med *302*:324, 1980.

47. Almy TP: Diverticular disease of the colon—the new look. Gastroenterology *49*: 109, 1965.

48. Burkitt DP, Walker ARP, Painter NS: Effect of dietary fiber in stools and transit times and its role in the causation of disease. Lancet *ii*: 1408, 1972.

49. Almy TP: The role of fiber in the diet. Curr Conc Nutr *4*:155, 1976.

50. Whiteway J, Morson BC: Pathology of the ageing—Diverticular disease. Clin Gastroenterol *14*:829, 1985.

51. Watters DA, Smith AN: Strength of the colon wall in diverticular disease. Br J Surg *77*:257, 1990.

52. Kourtesis GJ, Williams RA, Wilson SE: Acute diverticulitis: Safety and value of contrast studies in predicting need for operation. Aust NZ J Surg 58:801, 1988.

53. Smith TR, Cho KC, Morehouse HT, Kratka PS: Comparison of computed tomography and contrast enema evaluation of diverticulitis. Dis Colon Rectum 33:1, 1990.

54. Balthazar EJ, Megibow A, Schinella RA, Gordon R: Limitations in the CT diagnosis of acute diverticulitis: Comparison of CT, contrast enema, and pathologic findings in 16 patients. AJR 154:281, 1990.

55. Feczko PJ, Nish AD, Craig BM, Simms SM: Acute diverticulitis in patients under 40 years of age—Radiologic diagnosis. AJR 150:1311, 1988.

56. Mayo WJ, Wilson LB, Griffin HZ: Acquired diverticulitis of the large intestine. Surg Gynec Obstet 5:8, 1907.

57. Neff CC et al: Diverticular abscesses: Percutaneous drainage. Radiology 163:15, 1987.

58. Glick SN: Colonic imaging. Curr Opin Gastroenterol 7:46, 1991.

59. Johnston JH Jr: Diverticular disease of the colon. In Hardy JD (ed): Rhoads Textbook of Surgery. Principles and Practice, Fifth Edition. Philadelphia, JB Lippincott Co., 1977.

60. Beart RW Jr, Navatvongs S, Wolff B: The colon, rectum, and anus. In Nova PF (ed): Operative Surgery. Principles and Techniques. Philadelphia, 1990, WB Saunders Co, p. 616.

61. Imbembo AL, Bailey RW: Diverticular disease of the colon. In Sabiston DC (ed): Textbook of Surgery, Fourteenth Edition. Philadelphia, WB Saunders Co., 1991, p. 917.

62. Ming SC, Fleischner FG: Diverticulitis of the sigmoid colon: Reappraisal of pathology and pathogenesis. Surgery 58:627, 1965.

63. Hughes LE: Postmortem survey of diverticular disease of the colon. I. Diverticulosis and diverticulitis. Gut 10:336, 1969.

64. Naitove A, Almy TP: Diverticular disease of the colon. In Sleisenger MH, Fordtran JS (eds): Gastrointestinal Disease. Pathophysiology, Diagnosis, Management, Fourth edition. Philadelphia, WB Saunders Co, 1989, p. 1419.

65. Schuster MM: Diverticulosis and diverticulitis. In Paulson M (ed): Gastroenterologic Medicine. Philadelphia, Lea & Febiger, 1969, p. 1518.

66. de la Vega JM, Gonzalez JN, de Leon AP: Colonic diverticula. In Bockus HL (ed): Gastroenterology, Second Edition, Vol. II. Philadelphia, WB Saunders, 1964, p. 931.

67. Boles RS, Jordan SM: The clinical significance of diverticulosis. Gastroenterology 35:579, 1958.

68. Burkitt DP: Epidemiology of cancer of the colon and rectum. Cancer 28:3, 1971.

69. Reddy BS: Diet and colon cancer: Evidence from human and animal model studies. In Reddy BS, Cohen LA (eds): Diet, Nutrition and Cancer: A Critical Evaluation, Vol I. Boca Raton, CRC Press, 1986, p. 47.

70. Brodribb AJ: Treatment of symptomatic diverticular disease with a high-fiber diet. Lancet i:664, 1977.

71. Reilly RW, Kirsner JB: Dietary fiber and the colon. In Glass GBJ (ed): Progress in Gastroenterology, Vol. III. New York, Grune and Stratton, 1977, p. 521.

72. Smithwick RH: Experiences with the surgical management of diverticulitis of the sigmoid. Ann Surg 115:969, 1942.

73. Bartlett JK, McDermott WV: Surgical treatment of diverticulosis of the colon. N Engl J Med 248:497, 1953.

74. Smithwick RH: Surgical treatment of diverticulitis of the sigmoid. Am J Surg 99:192, 1970.

75. Moseley RV, Ross FP: Sigmoid diverticulitis. Evaluation of current practice in a community hospital. Ann Surg 164:275, 1966.

76. Penfold JCB: Management of uncomplicated diverticular disease by colonic resection in patients at St. Mark's hospital, 1964–9. Br J Surg 60:695, 1973.

77. Eusebio EB, Eisenberg MM: Natural history of diverticular disease of the colon in young patients. Am J Surg 125:308, 1973.

78. Larson DM, Masters SS, Spiro HM: Medical and surgical therapy in diverticular disease. A comparative study. Gastroenterology 71:734, 1976.

79. Parks TG: Natural history of diverticular disease of the colon. Clin Gastroenterol 4:53, 1976.

Liver

17

Bile: A Historical Review of Studies on its Form and Function

ULRICH BEUERS AND JAMES L. BOYER

"Ich weiss, dass die Galle ein nothwendig Glied des Lebens, ein Balsam des Bluts und der Leber ist."

Johann B. van Helmont, 1683*

Bile has attracted the attention of physicians and researchers for more than 3500 years and was first mentioned in the Ebers Papyrus (circa 1550 B.C.) as a useful remedy and purge. For centuries, bile was regarded as a major constituent of the human body, essential for health when present in an appropriate amount, but also a source of anger and rage. However, by the 16th and 17th centuries, bile was thought to be of little use other than a refuge for the sewage of the body, until its digestive function was recognized during the last 300 years. Today's knowledge of the function and formation of bile, still far from complete, is based on observations and studies covering 2000 years. This chapter begins with observations, views, and myths of the ancient world and then describes the first experimental findings obtained in the 17th and 18th century and the subsequent application of the disciplines of chemistry, physiology, and histomorphology during the 19th century. It then concludes by focusing on the enormous growth of knowledge of bile formation and function during the 20th century. In view of the extensive contributions to this field over the years, this overview will inevitably be incomplete. We apologize to many authors, past and present, for the omission of numerous excellent studies.

THE ANCIENT WORLD

τὸ δὲ σῶμα τοῦ ἀνθρώπου ἔχει ἐν ἑαυτῷ αἷμα

καὶ φλέγμα καὶ χολὴν ξανθήν τε καὶ μέλαιναν

Corpus Hippocraticum, 4th to 5th century B.C.†

The existence of bile ("water") had already been mentioned in ancient Babylonian sources which focused on the liver as the seat of the soul. Early medical reports related vomiting of bile to a burning pain in the stomach. Jaundice was described as "when the body is yellow, yellow the face, and the flesh is trembling. . . ". The preSocratic philosophers in ancient Greece were among the first to reflect on the formation and function of bile ("chole"), and they believed that bile either originated in the liver

* "I know that bile is necessary for life, a balm for blood and liver." J. B. Van Helmont: Sechsfache Verdauung (German Edition). 1683; §37:269 (2).

† "The human body contains blood, phlegm, yellow and black bile." Corpus Hippocraticum. De natura hominis. Circa 5th century B.C.

or was a "juice of flesh." Anaxagoras of Klazomenae (500–430 B.C.) regarded bile as the source of numerous diseases when it flooded the lungs or the blood vessels.

The Corpus Hippocraticum, a collection of papers and books of the 5th and 4th century B.C., was obtained from medical schools in Greece and Southern Italy and gathered under the name of Hippocrates of Cos (ca. 460–377 B.C.), the founder of a humanistic and rational medicine. It gave detailed information about physiologic and pathophysiologic ideas and clinical observations of that time. The liver was regarded as the major organ of bile formation, and some sources thought that jaundice was explained by flooding of body and skin with bile caused by liver disease. Others thought that jaundice resulted from disassembly of humors of the body with yellow bile, the lightest fluid, rising to the skin. The Hippocratic concepts were based on the theory of four humors whose harmonious equilibrium in the human body was fundamental for health, a theory which assembled concepts of Heraclitus of Ephesus (circa 550–475 B.C.), Pythagoras of Samos (circa 580–489 B.C.), Empedocles of Agrigentum (circa 495–435 B.C.) and others. These humors represented the four basic elements (fire, water, earth, and air) and were characterized by opposing qualities (warm, cold, moist, and dry). Yellow bile was warm and dry, blood was warm and moist, phlegm was cold and moist, and black bile was cold and dry. An imbalance in the quantity of the fluids or a qualitative alteration of one of the fluids resulted in disease; a surplus of yellow bile or phlegm was the most common causes of disease. The fluids were assumed to be collected in four reservoirs, the gallbladder (yellow bile) which was regarded as the most differentiated reservoir, the spleen (black bile), the head (phlegm), and the heart (blood). The gallbladder, like the other reservoirs, was believed to suck its fluid, the yellow bile, like a cupping-glass out of the abdominal cavity—a concept that was perhaps the first functional view of bile formation. Feces and urine were regarded as physiologic excretory routes for yellow bile. The content of bile in feces, urine, saliva, menstrual blood, earwax, or mother's milk provided information about potential bile disturbances. When bile was presumed

to be in excess, the patient was treated with cholagogues like cabbage or honey water.

Plato (427–347 B.C.) thought that bile resulted from disintegrated flesh, and was yellow when formed from young flesh but black when formed from old flesh. He localized bile formation within as well as outside the liver.

Aristotle (384–322 B.C.) provided the first careful and detailed anatomic description of the bile duct system from different animal species and concluded that bile flow is limited to a specific net of vessels. He reduced the view of the Hippocratic school that bile is one of the principal constituting fluids of the body and ranked yellow and black bile with other useless excrements like feces and phlegm. Aristotle also denied a pathogenic role for bile as first claimed by Anaxagoras.

Diocles of Karystos, a contemporary of Aristotle, performed extended anatomic studies of liver and biliary tract and concluded that jaundice wᴗs the consequence of obstruction of the bile ducts. Many of the findings and thoughts of Aristotle and Diocles were appreciated only 2000 years later because the Corpus Hippocraticum and the theories of Galen dominated Western medical thought up to the 17th and 18th centuries.

Alexandria was the center of medical and biologic research of the Hellenistic period. There the development of scientific dissections of the human body as well as the first physiologic experiments in living animals led to a better understanding of human anatomy, pathology, physiology, and pathophysiology. Erasistratos (circa 300–250 B.C.) of Alexandria offered the first detailed hypothesis on bile formation and excretion. Based on anatomic studies of the liver tissue ("parenchyma"), which led to the description of a hepatic network of blood and bile vessels and the venous blood supply of the liver, Erasistratos claimed that the bile—in his eyes a useless and potentially harmful fluid, which may be part of the ingested food or a product of gastric digestion—was separated from other components of nutrition after transport from the stomach by way of the portal vein into the liver. In his view, the capillary sink of the liver separated the more viscous blood from the more fluid bile. Erasistratos reduced bile formation to a purely physical phenomenon explained by different sizes of hepatic venous capillaries and the smaller bile capillaries within the liver.

Throughout the period of the Roman Empire, major progress was made in many cultural and scientific fields. However, medical knowledge did not advance. In particular, knowledge of the function and formation of bile was almost negligible. Ruphos of Ephesos (circa 100 A.D.) and Arataeus of Cappadocia (circa 150 A.D.) described the existence of yellow and black bile, much like their Greek predecessors. Formation of yellow bile occurred within, but also outside, the liver. Black bile was equal to the dark component of blood.

Galen of Pergamon (circa 130–201 A.D.) was the single most productive physician and researcher of the ancient world, as reflected by the size of his medical writings. He created a unifying concept of human anatomy and physiology that summarized medical studies over a period of 700 years. Like those of Aristotle, his anatomic descriptions of gallbladder and bile ducts were based on comparative studies in different animal species. In his view, the liver was the organ of blood formation where resorbed "chylus" entered the liver by way of the portal vein and was transformed into red, watery blood and yellow and black bile, a process comparable to fermentation of wine. Red, watery blood then reached the vena cava, where water was extracted by the kidneys. Yellow bile, the light, foamy, and bitter component of the chylus, was sucked into the gallbladder and poured out into the intestine, where it stimulated intestinal contraction and defecation, cleaned the intestinal interior, and dyed the feces. Black bile, a heavy, soil-like component of the chylus, was sucked by the spleen and excreted into the stomach. Galen's model of bile formation, based on views and myths of several centuries, became dogma and was not refuted until 1500 years later (1–4).

THE MIDDLE AGES AND THE RENAISSANCE

All areas of life became dominated by a dogmatic Christian Church, which stifled creative scientific thinking during the Middle Ages. For 1300 years, no significant

progress occurred in the entire field of medicine. The concepts of Galen were delivered without change from one generation to the next, as was the Christian literature. After more than 1000 years, Leonardo da Vinci (1452–1519) and Andreas Vesalius (1514–1564) were among the first to re-establish scientific thinking when they performed their extensive studies on liver anatomy and physiology (2–4). However, despite their fundamental studies, the most lasting thought about the role of bile in human life of this period was not proclaimed by physician scientists but by William Shakespeare's Hamlet:

"It cannot be
But I am pigeon-livered and lack gall
To make oppression bitter, or ere this
I should ha' fatted all the region kites
With this slave's offal. Bloody, bawdy villain!"*

17TH AND 18TH CENTURY

"Bilis . . . cum aqua subacta vires gerit saponis, et solvit oleum, ut aquae misceatur."

Albrecht von Haller, 1764†

Johann Baptista Van Helmont (1579–1644) was the first to clearly recognize that digestion was an important function of bile, and introduced this idea based on chemical analysis and by comparison of bile formation in different animal species. In subsequent decades, the chemistry of bile was analyzed with available methods by many different investigators, including Francis Glisson (1597–1677), Franciscus Sylvius de la Boe (1614–1672), Marcello Malpighi (1628–1694), Johannes Bohn (1640–1718), and Hermann Boerhaave (1668–1738). These studies indicated that bile was a water-soluble, soap-like, alkaline fluid that reacted with different color indicators. The process of bile formation was mainly explained by mechanical filtration within the liver, a theory which dated back to Erasistratos almost 2000 years earlier. The idea that bile was formed in the gallbladder (Syl-

---

* Shakespeare W. Hamlet, Prince of Denmark: II; ii:561–565. Published 1604 (4).

† "Bile has the properties of soap when it is mixed with water and it solves fat in water." A. von Haller. Elementa physiologica corporis humani VI. 1764 (2).

vius de la Boe) was opposed by animal experiments of Marcello Malpighi (1666), Johann Bohn (1686), and Giuseppe Zambeccari (1680), who demonstrated that bile was formed in spite of ligation of the cystic bile duct or extirpation of the gallbladder. The secretory pressure of bile was determined by Johann Georg Seeger (1739) in dogs at about 30 cm H_2O. Mauritius Reverhorst (1690) and Alfonso Borelli (1710) observed a marked difference between the amount of bile produced daily and the amount recovered in the feces and proposed the existence of a "motus circularis bilis," the enterohepatic circulation.

The "Elementa Physiologica Corporis Humani" of Albrecht von Haller (1764) represented the first detailed synthesis of anatomy and physiology since Galen's work 1600 years earlier, and described the functions of bile as (1) forming fat-water emulsions in the intestine to facilitate resorption of nutrients, in particular fatty contents, (2) neutralizing acids in the intestine, and (3) stimulating intestinal motility.

The last 30 years of the 18th century were characterized by considerable progress in the chemical analysis of bile. Bile salt crystals (Robert Ramsay, 1757) and cholesterol crystals (Benjamin Gottlob Friedrich Conradi 1775) were identified. The work of F.P.L. Poulletier de la Salle (1719–1787), Louis Claude Cadet (1731–1799) and Friedrich Albrecht Carl Gren (1760–1798) and his own extensive studies allowed Antoine Francois Fourcroy (1755–1809) to conclude in his "système des connaissances chimiques" (1801) that bile was an alkaline soaplike fluid composed of (1) water, (2) sodium, (3) an oily substance bound to sodium (bile acids), (4) a coloring substance (bilirubin), (5) a bitter-smelling oily substance (bile acids), (6) an animal coagulating substance, (7) a sugar, (8) and several salts, ferrumoxide (2–4).

19TH AND 20TH CENTURY

"Il est peu de substances qui aient autant attiré l'attention des chimistes que la bile. . ."

H. Demarcay, 1838*

* "There exist few substances which have attracted the attention of chemists like bile has. . ." C. Demarcay: De la nature de la bile. Ann Chem Phys (Paris) 67:177, 1838 (2).

Studies on bile formation and function performed and published during the last decades of the 18th century represented the start of a new era of enormous growth in anatomic, physiologic, and pathophysiologic knowledge. The diversity of excellent studies makes a comprehensive review difficult. Therefore, only selected areas will be reviewed.

Components of Bile

Bile Pigment

Chemistry and Metabolism. The bile pigment, visible as jaundice in patients with liver and bile duct disease, was well known to physicians for more than 2000 years. A yellow pigment was first mentioned as one of several components of bile by Fourcroy (1801) and Thenard (1806). Tiedemann and Gmelin (1824) were the first to describe a chemical reaction for the detection of the bile pigment, the classic "Gmelin reaction," an oxidation of bilirubin with nitric acid. Using this method, they detected bile pigment not only in bile, but also in the urine and chylus of bile duct-ligated dogs. In addition, Gmelin described a change in color from yellow-brown to green when bile was exposed to oxygen, but not in its absence, and correctly concluded that this bile pigment existed in a reduced, brown-yellow form (later called bilirubin) or an oxidized, green form (later called biliverdin). However, he was not the first to describe color changes of bile; they had been observed in bile exposed to air or acids and recorded more than 1500 years before by Galen. Berzelius (1840) characterized further properties of the bile pigment and described biliverdin. R. Virchow (1847) was the first to assume a similarity between blood pigment and bile pigment when he identified hematoidin crystals in a brain extravasate that reminded him of bile pigment crystals. His theory was confirmed 76 years later when H. Fischer (1923) (5) proved the identity of crystalline bilirubin and hematoidin by crystallography. Heintz (1851) isolated the yellow bile pigment and its green oxidation product from bile; Frerichs and Staedeler (1856) and Kuehne (1858) isolated these pigments from urine. Valentiner (1859) succeeded in precipitating bile pigment in its crystalline form using chloroform and was able to recognize similar appearance of bile and blood pigment crystals. Finally, F. Staedeler (1863) named his brown bile pigment "bilirubin" (bile red), a term that superseded former and later names like "cholephyrrhine" (Berzelius, 1840), "biliphaenin" (Simon, 1845), or "cholophaeine" (Thudichum, 1868). M. Jaffé (1868) isolated and characterized a similar substance from human urine, which he named "urobilin." Vanlair and Masius (1871) identified "stercobilin" in the feces. A number of additional metabolites were described and named during the following decades. However many of those were found to be artefacts in an extensive and brilliant chemical analysis of bilirubin and its metabolites performed by H. Fischer (1911) (6). In 1933, Siedel and Fischer (7) succeeded in determining the chemical structure of bilirubin, and in 1942, H. Fischer and H. Plieninger (8) were the first to synthesize the bilirubin molecule containing four pyrrole rings linked by three carbon bridges in an open chain structure.

The site of bilirubin formation was a matter of interest and controversy for almost a century. J. Mueller (1844) observed that bile pigment did not accumulate in serum of frogs after hepatectomy, and concluded that the liver was the only source of bilirubin. In contrast, R. Virchow (1847) emphasized the appearance of hemolytic jaundice in patients in the absence of liver disease. Support for the hepatic formation of bile pigment came 40 years later from Minkowski and Naunyn (1886), who treated animals with arsenic which induced severe jaundice. Jaundice was not observed if the liver was first removed ("Ohne Leber kein Ikterus"—"without the liver, no icterus"). The role of the reticuloendothelial system (RES) in the formation of bilirubin was first considered by Loewit (1889), who injected hemoglobin and found bile pigment and iron in hepatic sinusoidal cells (Kupffer cells), but not in hepatocytes. Aschoff and coworkers (1913) (9) confirmed the potential role of the RES in bilirubin formation by repeating the experiments of Minkowski and Naunyn. However, they focused on changes in the appearance of the Kupffer cells after exposure of their animals to arsenic and detected accumulation of iron and bile pigment in these cells. In addition, they

could prevent the appearance of jaundice in their arsenic-treated animals by pretreating them with colloidal silver to specifically block RES function. The exclusive role of the liver in the formation of bilirubin was finally disproved by Mann and coworkers (1924) (10), who clearly showed that bilirubin could also be formed in dogs in extrahepatic tissues after removal of the liver.

P. Ehrlich (1883) had demonstrated that bilirubin could react with diazo substances and form a colored reaction product. Based on this finding, Hijmans van den Bergh (1913) succeeded in developing a sensitive colorimetric assay for the determination of bilirubin in serum (11). It was necessary to pretreat serum with alcohol to extract all bilirubin as part of the assay. Van den Bergh then observed (1918) that a portion of bilirubin in serum could be determined without prior alcoholic extraction, and that the serum levels of this bilirubin were increased in patients with bile duct obstruction (12). He concluded that bilirubin in serum exists in two distinct forms, the "direct" (detectable without prior alcoholic extraction) hepatic bilirubin and the "indirect" (detectable only after prior alcoholic extraction from serum) anhepatic bilirubin. In addition, he found higher levels of bilirubin in venous serum of the spleen, suggesting that the reticuloendothelial system played a role in the formation of bilirubin as had been suggested earlier by Aschoff's group. Further evidence for at least two different types of bilirubin came from differences in solubility of bilirubin in hemolytic as compared to hepatic icterus (Grunenberg, 1923) (13) and from differences in the absorption spectra (Davis and Sheard, 1937) (14).

In 1937, Eppinger summarized the accumulated knowledge on chemistry and metabolism of bilirubin in his handbook of liver diseases (15) and referred, in particular, to the extensive studies of Hans Fischer, Hijmans van den Bergh (both Nobel laureates), and Ludwig Aschoff: Bilirubin is formed from hemoglobin in the RES and is transported to the liver, where it is transferred from its protein-bound form to its free form, which is excreted into bile. The chemical difference between direct and indirect bilirubin was long believed to be the protein binding of the indirect form which, in fact, is more tightly bound to serum albumin than the direct form and is not dialyzable, as opposed to the direct form. Not until 1953, when two protein-free bilirubin fractions were isolated from cholestatic serum by reverse-phase partition chromatography was it clear that protein binding could not account for differences in indirect- and direct-reacting bilirubin (Cole and Lathe 1953) (16). Simultaneous studies of Schmid (1956, 1957), Talefant (1956), and Billing et al. (1957) (17–21) demonstrated that bilirubin was converted to mono- and diglucuronide esters in the liver with uridine diphosphate (UDP) glucuronic acid as the donor (Schmid et al., 1957, Lathe and Walker 1958) (22,23). The site of glucuronidation was subsequently localized to the endoplasmic reticulum, and ultimately the responsible enzyme was found to be one single isoform of a UDP-glucuronyltransferase (Lathe and Walker 1957, Roy Chowdhury 1986) (24–26).

Nearly 30 years later, a third type of serum bilirubin was identified by Lauff and coworkers (1981) (27). This was covalently bound to albumin and was detected by Weiss and coworkers (1983) in cholestatic liver disease, but not in hemolytic jaundice (28). This derivative, which is probably a bilirubin glucuronide, was initially suspected by Kuenzle and coworkers (1966) (29). In bile, low amounts of glucose and xylose conjugates also are detected (Fevery, 1972) (30).

For a long time, the lipophilicity of unconjugated bilirubin was poorly understood because this property appeared to contradict the linear structure of the molecule as described by Fischer and Plieninger 1942 (8). Fog and Jellum (1963) suggested that strong intramolecular hydrogen bonding might provide an explanation (31), and this was first demonstrated by Bonnett and coworkers using x-ray analysis (1976) (32).

Bilirubin was recognized as a product of hemoglobin degradation for decades before it was established that degradation of nonerythrocyte heme molecules, mostly of hepatic and renal origin, also contributed to the formation of total bilirubin by approximately 30% (Robinson 1972, Berk et al., 1976) (33,34). Purification (Burchell 1980) (35) and molecular cloning (Ritter et al., 1991; Wooster et al., 1991) (36,37) of the UDP glucuronyltransferase responsible for

conjugation of bilirubin in the hepatocyte represent important steps for the understanding of bilirubin metabolism.

Transport. The mechanism of transport from blood to bile of organic anions like bilirubin, and bile acids and other biliary components has been of more recent interest during the last 20 years as new investigative techniques have become available. Hepatic uptake of bilirubin is carrier-mediated and saturable, but the rate of transport is far below the physiologic transport maximum under physiologic conditions and therefore hepatic uptake is not rate limiting for the excretion of bilirubin (Goresky 1975, Scharschmidt 1975, Paumgartner 1976) (38–40). Unconjugated and conjugated bilirubin seem to share the same multispecific organic anion transporter in the basolateral (sinusoidal) membrane of the hepatocyte and thus compete with other organic anions. The transport is bidirectional (Scharschmidt 1975, Berk 1969) (39,41). After transport across the membrane, bilirubin is mainly bound to a cytosolic binding protein ligandin, also called glutathione-S-transferase or Y protein (Levi et al. 1969) (42), a 47 kDa basic protein (Bhargava et al. 1980) (43) which forms up to 5% of soluble protein of the human liver. Ligandin is not directly involved in the uptake process of bilirubin across the basolateral membrane (Wolkoff, 1979) (44). Whether ligandin facilitates diffusion of bilirubin between plasma membrane and endoplasmic reticulum or decreases the efflux of bilirubin back into the plasma, remains unclear. Bilirubin molecules may partly bypass the cytosolic compartment and binding to ligandin or other binding proteins by partitioning into intracellular membranes and undergoing membrane-membrane transport (Whitmer 1984) (45).

Glucuronidation within the endoplasmic reticulum (see previous text) precedes the efficient and rapid transport of conjugated bilirubin to the canalicular membrane which occurs by two major pathways: (1) a microtubule-dependent, colchicine-inhibitable vesicular pathway (Crawford 1988) (46); (2) a microtubule-independent pathway in which bilirubin glucuronides are probably bound to binding proteins (Wolkoff 1978; see previous text) (47).

The final step involves excretion of bilirubin glucuronides across the canalicular membrane into bile and is the rate-limiting step (Goresky 1975) (50). This transport step appears to be mediated by an ATP-driven multiple organic anion transporter and occurs against a concentration gradient within the canalicular lumen (Kitamura 1990) (48).

Bile Acids

Structure. Fourcroy, in his "système des connaissances chimiques" (1801), put forth one of the first chemical analyses of bile components. These substances included water, sodium, an oily substance bound to sodium, a coloring substance, and a bitter-smelling, oily substance. The oily substances probably represented bile acids. Another early chemical investigation of bile composition was performed by L. J. Thenard (1806). By exposing ox bile to acids and bases and performing alcoholic extractions, he was able to separate three groups of substances, which he called "pikromel" (presumably unpure taurocholic acid), "bile resin" (presumably unpure glycocholic acid), and a yellow substance (presumably bilirubin). J. J. Berzelius, one of the outstanding chemists of the 19th century, published a report on bile analysis in 1808 and described a single bile substance, "bilin" (presumably a mixture of bile acids). The beginning of bile acid chemistry is connected to the name of L. Gmelin, a chemist from Heidelberg, who in cooperation with the anatomist Tiedemann, published an extensive study on digestive functions including a detailed chemical analysis of bile. He confirmed Fourcroy's and Thenard's report of a yellow substance (bilirubin), Thenard's pikromel and bile resin, and Chevreul's bile fat (cholesterine-cholesterol). In addition, he isolated a substance which he first called bile asparagine, but which later was called taurine because it was found in ox bile (tauros = ox), but not in pig bile. Also, he was the first to succeed in reasonably purifying one major substrate of bile which he called cholsäure (cholic acid according to its acid-like properties and its isolation from bile, chole = bile). His cholic acid presumably represented glycocholic acid. In 1838, Demarcay, a coworker of Liebig in Giessen, stated that 90% of the bile weight corresponds to a sodium soap (the bile salts). He identified taurine as a component bound to this sodium soap and described a new bile acid, which he called choleinsäure (choleinic acid), presumably taurocholic acid. The term "bile acid" was introduced by Liebig (1843). Berzelius, who was in competition with Liebig's group for decades, added 12 more biliary substances to the literature. Another fundamental work was published by A. Strecker in 1848. In it he described for the first time the purification of two major bile acids coupled to sodium from ox bile, one of them with nitrogen, but without sulfur (glycocholic acid), and the other one with sulfur, but without nitrogen (taurocholic acid). He was also able to show that glykochol (glycine) and cholalsäure (cholic acid) formed his cholic acid (glycocholic acid). In 1862, Kolbe elucidated the structure of taurine and synthesized taurine in vitro. In 1885, Latschinoff described another choleinsäure, which 30 years later was identified by H. Wieland as being composed of eight molecules of deoxycholic acid and one molecule of a fatty acid (49). Mylius, in 1886, identified deoxycholic acid in rotten cow bile and characterized the loss of an oxygen atom in comparison to cholic acid. F. Pregl (1902) demonstrated that deoxycholic acid was part of normal bile (50). O. Hammarsten (1902) isolated an "Ursocholeinische Säure" from polar bear bile, which presumably represented chenodeoxycholic acid (51). H. Fischer (1911) was the first to identify lithocholic acid in cow bile, before Windaus et al. (1924) and Wieland and Reverey (1924) described chenodeoxycholic acid (or "anthropodeoxycholic acid") in bile (52,53) which presumably had first been isolated by Marsson (1849), Heintz and Wislicenus (1859), and Hammarsten (1902) presented under different names. Finally, ursodeoxycholic acid was isolated first from bile of black bears by Shoda (1927) (54) and structurally characterized by Iwasaki (1936) (55). Windaus and Wieland, in a close collaboration, were able to elucidate the approximate structure of cholesterol and several bile acids. For this work, they were awarded the Nobel Prize in 1928 and 1929, respectively (56,57).

Until 1950, quantitative bile acid analysis was performed with colorimetric methods.

Separation of bile acids was then improved by use of reversed phase partition chromatography (Bergstroem and Sjoevall, 1951) (58), countercurrent chromatography (Ahrens and Craig, 1952) (59), and thin-layer and gas-liquid chromatography (Grundy et al., 1965) (60). Further insight into the molecular structure of bile acids has been achieved by application of mass spectrometry (Bergstroem et al., 1958; Lawson and Setchell, 1988) (61,62).

Simple and rapid methods for quantitative analysis of bile acids were then developed: (1) an enzymatic assay based on the oxidation of the 3-hydroxy group by a 3-hydroxysteroid dehydrogenase, first introduced by Iwata and Yamasaki (1964) (63); and (2) a radioimmunoassay, first developed for the determination of cholic acid conjugates by Hofmann et al. (1973) (64).

Application of these and other methods allowed rapid growth in the understanding of bile acid metabolism. Beside amidation of bile acids, further conjugation reactions were detected, such as glucuronidation (Back et al., 1974; Froehling and Stiehl, 1976), sulfation (Palmer, 1967), glucosidation (Matern et al., 1984), or N-acetylglucosaminidation (Marschall et al., 1989) (65–69).

Windaus and Neukirchen, in 1919, described the in vitro formation of cholanic acid (cholic acid) from cholesterol, an important finding for the understanding of bile acid synthesis (70). Bloch et al. (1943), by application of deuterium-labeled cholesterol, were able to show that cholic acid is derived from cholesterol in vivo (71). Already, 90 years earlier, studies performed by Moleschott (1853) had suggested that the liver is the only site of bile acid synthesis because no bile acids were detected in anhepatic frogs. Moleschott's findings were confirmed by Bollman and Mann (1936) in anhepatic dogs (72). Application of radiolabeled cholic acid allowed the first determination of turnover, synthesis rate and pool size of this bile acid in man (Lindstedt, 1957; Bergstroem, 1962) (73–74). It was observed that deoxycholic acid was not formed in the liver, but rather by intestinal bacteria (Lindstedt and Sjoevall, 1957) (75) with the cecum as a major site of biotransformation (Norman and Sjoevall, 1958) (76). Regulation of bile acid synthesis by feedback inhibition (Eriksson, 1957; Shefer et al., 1970; Vlah-

cevic et al., 1991) was elucidated (77–79). The rate-limiting enzyme, cholesterol 7α-hydroxylase, was characterized as a specific cytochrome P450 isozyme of the smooth endoplasmic reticulum of the hepatocyte (Myant and Mitropoulos, 1977) (80). The purification and cloning of this key enzyme of bile acid synthesis (and of elimination of cholesterol from the body) have been reported (Noshiro et al., 1989) (81).

Transport. The possibility that bile acids underwent an enterohepatic circulation was postulated from the 17th century. Early methods to detect bile products allowed Bidder and Schmidt (1852) and Hoppe-Seyler (1863) to perform studies in feces, where they found only low amounts of bile products. They concluded, in agreement with their predecessors, Reverhorst (1690) and Borelli (1710), that these findings could be explained only by intestinal absorption of bile and resecretion by the liver. The hypothesis of an enterohepatic circulation of bile was finally proved by studies in bile fistula dogs performed by Schiff (1870) and Whipple and Smith (1928, 1930) who observed a marked choleresis from the bile fistula after feeding bile to these animals (82).

The uptake of bile acids by the intestinal mucosa, a prerequisite for an enterohepatic circulation, was studied mostly in the 20th century. The first study describing ileal but not duodenal absorption of glyco- and taurocholic acid was reported in dogs in 1878 by Tappeiner. His findings were confirmed half a century later by Frölicher (1936) (83). The specific role of the ileum for bile acid absorption remained unclear for 30 more years. Then, Lack and Weiner (1961) proved the existence of specific bile acid binding sites in the distal ileum (84). Borgstroem (1963) demonstrated that the ileum represented the site of bile acid resorption (85). In another critical study, Dietschy (1966) showed that unconjugated bile acids were passively absorbed in the jejunum, whereas conjugated bile acids were actively taken up by the ileum (86). Together, these findings established the existence of an enterohepatic circulation of bile acids which had been hypothesized almost 300 years earlier based on a series of simple, but elegantly designed experiments.

The hepatic transport of bile acids has received increasing study during the last 20 years. Basic studies for the understanding of the hepatic uptake of bile acids were performed by Reichen and Paumgartner in the perfused rat liver (1975, 1976), by Glasinovic and coworkers in the dog (1975), and by Schwartz and coworkers (1975) and Anwer and coworkers (1977) in isolated rat hepatocytes (87–91). These, as well as further studies by Anwer and Hegner (1978) and Scharschmidt and Stephens (1981), clearly demonstrated sodium-dependent saturable uptake for taurocholate (92,93). Whether this Na^+-dependent uptake of taurocholate is electroneutral (Scharschmidt and Stephens, 1981, Duffy et al., 1983) or electrogenic (Fitz and Scharschmidt, 1987) remains unclear (93–95). These studies also showed that bile acid uptake is not the rate-limiting step in the transport across the hepatocyte, and that the K_m of 15 to 50 μM for the Na^+-dependent uptake of taurocholate allows unhindered uptake under physiologic conditions. Hardison et al. (1984) and Anwer et al. (1985) provided evidence that the charge and length of the side chain as well as the number of hydroxyl groups of the steroid nucleus determined the affinity of bile acids for the carrier (96,97). Photoaffinity labeling techniques performed by Buscher and coworkers (1986) and use of monoclonal antibodies by Ananthanarajanan, von Dippe, and Levy (1988) suggested that a 48–49 kDa protein of the sinusoidal membrane was identical with the Na^+-dependent bile acid transporter of the hepatocyte (98,99). However, an Na^+-dependent bile acid transporter has been cloned and sequenced from rat liver by Hagenbusch and coworkers using an oocyte expression system (1991) and has been identified as a glycoprotein with a molecular weight of approximately 39 kDa (100). This gene product has evolved in mammals but not in lower vertebrates (Boyer et al., 1993) (101).

An additional Na^+-independent bile acid uptake system also has been demonstrated by Anwer and Hegner (1978) and Van Dyke and coworkers (1982) (92,102). Photoaffinity labeling studies performed by Kramer, Kurz and coworkers (1982), and von Dippe and Levy (1983) suggested that a 54 kDa glycoprotein might function as a Na^+-independent carrier for bile acids and other organic anions on the sinusoidal/basolateral membrane of the hepatocyte (103,104). However, cloning and sequence analysis of a Na^+-independent organic anion transporter by Jacquemin and coworkers revealed a molecular weight of about 75 kDa for this glycoprotein (1992) (105).

In addition to carrier-mediated bile acid transport, uptake of unpolar, mostly unconjugated, more hydrophobic bile acids by means of nonionic diffusion also may occur (Van Dyke et al., 1982) (102). The intracellular transport of bile acids has been the subject of studies during recent years, but the mechanism is far from being elucidated. Under basic conditions, intracellular bile acid concentrations have been broadly estimated to be about 200 μM (Okishio and Nair, 1966) (106). Most of these bile acids are bound to proteins which may be partially identical to those mentioned previously for bilirubin and include a 14 kDa Z protein, a 33 kDa Y′ protein with 3a-hydroxysteroid dehydrogenase activity, and a 45 kDa ligandin with glutathione transferase activity (see Stolz et al., 1989) (107). Microtubule-dependent vesicular transport of bile acids is of minor (<10%) importance for physiologic rates of bile acid transport. However, exposure of hepatocytes to higher bile acid loads leads to a quantitative change of the transcellular transport mechanism where transcytotic vesicles play a major role (≥50%) in bile acid transport (Crawford et al., 1988; Erlinger, 1990) (46,108). Trafficking of bile acids through different compartments of the cell, including endoplasmic reticulum (Suchy et al., 1983) and Golgi membranes (Lambri et al., 1988), also may play a physiologic role in the transcellular transport of bile acids (109,110).

Canalicular secretion has been assumed to be the rate-limiting step for bile acid traffic across the liver cell, and therefore is a key determinant of bile acid-induced bile flow. Using photoaffinity labeling techniques developed by Fricker, Kurz, and colleagues (1987), Meier and coworkers (1987) have identified and isolated a 100 kDa protein which is exclusively localized to the canalicular membrane (111–113). This protein may represent a putative canalicular bile acid carrier, as shown by reconstitution studies in liposomes (Ruetz et al., 1988).

The driving force for the secretion of bile acids across the canalicular membrane against a concentration gradient also has not yet been completely determined. Graf and coworkers (1984) showed in hepatocyte couplets that a potential difference of about -25 to -35 mV exists between the canaliculus (-5 mV) and the interior of the cells (-30 to -40 mV), which would allow a potential-driven, three- to four-fold concentration gradient of bile acid anions between the cell and the canalicular lumen (114). This assumption was confirmed by Inoue and coworkers (1984) and Meier and coworkers (1984), who provided evidence for a potential-driven, carrier-mediated bile acid transport (in canalicular membrane vesicle preparations) (115,116). Weinman and colleagues (1989, 1993) provided direct evidence in hepatocyte couplets that bile acid excretion and bile acid-dependent bile secretion could be stimulated by the membrane potential (117,118). However, factors in addition to the electrical potential are necessary to explain the 10- to 100-fold concentration gradient for bile acids in the canaliculus. Several groups have recently provided evidence that ATP might be an additional driving force for carrier-mediated transport of bile acids across the canalicular membrane (119–122). Finally, vesicular exocytosis as the last step of the microtubule-dependent, transcytotic vesicular pathway also may contribute to the regulation of bile acid secretion by as yet unknown factors (Crawford et al. 1988, Erlinger 1990) (46,108).

The studies of Schiff in 1870 in dogs with a bile fistula not only provided evidence for an enterohepatic circulation of bile acids, but also showed that bile ingestion produced a marked choleresis, demonstrating the bile-forming potency of major bile components, e.g. the bile acids. The concept that bile flow is stimulated by the transport of osmotically active organic anions was first clearly enunciated by I. Sperber (1959,1965) (123,124). The concept of "bile acid dependent flow" (BADF) and "bile acid independent flow" (BAIF) was then established to distinguish the different osmotic driving forces for bile production. Studies in different animal species (Wheeler et al., 1968; Preisig et al., 1962; Forker, 1968; Strasberg et al., 1975, 1982) revealed marked species differences with regard to the rates of BADF and BAIF (125–129). In humans, bile acids account for about one third (circa 200 mL daily) of total daily bile flow as determined by Boyer and Bloomer (1975) in cholecystectomized bile fistula patients (130). Thus, the mechanism of bile formation is generally assumed to occur by osmotic filtration induced by the active transport of bile acids and other impermeant anions into the canalicular space, resulting in the passive diffusion of water and small electrolytes across the canalicular membrane and tight junctions.

Other Organic Anions

The contribution of organic anions other than bile acids to the formation of bile has been intensely studied during the last decade. A multispecific anion exchanger system with a molecular weight of about 54 to 55 kDa as determined by photo-affinity labeling techniques has been characterized in basolateral membrane preparations independently by different groups (Cheng and Levi, 1980; Kramer et al., 1982; Ziegler et al., 1982) (131–133). It is yet unclear whether this carrier system represents only one distinct protein complex or a family of isoforms with an overlapping substrate specificity and similar molecular structure and weight which may transport a wide array of different organic and inorganic anions including bilirubin, sulfobromophthalein (BSP), indocyanin green, succinate, oxalate, sulfate, and many others (Berk et al., 1987) (134). Transport has been shown to be independent of Na^+ ions, but (at least for bilirubin and BSP) dependent on Cl^- (Wolkoff et al., 1987; Potter et al., 1987) (135,136). OH^- ions also may function as counterions for anion uptake across the basolateral membrane (Hugentobler and Meier, 1986) (137). Recently, functional expression cloning of a Cl^--dependent BSP uptake system has been reported in a Xenopus laevis oocyte expression system (Jacquemin et al., 1991) (138) which, however, revealed a molecular weight of about 75 kDa (Jacquemin et al., 1992) (105). It remains to be determined whether this transporter is structurally related to the 54 kDa transport system previously identified by photolabeling techniques.

Cytosolic bilirubin binding proteins (see previous text) also may be involved in the binding of other organic anions. Biliary excretion of organic anions such as BSP or bilirubin is mediated by a multispecific ATP-dependent transport mechanism distinct from the potential- and ATP-dependent bile acid transporters. This conclusion is based on observations in patients with the Dubin-Johnson syndrome, in mutant Corriedale sheep, and in mutant TR$^-$ rats and GH rats (Jansen et al., 1985; Kuipers et al., 1989) (139,140). In these genetic mutants, impairment of bilirubin, BSP and glutathione excretion occurs with only minor or no disturbances in bile acid excretion (Kitamura 1990) (141).

Glutathione (GSH) is a major candidate for the formation of bile acid-independent bile flow. Glutathione is formed within the hepatocyte and transported by means of an ATP-dependent carrier system deficient in TR$^-$ and GH mutant rats and may contribute significantly although not exclusively to bile acid-independent bile flow in the perfused rat liver (Ballatori et al., 1988, 1989). GSH is metabolized in bile to glutamate, cystine, and glycine, which are reabsorbed back across the canalicular and bile duct epithelium by separate transport mechanisms to varying degrees dependent on the species (142,143). This cholehepatic shunt mechanism has been demonstrated previously for glucose (Guzelian and Boyer, 1974) (144) and postulated for several unconjugated bile acids (Yoon, Hofmann et al. 1986) (145).

Organic Cations

The mechanism of hepatic transport and excretion of organic cations into bile is poorly understood. Evidence from studies in basolateral membrane vesicles suggests that organic cations are taken up into the cell by means of a saturable, energy-dependent, Na$^+$-independent transport mechanism which uses H$^+$ as a counterion (Moseley et al., 1990) (146). Larger cations may be taken up by a distinct endocytic vesicular pathway (Braakman et al., 1989) (147). Canalicular excretion of organic cations may be mediated by an ATP-dependent transmembrane glycoprotein, the "multidrug resistance gene product" or Gp 170. The substrate specificity of this transporter is broad

(Kamimoto et al., 1989), although its endogenous substrate has not yet been determined (148).

Proteins

Bile contains numerous specific proteins, which vary with the species studied. Most serum proteins are found in bile but only in minute amounts. However, some high molecular weight proteins such as secretory IgA, hemoglobin-haptoglobin, or transferrin are enriched in bile (Mullock et al., 1980; Hinton et al., 1980; Jones et al., 1982) (149–151). These proteins are transported into bile by way of endocytotic vesicles (Renston et al., 1980; Hoppe et al., 1985) (152,153) across the hepatocytes (IgA in rat) or bile duct epithelial cells (IgA in man). Lysosomal and canalicular membrane enzymes are found in bile in considerable amounts (LaRusso and Fowler, 1979) (154).

Lipids

Bile is the major route for excretion of cholesterol, a substance of such importance that 13 Nobel prizes have been awarded for exceptional work on this molecule. Cholesterol was originally thought to be a compound found only in bile. Chemical analysis of gallstones led to the detection of cholesterol by Conradi (1775) and Poulletier de la Salle (1777). It was described as a substance soluble in alcohol, forming small crystalline leaves. Chevreul, who worked during the second and third decade of the 19th century on the physicochemical properties of fat derivatives, further characterized and named this gallstone-derived fat ("Je nommerai cholestérine, de "chole," bile, et "stereos," solid, la substance cristallisée des calculs biliaires humains. . ." ME Chevreul, Ann Chim Phys 2:346, 1816). Chevreul was also the first to detect cholesterol in human bile (1824). However, the role of cholesterol as a specific bile fat was questioned when it was detected in other human tissues (Couerbe 1835, Moleschott 1855). The structural similarity of cholesterol and bile acids was first noted by Redtenbacher (1846) and by Wislincenius and Moldenhauer (1868), who described the double bonding in cholesterol as the characteristic difference from bile acids. Mauthner and Suida (1894) characterized the cyclic structure of the molecule and its content of 27 carbon atoms. The final elucidation of the molecular structure of cholesterol was achieved by Adolf Windaus, who, between 1903 and 1927, published a series of papers that not only described its definitive molecular structure, but also demonstrated the in vitro transformation of cholesterol into a bile acid, and published the first quantitative determination of cholesterol and the separation of cholesterol esters (155,156). Gamble and Blackfan (1920) provided evidence that this lipid is synthesized by the human body by balancing uptake and output of cholesterol in human newborns (157). Nomura (1924) concluded that synthesis of cholesterol is not limited to the liver by detecting a cholesterase in different organ extracts (158). The key role of the liver in cholesterol metabolism had been emphasized earlier by Backmeister and Havers (1910), who measured cholesterol secretion into bile and concluded that the elimination of cholesterol was a key function of the liver (159). The central role of the liver in cholesterol synthesis and its elimination in bile, either in unesterified form (50%) or after transformation to bile acids (50%), was subsequently confirmed by numerous studies.

Lecithin (phosphatidylcholine) is quantitatively the most important lipid in bile and represents more than 95% of biliary phospholipids. Bile lecithin is characterized by an unusual fatty acid pattern, predominantly palmitoyl-linoleyl and palmitoyl-oleyl lecithin (Balint et al., 1965, Yousef and Fisher, 1975) (160,161). The physicochemical properties of lipids in bile, the origin of biliary lipids, and the mechanism of lipid secretion into bile have been elucidated only in the last two decades and are beyond the scope of this review. Extensive work has been performed by D. M. Small, M. C. Carey, and others on the physicochemistry of bile lipids (Small et al. 1966; Carey 1985; Carey and Lamont, 1992) (162–164). Cholesterol and lecithin overcome their agueous insolubility by aggregating in bile into mixed lipid micelles with bile acids. Cholesterol exceeds its solubility in bile by a factor of 2000. These micelles form mixed bilayer disks, characterized by hydrodynamic radii of about 13 to 21 A (Mazer and Carey 1980, Reuben et al., 1982) (165,166) and by a fixed stoichiometry between lipids and bile acids

(e.g., lecithin/bile acids 1.3 to 2.0). The excretion of lipids into bile is coupled to the excretion of micelle-forming bile acids and seems to be independent of hepatic lipid synthesis (Turley and Dietschy 1979, Schwartz et al. 1978, Robins and Brunengraber 1982) (167–169). The mechanism of lipid excretion is not yet understood. Under physiologic conditions, lipid secretion is closely linked to secretion of micelle-forming bile acids exerting an almost linear relationship (see Carey and Calahane, 1982) (170). Numerous organic anions (Apstein and Robbins, 1982), microtubule inhibitors (Gregory et al., 1978), and inducers of the mixed function oxidase system such as phenobarbital (Redinger and Small, 1973) uncouple this secretory linkage between lipids and bile acids (171–173). Recent evidence suggests that microtubule-dependent intracellular transport may play an important role in biliary lipid secretion (Crawford et al., 1988, 1991) (46,174).

Electrolytes, Inorganic Ions

The high amount of sodium in bile was first detected by Cadet and by Roederer and Speilmann who, in 1767, found sodium precipitations when different acids were added to bile samples. Inorganic electrolytes account for the major osmotic activity in bile (Moore and Dietschy, 1964) (175) since other compounds like bile acids and lipids are associated in mixed micelles or self aggregates (Wheeler and Ramos, 1960) (176). Today it is known that sodium, like other electrolytes, e.g., potassium, calcium, magnesium, chloride, bicarbonate, or phosphate, is present at similar concentrations in bile and serum (Cook et al., 1952; Brauer, 1956; for review see Boyer, 1987) (177–179). The mechanisms of solute transport from serum to bile have evolved only during the last two decades and still are incompletely understood. A short overview on major transport systems is given.

Na^+. Many transport systems involving Na^+ have been identified in hepatocellular plasma membranes; most are coupled to the uptake of other solutes, and one provides a mechanism for Na^+ extrusion. A Na^+-dependent, basolateral bile acid uptake system has been described in detail previously (see Transport). Evidence for a basolateral Na^+/HCO_3^- cotransport system has recently been obtained by Renner et al. (1989) in membrane vesicles, and by Gleeson et al. (1989) and Fitz et al. (1989) in isolated hepatocytes (180–182). This transporter may be of key importance for the hepatocyte in counteracting an acid load, and may play a role in volume regulation (Corasanti et al., 1990) (183). An Na^+/H^+ antiport with similar functions, i.e., pH and volume regulation, also has been demonstrated on the basolateral membrane in vesicles (Arias and Forgac, 1984; Moseley et al., 1986), in isolated hepatocytes (Renner et al., 1989) and hepatocyte couplets (Henderson et al., 1987) (180,184–186). Finally, a Na^+-dependent, saturable uptake system for unesterified fatty acids localized to the basolateral membrane has been identified by Stremmel and coworkers (1986, 1987) (187,188). An electrogenic, inward-directed, Na^+-dependent carrier for neutral amino acids has been identified in hepatocytes by Fehlmann et al. (1979) and Kristensen (1980), and an Na^+-glucose cotransporter has been detected in a subgroup of hepatocytes localized around the terminal hepatic venules (Tal et al., 1990) (189–191).

The Na^+ uptake systems are counterbalanced by a Na^+/K^+ ATPase, which was characterized and cytochemically localized to the basolateral membrane by Blitzer and Boyer in 1978 (192). Na^+/K^+ ATPase exchanges three Na^+ ions (outwardly directed) for two K^+ ions (inwardly directed) and thereby establishes a chemical gradient across the membrane, which is the major driving force for the other Na^+-dependent transport systems and establishes a negative intracellular potential (-35 to $-40\,mV$) for the hepatocyte (see the electrophysiologic studies performed by Graf et al. (1987) and Weinman et al. (1989, 1993) (117,118,193).

No transport systems have yet been identified in the canalicular membrane that extrude Na^+, indicating that transcellular transport of Na^+ into bile is highly unlikely to be a major source of biliary Na^+. Studies by Graf and Peterlik (1975) in the perfused rat liver suggested that 95% of biliary Na^+ is derived from serum by way of a paracellular route across cation-permeable tight junctions (194).

K^+. Uptake of K^+ by means of Na^+/K^+ ATPase is counterregulated by outward flux by a basolateral K^+ conductance pathway as identified by Graf et al. (1987) (193). Like Na^+, K^+ is transported into bile primarily via a paracellular route as first reported by Brauer (1956; see also Graf and Peterlik, 1975) (178,194).

Ca^{++}. Regulation of intracellular Ca^{++} concentrations is critically important for the regulation of multiple cell activities. Ca^{++} is essential for bile formation because removal of perfusate Ca^{++} results in cholestasis in the isolated perfused rat liver (Anwer et al., 1975; Reichen et al., 1975) (195,196). Little information exists in regard to mechanisms of Ca^{++} entry into the hepatocyte across the sinusoidal membranes. In addition to passive Ca^{++} influx in the resting cell (Mauger et al., 1984 and references) (197), Ca^{++} channels (still poorly defined) are regulated by hormones and receptor-independent Ca^{++} agonists. Extrusion of Ca^{++} across the plasma membrane occurs via a Ca^{++}-ATPase (Pavoine et al., 1987), a putative Na^+/Ca^{++} exchanger (Shanne and Moore, 1986), and Ca^{++}/H^+ exchanger (Kraus-Friedmann et al., 1982), although the physiologic relevance of the latter two exchangers is not clear (Lidowsky et al., 1989) (198–201). It also is uncertain whether Ca^{++} is extruded across the canalicular membrane into bile. Ca^{++} probably enters bile paracellularly. Whether Ca^{++} enters bile predominantly by the paracellular route must be questioned in view of recent studies of Bygrave and coworkers (1992) (202), which show that conjugated ursodeoxycholic acid, a potent Ca^{++} agonist in the hepatocyte (Beuers et al., 1993) (203), can stimulate Ca^{++} extrusion into bile. Ca^{++} gradients of $1:10000$ must be maintained between cytosol and the extracellular milieu for regulation of numerous hepatocyte functions to occur and to maintain hepatocyte viability. Thus, additional mechanisms exist within the cell for the storage of Ca^{++} in compartments of the endoplasmic reticulum. An ATP-driven Ca^{++} pump in the membrane of the endoplasmic reticulum is of primary importance (Spamer et al., 1987) (204). It is beyond the scope of this review to discuss the role of Ca^{++} in cell function in more detail but this subject will continue to be of considerable interest in future years.

Cl^-. Cl^- moves across the basolateral and canalicular membranes through Cl^- channels by passive diffusion according to electrochemical driving forces (Graf and co-workers, 1987) (193). In addition, a Cl^-/HCO_3^- antiport system has been identified and characterized by Meier and coworkers (1985) (205) which is localized exclusively to the canalicular membrane. Recent evidence suggests that this transporter is the major acid-loading mechanism in hepatocytes (Benedetti et al., 1992) and is regulated by insertion of vesicles in the canalicular membrane by microtubule-dependent pathways (Beneditti et al., 1993) (206,207).

HCO_3^-. Bicarbonate concentrations in bile are comparable to serum. Bicarbonate replacement results in reduction of bile acid-independent bile formation in the perfused rat liver (Hardison et al., 1981; Van Dyke et al., 1982; Anwer and Hegner, 1983) (208–210). Hepatocellular uptake of HCO_3^- occurs by means of a basolateral Na^+/HCO_3^- cotransport system, whereas canalicular secretion is mediated by means of a Cl^-/HCO_3^- antiport system. Both exchangers help maintain pH_i and may play a role in cell volume regulation. HCO_3^- is secreted into bile by hepatocytes as well as bile duct epithelial cells. Their relative contributions vary with the species.

Functional Aspects and the Actual Concept of Bile Formation

Major functions of bile have been described in previous paragraphs. Historically, bile was initially regarded by the Corpus Hippocraticum as well as Galen of Pergamon as a major constituent of the human body affecting health and disease. Bile then became increasingly seen as a useless excrement ("cloaca sordium et superfluitatum," J. B. Van Helmont) before J. B. Van Helmont and A. von Haller among others in the 17th and 18th century first pointed out its potential digestive function.

Today, in addition to its role in facilitating intestinal digestion and absorption of fats, vitamins, or heavy metals (e.g., Ca^{++}, Fe^{++}), bile functions to excrete cholesterol and other lipid-soluble organic compounds with a molecular weight generally exceeding 300 Da, as well as heavy metals, and IgA. The latter is a process of functional importance for small intestine immunity.

Modern concepts of the mechanisms of hepatic bile formation developed following Sperber's observations in the 1950s that bile flow was stimulated by the excretion of osmotically active organic anions (123,124). These findings gave rise to the present concept that bile is formed by a process of osmotic filtration. Since that time, efforts have been directed at elucidating the transport mechanisms responsible for generating the osmotic gradients between blood and bile necessary for promoting this secretion.

For the next two decades, transport systems for organic and inorganic solutes were identified in liver plasma membranes and assigned specific domains in the basolateral and/or canalicular regions of the hepatocyte. These studies were facilitated by immunohistochemical and cytochemical techniques and by the development of techniques to separate canalicular membranes from plasma membrane fractions (Meier et al., 1984; Inoue et al., 1984) (115,116).

The concept that hepatocytes were highly polarized cells that generated secretion like classic epithelial cells (Boyer, 1980) (211) evolved once it was discovered that Na^+, K^+-ATPase was present on the basolateral rather than the canalicular domain (Blitzer and Boyer, 1978) (192). This observation led to the realization that the driving forces for solute transport into bile were first provided by the activity of the Na^+ pump, which created inwardly directed Na^+ gradients. These Na^+ gradients were then coupled to solute entry mechanisms, such as the Na^+-dependent bile acid transporter. Excretion of osmotically active organic solutes (bile acids and other solutes) into bile could occur either through electrical potential driven mechanisms, by exocytosis, or as recently discovered, by ATP-dependent transport mechanisms (Arias, 1993) (212) at the canalicular membrane. The development of the isolated rat hepatocyte couplet, a polarized bile secretory unit in cell culture (Oshio and Phillips 1981, Graf et al. 1984, Boyer 1993) (114,213,214) provided a model from which direct proof for many of these concepts could be obtained and which have been reinforced by a large number of experimental studies from many laboratories.

The role of the bile ducts in bile formation only recently has been studied in similar detail. Although it was known that bile flow could be stimulated by the hormone secretin since its discovery by Bayliss and Starling (1902) (215), neither the site nor the composition of the secretion was determined until the studies of Wheeler (1968), who used inert solute to discriminate between hepatocyte and bile duct bile and demonstrated that secretin stimulated bicarbonate-rich watery secretion from the bile duct epithelium (126). The mechanism of the secretin effect has recently been elucidated following the development of techniques for isolating bile duct epithelial cells (Sirica et al., 1990) (216). Secretin binds to receptors on bile duct cells, leading to an increase in intracellular cyclic AMP (Lenzen et al., 1990) (217), which in turn opens Cl^- conductive pathways on the luminal membrane that share homology with the CFTR gene product, which is defective in patients with cystic fibrosis (Fitz et al., 1993; Alvaro et al., 1993) (218,219). The opening of Cl^- channels then facilitates the increased cycling of a Cl^-/HCO_3^- exchanger, leading to the exchange of HCO_3^- for Cl^- anions in bile. Because Cl^- anions are recycled into bile by conductive mechanisms, bile flow is stimulated and is enriched in HCO_3^-.

Like all scientific progress, knowledge of the formation and composition of bile over many centuries has been critically dependent on the discovery of new technologies which, when adopted, have led to greater understanding of its form and function.

REFERENCES

All sources covering the period from 1550 B.C. to 1900 A.D. are given in references 1 to 4. We are indebted to N. Mani (1,2), F. H. Franken (3), and T. S. and P. S. Chen (4). Their extensive and excellent overviews on the history of hepatology provided us with the historic background given in this review. Starting with reference 5, papers published during the 20th century are cited.*

* Z. Physiol. Chem. = Hoppe-Seyler's Z. Physiol. Chem.

1. Mani N: Die historischen Grundlagen der Leberforschung. I. Die Vorstellungen über Anatomie, Physiologie und Pathologie in der Antike. Basel (Switzerland), Benno Schwabe & Co. Verlag, 1959.
2. Mani N: Die historischen Grundlagen der Leberforschung. II. Die Geschichte der Leberforschung von Galen bis Claude Bernard. Basel (Switzerland), Schwabe & Co. Verlag, 1967.
3. Franken FH: Die Leber und ihre Krankheiten. Zweihundert Jahre Hepatologie. Stuttgart (Germany), Ferdinand Enke Verlag, 1968.
4. Chen TS, Chen PS: Understanding the liver. A history. Westport (Connecticut), Greenwood Press, 1984.
5. Fischer H, Reindel F: Über Hämatoidin. Z Physiol Chem *127*:299, 1923.
6. Fischer H: Zur Kenntnis der Gallenfarbstoffe. Z Physiol Chem *73*:204, 1911.
7. Siedel W, Fischer H: Über die Konstitution des Bilirubins, Synthesen der Neo- und der Iso-Neoxanthobilirubinsäure. Z Physiol Chem *214*:145, 1933.
8. Fischer H, Plieninger H: Synthese des Biliverdins (Uteroverdins) und Bilirubins, der Biliverdine XIIIα und IIIα sowie der Vinylneoxanthosäure. Z Physiol Chem *274*:231, 1942.
9. Aschoff L, Kiyono K: Ein Beitrag zur Lehr von den Makrophagen. Verhandl Dtsch Ges Pathol *16*:107, 1913.
10. Mann FC et al.: Formation of bile pigment after total removal of the liver. Am J Physiol *69*:393, 1924.
11. Hijmans van den Bergh AA, Snapper J: Die Farbstoffe des Blutserums. Dtsch Arch Klin Med *110*:540, 1913.
12. Hijmans van den Bergh AA: Der Gallenfarbstoff im Blute. Leiden, The Netherlands, SC van Doesburgh, 1918.
13. Grunenberg K: Über die Chloroformlöslichkeit des Bilirubins. Z Ges Exp Med *35*:128, 1923.
14. Davis GE, Sheard C: Absorption spectra of direct and indirect reacting types of serum bilirubin. J Lab Clin Med *23*:22, 1937.
15. Eppinger H: Die Leberkrankheiten. Vienna, J Springer, 1937.
16. Cole PG, Lathe GH: The separation of serum pigments giving the direct and indirect van den Bergh reaction. J Clin Pathol *6*:99, 1953.
17. Schmid R: Direct reacting bilirubin, bilirubin glucuronide in serum, bile and urine. Science *124*:76, 1956.
18. Billing BH, Cole PG, Lathe GH: The excretion of bilirubin as a diglucuronide giving the direct van den Bergh reaction. Biochem J *65*:774, 1957.

19. Talefant E: Properties and composition of the bile pigments giving a direct diazo reaction. Nature *178*:312, 1956.

20. Billing BH: Twenty-five years of progress in bilirubin metabolism. Gut *19*:481, 1978.

21. Schmid R, Hammaker L, Axelrod J: The enzymatic formation of bilirubin glucuronide. Arch Biochem Biophys *70*:285, 1957.

22. Schmid R: The identification of direct reacting bilirubin as bilirubin glucuronide. J Biol Chem *229*:881, 1957.

23. Lathe GH, Walker M: The synthesis of bilirubin glucuronide in animal and human liver. Biochem J *70*:705, 1958.

24. Lathe GH, Walker W: An enzyme defect in human neonatal jaundice and in Gunn's strain of jaundiced rats. Biochem J *67*:9P, 1957.

25. Roy Chowdhury J et al.: Isolation and characterization of multiple forms of rat liver UDP-glucuronate glucuronyltransferase. Biochem J *233*:827, 1986.

26. Crawford JM, Hauser SC, Gollan JL: Formation, metabolism, and transport of bile pigments: A status report. Semin Liver Dis *8*:105, 1988.

27. Lauff JJ, Kasper ME, Ambrose RT: Separation of bilirubin species in serum and bile by high-performance reversed-phase liquid chromatography. J Chromatogr *226*:391, 1981.

28. Weiss JS et al.: The clinical importance of a protein-bound fraction of serum bilirubin in patients with hyperbilirubinemia. N Engl J Med *309*:147, 1983.

29. Kuenzle CC, Sommerhalder M, Ruttner JR, Maier C: Separation and quantitative estimation of four bilirubin fractions from serum and three bilirubin fractions from bile. J Lab Clin Med *67*:294, 1966.

30. Fevery J et al.: Bilirubin conjugates in bile of man and rat in the normal state and in liver disease. J Clin Invest *51*:2482, 1972.

31. Fog J, Jellum E: Structure of bilirubin. Nature *198*:88, 1963.

32. Bonnett R, Davies JE, Hursthouse MB: Structure of bilirubin. Nature *262*:326, 1976.

33. Robinson SH: Formation of bilirubin from erythroid and non-erythroid sources. Semin Hematol *9*:43, 1972.

34. Berk PD et al.: A new approach to quantitation of the various sources of bilirubin in man. J Lab Clin Med *87*:767, 1976.

35. Burchell B: Isolation and purification of bilirubin UDP-glucuronyl-transferase from rat liver. FEBS Lett *111*:131, 1980.

36. Wooster R et al.: Cloning and stable expression of the human liver phenol/bilirubin: UDP-glucuronosyltransferase cDNA family. Biochem J *278*:465, 1991.

37. Ritter JK, Crawford JM, Owen IS: Cloning of two human liver bilirubin UDP-glucuronosyl-transferase cDNAs with expression in COS-1 cells. J Biol Chem *266*:1043, 1991.

38. Goresky CA: The hepatic uptake process: Its implications for bilirubin transport. *In* Goresky CA, Fisher MM (eds): Jaundice. New York, Plenum Press, 1975, p. 159.

39. Scharschmidt BF, Waggoner JG, Berk PD: Hepatic organic anion uptake in the rat. J Clin Invest *56*:1280, 1975.

40. Paumgartner G, Reichen J: Kinetics of hepatic uptake of unconjugated bilirubin. Clin Sci Molec Med *51*:169, 1976.

41. Berk PD et al.: Studies of bilirubin kinetics in normal adults. J Clin Invest *48*:2176, 1969.

42. Levi AG, Gatmainan Z, Arias IM: Two hepatic cytoplasmic protein fractions, Y and Z, and their possible role in the hepatic uptake of bilirubin, sulfobromophthalein, and other anions. J Clin Invest *48*:2156, 1969.

43. Bhargava MM et al.: Structural, catalytic, binding and immunological properties associated with each of the two subunits of rat liver ligandin. J Biol Chem *233*:718, 1980.

44. Wolkoff AW et al.: Role of ligandin in transfer of bilirubin from plasma into liver. Am J Physiol *236*:E638, 1979.

45. Whitmer DI, Ziurys JC, Gollan JL: Hepatic microsomal glucuronidation of bilirubin in unilamellar liposomal membranes. Implications for intracellular transport of lipophilic substrates. J Biol Chem *259*:11969, 1984.

46. Crawford JM, Berken CA, Gollan JL: Role of the hepatocyte microtubular system in the excretion of bile salts and biliary lipid: Implications for intracellular vesicular transport. J Lipid Res *29*:144, 1988.

47. Wolkoff AW et al.: Hepatic accumulation and intracellular binding of conjugated bilirubin. J Clin Invest *61*:142, 1978.

48. Kitamura T et al.: Defective ATP-dependent bile canalicular transport of organic anions in mutant (TR) rats with conjugated hyperbilirubinemia. Proc Natl Acad Sci USA *87*:3557, 1990.

49. Wieland H, Sorge H: Zur Kenntnis der Choleinsäure. Z Physiol Chem *97*:1, 1916.

50. Pregl F: Über Isolierung von Desoxycholsäure und Choalsäure aus frischer Rindergalle und über Oxydationsprodukte dieser Säuren. S ber Acad Wiss, Wien, math.-naturw.K1. *111(2b)*:1024, 1902.

51. Hammarsten O: Untersuchungen über die Gallen einiger Polarthiere. Z Physiol Chem *36*:525, 1902.

52. Windaus H et al.: Über die Cheno-desoxycholsäure. Z Physiol Chem *140*:177, 1924.

53. Wieland H, Reverey G: Untersuchungen

über die Gallensäuren. 21.Mitteilung. Zur Kenntnis der menschlichen Galle 1. Z Physiol Chem *140*:186, 1924.

54. Shoda M: Über die Ursodesoxycholsäure aus Bärengallen und ihre physiologische Wirkung. J Biochem 7:505, 1927.

55. Iwasaki T: Über die Konstitution der Ursodesoxycholsäure. Z Physiol Chem *244*:181, 1936.

56. Wieland H: Die Chemie der Gallensäuren. Z Angew Chemie *42*:421, 1929.

57. Windaus A: Constitution of sterols and their connection with other substances in nature. *In* Nobel Lectures in Chemistry. Amsterdam, Elsevier, 1977, p. 105.

58. Bergström S, Sjövall J: Separation of bile acids with reversed phase partition chromatography. Acta Chem Scand 5:1267, 1951.

59. Ahrens EH, Craig LC: The extraction and separation of bile acids. J Biol Chem *195*:763, 1952.

60. Grundy SM et al.: Quantitative isolation and gas-liquid chromatographic analysis of total fecal bile acids. J Lipid Res 6:397, 1965.

61. Bergström S et al.: Mass spectrometric studies on bile acids and other steroid derivatives. Acta Chem Scand *12*:1349, 1958.

62. Lawson AM, Setchell KDR: Mass spectrometry of bile acids. *In* Setchell KDR, Kritchevsky D, Nair PP (eds): The Bile Acids. Vol. IV. New York, Plenum Press, 1988, p. 167.

63. Iwata T, Yamasaki K: Enzymatic determination and thin-layer chromatography of bile acids in blood. J Biochem 56:424, 1964.

64. Simmonds WJ, Korman MG, Go VLW, Hofmann AF: Radioimmunoassay of conjugated cholyl bile acids in serum. Gastroenterology 65:705, 1973.

65. Back P, Spaczynski K, Gerok W: Bile salt glucuronides in urine. Hoppe Seyler's Z Physiol Chem *355*:749, 1974.

66. Fröhling W, Stiehl A: Bile salt glucuronides: Identification and quantitative analysis in the urine of patients with cholestasis. Eur J Clin Invest 6:67, 1976.

67. Palmer RH: The formation of bile acid sulfates: A new pathway of bile acid metabolism in humans. Proc Natl Acad Sci USA 58:1047, 1967.

68. Matern H, Matern S, Gerok W: Formation of bile acid glucosides by a sugar nucleotide-independent glucosyltransferase isolated from human liver microsomes. Proc Natl Acad Sci USA *81*:7036, 1984.

69. Marschall HU et al.: N-Acetylglucosaminides. A new type of bile acid conjugate in man. J Biol Chem *264*:12989, 1989.

70. Windaus A, Neukirchen K: Die Umwandlung des Cholesterins in Cholansäure. Ber Dtsch Chem Ges *52B*:1915, 1919.

71. Bloch K et al.: The biological conversion of cholesterol to cholic acid. J Biol Chem *149*:511, 1943.

72. Bollman JL, Mann FC: The influence of the liver in the formation and destruction of bile salts. Am J Physiol *116*:214, 1936.

73. Lindstedt S: The turnover of cholic acid in man. Bile acids and steroids. Acta Physiol Scand *40*:1, 1957.

74. Bergström S: Metabolism of bile acids. Fed Proc *21*:28, 1962.

75. Lindtstedt S, Sjövall J: On the formation of deoxycholic acid from cholic acid in the rabbit. Acta Chem Scand *11*:421, 1957.

76. Norman A, Sjövall J: On the transformation and enterohepatic circulation of cholic acid in the rat: Bile acids and steroids. J Biol Chem *233*:872, 1958.

77. Eriksson S: Biliary excretion of bile acids and cholesterol in bile fistula rats: Bile acids and steroids. Proc Soc Exp Biol Med *94*:578, 1957.

78. Shefer S et al.: Biochemical site of regulation of bile acid synthesis in the rat. J Lipid Res *11*:404, 1970.

79. Vlahcevic ZR, Heuman DM, Hylemon PB: Regulation of bile acid synthesis. Hepatology *13*:590, 1991.

80. Myant NB, Mitropoulos KA: Cholesterol 7α-hydroxylase. J Lipid Res *18*:135, 1977.

81. Noshiro M, Nishimoto M, Morohashi K, Okuda K: Molecular cloning of cDNA for cholesterol 7α-hydroxylase from rat liver microsomes. FEBS Lett *257*:97, 1989.

82. Whipple GH, Smith HP: Bile salt metabolism. Liver injury and liver stimulation. J Biol Chem *89*:727, 1930.

83. Frölicher E: Die Resorption von Gallensäuren aus verschiedenen Dünndarmabschnitten. Biochem Z *283*:273, 1936.

84. Lack L, Weiner IM: In vitro absorption of bile salts by small intestine of rats and guinea pigs. Am J Physiol *200*:313, 1961.

85. Borgström B et al.: The site of absorption of deconjugated bile salts in man. Gastroenterology *45*:229, 1963.

86. Dietschy JM et al.: Bile acid metabolism: 1. Studies on the mechanism of intestinal transport. J Clin Invest *45*:832, 1966.

87. Reichen J, Paumgartner G: Kinetics of taurocholate uptake by the perfused rat liver. Gastroenterology *68*:132, 1975.

88. Reichen J, Paumgartner G: Uptake of bile acids by perfused rat liver. Am J Physiol *231*:734, 1976.

89. Glasinovic JC, Dumont M, Duval M, Erlinger S: Hepatocellular uptake of taurocholate in the dog. J Clin Invest *55*:419, 1975.

90. Schwartz LR et al.: Uptake of taurocholic acid into isolated rat liver cells. Eur J Biochem 55:617, 1975.

91. Anwer MS et al.: Cholic acid uptake in isolated rat hepatocytes. Z Physiol Chem 358:543, 1977.

92. Anwer MS, Hegner D: Effect of Na on bile acid uptake by isolated rat hepatocytes. Evidence for a heterogenous system. Z Physiol Chem 359:181, 1978.

93. Scharschmidt BF, Stevens JE: Transport of sodium, chloride, and taurocholate by cultured rat hepatocytes. Proc Natl Acad Sci USA 78:986, 1981.

94. Duffy MC, Blitzer BL, Boyer JL: Direct determination of the driving forces for taurocholate uptake into rat liver plasma membrane vesicles. J Clin Invest 72:1470, 1983.

95. Fitz G, Scharschmidt BF: Regulation of hepatocyte membrane potential in vivo: The effects of glucagon, fasting, and alanine on taurocholate transport. Am J Physiol 253:G56, 1987.

96. Hardison WGM, Bellentani S, Heasley V, Shellhammer D: Specificity of a Na^+-dependent taurocholate transport site in isolated rat hepatocytes. Am J Physiol 246:G477, 1984.

97. Anwer MS et al.: Influence of side-chain charge on hepatic transport of bile acids and bile acid analogues. Am J Physiol 249:G479, 1985.

98. Buscher HP et al.: Hepatic transport system for bile salt: localization and specificity. In Paumgartner G, Gerok W (eds): Bile Acids and Cholesterol in Health and Disease. Lancaster, UK, MTP Press, 1977, p. 95.

99. Ananthanarayanan M, von Dippe P, Levy D: Identification of the hepatocyte Na^+-dependent bile acid transport protein using monoclonal antibodies. J Biol Chem 263:8338, 1988.

100. Hagenbuch B, Steiger B, Meier PJ: Functional expression cloning and characterization of the hepatocyte Na^+/bile acid cotransport system. Proc Natl Acad Sci USA 88:10629, 1991.

101. Boyer JL et al.: Phylogenic and ontogenic expression of hepatocellular bile acid transport. Proc Natl Acad Sci USA 90:435, 1993.

102. Van Dyke RW, Stephens JE, Scharschmidt BF: Effect of ion substitution on bile acid-dependent and bile acid-independent bile formation by the isolated perfused rat liver. J Clin Invest 70:505, 1982.

103. Kramer W et al.: Bile salt-binding polypeptides in plasma membranes of hepatocytes revealed by photoaffinity labelling. Eur J Biochem 129:13, 1982.

104. Von Dippe P, Levy D: Characterization of the bile acid transport system in normal and transformed hepatocytes. J Biol Chem 258:8896, 1983.

105. Jacquemin E et al.: Cloning and expression of cDNA encoding the chloride dependent sulfobromophthalein (BSP) uptake system of rat liver [Abstract]. Hepatology 16:89A, 1992.

106. Okishio T, Nair PP: Studies on bile acids. Some observations on the intracellular localization of major bile acids in rat liver. Biochemistry 5:3662, 1966.

107. Stolz A, Takikawa H, Ookhtens M, Kaplowitz N: The role of cytoplasmic proteins in hepatic bile acid transport. Annu Rev Physiol 51:161, 1989.

108. Erlinger S: Role of intracellular organelles in the hepatic transport of bile acids. Biomed Pharmacother 44:409, 1990.

109. Suchy FJ et al.: Intracellular bile acid transport in rat liver as visualized by electron microscope autoradiography using a bile acid analogue. Am J Physiol 245:G681, 1983.

110. Lambri Y et al.: Immunoperoxidase localization of bile salts in rat liver cells. Evidence for a role of the Golgi apparatus in bile salt transport. J Clin Invest 82:1173, 1988.

111. Fricker G, Schneider S, Gerok W, Kurz G: Identification of different transport systems for bile salts in sinusoidal and canalicular membranes of hepatocytes. Biol Chem Hoppe-Seyler 368:1143, 1987.

112. Ruetz ST et al.: Isolation and characterization of the putative canalicular bile salt transport system of rat liver. J Biol Chem 262:11324, 1987.

113. Ruetz ST, Hugentobler G, Meier PJ: Functional reconstitution of the canalicular bile salt transport system of rat liver. Proc Natl Acad Sci USA 85:6147, 1988.

114. Graf J, Gautam A, Boyer JL: Isolated rat hepatocyte couplets: A primary secretory unit for electrophysiologic studies of bile secretory function. Proc Natl Acad Sci USA 81:6516, 1984.

115. Inoue M, Kinne R, Tran T, Arias IM: Taurocholate transport by rat liver canalicular membrane vesicles. J Clin Invest 73:659, 1984.

116. Meier PJ, Meier-Abt ASt, Barrett C, Boyer JL: Mechanisms of taurocholate transport in canalicular and basolateral rat liver plasma membrane vesicles. J Biol Chem 259:10614, 1984.

117. Weinman SA, Graf J, Boyer JL: Voltage-driven taurocholate-dependent secretion in isolated hepatocyte couplets. Am J Physiol 256:G826, 1989.

118. Weinman SA, Graf J, Veith C, Boyer JL: Electroneutral uptake and electrogenic secretion of a fluorescent bile salt by rat hepatocyte couplets. Am J Physiol *264*:G220, 1993.

119. Nishida T, Gatmaitan Z, Che M, Arias IM: Rat liver canalicular membrane vesicles contain an ATP-dependent bile acid transport system. Proc Natl Acad Sci USA *88*: 6590, 1991.

120. Müller M et al.: ATP-dependent transport of taurocholate across the hepatocyte canalicular membrane mediated by a 110 kDa glycoprotein binding ATP and bile salt. J Biol Chem *266*:18920, 1991.

121. Adachi Y et al.: ATP-dependent taurocholate transport by rat liver canalicular membrane vesicles. Hepatology *14*:655, 1991.

122. Stieger B, O'Neill B, Meier PJ: ATP-dependent bile salt transport in canalicular rat liver plasma membrane vesicles. Biochem J *284*:67, 1992.

123. Sperber I: Secretion of anorganic anions in the formation of urine and bile. Pharm Rev *11*:109, 1959.

124. Sperber I: Biliary secretion of organic anions and its influence on bile flow. *In* Taylor W (ed.): The Biliary System. Oxford, UK, Blackwell Scientific Publication, 1965, p. 457.

125. Preisig R, Cooper HL, Wheeler HO: The relationship between taurocholate secretion rate and bile production in the unanesthetized dog during cholinergic blockade and during secretin administration. J Clin Invest *41*:1152, 1962.

126. Wheeler HO, Ross ED, Bradley SE: Canalicular bile production in dogs. Am J Physiol *214*:866, 1968.

127. Forker EL: Bile formation in guinea pigs: Analysis with inert solutes of graded molecular radius. Am J Physiol *215*:56, 1968.

128. Strasberg SM et al.: Analysis of the components of bile flow in the rhesus monkey. Am J Physiol *228*:115, 1975.

129. Strasberg SM, Ilson RG, Petrunka CN: 14C-Erythritol clearance and canalicular bile acid independent flow in the baboon. Am J Physiol *242*:G475, 1982.

130. Boyer JL, Bloomer JR: Canalicular bile secretion in man: Studies utilizing the biliary clearance of ^{14}C-mannitol. J Clin Invest *54*: 773, 1974.

131. Cheng S, Levy D: Characterization of the anion transport system in hepatocyte plasma membranes. J Biol Chem *255*:2637, 1980.

132. Ziegler K, Frimmer M, Möller W, Fasold H: Chemical modification of membrane proteins by brominated taurodehydrocholate in isolated hepatocytes; relationship to the uptake of cholate and phalloidin and to the sensitivity of hepatocytes to phalloidin. Naunyn-Schmiedeberg's Arch Pharmacol *319*:254, 1982.

133. Kramer W et al.: Bile salt-binding polypeptides in plasma membranes of hepatocytes revealed by photoaffinity labeling. Eur J Biochem *129*:13, 1982.

134. Berk PD, Potter BJ, Stremmel W: Role of plasma membrane ligand-binding proteins in the hepatocellular uptake of albumin-bound organic anions. Hepatology *7*:165, 1987.

135. Wolkoff AW et al.: Influence of Cl$^-$ on organic anion transport in short-term cultured rat hepatocytes and isolated perfused rat liver. J Clin Invest *79*:1259, 1987.

136. Potter BJ et al.: The kinetics of sulfobromophthalein uptake by rat liver sinusoidal vesicles. Biochim Biophys Acta *898*:159, 1987.

137. Hugentobler G, Meier PJ: Multispecific anion exchange in basolateral (sinusoidal) rat liver plasma membrane vesicles. Am J Physiol *251*:G656, 1986.

138. Jacquemin E et al.: Expression of the hepatocellular chloride-dependent sulfobromophthalein uptake system in Xenopus laevis oocytes. J Clin Invest *88*:2146, 1991.

139. Jansen PLM, Peters WH, Lamers WH: Hereditary chronic conjugated hyperbilirubinemia in mutant rats caused by defective heptic anion transport. Hepatology *5*:573, 1985.

140. Kuipers F et al.: Defective biliary secretion of bile acid 3-0-glucuronides in rats with hereditary conjugated hyperbilirubinemia. J Lipid Res *30*:1835, 1989.

141. Kitamura T et al.: Defective ATP-dependent bile canalicular transport of organic anions in mutant (TR−) rats with conjugated hyperbilirubinemia. Proc Natl Acad Sci USA *87*:3557, 1990.

142. Ballatori N, Truong AT: Relation between biliary glutathione excretion and bile acid-independent bile flow. Am J Physiol *256*: G22, 1989.

143. Ballatori N, Jacob R, Barrett C, Boyer JL: Biliary catabolism of glutathione and differential reabsorption of its amino acid constituents. Am J Physiol *254*:G1, 1988.

144. Guzelian P, Boyer JL: Glucose reabsorption from bile: Evidence for a biliohepatic circulation. J Clin Invest *53*:526, 1974.

145. Yoon YB et al.: Effect of side-chain shortening on the physiologic properties of bile acids: Hepatic transport and effect on biliary secretion of 23-nor-ursodeoxycholate in rodents. Gastroenterology *90*:837, 1986.

146. Moseley RH, Morrissette J, Johnson TR: Transport of N^1-methylnicotinamide by organic cation-proton exchange in rat liver membrane vesicles. Am J Physiol *259*: G973, 1990.

147. Braakman I et al.: Vesicular uptake system for the cation lucigenin in the rat hepatocyte. Molec Pharmacol *36*:537, 1989.

148. Kamimoto Y, Gatmaitan Z, Hsu J, Arias IM: The function of Gp170, the multidrug resistance gene product in rat liver canalicular membrane vesicles. J Biol Chem *264*: 11693, 1989.

149. Mullock BM et al.: Distribution of secretory component in hepatocytes and its mode of transfer into bile. Biochem J *190*: 819, 1980.

150. Hinton RH, Dobrota M, Mullock BM: Haptoglobin-mediated transfer of haemoglobin from serum into bile. FEBS Lett *112*:247, 1980.

151. Jones AL, Renston RH, Burwen SJ: Uptake and intracellular disposition of plasma-derived proteins and apoproteins by hepatocytes. Progr Liver Dis *8*:51, 1982.

152. Renston RH, Jones AL, Christiansen WD, Hradek GT: Evidence for a vesicular transport mechanism in hepatocytes for biliary secretion of immunoglobulin A. Science *208*:1276, 1980.

153. Hoppe CA, Connolly TP, Hubbard AL: Transcellular transport of polymeric IgA in the rat hepatocyte: Biochemical and morphological characterization of the transport pathway. J Cell Biol *101*:2113, 1985.

154. LaRusso NF, Fowler S: Coordinate secretion of acid hydrolases in rat bile. J Clin Invest *64*:948, 1979.

155. Windaus A: Über Cholesterin. Ber dtsch chem Ges Berlin *37*:3699, 1904.

156. Windaus A: Über die quantitative Bestimmung des Cholesterins und der Cholesterinester in einigen normalen und pathologischen Nieren Z Physiol Chem *65*:110, 1910.

157. Gamble JJ, Blackfan KD: Evidence indicating a synthesis of cholesterol by infants. J Biol Chem *42*:401, 1920.

158. Nomura T: Zur Frage der Cholesterase im Blutserum und in Organextrakten. Tohoku J Exper Med *4*:677, 1924.

159. Backmeister A, Havers K: Untersuchungen über Cholesterinausscheidung in die menschliche Galle. Biochem Z *26*:233, 1910.

160. Balint JA, Kyriakides EC, Spitzer HL, Morrison ES: Lecithin fatty acid composition in bile and plasma of man, dogs, rats, and oxen. J Lipid Res *6*:96, 1965.

161. Yousef I, Fisher MM: In vitro effect of free bile acids on the bile canalicular membrane phospholipids in the rat. Can J Biochem *54*: 1040, 1975.

162. Small DM, Bourges M, Dervichian DG: Ternary and quaternary aqueous systems containing bile salt, lecithin, and cholesterol. Nature *211*:816, 1966.

163. Carey MC: Physical-chemical properties of bile acids and their salts. *In* Danielsson H, Sjövall J (eds.): Sterols and bile acids. Amsterdam, Elsevier, 345, 1985.

164. Carey MC, Lamont JT: Cholesterol gallstone formation. 1. Physical chemistry of bile and biliary lipid secretion. Progr Liver Dis *10*:139, 1992.

165. Mazer NA, Carey MC: Quasielastic light scattering studies of aqueous biliary lipid systems: Cholesterol solubilization and precipitation in model bile solutions. Biochemistry *19*:601, 1980.

166. Reuben A, Howell KE, Boyer JL: Effects of taurocholate on the size of mixed lipid micelles and their associations with pigment and proteins in rat bile. J Lipid Res *23*:1039, 1982.

167. Turley SD, Dietschy JM: Regulation of biliary cholesterol output in the rat: Dissociation from the rate of hepatic cholesterol synthesis, the size of the hepatic cholesteryl ester pool, and the hepatic uptake of chylomicron cholesterol. J Lipid Res *20*: 923, 1979.

168. Schwartz CC et al.: Multicompartmental analysis of cholesterol metabolism in man: characterization of the hepatic bile acid and biliary cholesterol precursor sites. J Clin Invest *61*:408, 1978.

169. Robins SJ, Brunengraber H: Origin of biliary cholesterol and lecithin in the rat: Contribution of new synthesis and preformed hepatic stores. J Lipid Res *23*:604, 1982.

170. Carey MC, Calahane MJ: Enterohepatic circulation. *In* Arias IM, et al. (eds.): The liver: Biology and Pathobiology. New York, Raven Press, 1988, p. 573.

171. Apstein MD, Robbins SJ: Effect of organic anions on biliary lipids in the rat. Gastroenterology *83*:1120, 1982.

172. Gregory DH, Vlahcevic ZR, Prugh MF, Swell T: Mechanism of secretion of biliary lipids: Role of a microtubular system in hepatocellular transport of biliary lipids in the rat. Gastroenterology *74*:93, 1978.

173. Redinger RN, Small DM: Primate biliary physiology. VIII. The effect of phenobarbital upon bile salt synthesis and pool size, biliary lipid secretion and bile composition. J Clin Invest *52*:161, 1973.

174. Crawford JM, Gollan JL: Transcellular transport of organic anions in hepatocytes:

Still a long way to go. Hepatology *14*:192, 1991.

175. Moore EW, Dietschy JM: Na and K activity coefficients in bile and bile salts determined by glass electrodes. Am J Physiol *206*:1111, 1964.

176. Wheeler HO, Ramos OL: Determinants of the flow and composition of bile in the unanesthetized dog during constant infusions of sodium taurocholate. J Clin Invest *39*: 161, 1960.

177. Cook DL, Lawler CA, Calvin LD, Green DM: Mechanisms of bile formation. Am J Physiol *171*:62, 1952.

178. Brauer RW: Mechanisms of bile secretion. JAMA *150*:1462, 1956.

179. Boyer JL: Mechanisms of bile secretion and hepatic transport. *In* Andreoli TE, Hoffman JF, Fanestil DD, Schultz SG (eds): Membrane Transport Processes in Organized Systems. New York, Plenum Medical Book Company, 1987, p. 225.

180. Renner EL et al.: Rat hepatocytes exhibit basolateral Na^+/HCO_3^- cotransport. J Clin Invest *84*:312, 1989.

181. Gleeson D, Smith ND, Boyer JL: Bicarbonate-dependent and independent intracellular pH regulatory mechanisms in rat hepatocytes. J Clin Invest *84*:312, 1989.

182. Fitz JG, Persico M, Scharschmidt BF: Electrophysiological evidence for Na^+-coupled bicarbonate transport in cultured rat hepatocytes. Am J Physiol *256*:G491, 1989.

183. Corasanti JG, Gleeson D, Boyer JL: Effects of osmotic stresses on isolated rat hepatocytes. II. Modulation of intracellular pH. Am J Physiol *258*:G290, 1990.

184. Arias IM, Forgac M: The sinusoidal domain of the plasma membrane of rat hepatocytes contains an amiloride-sensitive Na^+/H^+ antiport. J Biol Chem *259*:5406, 1984.

185. Moseley RH, Meier PJ, Aronson PS, Boyer JL: Na-H exchange in rat liver basolateral but not canalicular plasma membrane vesicles. Am J Physiol *250*:G35, 1986.

186. Henderson RM, Graf J, Boyer JL: Na-H exchange regulates intracellular pH in isolated rat hepatocyte couplets. Am J Physiol *252*:G109, 1987.

187. Stremmel W, Strohmeyer G, Berk PD: Hepatocellular uptake of oleate is energy dependent, sodium linked, and inhibited by an antibody to a hepatocyte plasma membrane fatty acid binding protein. Proc Natl Acad Sci *83*:3584, 1986.

188. Stremmel W: Translocation of fatty acids across the basolateral rat liver plasma membrane is driven by an active potential-sensitive sodium-dependent transport system. J Biol Chem *262*:6284, 1987.

189. Kristensen LO: Energization of alanine transport in isolated rat hepatocytes. J Biol Chem *255*:5236, 1980.

190. Fehlmann M et al.: Regulation of amino acid transport in the liver. J Biol Chem *254*: 401, 1979.

191. Tal M, Schneider DL, Thorens B, Lodish BF: Restricted expression of the erythroid/brain glucose transporter isoform to perivenous hepatocytes in rats. J Clin Invest *86*: 986, 1990.

192. Blitzer BL, Boyer JL: Cytochemical localization of Na^+, K^+-ATPase in the rat hepatocyte. J Clin Invest *62*:1104, 1978.

193. Graf J et al.: Cell membrane and transepithelial voltages and resistances in isolated rat hepatocyte couplets. J Membr Biol *95*: 241, 1987.

194. Graf J, Peterlik M: Mechanism of transport of inorganic ions into bile. *In* Taylor W (ed): The Hepatobiliary System—Fundamental and Pathological Mechanisms. New York, Plenum Press, 1975, p. 43.

195. Reichen J, Berr F, Le M, Warren GH: Characterization of calcium deprivation-induced cholestasis in the perfused rat liver. Am J Physiol *249*:G48, 1985.

196. Anwer MS, Clayton LM: Role of extracellular Ca^{++} in hepatic bile formation and taurocholate transport. Am J Physiol *249*: G711, 1985.

197. Mauger JP, Poggioli J, Guesdon F, Claret M: Noradrenaline, vasopressin and angiotensin increase Ca^{++} influx by opening a common pool of Ca^{++} channels in isolated rat liver cells. Biochem J *221*:121, 1984.

198. Pavoine C, Lotersztajn S, Mallat A, Pecker F: The high affinity $(Ca^{++}-Mg^{++})$-ATPase in liver plasma membranes in a Ca^{++} pump. J Biol Chem *262*:5113, 1987.

199. Shanne FAX, Moore L: Liver plasma membrane calcium transport. Evidence for a Na^+ dependent Ca^{++} flux. J Biol Chem *261*:9886, 1986.

200. Kraus-Friedmann N, Biber J, Murer H, Carafoli E: Calcium uptake in isolated hepatic plasma membrane vesicles. Eur J Biochem *129*:7, 1982.

201. Lidovsky SD, Xie MH, Scharschmidt BF: Na^+-Ca^{++} exchange in cultured rat hepatocytes: Evidence against a role in cytosolic Ca^{++} regulation or signaling. Am J Physiol *259*:G56, 1990.

202. Hamada Y et al.: Acute effects of cholestatic and choleretic bile salts on vasopressin- and glucagon-induced hepatobiliary calcium fluxes in the perfused rat liver. Biochem J *283*:575, 1992.

203. Beuers U, Nathanson M, Boyer JL: Effects of tauroursodeoxycholic acid on cytosolic

Ca^{++} signals in isolated rat hepatocytes. Gastroenterology *104*:604, 1993.

204. Spamer C, Heilmann C, Gerok W: Ca^{++}-activated ATPase in microsomes from human liver. J Biol Chem *262*:7782, 1987.

205. Meier PJ et al.: Evidence for carrier-mediated chloride/bicarbonate exchange in canalicular rat liver plasma membrane vesicles. J Clin Invest *75*:1256, 1985.

206. Benedetti A et al.: Cl$^-$-HCO$_3^-$ exchanger in isolated rat hepatocytes: Role in regulation of intracellular pH. Am J Physiol *261*: G512, 1991.

207. Benedetti A, Strazzabosco M, Boyer JL: Cellular regulation of Cl$^-$/HCO$_3$ exchange activity by HCO$_3^-$, cAMP and colchicine in isolated rat hepatocytes (Abstract). Hepatology *12*:887, 1990.

208. Hardison WGM, Wood CA: Importance of bicarbonate in bile salt independent fraction of bile flow. Am J Physiol *235*:E158, 1981.

209. Van Dyke RW, Stephens JE, Scharschmidt BF: Effects of ion substitution on bile acid-dependent and -independent bile formation by rat liver. J Clin Invest *70*:505, 1982.

210. Anwer MS, Hegner D: Role of inorganic electrolytes in bile acid-independent canalicular bile formation. Am J Physiol *244*: G116, 1983.

211. Boyer JL: New concepts of mechanisms of hepatocyte bile formation. Physiol Rev *60*: 303, 1980.

212. Arias IM et al.: The biology of the bile canaliculus, 1993. Hepatology *17*:318, 1993.

213. Oshio C, Phillips MJ: Contractility of bile canaliculi: Implications for liver function. Science *212*:1041, 1981.

214. Boyer JL: Isolated rat hepatocyte couplets: A model for the study of bile secretory function. *In* Tavoloni N, Berk PD (eds): Hepatic Transport and Bile Secretion. New York, Raven Press, 597, 1993.

215. Bayliss MW, Starling EH: The mechanism of pancreatic secretion. J Physiol *28*:325, 1902.

216. Sirica AE, Mathis GA, Sano N, Elmore LW: Isolation, culture, and transplantation of intrahepatic biliary epithelial cells and oval cells. Pathobiology *58*:44, 1990.

217. Lenzen R, Alpini G, Tavoloni N: Secretin stimulates bile ductular secretory activity through the cAMP system [Abstract]. Hepatology *12*:890, 1990.

218. Fitz G et al.: Regulation of membrane chloride currents in rat bile duct epithelial cells. J Clin Invest *91*:319, 1993.

219. Alvaro D, Cho WK, Mennone A, Boyer JL: Effect of secretin on intracellular pH regulation in isolated rat bile duct epithelial cells. J Clin Invest *92*:1314, 1993.

18

Viral Hepatitis

JULES L. DIENSTAG

The understanding of viral hepatitis has evolved more rapidly in the last 30 years than at any other time in history, and the pace has quickened dramatically during the last two decades. Before this period, progress was limited, punctuated by rare, episodic advances, and hindered by false turns and misconceptions. Not long ago, all forms of jaundice were believed to be caused by mucus plugging of the distal common bile duct resulting from inflammation of the duodenal mucosa ("catarrhal" jaundice), despite the fact that epidemics of jaundice, following patterns common to other contagions, were recognized in the Middle Ages. During the early 20th century, pathologic examination of livers from patients with "epidemic" jaundice showed that the primary process was inflammation of the liver. Advances in laboratory tests associated with liver inflammation and injury (1,2) and the introduction of percutaneous liver biopsy in the middle of the 20th century (3,4) secured the notion that outbreaks of jaundice were the result of hepatitis.

Although several critical thinkers in the early 20th century interpreted outbreaks of jaundice after injection therapy (such as the 1883 outbreak of jaundice in Bremen shipyard workers vaccinated with human lymph against smallpox (5)) and in military troops to support an infectious cause, firm conclusions about the role of infectious agents in epidemics of jaundice were not reached until the years of World War II. During those years, two seminal observations established beyond any doubt that epidemics of jaundice were caused by a filterable infectious agent (a virus):

1. Large outbreaks of hepatitis in military personnel immunized with yellow fever vaccine were attributed to contamination of the vaccine by an agent in the serum used to supplement virus culture medium (6–8).

2. Viral hepatitis was transmitted to volunteers (9–11).

Many investigators from countries all over the world contributed to the growth of knowledge about viral hepatitis, in both the early period of limited progress and the more recent period of extraordinary advances. Standing out are a number of landmark observations and investigations whose impact has been profound. These are summarized in the following sections.

STUDIES AT THE WILLOWBROOK STATE SCHOOL

Krugman and his colleagues were not the first to study viral hepatitis in an institutional setting or to conduct human transmission experiments, and much of what they learned was based on earlier observations made by others. Most authorities would agree, however, that the modern era of hepatitis virology began with the elegant and meticulous studies conducted in the late 1950s and 1960s by Krugman at the Willowbrook State School in Staten Island, New York. Asked to study and attempt to control the high frequency of measles at this institution for the mentally handicapped, Krugman and his colleagues recognized quickly that viral hepatitis was much more of a problem; most of the newly admitted children acquired viral hepatitis within the first 6 to 12 months there. Although current standards of research ethics would not have permitted these studies in mentally handicapped persons, the studies undertaken adhered scrupulously to accepted ethical standards of the era and were approved by official review bodies with jurisdiction over human investigation. These studies established definitively that there were two, immunologically distinct, hepatitis viruses, hepatitis A and B, with different incubation periods and different primary modes of transmission. The serum of one child (whose initials were MS and who had two bouts of acute hepatitis) became reference materials for later studies of hepatitis A virus, called MS-1, and hepatitis B virus, called MS-2. Hepatitis A virus (HAV) was confirmed to be readily transmitted by personal contact and fecal-oral spread; hepatitis B virus (HBV) was confirmed to be much less infectious under these circumstances but still transmitted, inefficiently to be sure, by oral ingestion. These studies established the efficacy of immunoprophylaxis with immune globulin of hepatitis A, and the demonstration that boiled MS-2 serum inoculated into susceptible persons could prevent subsequent challenge with hepatitis B laid the intellectual foundation for the first-generation, plasma-derived hepatitis B vaccine developed in the 1970s. Carefully pedigreed clinical materials derived from these studies proved crucial to those who developed specific serologic tests of HBV and HAV antigens and antibodies (12–15).

IDENTIFICATION AND CHARACTERIZATION OF HEPATITIS B VIRUS

Discovery of "Australia Antigen."

The most seminal observation leading to the discovery of HBV and establishing the foundation for the immunologic and biochemical characterization of HBV and all the other hepatitis viruses was the discovery by Blumberg and his colleagues of Australia antigen, the envelope protein of HBV. Blumberg did not set out to identify hepatitis B. Instead, he was a geneticist searching for protein polymorphisms, i.e., the occurrence of variants of common genetic traits, such as blood groups. Based on the hypothesis that multiply transfused persons would have been exposed to protein antigens different from their own, he and his coworkers used serum from persons who had received transfusions as a probe for protein antigens in the serum of other persons. This approach led to the detection of an immunoprecipitin line in agar gel between the serum of a multitransfused hemophiliac and an Australian aborigine (16). Initially, the high frequencies of this antigen in the serum of patients with leukemia and Down syndrome led Blumberg and his colleagues to suggest that the Australia antigen was a leukemia antigen or related to the cause of leukemia (a disease more common in Down syndrome). Ultimately, however, the detection of this antigen in the serum of patients with viral hepatitis and the acquisition of the antigen in serum by a technician working in Blumberg's laboratory who had a clinically mild case of acute viral hepatitis led to the conclusion that Australia antigen was a marker of viral hepatitis (17). Independently, Prince and his colleagues found an antigen, which they labeled serum hepatitis (SH) antigen, in the serum of patients with transfusion-associated hepatitis (18). The Australia antigen and SH antigen were one and the same, and the association between Australia antigen and "serum" hepatitis was confirmed by others (19).

Following these observations came numerous reports associating Australia antigen with hepatitis B, with acute and chronic hepatitis, and with an asymptomatic hepatitis B carrier state. As a serologic marker for HBV infection, Australia antigen was used to distinguish between cases of hepatitis B, with a positive test, and cases of hepatitis A, with a negative test. Because hepatitis viruses had not been cultivated, and because animal models had not yet been discovered, this first serologic "handle" with which to study viral hepatitis had a profound impact on future research. An exhaustive effort was launched in many laboratories to characterize this viral protein. More sensitive test methods, including radioimmunoassay and enzyme immunoassay, were applied to the detection of this viral protein, and the search for other viral markers led to the discovery of the other antigens of hepatitis B. When data supported the identity of Australia antigen as the outer envelope protein of HBV, the nomenclature hepatitis B surface antigen (HBsAg) was adopted. For his serendipitous discovery of the envelope protein of HBV, Blumberg was awarded the 1976 Nobel Prize in Medicine.

Further Characterization of HBV

The application of serologic, immunologic, electron microscopic, immunohistochemical, and biophysical techniques led to the identification of the 42-nm hepatitis B virion (20), with its HBsAg envelope and its internal 27-nm nucleocapsid core, expressing hepatitis B core antigen (HBcAg) (21). Hepatitis B surface antigen was expressed also on smaller, 22-nm spherical and tubular particles associated with HBV—noninfectious, excess virus coat protein. In the infancy of molecular virology, HBV was found to be a DNA virus (22) and to have an endogenous, DNA-dependent DNA polymerase (23). Within a short time, the entire DNA genome of HBV was characterized and cloned. Early in the 1970s, subtypes of HBV were defined by simple immunodiffusion techniques, and subtype distinctions were pursued further at the molecular level with the introduction of gene cloning and sequencing techniques.

In a few instances, preliminary reports of a new finding were so counterintuitive that they were not readily accepted. One of these was the discovery of a third HBV antigen, HBeAg. Magnius and Espmark (24) identified this new antigen-antibody system by agar-gel immunodiffusion in HBsAg-positive serum samples. Many authorities were skeptical, however, given the fact that no such marker was detected during the exhaustive work of others in this area. In fact, several years elapsed before this third antigen-antibody system was accepted and found to represent a soluble protein, a component of the nucleocapsid core; its presence in the circulation correlated with a high level of HBV replication and infectivity (25). Ultimately, molecular virologic techniques showed that HBeAg was coded for by the gene for the nucleocapsid and, unlike HBcAg, was a secreted protein (see subsequent text). This viral marker, which was dismissed initially as an artifact, has become an important clinical marker of relative virus replication correlating with infectivity and liver injury.

Clinical Features of Hepatitis B

The availability of precise serologic tools for the study and diagnosis of hepatitis B provided new clinical insights about the disease and its pathogenesis. This agent was found to be associated with several immune complex disorders, including a prodromal dermatitis-arthritis syndrome, glomerulonephritis, and generalized vasculitis (26). In addition, the availability of serologic markers on a broad epidemiologic scale and the application of probes for HBV DNA to hepatic tissue revealed an undeniable link between HBV and hepatocellular carcinoma (HCC), the most common malignancy (27–30). This link was cemented by the observation of HCC in other species with viruses similar to HBV (i.e., other hepadnaviruses, see below) (31). Scientists today are still attempting to understand the factors that contribute to the oncogenicity of HBV.

Pathogenesis of Hepatitis B

Although immune-complex-induced vasculitis has been shown to account for the extrahepatic manifestations of acute and chronic hepatitis B, the pathogenesis of liver injury associated with this virus remains incompletely understood. The factors that distinguish persons who recover from those who do not have not been elucidated; however, based on in-depth studies of viral markers and immunologic responses—limited as they may be by the inadequacy of in vitro tools—most would conclude that HBV is not cytopathic but destroys liver cells through cell-mediated mechanisms. Current data support the hypothesis that cytolytic T cells directed at the nucleocapsid protein, HBcAg, rather than the envelope protein, HBsAg, are responsible for liver cell injury in patients with hepatitis B (32). The availability of sensitive probes for HBV antigens and DNA has unearthed the presence of HBV in lymphocytes, among other extrahepatic reservoirs (33,34). This observation may indicate that HBV has a potential direct effect on immunologic responsiveness.

Despite the evidence in favor of HBcAg as the target of cytolytic T cells, attention to HBsAg as a potential target has been resurrected by the elegant experiments of Chisari and his colleagues, demonstrating hepatocellular injury in *transgenic mice* expressing HBsAg (35–38). The use of transgenic mice is likely to become a valuable model system with which to study other features of HBV and its pathogenesis.

Observations about the pathogenesis of hepatitis B have derived from unusual, unexpected sources. Another observation that points towards the importance of HBsAg in the pathogenesis of liver cell injury derives from observations gleaned from patients who have undergone liver transplantation for end-stage chronic hepatitis B. In contrast to immunocompetent persons, liver transplant recipients receive immunosuppressive drugs, which affect not only their ability to reject the new organ but also their capacity to mount an immune response to virus-infected hepatocytes. In a proportion of such patients, rapidly progressive liver injury ensues, apparently, in the absence of an immunologic component. In these patients, an unusual pathologic lesion, *"fibrosing cholestatic hepatitis,"* has been observed with ultrastructural features, suggesting that the cell becomes choked with vast quantities of HBsAg (39). This, under certain circumstances, HBV appears to have the potential to be directly cytopathic. Further study of this interesting lesion is likely to shed additional light on the pathogenesis of hepatitis B even in immunocompetent persons.

Important insights with potential clinical relevance have come from studies of *genetic regulation of immune responses to HBV proteins*. Milich and his colleagues have meticulously dissected out components of the immune response to HBV proteins in mice (40). These elegant studies have demonstrated a genetically determined hierarchy of immune responsiveness to HBsAg, independent of the genetic control over immune responsiveness to proteins of the product of the pre-S genes, upstream of the gene for HBsAg (the S gene region) (41–43). If the same is true for humans, then persons who do not respond to HBsAg in

hepatitis B vaccine theoretically might respond to a vaccine made with pre-S proteins. Similarly, these investigators have shown that the murine T-cell immune response to HBcAg can provide help for the production of antibody to HBsAg (44), which may explain why vaccine nonresponders (exposed exclusively to HBsAg) have a normal immune response if infected with HBV (which includes exposure to both HBsAg and HBcAg). This observation also suggests that, in future vaccines, HBcAg should not be overlooked as a potential immunogen. Milich and colleagues also have used the transgenic mouse model to study immune responsiveness to HBeAg and have shown that in utero exposure to HBeAg induces T-cell tolerance to HBeAg as well as HBcAg (45). These observations may help explain the profound level of immunologic tolerance to HBV in children born to HBsAg-positive, HBeAg-positive mothers. These exciting studies have attracted the interest of the investigative community and are likely to have an important impact in the future.

Epidemiologic Features of Hepatitis B

Substantial new information has been generated by the application of the entire panoply of serologic tools to a reanalysis of the epidemiology of hepatitis B. Many cases that had been labeled "infectious" hepatitis turned out to be caused by HBV, and most cases of "serum" hepatitis were found to be unrelated to HBV. Recognition of the existence of "non-B" cases of "serum" hepatitis was one of the crucial discoveries pointing towards the existence of "non-A, non-B" hepatitis (see subsequent text). Currently, we recognize that the most important modes of HBV transmission are perinatal, sexual, and percutaneous (exposure to contaminated blood, blood products, needles, and other instruments). Unfortunately, approximately 30% of all cases of acute hepatitis B occur in persons with no recognized or admitted risk factor. Unearthing the source of these infections remains a challenge for the future. Although other non-virus-specific changes in blood procurement policies had an impact on the occurrence of hepatitis B after transfusion, the discovery of Australia antigen paved the way for ever more sensitive screening of donor blood for HBV and for the ultimate near elimination of hepatitis B as a transfusion-transmitted disease.

HEPATITIS B VACCINE

As described previously, Krugman (15) showed that boiling serum containing HBV could inactivate the virus without destroying its antigenicity and that such material injected into susceptible hosts could protect them from infection with live virus. This important observation laid the intellectual foundation for the development of a hepatitis B vaccine derived from human plasma. At the time, HBV could not be cultivated in vitro, and molecular cloning techniques were no more than a pipe dream; therefore, the then conventional and now contemporary, molecular approaches to vaccine production were not possible. Studies of the properties of HBV indicated that the small, spherical 22-nm spherical particles (devoid of nucleic acid and noninfectious) could be separated biophysically from intact, infectious virions (46,47). Therefore, if an immune response to these HBsAg-expressing particles could induce antibody to HBsAg (anti-HBs), the protective antibody, in susceptible hosts, a "subunit" vaccine prepared from these particles could be developed by relying for a source of viral protein not on in vitro cultivation but, instead, on plasma obtained from hepatitis B carriers. This concept was actually patented (48), then developed in parallel programs by Purcell and Gerin at the National Institutes of Health and by Hilleman and colleagues at Merck Sharp & Dohme Research Laboratories. Comparable programs were instituted in Europe as well. The development of this unconventional vaccine required exhaustive purification of the small 22-nm HBsAg particles of HBV, multistep inactivation procedures, and extensive testing for safety and immunogenicity in chimpanzees before testing in humans could begin in the late 1970s. The plasma-derived vaccine developed by Merck was tested in a double-blind, placebo-controlled trial in a high-risk population (promiscuous homosexual men) by Szmuness and his colleagues at the New York Blood Center (49). Among those re-

sponding to the vaccine by acquiring anti-HBs, the vaccine was essentially 100% effective in preventing acute hepatitis B; vaccine safety was established as well in that landmark study. The efficacy of plasma-derived vaccines was confirmed in studies of other high-risk populations in the United States and Europe, and the vaccine was licensed in 1981, then released commercially in 1982. Development of an effective hepatitis B vaccine, without the benefit of in vitro cultivation of the virus, within approximately 15 years of the discovery of Australia antigen was hailed as one of the major medical-science breakthroughs of the time.

No sooner had the first-generation, plasma-derived vaccine been released than development of a second-generation vaccine was pursued, based on recombinant DNA technology. Advances in molecular virology had progressed to the point at which large-scale viral protein or particle synthesis in recombinant bacteria or yeast became feasible, and a recombinant-yeast hepatitis B vaccine was the first such genetically engineered product to reach clinical application and commercial release. Comparable in immunogenicity and efficacy to the plasma-derived hepatitis B vaccine (50), and devoid of the imagined but never-realized dangers of a plasma-derived vaccine, recombinant hepatitis B vaccines supplanted plasma-derived vaccines by the end of the 1980s.

Today, HBV can be propagated in vitro (33), and there are potential alternative approaches to development of genetically engineered hepatitis B vaccines (51–57), many based on ingenious applications of molecular virology. Ultimately, one or more of these methods may emerge as the technology of the next generation of hepatitis B vaccines. With current and future vaccines, the potential exists for interrupting the vicious cycle of maternal-neonatal transmission of hepatitis B, of reducing or even eliminating hepatitis B as a public health problem, and the exciting concept of preventing hepatocellular carcinoma by vaccination.

Public Health Failure

Because the development of hepatitis B vaccines was hailed as a scientific breakthrough, few would have predicted that hepatitis B immunization policy would turn out to be substantially less than a public health success. Since the introduction of the first-generation hepatitis B vaccine in the early 1980s, the frequency of hepatitis B has not decreased but has continued to climb; no more than a small proportion of those targeted within high-risk groups have actually been vaccinated; and approximately 30 percent of new hepatitis B cases occur in persons not identified as belonging to high risk groups. Thus, the current approach of vaccinating persons within high risk groups has had a limited impact. Therefore, an alternative approach to overcome these unanticipated obstacles, universal vaccination in childhood has been recommended (58).

Genetic Nonresponsiveness to Hepatitis B Vaccine

The introduction of hepatitis B vaccines has had another unintended but important consequence. Among immunocompetent recipients of hepatitis B vaccine, 2.5 to 5% are incapable of responding by mounting an antibody response. Examples of genetic nonresponsiveness to specific antigens had long been recognized in mice, and nonresponsiveness to HBsAg in mice already had been shown to be genetically determined (42,43). The recognition of a subset of normal adults who failed to respond to hepatitis B vaccine led to the hypothesis that what was true for inbred strains of mice applied as well to outbred humans. Indeed, nonresponsiveness in humans to hepatitis B vaccine has been shown to be genetically determined (59–61), the first demonstration of such genetic control over immunologic responsiveness in humans. Who would have predicted that the development of hepatitis B vaccine would have "opened the door" to a new and important field of inquiry in human genetics?

ANIMAL MODELS FOR VIRAL HEPATITIS

Almost every major advance in hepatitis research has relied directly or indirectly at some point on the availability of suitable animal models. Unfortunately, common laboratory animals are not susceptible to human hepatitis viruses. Although several nonhuman primate species are susceptible to one or more of the hepatitis viruses, the most reliable animal model and suitable animal host has been the chimpanzee. Substantial progress in understanding the biology of all five known human hepatitis viruses was achieved by studying experimental infection in chimpanzees (62–67). For example, this animal model provided a tool to study chronic hepatitis B (68) and to document the potential infectivity of semen and saliva (69). The chimpanzee was instrumental in the development of hepatitis B vaccine, and pedigreed high-level infectious chimpanzee plasma provided the material from which hepatitis C virus was identified and characterized (70).

The importance of the marmoset model for hepatitis A virus infection (71,72) and of cynomolgus macaques for the study of hepatitis E virus (73,74) is addressed in subsequent text.

Other Hepadnaviruses

One of the most startling and provocative discoveries of the late 1970s and early 1980s was the occurrence in nature of viruses that shared morphologic, genomic, and biologic features with human HBV. Woodchuck hepatitis virus (31), ground squirrel hepatitis virus (75), and duck hepatitis B virus (76) were found to have the same three morphologic particles as HBV; the same envelope(s), particulate (c) and soluble (e) nucleocapsid antigens; the same genomic structure and organization; the same hepatotropism and association with acute and chronic liver injury; the same modes of transmission; and the same potential for hepatocarcinogenicity (77–79). As a group, these viruses and HBV have been designated as the family Hepadnaviridae. Although genomic and antigenic homology among the hepadnaviruses is limited, detailed studies of the structure and replicative strategy of the nonhuman hepadnaviruses provided invaluable information about HBV and demonstrated that, in all these viruses, the mechanism of virus replication was reminiscent of that in RNA-containing retroviruses (80–85). The availability of these animal models for HBV, as well as others more recently described, continue to provide new information about the pathophysiology of hepatitis B.

Transgenic Mice

As noted previously, Chisari and his colleagues have pioneered the development of transgenic mice for the study of hepatitis B (35,36). These mice, which have had HBV DNA introduced and integrated into their genomes, express HBV proteins, and they can be engineered to express a specific antigen of interest. Chisari already has shown that isolated expression of HBsAg can be associated with liver injury in these mice, challenging to some extent the now well-established hypothesis that HBcAg is the target of cell-mediated immunologic injury in hepatocytes infected with HBV. Studies of HBV in transgenic mice will allow the dissection of immunologic responses to individual HBV antigens, and the hepatocarcinogenicity of HBV also can be studied by creating transgenic mice into which oncogenes or tumor regulatory genes can be expressed with HBV DNA.

APPLICATION OF MOLECULAR BIOLOGY TO VIRAL HEPATITIS

From the isolation, characterization, and cloning of the HBV genome (22,80,84–93) and its eventual transfection in in vitro systems (33) have come both conceptual and practical advances in understanding and controlling viral hepatitis. HBV DNA in blood and liver tissue has been detected in patients with hepatitis B and hepatocellular carcinoma, even, sometimes, in the absence of typical serum HBV markers (29,94,95). Studies of HBV DNA in extrahepatic tissues have demonstrated the presence of the virus outside the liver (96). Tests for HBV DNA can be applied to the clinical evaluation of patients with hepatitis B and to monitoring during and after antiviral therapy (97), and recombinant viral antigens are now used routinely for diagnostic assays. In the field of viral hepatitis, one of the most important practical applications of molecular biology has been the development of recombinant hepatitis B vaccines (50,98,99). Most of the novel suggestions for vaccine development techniques, such as synthetic

peptides and production of HBV antigens in other recombinant vectors, rely on molecular biological approaches. These may provide vaccines of the future.

The important contributions of molecular biology to the study of hepatitis viruses besides HBV are summarized below.

Genetic Variants

An important observation derived from molecular studies of hepatitis viruses is their genomic heterogeneity. The hepatitis C virus genome varies so substantially among isolates that confusion reigns over the number of discrete viral strains (100,101). Recent attention has been focused on several genetic variants of HBV. An escape mutant, in which a single amino acid substitution occurs in the immunodominant, group-common *a* determinant of HBsAg, has been recognized rarely after active and passive immunization against hepatitis B (102,103). Such mutant HBV is not neutralized by vaccine-induced or passively infused anti-HBs. Although these genomic changes are not known to be common after vaccination, their rare occurrence demands a careful re-evaluation of immunoprophylaxis strategies. In another important category of HBV genetic variants, a single base-pair mutation in the pre-core region of the C gene results in a stop codon, which prevents the translation of HBeAg (102,104, 105). In patients infected with this variant, HBV DNA can be detected, but HBeAg cannot. Unlike patients with wild-type HBV, in whom loss of circulating HBeAg is associated with the loss of circulating HBV DNA and a marked reduction in infectivity and liver injury, in patients with pre-core HBV mutants, circulating HBV DNA, high infectivity, and severe liver injury can occur without detectable HBeAg. Understanding of the overall pathophysiologic and clinical import of such mutations, impossible before the application of molecular biology to studies of HBV, will occupy clinical investigators in the coming decade and beyond.

DISCOVERY OF HEPATITIS A VIRUS

Despite the careful characterization of HAV during human transmission studies such as those at Willowbrook (12) and derivative studies at the federal prison in Joliet, Illinois (106), despite the demonstration that marmoset monkeys could serve as susceptible hosts for experimental infection (71,72,107), progress in hepatitis A research was limited until 1973, when Feinstone, Kapikian, and Purcell visualized 27-nm hepatitis A virus particles by immune electron microscopy (108). Shortly thereafter, and independently, Provost and Hilleman and colleagues identified HAV particles in livers of marmosets with experimentally induced hepatitis A (109). These breakthroughs led rapidly to biophysical and biochemical characterization of the virus, to simple serologic tests, to a re-analysis of the epidemiology of hepatitis A, to the preparation of a crude vaccine based on inactivated virus obtained from marmoset liver (110), and to in vitro cultivation of the virus (111). Later, the molecular characterization of the genome was accomplished (112–115). Based on a more complete characterization of HAV and its nucleotide and amino acid sequences, this agent, which was classified provisionally as enterovirus type 72, has now been assigned to a new genus and classified as a heparnavirus (116). The ultimate goal of the study of infectious agents is to prevent infection and reduce the health threat of disease. As a result of the progress in hepatitis A virology that followed the detection of HAV in 1973, commercial release of killed hepatitis A vaccines that are immunogenic, effective, and safe is imminent (117). This age-old scourge is about to be conquered.

DISCOVERY OF HEPATITIS D (DELTA) VIRUS

The existence of the delta agent, or hepatitis D virus (HDV), would never have been predicted on the basis of knowledge of the other hepatitis viruses or other mammalian viruses. In this sense, its discovery stands as one of the ground-breaking developments in hepatitis virus research. Rizzetto and colleagues in Turin, Italy (118) were studying immunohistochemical features of hepatitis B but found an immunofluorescence reactivity that was distinct from known HBV antigen-antibody systems.

This antigen was detectable exclusively in hepatocyte nuclei from patients with hepatitis B, and Rizzetto et al. demonstrated that this antigen was distinct from HBsAg and HBeAg as well as from HBcAg, the expected nuclear staining antigen in hepatitis B. The detection of this antigen, labeled delta (d), was more common in patients with the more severe forms of chronic hepatitis B. Some investigators might have been quick to dismiss this reactivity as an artifact, as, no doubt, would reviewers of a manuscript describing these inexplicable findings. To his credit, Rizzetto pursued this new immunologic reactivity, and to their credit, investigators at the National Institutes of Health provided the technical expertise and environment for Rizzetto to investigate the meaning of the delta antigen-antibody system. This collaboration led to the unraveling of a remarkable biologic phenomenon.

After delta antigen was purified from the liver of an Italian patient, a sensitive radioimmunoassay was developed for delta antigen and antibody (119), the antigen was characterized, and clinical and epidemiologic investigations were launched. Transmission to chimpanzees was another important ingredient in unraveling this mystery (66,120). These efforts demonstrated that the delta antigen was the internal nucleocapsid protein of a small, 35 to 37 nm, defective RNA virus which was encapsidated by an envelope of HBsAg derived from the requisite simultaneous HBV infection. The delta agent requires the helper function of HBV—or other hepatitis viruses (121)—to support its replication and assembly into intact virions; therefore, delta hepatitis can occur only in conjunction with HBV infection, as either a simultaneous acute coinfection or a superinfection in a patient already chronically infected with HBV (122–124). As noted, clinically, infection with HDV is associated with the more serious outcomes of hepatitis B, such as severe chronic active hepatitis, end-stage cirrhosis, and fulminant hepatitis (124). Epidemiologically, infection with HDV is concentrated in Mediterranean countries, where transmission through personal contact is important; in lower-frequency regions, such as North America and northern and western Europe, HDV infection tends to remain confined primarily, albeit not exclusively, within subpopulations with intense blood exposure, such as hemophiliacs and intravenous drug users (123). Large outbreaks of HDV superinfection have been recorded episodically in South America, and outbreaks of co-infection have occurred in nonendemic areas of the United States—both with a high mortality. This agent tends to exploit human behaviors and population shifts for its amplification. For example, in nonendemic countries, introduction of HDV into populations of previously unexposed drug users has been shown to spread rapidly within the drug-using community; when this occurs, infection is introduced, probably through sexual contact, into the nondrug-using community as well (125). Ironically, population migrations in Italy during the early 1970s provided the serendipitous circumstances that allowed Rizzetto to "stumble upon" the existence of HDV. During that period, northward migration from southern Italy, where HDV is endemic, to more industrialized northern Italy, where HDV had been much less common, led to a sustained outbreak of delta infection in the north, maintained by person-to-person spread (126).

When molecular virologic techniques were applied to the study of HDV, the genomic structure of the virus was elucidated. It has a circular, single-stranded RNA that has extensive internal complementarity, affording it a very rigid, rod-like conformation. An antigenomic strand can be detected in clinical materials, and it is the antigenomic strand that codes for delta antigen (127–129). The structure and replication of HDV are similar to those of plant viroids, virusoids, and satellite viruses (128). An inviting hypothesis is that HDV evolved from a plant virus.

The absolute reliance on HBV for its replication has another important implication for prevention of HDV. Persons immune to HBV as a result of either previous infection and recovery or active immunization with hepatitis B vaccine are not susceptible to HDV infection. Therefore, vaccination against hepatitis B should protect as well against hepatitis D. Unfortunately, for persons already infected with HBV, no hepatitis D vaccine is available to prevent HDV superinfection.

After a decade of data supporting the absolute requirement of concomitant HBV infection for successful HDV infection, more recent observations suggest that, under certain circumstances, HDV can replicate without HBV. Human HDV has been cultivated in vitro in woodchuck hepatocyte cultures. In this system, intracellular HDV replication can be demonstrated in the absence of hepadnavirus coinfection (130). Similarly, in patients who undergo liver transplantation for end-stage hepatitis D, recurrence of HDV without HBV has been observed, but virus-induced liver injury requires recurrence of both infections (131). Therefore, HDV does require HBV infection for extracellular assembly and pathogenicity, but intracellular and nonpathogenic isolated HDV infection can occur.

DISCOVERY OF HEPATITIS C VIRUS

Until the early 1970s, conventional wisdom held that there were only two human hepatitis viruses. Certainly, the careful studies by Krugman and colleagues (12) demonstrated unequivocally that hepatitis A and B viruses accounted for all the cases of hepatitis at the Willowbrook State School. In the late 1960s and early 1970s, however, important transitions were occurring in blood banking that were destined to suggest the existence of other viral hepatitis agents. In 1971 Australia antigen was introduced as a screening test for donated blood. For at least a decade before this change in blood banking, commercially donated blood was recognized to be more likely than voluntarily donated blood to transmit hepatitis to blood recipients (132–134). Therefore, as the 1960s were ending and the 1970s were beginning, the conversion had begun to an all-volunteer blood-donor pool. When HBsAg-reactive and commercial donors were excluded, however, there was only a 25% reduction in the frequency of hepatitis after transfusion (135). At the time, these residual cases could have been the result of the insensitivity of the available assays for HBsAg, but even the most sensitive tests for hepatitis B could not prevent most cases of transfusion-associated hepatitis. Therefore, these non-B cases after transfusion were attributed by some authorities to hepatitis A; however, the long incubation period for hepatitis after transfusion was not at all characteristic for hepatitis A (136).

When, in 1973, a test became available to identify hepatitis A serologically (108), application of this test to cases of transfusion-associated hepatitis demonstrated convincingly that HAV was not involved at all (137). This was the seminal observation, later confirmed many times over, as reviewed elsewhere (138), that documented the existence of another important hepatitis virus, responsible for almost all cases of hepatitis after transfusion. Because very sensitive and sophisticated approaches were available in the early 1970s to identify viral antigens, antibodies, and particles, investigators believed that the discovery of "hepatitis C" was imminent. In the interim, they designated these cases as "non-A, non-B" hepatitis (137,139). This brief "interim" turned into a 15-year quest that was not completed until a novel molecular cloning technique was finally successful in the late 1980s (70).

During the approximately 15 years between the recognition of "non-A, non-B" hepatitis and the discovery of hepatitis C virus (HCV), many putative hepatitis C agents were described, but none could be confirmed (140). During this period, however, detailed epidemiologic investigations demonstrated the modes of transmission of this blood-borne agent; careful clinical studies showed that the frequency of chronic hepatitis was approximately 50% after acute non-A, non-B hepatitis and that cirrhosis ensued over the course of a decade in approximately 20% of those with chronic transfusion-associated hepatitis; the chimpanzee was found to be an excellent animal model for non-A, non-B hepatitis; cross-challenge experiments in chimpanzees even suggested that there might be more than a single non-A, non-B hepatitis agent; and, in the absence of virus-specific serologic tests, "surrogate" markers—alanine aminotransferase (ALT) and antibody to the core antigen of HBV (anti-HBc)—were shown to be associated with a higher risk of non-A, non-B hepatitis transmission from blood donor to recipient and were introduced as blood donor screening tests. Most of these advances are reviewed elsewhere (141,142).

Several important observations about the agent of non-A, non-B hepatitis derived from infectivity studies in chimpanzees. The agent was found to be chloroform-sensitive and to fall into the size range of approximately 30 to 60 nm, suggesting that it was a small lipid-enveloped virus (143–145). In addition, titration studies of various inocula in chimpanzees demonstrated that viremia was limited in some cases ($\leq 1:10^2$) but $>1:10^6$ in others (146,147). During the 1970s, while the search for non-A, non-B hepatitis agents was intense, molecular biology was advancing rapidly; recombinant DNA and cloning techniques were developed. In the 1980s, these techniques were applied to the cloning of human genes, such as those for insulin and interferon, and to viral genes, such as those of HBV and HAV, and their gene-product proteins were expressed in bacteria, yeast, and mammalian cells (148). By 1983, techniques were developed that would allow molecular screening of complementary DNA (cDNA) libraries with antibody probes (149). With these techniques, with high-titer chimpanzee inocula, and with serum from a patient with chronic non-A, non-B hepatitis as an antibody probe, investigators at the Chiron Corporation set out on what amounted to a genetic fishing expedition to accomplish what had never been done before—to identify a viral agent by molecular cloning, despite the fact that the virus had not been cultivated, that serologic assays for its antigens and antibodies had not been developed, and that its nucleic acid and protein sequences were not known (148).

These investigators chose a chimpanzee plasma with a known high infectivity titer (10^6 chimpanzee infectious doses per mL), extracted all the nucleic acid from a plasma pellet, and reverse-transcribed all the nucleic acids with random primers to cDNA. Restriction enzymes were used to cleave the cDNAs, and a cDNA library was constructed by inserting gene fragments into bacteriophage GT-11. These were expressed in Escherichia coli, and the individual clones were expanded. Serum from a patient with chronic non-A, non-B hepatitis, a serum assumed to contain antibodies to non-A, non-B virus proteins, was used as a probe to locate virus-specific proteins elaborated as the translation product of the bacterial clones. Screening approximately 1 million clones, they identified one, finally, a 155-base-pair cDNA clone that expressed a protein that reacted with the antibody probe (serum from a patient with chronic non-A, non-B hepatitis) but not with preillness serum from a patient with non-A, non-B hepatitis (70). Genetic specificity of the clone was established, as was the sensitivity and specificity of an immunoassay for antibody to the agent constructed by using as an antigen a 363-amino acid polypeptide gene product of the cloned genome (70,150).

This remarkable breakthrough ended years of frustration and led rapidly to characterization of HCV as a 9400 base-pair RNA virus with multiple genotypes and properties similar to those of flaviviruses, pestiviruses, and plant potyviruses (70,100,101,151). First-generation and second-generation immunoassays have been introduced as blood-donor -screening and clinical-diagnostic tests (150,152–154); a test to identify HCV RNA by genetic amplification (polymerase chain reaction) has been developed (155); modes of transmission have been redefined (156), including the demonstration that perinatal and sexual transmission are very unlikely (157–160) and that a third of cases cannot be linked to any recognized mode of spread (161); the high frequency of chronic hepatitis following acute hepatitis C was confirmed, and protracted viremia was shown to persist even in patients who had recovered biochemically and clinically from acute hepatitis C (162). Despite the high frequency of chronic disease after acute HCV infection, long-term follow-up observations of patient cohorts with transfusion-associated non-A, non-B hepatitis who were studied initially in the 1970s revealed that mortality over an 18-year period was not increased compared to that in a control group of transfused patients in whom non-A, non-B hepatitis did not develop (163). Another unanticipated observation that emerged after the introduction of serologic assays for HCV infection was the association in some cases between hepatitis C and a type of autoimmune chronic active hepatitis (164,165), and the association between cirrhosis secondary to chronic hepatitis C and hepatocellular carcinoma was firmly established (166–169).

Perhaps the most striking and disturbing new revelation about HCV derives from serologic and virologic reinterpretation of cross-challenge studies in chimpanzees. Before the availability of serologic markers for HCV, evidence generated in such studies suggested that there were two distinct non-A, non-B hepatitis agents between which heterologous immunity did not exist, as reviewed elsewhere (170). Farci and colleagues (171) at the National Institutes of Health found, however, that virologic evidence of *reinfection* occurred in chimpanzees challenged twice with the *same* inoculum! Therefore, two distinct bouts of acute non-A, non-B hepatitis in a chimpanzee infected experimentally with different inocula cannot be interpreted to support the existence of two non-A, non-B agents. Moreover, the lack of protective immunity against reinfection established definitively in these experiments, not to mention marked strain differences among isolates (100,101), raise serious doubts that a vaccine against hepatitis C can be developed.

During the last two decades, concepts about what used to be called blood-borne non-A, non-B hepatitis, and which we know now to be hepatitis C predominantly, if not exclusively, have been molded and reshaped. Although the frequency of hepatitis C has been reduced dramatically after transfusion (153,154), overall, the frequency of hepatitis C has not fallen, primarily because of recorded increases in cases among intravenous drug users (161). This virus will remain a challenge for the immediate future, until strategies can be developed for its prevention.

DISCOVERY OF HEPATITIS E VIRUS

At a time when only two hepatitis viruses were recognized, all cases attributed to fecal-oral transmission were believed to be caused by hepatitis A virus. In December, 1955, a large common-source epidemic of water-borne hepatitis occurred in Delhi, India (172). Because this epidemic occurred in adults in a developing country, who should have been immune to hepatitis A, Melnick, who investigated the outbreak, concluded that the Delhi epidemic demonstrated that immunity to hepatitis A could be overwhelmed by a massive inoculum (173). For 25 years, the Delhi epidemic was felt to have been caused by hepatitis A, but serologic re-evaluation demonstrated ultimately that neither HBV nor HAV were involved (174). This realization generated interest in this type of hepatitis, which was labeled enteric or epidemic non-A, non-B hepatitis. Although this type of hepatitis was similar in mode of transmission and in the absence of chronicity to hepatitis A, many features distinguished the two. The mean incubation period, 40 days, was longer than that for hepatitis A; the age distribution, 20 to 40 years, was atypical for hepatitis A; the absence of secondary cases in households was very unusual for hepatitis A; cholestasis was a common histologic feature, unlike the case for hepatitis A; and fulminant hepatitis occurred in approximately 10%, primarily in pregnant women, also highly unusual for hepatitis A.

Similar outbreaks and sporadic cases have been reported from the Indian subcontinent, Asia, Africa, and Mexico. Like the other hepatitis viruses, hepatitis E can be transmitted experimentally in chimpanzees (67) and volunteers (175) and can be visualized by immune electron microscopy (176). Cynomolgus macaques have proven to be an excellent animal model for infection with this virus (73), and the availability of clinical material from experimentally infected macaques was instrumental in isolation and characterization of the genome by molecular cloning from infected bile (74,177). Hepatitis E virus (HEV) is now recognized to be a 32–34 nm nonenveloped virus with a 7600 base-pair RNA genome. Its classification is not complete, but it probably belongs in the alpha virus-like subgroup of positive-stranded RNA viruses that includes rubella. Simple serologic tests now have been developed (178,179), but they remain to be broadly distributed for routine diagnostic use. To date, domestic cases of hepatitis E in the United States have not been recorded; all documented cases in the United States have been imported from endemic countries. Nevertheless, up to 2% of blood donors in a typical American city have circulating anti-HEV (179). Now that the necessary serologic tools are to made available, a more thorough epidemiologic characterization of hepatitis E will emerge.

Finally, now that the virus has been identified and cloned, the potential for a vaccine exists. The question remains whether this agent, like HAV, can be cultivated, or whether a recombinant vaccine will be necessary. Certainly, the geographic distribution of HEV infection will have to be delineated before decisions can be made about target populations for vaccination.

ANTIVIRAL THERAPY

Although progress in understanding viral hepatitis accelerated during the latter part of the 20th century, most clinical attention was focused on diagnosis and prevention. Once corticosteroids were established as effective therapy for severe chronic active hepatitis (180), however, corticosteroids were applied to the treatment of patients with chronic viral hepatitis. By the end of the 1970s, however, clinical observations suggested that such therapy was not helpful for patients with hepatitis B (181) and actually increased the level of HBV replication (182,183). When corticosteroids were tested prospectively in controlled trials of patients with HBsAg-positive chronic active hepatitis, this therapy was found to be not only ineffective but also deleterious (184–186). At a molecular level, HBV DNA was found to contain a glucocorticoid-responsive element, or receptor, which increases the activity of the HBV enhancer, which in turn increases HBV replication (187,188). These observations led to the abandonment of steroids as therapy for chronic active hepatitis B.

In the mid-1970s, interferon, with recognized antiviral properties, was difficult to obtain and in short supply. Merigan and Robinson were able to obtain a limited amount of leukocyte interferon and to test it in a small group of patients with chronic active hepatitis B. They found that markers of HBV replication were inhibited by interferon, thus launching the antiviral era for chronic hepatitis (189). Many small, mostly uncontrolled trials followed, which cumulatively suggested that long-term low-dose therapy was more effective and associated with fewer side effects than short-duration, high-dose therapy (190). Ultimately, more definitive trials during the 1980s with recombinant interferon alpha demonstrated unequivocally that interferon was effective for 30 to 40% of patients with chronic hepatitis B (97,191). The wider availability in the 1980s of tests for markers of HBV replication contributed to the progress of antiviral therapy.

Other antivirals, such as adenine arabinoside, which is a more potent inhibitor of HBV replication than interferon, were disappointing (192,193); however, a combination of corticosteroid withdrawal followed by interferon was effective (97,194). Although corticosteroids used conventionally for long-term therapy are deleterious in hepatitis B, their effect on the interaction between the virus and its host can be exploited for the benefit of the patient, based on the following hypothetical explanation. During steroid therapy, the level of HBV DNA increases (a direct effect of steroids on HBV replication) while cell-mediated lysis of virus-infected hepatocytes is suppressed (an effect of the immunosuppressive, anti-inflammatory effect of steroids on lymphocyte function). Withdrawal of steroid abruptly, however, reverses these trends. Levels of HBV DNA plummet as the steroid stimulus is withdrawn, and cytolytic T cell activity is restored. When cytolytic T cell activity resumes, these cytolytic T cells encounter hepatocytes rich in membrane expression of HBV antigen(s), an effect of the enhancement of HBV replication during the period of steroid therapy. Clinically, this appears as an acute hepatitis-like exacerbation, and such a change in aminotransferase activity occurs regularly also in patients treated with interferon alone (which, based on this observation, is believed to have both an antiviral and immunostimulatory effect in hepatitis B) and in patients who seroconvert spontaneously from replicative (detectable circulating HBeAg and HBV DNA) to nonreplicative (undetectable HBeAg and HBV DNA) HBV infection. Although corticosteroid withdrawal alone has not been demonstrated convincingly to be effective or safe, in combination with antiviral therapy, it appears to be a promising approach.

An important lesson from studies with interferon alone, interferon with steroid withdrawal, and other antivirals is that effective antiviral therapy in chronic hepatitis B requires a balance between a direct antiviral effect and an enhancement of the cell-mediated immune response to HBV-infected hepatocytes. Studies are now in progress to test the value of immunologic stimulation alone, for example with thymosin (195). Similarly, other antivirals, even those more potent than interferon, may require concomitant treatment with another agent such as interferon, interleukin, or steroid withdrawal to stimulate the immune system appropriately.

As the benefit of interferon in chronic hepatitis B was being pursued, Hoofnagle and colleagues at the National Institutes of Health postulated that hepatitis C, too, might be susceptible to antiviral therapy with interferon. A pilot uncontrolled trial, completed in 1986, demonstrated that aminotransferase activity and histologic activity improved in eight of 10 patients (196). Thus, even before HCV had been identified, investigators had established a beachhead in the effort to establish effective therapy for chronic hepatitis C. Larger, controlled trials followed and established the efficacy of interferon alpha in chronic hepatitis C (197,198).

Interferon does not work for everyone with chronic hepatitis B and C, and its efficacy for chronic hepatitis D remains to be established. Much remains to be learned, better regimens need to be evaluated, new antivirals need to be tested, and predictive factors for responsiveness need to be defined. On the other hand, these early successes portend a new era of antiviral therapy for chronic viral hepatitis; many new advances are anticipated as the 20th century draws to a close.

CONCLUSION

A recurring theme in the evolution of hepatitis research becomes apparent from a review of the advances that have occurred since the 1960s. Progress remained slow until tools were developed for virus detection. Discovery of the Australia antigen by immunodiffusion launched intensive hepatitis B research, as did the discovery of HAV antigen by immune electron microscopy and the discovery of HCV and HEV by molecular techniques. Ironically, such a sophisticated array of virologic tools has been inadequate to determine whether other hepatitis agents exist beyond hepatitis A through E. Still, with adequate serologic and virologic techniques, and with the availability of animal models, investigators are limited only by the extent of their initiative and imagination.

REFERENCES

1. Hanger FM: Serological differentiation of obstructive from hepatogenous jaundice by flocculation of cephalin-cholesterol emulsion. J Clin Invest *18*:261, 1939.
2. Karmen A, Wroblewski F, LaDue JS: Transaminase activity in human blood. J Clin Invest *34*:126, 1955.
3. Roholm K, Iversen P: Changes in the liver in acute epidemic hepatitis (catarrhal jaundice) based on 38 aspiration biopsies. Acta Pathol Microbiol Scand *16*:29, 1939.
4. Menghini G: One-second needle biopsy of the liver. Gastroenterology *35*:190, 1958.
5. Lurman A: Eine icterusepidemie. Berlin Klin Wschr *22*:20, 1885.
6. Findlay GM, MacCallum FO, Murgatroyd F: Observations bearing on the aetiology of infective hepatitis (so-called epidemic catarrhal jaundice). Trans Roy Soc Trop Med Hyg *32*:575, 1939.
7. MacCallum FO: Historical perspectives: 1971 international symposium on viral hepatitis. Can Med Assoc J *106*:423, 1972.
8. MacCallum FO: Early studies of viral hepatitis. Br Med Bull *28*:105, 1972.
9. Voegt H: Zur aetiologie der hepatitis epidemica. Munchener Medizinische Wochenschrift *89*:76, 1942.
10. MacCallum FO, Bradley WH: Transmission of infective hepatitis to human volunteers. Lancet *ii*:228, 1944.
11. Paul JR et al.: Transmission experiments in serum jaundice and infectious hepatitis. JAMA *128*:911, 1945.
12. Krugman S, Giles JP, Hammond J: Infectious hepatitis: Evidence for two distinctive clinical, epidemiological, and immunological types of infection. JAMA *200*:365, 1967.
13. Krugman S, Giles JP, Hammond J: Hepatitis virus: Effect of heat on the infectivity and antigenicity of the MS-a and MS-2 strains. J Infect Dis *122*:432, 1970.
14. Krugman S, Giles JP: Viral hepatitis: New light on an old disease. JAMA *212*:1019, 1970.
15. Krugman S, Giles JP, Hammond J: Viral hepatitis, type B (MS-2 strain): Studies on active immunization. JAMA *217*:41, 1971.
16. Blumberg BS, Alter HJ, Visnich S: A "new" antigen in leukemic sera. JAMA *191*:541, 1965.
17. Blumberg BS et al.: A serum antigen (Australia antigen) in Down's syndrome, leukemia and hepatitis. Ann Intern Med *66*:924, 1967.
18. Prince AM: An antigen detected in the blood during the incubation period of serum hepatitis. Proc Natl Acad Sci USA *60*:814, 1968.
19. Okochi K, Murakami S: Observations on Australia antigen in Japanese. Vox Sang *15*:374, 1968.
20. Dane DS, Cameron CH, Briggs M: Virus-like particles in serum of patients with Australia-antigen-associated hepatitis. Lancet *i*:695, 1970.
21. Almeida JD, Rubinstein D, Stott EJ: New antigen-antibody system in Australia-antigen-positive hepatitis. Lancet *ii*:1225, 1971.
22. Robinson WS, Clayton DA, Greenman RL: DNA of human hepatitis B virus candidate. J Virol *14*:384, 1974.
23. Kaplan PM et al.: DNA polymerase associated with human hepatitis B antigen. J Virol *12*:995, 1973.
24. Magnius LO, Espmark A: A new antigen complex co-occurring with Australia antigen. Acta Pathol Microbiol Scand (B) *80*:335, 1972.
25. Magnius LO et al.: A new antigen-antibody system: Clinical significance in long-term carriers of hepatitis B surface antigen. JAMA *231*:356, 1975.
26. Dienstag JL: Hepatitis B as an immune complex disease. Semin Liver Dis *1*:45, 1981.
27. Szmuness W: Hepatocellular carcinoma and the hepatitis B virus: Evidence for a causal association. Prog Med Virol *24*:40, 1978.
28. Beasley RP et al.: Hepatocellular carcinoma and hepatitis B virus: A prospective study of 22,707 men in Taiwan. Lancet *ii*:1129, 1981.
29. Shafritz DA et al.: Integration of hepatitis B virus DNA into the genome of liver cells in chronic liver disease and hepatocellular carcinoma: Studies in percutaneous liver biopsies and post-mortem tissue specimens. N Engl J Med *305*:1067, 1981.
30. Popper H, Shafritz DA, Hoofnagle JH: Relation of the hepatitis B virus carrier state to hepatocellular carcinoma. Hepatology *7*:764, 1987.
31. Summers J, Smolec JM, Snyder R: A virus similar to human hepatitis B virus associated with hepatitis and hepatoma in woodchucks. Proc Natl Acad Sci USA *75*:4533, 1978.
32. Mondelli M et al.: Specificity of T lymphocyte cytotoxicity to autologous hepato-

cytes in chronic hepatitis B virus infection: Evidence that T cells are directed against HBV core antigen expressed on hepatocytes. J Immunol *129*:2773, 1982.

33. Romet-Lemonne JL et al.: Hepatitis B virus infection in cultured human lymphoblastoid cells. Science *221*:667, 1983.

34. Yoffe B et al.: Hepatitis B virus DNA in mononuclear cells and analysis of cell subsets for the presence of replicative intermediates of viral DNA. J Infect Dis *153*:471, 1986.

35. Chisari FV et al.: A transgenic mouse model of the chronic hepatitis B surface antigen carrier state. Science *230*:1157, 1985.

36. Chisari FV et al.: Structural and pathological effects of hepatitis B virus large envelope polypeptide synthesis in transgenic mice. Proc Natl Acad Sci USA *84*:6909, 1987.

37. Moriyama T et al.: Hepatitis B surface antigen-specific antibody and T cell-mediated hepatocellular injury in hepatitis B virus transgenic mice. *In* Hollinger FB, Lemon SM, Margolis HS (eds). Viral hepatitis and liver disease. Baltimore, Williams & Wilkins, 1991, p. 282.

38. Moriyama T et al.: Immunobiology and pathogenesis of hepatocellular injury in hepatitis B virus transgenic mice. Science *248*:361, 1990.

39. Davies SE et al.: Hepatic histological findings after transplantation for chronic hepatitis B virus infection, including a unique pattern of fibrosing cholestatic hepatitis. Hepatology *13*:150, 1991.

40. Milich DR: Immune response to hepatitis B virus proteins: Relevance of the murine model. Semin Liver Dis *11*:93, 1991.

41. Milich DR et al.: Distinct H2-linked regulation of T-cell responses to the pre-S and S regions of the same hepatitis B surface antigen polypeptide allows circumvention of nonresponsiveness to the S region. Proc Natl Acad Sci USA *82*:8168, 1985.

42. Milich DR, Chisari FV: Genetic regulation of the immune response to hepatitis B surface antigen (HBsAg). I. H-2 restriction of the murine humoral immune response to the *a* and *d* determinants of HBsAg. J Immunol *129*:320, 1982.

43. Milich DR, Lerous-Roels G, Chisari FV: Genetic regulation of the immune response to hepatitis B surface antigen (HBsAg). II. Qualitative characteristics of humoral immune response to the *a, d,* and *y* determinants of HBsAg. J Immunol *130*:1395, 1983.

44. Milich DR et al.: Antibody production to the nucleocapsid and envelope of the hepatitis B virus primed by a single synthetic T cell site. Nature *329*:547, 1987.

45. Milich DR et al.: Is a function of the secreted hepatitis B e antigen to induce immunologic tolerance *in utero?* Proc Natl Acad Sci USA *87*:6599, 1990.

46. Gerin JL et al.: Biophysical properties of Australia antigen. J Virol *4*:763, 1969.

47. Gerin JL, Holland PV, Purcell RH: Australia antigen: Large-scale purification from human serum and biochemical studies of its protein. J Virol *7*:569, 1971.

48. Lustbader ED, London WT, Blumberg BS: Study design for a hepatitis B vaccine trial. Proc Natl Acad Sci USA *73*:955, 1976.

49. Szmuness W et al.: Hepatitis B vaccine: Demonstration of efficacy in a controlled clinical trial in a high-risk population in the United States. N Engl J Med *303*:833, 1980.

50. Scolnick EM et al.: Clinical evaluation in healthy adults of a hepatitis B vaccine made by recombinant DNA. JAMA *251*:2812, 1984.

51. Purcell RH, Gerin JL: Prospects for second and third generation hepatitis B vaccines. Hepatology *5*:159, 1985.

52. Kennedy RC et al.: Anti-idiotypic antibody vaccine for type B viral hepatitis in chimpanzees. Science *232*:220, 1986.

53. Moss B et al.: Live recombinant vaccinia virus protects chimpanzees against hepatitis B. Nature *311*:67, 1984.

54. Morin JE et al.: Recombinant adenovirus induces antibody response to hepatitis B virus surface antigen in hamsters. Proc Natl Acad Sci USA *84*:4626, 1987.

55. Kniskern PJ et al.: A candidate vaccine for hepatitis B containing the complete viral surface protein. Hepatology *8*:82, 1988.

56. Wu JY et al.: Expression of immunogenic epitopes of hepatitis B surface antigen with hybrid flagellin proteins by a vaccine strain of Salmonella. Proc Natl Acad Sci USA *86*:4726, 1989.

57. Rutgers T, Hauser P, DeWilde M: Potential future recombinant vaccines, *In* Ellis RW (ed): Hepatitis B Vaccines in Clinical Practice. New York, Marcel Dekker, 383, 1993.

58. Alter MJ et al.: The changing epidemiology of hepatitis B in the United States: Need for alternative vaccination strategies. JAMA *263*:1218, 1990.

59. Craven DE et al.: Nonresponsiveness to hepatitis B vaccine in health care workers: Results of revaccination and genetic typings. Ann Intern Med *105*:137, 1986.

60. Alper CA et al.: Genetic prediction of nonresponse to hepatitis B vaccine. N Engl J Med *321*:708, 1989.

61. Kruskall MS et al.: The immune response to hepatitis B vaccine in humans: Inheritance patterns in families. J Exp Med *175*:495, 1992.

62. Barker LF et al.: Transmission of type B viral hepatitis to chimpanzees. J Infect Dis *127*:648, 1973.

63. Dienstag JL et al.: Experimental infection of chimpanzees with hepatitis A virus. J Infect Dis *132*:532, 1975.

64. Alter HJ et al.: Transmissible agent in non-A, non-B hepatitis. Lancet *i*:459, 1978.

65. Tabor E et al.: Transmission of non-A, non-B hepatitis from man to chimpanzee. Lancet *i*:463, 1978.

66. Rizzetto M et al.: Transmission of the hepatitis B virus-associated delta antigen to chimpanzees. J Infect Dis *141*:590, 1980.

67. Arankalle VA et al.: Aetiological association of a virus-like particle with enterically transmitted non-A, non-B hepatitis. Lancet *i*:550, 1988.

68. Shouval D et al.: Chronic hepatitis in chimpanzee carriers of hepatitis B virus: Morphologic, immunologic, and viral DNA studies. Proc Natl Acad Sci USA *77*:6147, 1980.

69. Alter HJ et al.: Transmission of hepatitis B to chimpanzees by hepatitis B surface antigen-positive saliva and semen. Infect Immun *16*:928, 1977.

70. Choo Q-L et al.: Isolation of a cDNA clone derived from a blood-borne non-A, non-B viral hepatitis genome. Science *244*:359, 1989.

71. Deinhardt F et al.: Studies of the transmission of human viral hepatitis to marmoset monkeys. I. Transmission of disease, serial passages, and description of liver lesions. J Exp Med *125*:673, 1967.

72. Holmes A et al.: Hepatitis in marmosets: Induction of disease and coded specimens. Science *165*:816, 1969.

73. Bradley DW et al.: Enterically transmitted non-A, non-B hepatitis: Serial passage of disease in cynomolgus macaques and tamarins and recovery of disease-associated 27- to 34-nm viruslike particles. Proc Natl Acad Sci USA *84*:6277, 1987.

74. Reyes GR et al.: Isolation of a cDNA from the virus responsible for enterically transmitted non-A, non-B hepatitis. Science *247*:1335, 1990.

75. Marion PL et al.: A virus in Beechey ground squirrels that is related to hepatitis B virus of humans. Proc Natl Acad Sci USA *77*:2941, 1980.

76. Mason WS, Seal G, Summers J: Virus of Pekin ducks with structural and biological relatedness to human hepatitis B virus. J Virol *36*:829, 1980.

77. O'Connell AP, Urban MK, London WT: Naturally occurring infection of Pekin duck embryos by duck hepatitis B virus. Proc Natl Acad Sci USA *80*:1703, 1983.

78. Yokosuka O et al.: Duck hepatitis B virus DNA in liver and serum of Chinese ducks: Integration of viral DNA in a hepatocellular carcinoma. Proc Natl Acad Sci USA *82*:5180, 1985.

79. Popper H et al.: Hepatocarcinogenicity of the woodchuck hepatitis virus. Proc Natl Acad Sci USA *84*:866, 1987.

80. Tiollais P, Charnay P, Vyas GN: Biology of hepatitis B virus. Science *213*:406, 1981.

81. Summers J, Mason WS: Replication of the genome of a hepatitis B-like virus by reverse transcription of an RNA intermediate. Cell *29*:403, 1982.

82. Summers J, Mason WS: Properties of the hepatitis B-like viruses related to their taxonomic classification. Hepatology *2*:61, 1982.

83. Miller RH, Robinson WS: Common evolutionary origin of hepatitis B virus and retroviruses. Proc Natl Acad Sci USA *83*:2531, 1986.

84. Seeger C, Ganem D, Varmus HE: Biochemical and genetic evidence for the hepatitis B virus replication strategy. Science *232*:477, 1986.

85. Miller RH et al.: Compact organization of the hepatitis B virus genome. Hepatology *9*:322, 1989.

86. Summers J, O'Connell A, Millman I: Genome of hepatitis B virus: Restriction enzyme cleavage and structure of the DNA isolated from Dane particles. Proc Natl Acad Sci USA *72*:4597, 1975.

87. Burrell CJ et al.: Expression in Escherichia coli of hepatitis B virus DNA sequences cloned in plasmid pBR322. Nature *279*:43, 1979.

88. Sninsky JJ et al.: Cloning and endonuclease mapping of the hepatitis B viral genome. Nature *279*:346, 1979.

89. Valenzuela P et al.: Nucleotide sequence of the gene coding for the major protein of hepatitis B virus surface antigen. Nature *280*:815, 1979.

90. Galibert F et al.: Nucleotide sequence of the hepatitis B virus genome (subtype ayw) cloned in E. coli. Nature *281*:646, 1979.

91. Pasek M et al.: Hepatitis B virus genes and their expression in E. coli. Nature *282*:575, 1979.

92. Valenzuela P et al.: Synthesis and assembly of hepatitis B virus surface antigen particles in yeast. Nature *298*:347, 1982.

93. Charnay P et al.: Biosynthesis of hepatitis B virus surface antigen in Escherichia coli. Nature *286*:893, 1980.

94. Kim W et al.: Hepatitis B viral DNA in liver and serum of asymptomatic carriers. Proc Natl Acad Sci USA *79*:7522, 1982.

95. Brechot C et al.: State of hepatitis B virus DNA in hepatocytes of patients with hepatitis B surface antigen-positive and -negative liver disease. Proc Natl Acad Sci USA *78*:3906, 1981.

96. Elfassi E et al.: Evidence of extrachromosomal forms of hepatitis B viral DNA in a bone marrow culture obtained from a patient recently infected with hepatitis B virus. Proc Natl Acad Sci USA *81*:3526, 1984.

97. Perrillo RP et al.: A randomized, controlled trial of interferon alfa-2b alone and after prednisone withdrawal for the treatment of chronic hepatitis B. N Engl J Med *323*:295, 1990.

98. McAleer WJ et al.: Human hepatitis B vaccine from recombinant yeast. Nature *307*:178, 1984.

99. Petre J et al.: Development of a hepatitis B vaccine from transformed yeast cells. Postgrad Med J *63(Suppl 2)*:73, 1987.

100. Choo Q-L et al.: Genetic organization and diversity of the hepatitis C virus. Proc Natl Acad Sci USA *88*:2451, 1991.

101. Cha T-A et al.: At least five related, but distinct, hepatitis C viral genotypes exist. Proc Natl Acad Sci USA *89*:7144, 1992.

102. Carman WF et al.: Mutation preventing formation of hepatitis B e antigen in patients with chronic hepatitis B infection. Lancet *ii*:588, 1989.

103. McMahon G et al.: Genetic alterations in the gene encoding the major HBsAg: DNA and immunological analysis of recurrent HBsAg derived from monoclonal antibody-treated liver transplant patients. Hepatology *15*:757, 1992.

104. Brunetto MR et al.: A new hepatitis B virus strain in patients with severe anti-HBe positive chronic hepatitis B. J Virol *10*:258, 1990.

105. Carman WF, Thomas HC: Genetic variation in hepatitis B virus. Gastroenterology *102*:711, 1992.

106. Boggs JD et al.: Viral hepatitis: Clinical and tissue culture studies. JAMA *214*:1041, 1970.

107. Provost PJ et al.: Etiologic relationship of marmoset-propagated CR326 hepatitis A virus to hepatitis in man. Proc Soc Exp Biol Med *142*:1257, 1973.

108. Feinstone SM, Kapikian AZ, Purcell RH: Hepatitis A: Detection by immune electron microscopy of a virus-like antigen associated with acute illness. Science *182*:1026, 1973.

109. Provost PJ et al.: Physical, chemical and morphologic dimensions of human hepatitis A virus strain CR326. Proc Soc Exp Biol Med *148*:532, 1975.

110. Provost PJ, Hilleman MR: An inactivated hepatitis A virus vaccine prepared from infected marmoset liver. Proc Soc Exp Biol Med *159*:201, 1978.

111. Provost PJ, Hilleman MR: Propagation of human hepatitis A virus in cell culture in vitro. Proc Soc Exp Biol Med *160*:213, 1979.

112. Ticehurst JR et al.: Molecular cloning and characterization of hepatitis A virus cDNA. Proc Natl Acad Sci USA *80*:5885, 1983.

113. Baroudy BM et al.: Sequence analysis of hepatitis A virus cDNA coding for capsid proteins and RNA polymerase. Proc Natl Acad Sci USA *82*:2143, 1985.

114. Najarian R et al.: Primary structure and gene organization of human hepatitis A virus. Proc Natl Acad Sci USA *82*:2627, 1985.

115. Cohen JI et al.: Complete nucleotide sequence of an attenuated hepatitis A virus: Comparison with wild-type virus. Proc Natl Acad Sci USA *84*:2497, 1987.

116. Melnick JL: Properties and classification of hepatitis A virus. Vaccine *10 Suppl 1*:S24, 1992.

117. Werzberger A et al.: A controlled trial of formalin-inactivated hepatitis A vaccine in healthy children. N Engl J Med *327*:453, 1992.

118. Rizzetto M et al.: Immunofluorescence detection of new antigen-antibody system (s/anti-s) associated to hepatitis B virus in liver and in serum of HBsAg carriers. Gut *18*:997, 1977.

119. Rizzetto M, Shih JW-K, Gerin JL: The hepatitis B virus-associated d antigen: Isolation from liver, development of a solid-phase radioimmunoassay for d antigen and anti-d and partial characterization of d antigen. J Immunol *125*:318, 1980.

120. Rizzetto M et al.: d agent: Association of d antigen with hepatitis B surface antigen and RNA in serum of d-infected chimpanzees. Proc Natl Acad Sci USA *77*:6124, 1980.

121. Ponzetto A et al.: Transmission of the hepatitis B virus-associated d agent to the eastern woodchuck. Proc Natl Acad Sci USA *81*:2208, 1984.

122. Rizzetto M et al.: Incidence and significance of antibodies to delta antigen in hepatitis B virus infection. Lancet *ii*:986, 1979.

123. Rizzetto M, Purcell RH, Gerin JL: Epidemiology of HBV-associated delta agent: Geographical distribution of anti-delta and prevalence in polytransfused HBsAg carriers. Lancet *i*:1215, 1980.

124. Rizzetto M: The delta agent. Hepatology *3*:729, 1983.

125. Hansson BG et al.: Infection with delta agent in Sweden: Introduction of a new hepatitis agent. J Infect Dis *146*:472, 1982.

126. Smedile A et al.: Epidemiologic patterns of infection with the hepatitis B virus-associated delta agent in Italy. Am J Epidemiol *117*:223, 1983.

127. Wang K-S et al.: Structure, sequence and expression of the hepatitis delta (d) viral genome. Nature *323*:508, 1986.

128. Chen P-J et al.: Structure and replication of the genome of the hepatitis d virus. Proc Natl Acad Sci USA *83*:8774, 1986.

129. Bergmann KF, Gerin JL: Antigens of hepatitis delta virus in the liver and serum of humans and animals. J Infect Dis *514*:702, 1986.

130. Taylor J et al.: Replication of human hepatitis delta virus in primary cultures of woodchuck hepatocytes. J Virol *61*:2891, 1987.

131. Ottobrelli A et al.: Patterns of hepatitis delta virus reinfection and disease in liver transplantation. Gastroenterology *101*:1649, 1991.

132. Kunin CM: Serum hepatitis from whole blood: Incidence and relation to source of blood. Am J Med Sci *237*:293, 1959.

133. Allen JG et al.: Blood transfusions and serum hepatitis: Use of monochloroacetate as an antibacterial agent in plasma. Ann Surg *150*:455, 1959.

134. Walsh JH et al.: Posttransfusion hepatitis after open-heart operations: Incidence after administration of blood from commercial and volunteer donor populations. JAMA *211*:261, 1970.

135. Alter HJ et al.: Post-transfusion hepatitis after exclusion of commercial and hepatitis-B antigen-positive donors. Ann Intern Med *77*:691, 1972.

136. Prince AM et al.: Long-incubation posttransfusion hepatitis without serological evidence of exposure to hepatitis-B virus. Lance *ii*:241, 1974.

137. Feinstone SM et al.: Transfusion-associated hepatitis not due to viral hepatitis type A or B. N Engl J Med *292*:767, 1975.

138. Dienstag JL: Non-A, non-B hepatitis. I. Recognition, epidemiology, and clinical features. Gastroenterology *85*:439, 1983.

139. Alter HJ et al.: Clinical and serological analysis of transfusion-associated hepatitis. Lancet *ii*:838, 1975.

140. Alter HJ et al.: Non-A, non-B hepatitis: Its relationship to cytomegalovirus, to chronic hepatitis, and to direct and indirect test methods. *In* Szmuness W, Alter JH, Maynard JE (eds): Viral Hepatitis: 1981 International Symposium. Philadelphia, Franklin Institute Press, 1982, p. 279.

141. Dienstag JL: Non-A, non-B hepatitis. II. Experimental transmission, putative virus agents and markers, and prevention. Gastroenterology *85*:743, 1983.

142. Dienstag JL: Viral hepatitis in the compromised host. *In* Rubin RH, Young LS (eds): Clinical Approach to Infection in the Compromised Host. New York, Plenum Medical, 1983, p. 325.

143. Feinstone SM et al.: Inactivation of hepatitis B virus and non-A, non-B hepatitis by chloroform. Infect Immunol *41*:816, 1983.

144. Bradley DW et al.: Posttransfusion non-A, non-B hepatitis in chimpanzees: Physicochemical evidence that the tubule-forming agent is a small, enveloped virus. Gastroenterology *88*:773, 1985.

145. He L-F et al.: Determining the size of non-A, non-B hepatitis virus by filtration. J Infect Dis *156*:636, 1987.

146. Feinstone SM et al.: Non-A, non-B hepatitis in chimpanzees and marmosets. J Infect Dis *144*:588, 1981.

147. Bradley DW et al.: Non-A, non-B hepatitis: Toward the discovery of hepatitis C and E viruses. Semin Liver Dis *11*:128, 1991.

148. Overby LR: Hepatitis C virus: Strategies for discovery. *In* Hollinger FB, Lemon SM, Margolis HS (eds): Viral Hepatitis and Liver Disease. Baltimore, Williams & Wilkins, 1991, p. 356.

149. Young RA, Davis RW: Efficient isolation of genes by using antibody probes. Proc Natl Acad Sci USA *80*:1194, 1983.

150. Kuo G et al.: An assay for circulating antibodies to a major etiologic virus of human non-A, non-B hepatitis. Science *244*:362, 1989.

151. Houghton M et al.: Molecular biology of the hepatitis C viruses: Implications for diagnosis, development and control of viral disease. Hepatology *14*:381, 1991.

152. Alter HJ et al.: Detection of antibody to hepatitis C virus in prospectively followed transfusion recipients with acute and chronic non-A, non-B hepatitis. N Engl J Med *321*:1494, 1989.

153. Aach RD et al.: Hepatitis C virus infection in post-transfusion hepatitis: An analysis with first- and second-generation assays. N Engl J Med *325*:1325, 1991.

154. Donahue JG et al.: The declining risk of post-transfusion hepatitis C virus infection. N Engl J Med *327*:369, 1992.

155. Weiner AJ et al.: Detection of hepatitis C viral sequences in non-A, non-B hepatitis. Lancet *335*:1, 1990.

156. Genesca L, Esteban JI, Alter HJ: Blood-borne non-A, non-B hepatitis: Hepatitis C. Semin Liver Dis *11*:147, 1991.

157. Everhart JE et al.: Risk for non-A, non-B (type C) hepatitis through sexual or household contact with chronic carriers. Ann Intern Med *112*:544, 1990.

158. Osmond DH et al.: Risk factors for hepatitis C virus seropositivity in heterosexual couples. JAMA *269*:361, 1993.

159. Weinstock HS et al.: Hepatitis C virus infection among patients attending a clinic for sexually transmitted diseases. JAMA *269*: 392, 1993.

160. Reinus JF et al.: Failure to detect vertical transmission of hepatitis C virus. Ann Intern Med *117*:881, 1992.

161. Alter MJ et al.: Risk factors for acute non-A, non-B hepatitis in the United States and association with hepatitis C virus infection. JAMA *264*:2231, 1990.

162. Alter MJ et al.: The natural history of community acquired hepatitis C in the United States. N Engl J Med *327*:1899, 1992.

163. Seeff LB et al.: Long-term mortality after transfusion-associated non-A, non-B hepatitis. N Engl J Med *327*:1906, 1992.

164. Lenzi M et al.: Antibodies to hepatitis C virus in autoimmune liver disease: Evidence for geographical heterogeneity. Lancet *338*:277, 1991.

165. Lunel F et al.: Liver/kidney microsome antibody type 1 and hepatitis C virus infection. Hepatology *16*:630, 1992.

166. Kiyosawa K et al.: Interrelationship of blood transfusion, non-A, non-B hepatitis and hepatocellular carcinoma. Analysis by detection of antibody to hepatitis C virus. Hepatology *12*:671, 1990.

167. Colombo M et al.: Hepatocellular carcinoma in Italian patients with cirrhosis. N Engl J Med *325*:675, 1991.

168. Simonetti RG et al.: Hepatitis C virus infection as a risk factor for hepatocellular carcinoma in patients with cirrhosis: A case-control study. Ann Intern Med *116*:97, 1992.

169. Saito I et al.: Hepatitis C virus infection is associated with the development of hepatocellular carcinoma. Proc Natl Acad Sci USA *87*:6547, 1990.

170. Dienstag JL, Katkov WN, Cody H: Evidence for non-A, non-B hepatitis agents besides hepatitis C virus. *In* Hollinger FB, Lemon SM, Margolis HS (eds): Viral Hepatitis and Liver Disease, Baltimore, Williams & Wilkins, 1991, p. 349.

171. Farci P et al.: Lack of protection against reinfection with hepatitis C virus (HCV) in multiple cross-challenges of chimpanzees (abstract). Hepatology *14*:90, 1991.

172. Melnick JL: A water-borne urban epidemic of hepatitis. *In* Hartman FW, LoGrippo GA, Mateer JG, Barron J (eds): Hepatitis Frontiers, Boston, Little Brown, 1957.

173. Melnick J, Boggs JD: Human volunteer and tissue culture studies of viral hepatitis. Can Med Assoc J *106*:461, 1972.

174. Wong DC et al.: Epidemic and endemic hepatitis in India: Evidence for a non-A, non-B hepatitis virus aetiology. Lancet *ii*: 876, 1980.

175. Balayan MS et al.: Evidence for a virus in non-A, non-B hepatitis transmitted via the fecal-oral route. Intervirology *20*:23, 1983.

176. Ramalingaswami V, Purcell RH: Waterborne non-A, non-B hepatitis. Lancet *i*:571, 1988.

177. Koonin EV et al.: Computer-assisted assignment of functional domains in the nonstructural polyprotein of hepatitis E virus: Delineation of an additional group of positive-stranded RNA plant and animal viruses. Proc Natl Acad Sci USA *89*:8259, 1992.

178. Goldsmith R et al.: Enzyme-linked immunosorbent assay for diagnosis of acute sporadic hepatitis E in Egyptian children. Lancet *339*:328, 1992.

179. Dawson GJ et al.: Solid-phase enzyme-linked immunosorbent assay for hepatitis E virus IgG and IgM antibodies utilizing recombinant antigens and synthetic peptides. J Virol Methods *38*:175, 1992.

180. Summerskill WHJ, Korman MG, Ammon HV: Prednisone for chronic active liver disease. Dose titration, standard dose, and combination with azathioprine compared. Gut *16*:876, 1975.

181. Schalm SW et al.: Contrasting features and response to treatment of severe chronic active liver disease with and without hepatitis Bs antigen. Gut *17*:781, 1976.

182. Sagnelli E et al.: Serum levels of hepatitis B surface and core antigens during immunosuppressive treatment of HBsAg-positive chronic active hepatitis. Lancet *ii*:395, 1980.

183. Scullard GH et al.: Effects of immunosuppressive therapy on viral markers in chronic active hepatitis B. Gastroenterology *81*:987, 1981.

184. Lam KC et al.: Deleterious effect of prednisolone in HBsAg-positive chronic active hepatitis. N Engl J Med *304*:380, 1981.

185. Liaw Y-F et al.: A prospective trial of prednisolone combined with azathioprine in HBsAg-positive chronic active hepatitis. Hepatogastroenterology *30*:51, 1983.

186. Tygstrup N, Krag Andersen P, Juhl E: Steroids in chronic B-hepatitis: A randomized, double-blind, multinational trial on the effect of low-dose, long-term treatment on survival. Liver *6*:227, 1986.

187. Tur-Kaspa R et al.: Hepatitis B virus DNA contains a glucocorticoid-responsive element. Proc Natl Acad Sci USA *83*:1627, 1986.

188. Tur-Kaspa R et al.: The glucocorticoid receptor recognizes a specific nucleotide sequence in hepatitis B virus DNA causing increased activity of the HBV enhancer. Virology *167*:630, 1988.

189. Greenberg HB et al.: Effect of leukocyte interferon on hepatitis B virus infection in patients with chronic active hepatitis. N Engl J Med *295*:517, 1976.

190. Davis GL, Hoofnagle JH: Interferon in viral hepatitis: Role in pathogenesis and treatment. Hepatology *6*:1038, 1986.

191. Hoofnagle JH et al.: Randomized, controlled trial of recombinant human a-interferon in patients with chronic hepatitis B. Gastroenterology *95*:1318, 1988.

192. Hoofnagle JH et al.: Randomized controlled trial of adenine arabinoside monophosphate for chronic type B hepatitis. Gastroenterology *86*:150, 1984.

193. Garcia G et al.: Adenine arabinoside monophosphate (vidarabine phosphate) in combination with human leukocyte interferon in the treatment of chronic hepatitis B. Ann Intern Med *107*:278, 1987.

194. Perrillo RP et al.: Prednisone withdrawal followed by recombinant alpha interferon in the treatment of chronic type B hepatitis: A randomized, controlled trial. Ann Intern Med *109*:95, 1988.

195. Mutchnick MG et al.: Thymosin treatment of chronic hepatitis B: A placebo-controlled pilot trial. Hepatology *14*:409, 1991.

196. Hoofnagle JH et al.: Treatment of chronic non-A, non-B hepatitis with recombinant human alfa interferon. N Engl J Med *315*: 1575, 1986.

197. Davis GL et al.: Treatment of chronic hepatitis C with recombinant interferon alfa: A multicenter randomized, controlled trial. N Engl J Med *321*:1501, 1989.

198. Di Bisceglie AM et al.: Recombinant interferon alfa therapy for chronic hepatitis C: A randomized, double-blind, placebo-controlled trial. N Engl J Med *321*:1506, 1989.

19

Sclerosing Cholangitis

JOHN O. PHILLIPS, RUSSELL H. WIESNER, AND
NICHOLAS F. LaRUSSO

Sclerosing cholangitis is a clinical syndrome characterized by progressive fatigue and jaundice resulting from diffuse destruction of bile ducts. Primary sclerosing cholangitis is an idiopathic syndrome and should be distinguished from secondary sclerosing cholangitis, a similar clinical entity, but one with identifiable causes (Table 19–1). This chapter will focus principally on the primary variety of sclerosing cholangitis.

Primary sclerosing cholangitis (PSC) is a chronic cholestatic hepatobiliary disease characterized by inflammation and fibrosis of the bile ducts; PSC usually affects both the intrahepatic and extrahepatic biliary ductal systems and eventually leads to bile duct obliteration (1,2). Although it was thought to be an uncommon disease at the time of its first description over 100 years ago (3), advances in cholangiographic techniques have led to an increased awareness and diagnosis of PSC; indeed, PSC now represents one of the two most common adult cholestatic liver diseases, the other being primary biliary cirrhosis (PBC). The natural history of the disease is currently in evolution, but is generally thought to be one of slow but relentless progression to cirrhosis, portal hypertension, and hepatic failure. The disease may occur alone, but is more commonly found in association with inflammatory bowel disease (IBD), especially chronic ulcerative colitis (CUC) (1,2,4,5). The diagnosis of PSC relies on a constellation of clinical, biochemical, and radiographic findings; endoscopic retrograde cholangiography (ERCP) usually unequivocally establishes the diagnosis (6,7), assuming that secondary causes can be excluded. While evidence of biliary disease usually is detected on liver biopsy, the histopathologic findings associated with PSC are not necessarily diagnostic. Ludwig has proposed a classification scheme for PSC based on cholangiographic and histologic findings which are referred to as large-duct PSC, small-duct PSC and global PSC involving the entire biliary system (8,9). The criteria for these subtypes of PSC are listed in Table 19–2.

HISTORICAL PERSPECTIVES

Before the advent and widespread application of endoscopic and percutaneous transhepatic cholangiography, PSC was considered a rare disease, with only 100 documented cases in the English literature before 1980 (10). The diagnosis usually was made during laparotomy by palpation and biopsy of a fibrotic common bile duct (11,12). Although patients were treated by various surgical procedures in an attempt to improve biliary drainage, the efficacy of these surgical approaches was unclear because of the absence of controlled clinical trials (13,14).

The recognition of an association between PSC and IBD led to earlier diagnosis and an increased awareness of PSC, especially in patients with IBD and persistently elevated serum liver enzymes (4,15–20).

Table 19–1
Differential Diagnosis for Primary
Sclerosing Cholangitis

Secondary sclerosing cholangitis
  Choledocholithiasis
  Trauma
  Tumors
  Infections
  Congenital anomalies
  Ischemia
  Iatrogenic strictures
  Drugs/chemical irritants
  AIDS-associated cholangiopathy
Primary biliary cirrhosis
Idiopathic adulthood ductopenia
Chronic active hepatitis
Extrahepatic obstruction

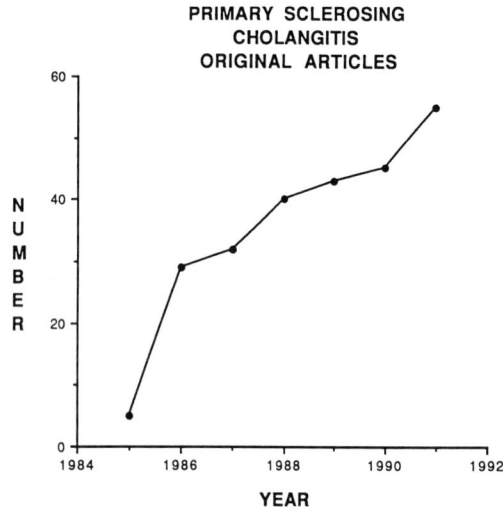

Fig. 19–1.   Number of publications devoted to PSC in the last decade.

Thus, in patients with IBD, hepatic histology was assessed and the term pericholangitis was coined to describe the hepatic histologic abnormalities associated with IBD (21). ERCP revealed that many, if not all, of these patients with IBD and pericholangitis had PSC (17).

Although endoscopic and percutaneous transhepatic cholangiography have had the greatest impact on the increased frequency of diagnosis of PSC, operative cholangiography was the first method to describe the classic "beaded" appearance of the ductal system in PSC (4). This radiologic procedure also revealed the patchy intrahepatic involvement of PSC, the decreased arborization of the biliary system, and the lack of marked dilatation of intrahepatic ducts proximal to extrahepatic strictures (4,22).

As ERCP techniques were refined and improved, PSC became largely a diagnosis confirmed by cholangiography (23). Abnor-

malities of the gallbladder, pancreas and isolated segments of the bile ducts also were demonstrated by ERCP and the criteria for the diagnosis of PSC were refined (24–26). As a result of both the increased availability of ERCP and an increased awareness of the disease, there has been a steady and dramatic increase in the diagnostic recognition of PSC (1). Figure 19–1 shows the increasing number of publications devoted to PSC in the last decade.

CLINICAL FEATURES

Clinical Presentation

Primary sclerosing cholangitis occurs primarily in young adult males and two thirds of patients are under the age of 45 at the

Table 19–2
Ductular Disease Classification for the Primary Sclerosing Cholangitis Syndrome*

Diagnostic Terminology	Cholangiography†	Liver Biopsy
Large-duct PSC (extrahepatic or intrahepatic)	Typical findings	Not diagnostic
Small-duct PSC (pericholangitis)	Not diagnostic	Typical findings
Combined large- and small-duct PSC (global PSC)	Typical findings	Typical findings

* Reproduced with permission from Ludwig J: Small-duct primary sclerosing cholangitis. Semin Liver Dis *11*:11, 1991.
† Usually by endoscopic retrograde cholangiopancreatography

time of diagnosis; 70% are men (1,2,27). Approximately 70% of patients have coexistent CUC, which is usually either quiescent or mildly severe (1,2,5,27–29). The gradual onset of progressive fatigue and pruritus, followed later by jaundice, is the most frequent symptomatic presentation that leads to the diagnosis of PSC. These symptoms may or may not be associated with acholic stools or choluria. Most symptomatic patients have had symptoms for an average of 2 years before diagnosis. However, some PSC patients with or without IBD present without signs or symptoms; instead, the disease is detected by the findings of a cholestatic biochemical profile of serum liver tests during a routine medical evaluation. Patients also may present with symptoms of recurrent bacterial cholangitis, but this usually occurs in PSC patients with previous biliary tract surgery such as choledochoenterostomy. Occasionally, patients present for the first time with complications from advanced cholestatic disease, including ascites or bleeding from gastroesophageal varices. Less common forms of presentation include: (1) discovery during laparotomy; (2) evaluation for recurrent fevers and septicemia; (3) IBD and a previous diagnosis of chronic idiopathic or autoimmune chronic hepatitis in a patient who fails to respond to immunosuppressive therapy; (4) previous proctocolectomy and ileostomy for CUC in patients who present with peristomal variceal bleeding; and (5) weight loss and steatorrhea caused by nontropical sprue or pancreatic exocrine insufficiency (44).

Most patients have some abnormality on physical examination including jaundice, hepatomegaly, or splenomegaly (1,2,27, 29–32). Less frequent physical findings include hyperpigmentation, xanthelasma, and xanthomas, signs more commonly associated with PBC (1,2,33). In patients with advanced stages of PSC, physical findings consistent with ascites as well as peripheral edema and stigmata of chronic liver disease including nail clubbing, spider angiomas, and palmar erythema may be present (1,2). Table 19–3 summarizes some of the general and specific complications of PSC.

Table 19–3
Complications Secondary to Primary Sclerosing Cholangitis

General
  Fatigue
  Pruritus
  Steatorrhea
  Hepatic osteodystrophy
  Fat soluble vitamin deficiency
  Cholangitis
  Portal hypertension
  Gastroesophageal varices
  Cirrhosis
  Hepatic failure
Specific
  Dominant stricture
  Cholelithiasis
  Peristomal varices following proctocolectomy for CUC
  Cholangiocarcinoma

Biochemical Characteristics

A biochemical picture of cholestatic liver disease usually is present with an elevated serum alkaline phosphatase in most patients. Although the level of elevation is usually more than five times the upper limit of normal, the serum alkaline phosphatase may rarely be normal (1,2,34). Most patients also have a modest increase in serum aminotransferase levels (33). Serum bilirubin is increased in over 50% of PSC patients at the time of diagnosis, but considerable fluctuation is common (1,33). High bilirubin levels suggest progression of disease, choledocholithiasis, the development of a benign dominant stricture, or the development of adenocarcinoma of the bile ducts. Serum copper levels and urinary copper excretion are increased in many PSC patients, abnormalities reflecting the cholestatic nature of the disease (35). Hepatic copper levels are frequently as high as those noted in Wilson's disease and PBC (35). Biosynthetic function of the liver, as measured by the serum albumin and the prothrombin time, usually is normal until the very advanced stages of the disease (1). Table 19–4 summarizes selected serum biochemical tests and the percentage of PSC patients with abnormal values at the time of diagnosis.

Serum markers for autoimmune diseases

Table 19–4
Biochemical Abnormalities in Primary
Sclerosing Cholangitis Patients at Time of
Diagnosis

Test	Percentage of Patients with Abnormal Results
Serum alkaline phosphatase	99
Serum aminotransferase	95
Serum bilirubin	65
Serum copper	50
Serum ceruloplasmin	75
Urine copper	65
Serum albumin	20
Prothrombin time	10

generally have not been helpful in the diagnosis of PSC. Serum antimitochondrial, antinuclear, and antismooth muscle antibodies and rheumatoid factor are absent in 90 to 95% of patients with PSC (1,2,4,33). Although a small percentage (<5%) of PSC patients have a positive antimitochondrial antibody, the titers are low (2,33). Others have reported higher prevalence rates of autoimmune antibody markers in PSC patients; however, no correlation between the patients' clinical status and the presence of circulating autoantibodies was observed (36). Serum IgM levels may be elevated in PSC but are not as high as those observed in PBC (2). Recent reports have shown that ~70% of PSC patients have anti-neutrophil nuclear and cytoplasmic antibodies (37,38). Although the identity of the antigenic markers is still unknown, these serologic tests merit further evaluation.

Histopathology

Virtually all patients with PSC have some histologic abnormality on liver biopsy (8,9). The hepatic histologic lesions characteristic of PSC is nonsuppurative obliterative cholangitis, a lesion characterized by a mixed inflammatory cell infiltrate in or near the damaged ductular epithelium. Ductular damage often is segmental with extensive concentric collagen deposition around ducts

(Fig. 19–2). PSC proceeds temporally through various histologic stages which are summarized in Table 19–5. Stage I is characterized by portal edema, inflammation and ductular proliferation. This stage may be indistinguishable from incomplete large duct obstruction from other causes or stage I PBC (9). Stage II disease reveals the presence of periportal fibrosis and inflammation, with or without ductular proliferation. Lymphocytic piecemeal necrosis may be present. In stage III disease, fibrous septa extend between adjacent portal tracts. Ductopenia becomes more prominent and piecemeal necrosis may become apparent. Stage IV disease is overt cirrhosis with irregular garland-shaped regenerative nodules. Near-complete loss of interlobular bile ducts is seen in tissue samples.

Radiologic Findings

The radiographic abnormalities seen in PSC are the most useful findings for diagnosis. ERCP is the method of choice to visualize the biliary tree in patients with suspected PSC (26). The cholangiographic findings include diffuse, multifocal annular strictures of the intrahepatic and extrahepatic biliary system with intervening segments of normal or slightly ectatic ducts, diverticular outpouchings, or short band-like strictures (Fig. 19–3). The cholangiographic changes

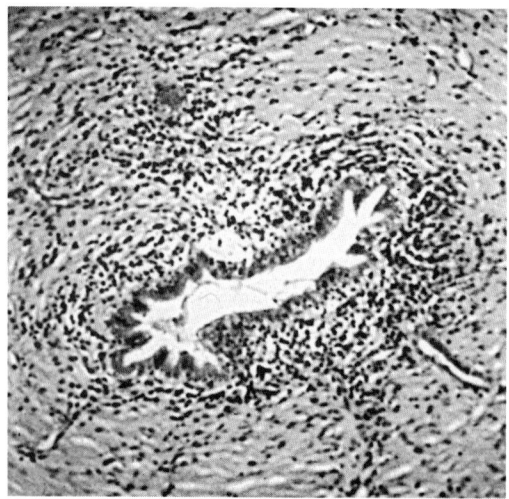

Fig. 19–2. Stained photomicrograph of a fibrous-obliterative lesion seen in PSC.

Table 19–5
Histologic Staging for Primary Sclerosing Cholangitis*

Stage I (portal stage)	Portal edema, inflammation and ductal proliferation; abnormalities do not extend beyond limiting plate
Stage II (periportal stage)	Periportal fibrosis, inflammation ± ductular proliferation; lymphocytic piecemeal necrosis may be present
Stage III (septal stage)	Fibrous septa extend between portal tracts; ductopenia more prominent; biliary piecemeal necrosis
Stage IV (cirrhotic stage)	Irregular regenerative nodules, ductular and piecemeal necrosis, loss of interlobular bile ducts

* Adapted with permission from Ludwig J: Surgical pathology of the syndrome of primary sclerosing cholangitis. Am J Surg Pathol *13*:43, 1989.

rarely are limited to the intrahepatic ducts, a situation referred to as intrahepatic sclerosing cholangitis. This entity represents a variant in the disease spectrum of PSC and can progress to the more global variety (9).

Other diffuse liver diseases including advanced cirrhosis, lymphoma, polycystic liver disease, metastatic cancer, and adeno-

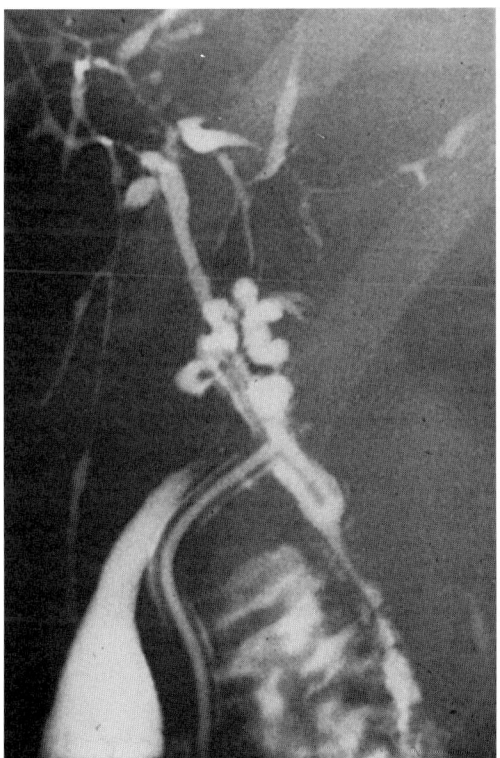

Fig. 19–3. Cholangiogram demonstrating the classic appearance of PSC on intrahepatic or extrahepatic bile ducts.

carcinoma of the bile ducts on occasion may be associated with cholangiographic abnormalities that overlap with those seen in PSC. However, the beaded appearance, pseudodiverticula, band strictures, and extrahepatic abnormalities produce a cholangiographic appearance, which is usually diagnostic of PSC. The greater radiographic challenge is to distinguish a benign dominant stricture from a superimposed cholangiocarcinoma in patients with PSC. The latter is suggested by certain cholangiographic features, including proximal ductal dilatation, mucosal irregularities, or nodular polyploid filling defects greater than 1 cm in diameter (39). Most commonly, the distinction cannot be made by radiographic findings only, and a biopsy of the lesion is required.

RELATIONSHIP WITH ULCERATIVE COLITIS

The relationship between PSC and IBD, especially CUC, is well documented (1,2,4,5,40–46). About 77% of PSC patients have coexistent CUC; Crohn's colitis and Crohn's ileocolitis are much less commonly associated with PSC (1,2,4,5). Table 19–6 summarizes reviews from various geographic locales which have evaluated the relationship between PSC and IBD. Several features regarding the association of PSC with CUC have been observed, including the following:

1. The diagnosis of CUC usually precedes PSC, but the symptoms of PSC may precede those of CUC.

Table 19–6
Frequency of Association of Inflammatory Bowel Disease in Patients with Primary Sclerosing Cholangitis

Author and Reference	Number of Patients	Expressed as Percentage of Total Number of Patients with IBD			
		IBD	PSC with		
			UC	CD	Unclassified
Chapman et al. (2)	29	72	72		
Wiesner and LaRusso (1)	50	54	48	6	
Sivak et al. (40)	13	85	77	8	
Lebovics et al. (41)	38	61	47	13	
Helzberg et al. (27)	53	62	58	4	
Aadland et al. (42)	45	100	82	13	5
Stockbrugger et al. (43)	44	98	82	5	21
Wiesner et al. (44)	174	71			
Rabinovitz et al. (45)	66	71	59	12	
Fausa et al. (46)	60	98	78	13	7

* Modified with permission from Fausa O et al.: Relationship of inflammatory bowel disease and primary sclerosing cholangitis. Semin Liver Dis *11*:31, 1991.
IBD: inflammatory bowel disease
UC: ulcerative colitis
CD: Crohn's disease

2. There is apparently no distinction between PSC patients with and without CUC.
3. The ulcerative colitis associated with PSC usually involves the entire colon with rectal sparing occurring in ~25% of patients and is more common in male PSC patients than in female PSC patients.
4. The CUC associated with PSC usually is clinically mild or quiescent.

The lack of correlation between hepatobiliary disease and colitic symptoms as well as the lack of effect of total proctocolectomy on the progression of liver disease in patients with PSC and CUC suggests that PSC is not a direct result of the CUC (47). However, until the etiology of PSC is better understood, the complex pathogenetic relationship of PSC and CUC will remain obscure.

DIAGNOSTIC CRITERIA

The diagnosis of PSC is based upon several criteria, including: (1) the absence of identifiable causes of sclerosing cholangitis (see Table 19–1); (2) an elevated (usually greater than twofold over normal) serum alkaline phosphatase, especially in a male patient with CUC; (3) hepatic histologic abnormalities as suggested by Ludwig (8,9) (see Table 19–5); and (4) the characteristic radiographic findings on cholangiogram (26). An abnormal cholangiogram remains the gold standard for the diagnosis of PSC, but the small-duct variant of PSC requires histologic confirmation because the cholangiogram in this subgroup of PSC patients may be normal (9).

DIFFERENTIAL DIAGNOSIS

The most important diagnostic test to establish the diagnosis of PSC is cholangiography. A retrograde route generally is preferred over a transhepatic route because the endoscopic approach usually is less uncomfortable and the rate of successful visualization of bile ducts is probably higher. The endoscopic approach also allows visualization of the pancreatic duct. The transhepatic cholangiogram may be the preferred route in patients with previous biliary tract surgery. A cholangiogram with the classic features of PSC and in the appropriate clinical setting usually is sufficient for the diagnosis of PSC; a liver biopsy is confirmatory but is not usually necessary for the diagnosis. Although liver biopsy may confirm the diagnosis, its primary value is to provide accurate histologic staging and to assist in predicting prognosis.

Other syndromes listed in Table 19–1 should be considered in the differential diagnosis of PSC. Secondary causes of sclerosing cholangitis which lead to extrahepatic biliary obstruction include biliary stone disease, trauma, tumors, ischemia, congenital anomalies, infections, and iatrogenic strictures. Causes of extrahepatic obstruction usually can be excluded by noninvasive imaging studies such as ultrasonography. Drugs which induce cholestasis such as estrogens, androgens, and phenothiazines, as well as drugs which lead to granuloma formation in the liver, also should be excluded. Rarely, cholangiocarcinoma may lead to sclerosis of the bile ducts and may mimic PSC; the more common problem, however, is the development of cholangiocarcinoma as a complication of PSC. Primary biliary cirrhosis also must be excluded, especially in middle-aged women with chronic cholestasis. An autoantibody to the M2 antigen is present in >95% of patients with PBC, but absent from virtually all patients with PSC (33). Cholangiograms also are distinctive in PBC, with either a normal appearance or decreased intrahepatic branching and normal extrahepatic bile ducts. A very rare syndrome distinct from PSC and PBC, termed idiopathic adulthood ductopenia, has been described (48). These patients usually are under 25 years of age, present with chronic cholestasis, and have ductopenia on liver biopsy but have normal cholangiograms, a negative antimitochondrial antibody, and no associated IBD. Last, an overlap syndrome may occur between PSC and idiopathic or autoimmune chronic active hepatitis. Thus, patients with chronic active hepatitis and either a cholestatic biochemical profile or IBD should have a cholangiogram to exclude PSC.

ETIOPATHOGENESIS

Association with Inflammatory Bowel Disease

Early efforts to identify the cause of PSC focused on the association of PSC with ulcerative colitis. This approach led to hypotheses that proposed increased absorption of luminal contents, including infectious agents or toxins, from a gastrointestinal mucosa with increased permeability. It was initially hypothesized that portal bacteremia from increased gastrointestinal permeability led to biliary tract inflammation (49,50). Subsequent studies failed to find significant bacteremia in the portal blood of patients undergoing surgery for severe colitis (51). In addition, portal phlebitis, which represents the histologic hallmark of portal bacteremia, is mild or absent in PSC patients, and bacterial cultures of liver biopsies are consistently negative for bacteria (52). What role inflammatory mediators, bacterial products, or immune cytokines produced in the colon might play in the etiology of PSC requires further study. The lack of correlation between the progression of PSC and IBD, coupled with the occurrence of PSC in the absence of IBD, as well as the lack of effect of proctocolectomy on the course of PSC, suggests no simple etiologic relationship between IBD and PSC. Despite these observations, the close association of PSC with CUC (i.e., 70% of patients with PSC have IBD) indicates an etiologic relationship, albeit currently obscure: between these two diseases.

In addition to portal bacteremia, other infectious agents have been implicated in the development of PSC. Both cytomegalovirus (CMV) and Reo virus type 3 have a tropism for biliary epithelium (53–57). The ability of Reo virus type 3 to induce cholangitis and biliary atresia in weanling mice has suggested a viral etiology for PSC (53,54). CMV can cause intrahepatic bile duct destruction, but large bile duct destruction has not been observed with this agent, and the histology of CMV infection in the liver is distinct from that in PSC; further, PCR has failed to demonstrate CMV-specific DNA in liver samples of patients with PSC (58). Hepatitis A, B and C have been excluded as etiologic agents for PSC (57).

Immunodeficiency states have been associated with intrahepatic sclerosing cholangitis (59,60). Whether the immunodeficiency reduces host defenses and allows bacteria, parasites or viruses, or their byproducts or inflammatory mediators, to cause hepatobiliary disease is unclear. Sclerosing cholangitis also has been linked to isolated cases of immunodeficiency states, including severe combined immunodeficiency, X-linked immunodeficiency, and angioblastic lymphadenopathy (61–64). Moreover, patients with acquired immunodeficiency syndrome (AIDS) also have been found to have abnormalities of the biliary system, resulting most commonly from infections caused by CMV, mycobacteria, cryptosporidium, or other opportunistic organisms (65).

Acquired Disease

It has been postulated that toxic bile acids generated by colonic bacteria in a diseased colon could lead to portal tract inflammation (66). However, studies have failed to show major abnormalities in bile acid metabolism in PSC patients with or without CUC (67–69).

Excess hepatic copper in PSC patients is well established, but it is unlikely that abnormalities in copper metabolism are important in the initiation of PSC (35). Elevated copper is found in other liver diseases characterized by cholestasis, suggesting that it is a consequence of the cholestatic process and not a primary event in PSC (70). Moreover, PSC progresses despite the ability of D-penicillamine to decrease hepatic copper content (71).

Vascular Disease

The bile ducts receive blood exclusively from the hepatic artery, which forms a rich peribiliary vascular plexus. Interruption of this blood supply leads to ischemic necrosis and the disappearance of bile ducts (72,73). The disappearance of large interlobular bile ducts has been noted during chronic allograft rejection after liver transplantation (74). Although some of the ductopenia may be secondary to immunologically mediated processes, some of the biliary damage may be caused by interruption of the vascular blood supply from thickening of the hepatic

arterioles. Nonetheless, the outcome is a syndrome with clinical, biochemical, radiologic, and histologic features similar to PSC.

Extrahepatic biliary disease similar to PSC also has been observed following infusion of the chemotherapeutic agent, 5-fluorodeoxyuridine, through the hepatic artery for hepatic metastasis from colorectal adenocarcinoma (75–78). This process causes small-vessel arteriopathy and probably leads to fibrosis and obliteration of the bile ducts (75–78). Although these data clearly demonstrate that ischemia can result in radiologic and histologic features similar to those seen in PSC, small and large vessel arteriopathy have not been observed in PSC, suggesting that a purely vascular basis for the pathogenesis of PSC is unlikely.

Genetics

Several lines of evidence suggest a genetic predisposition to the development of PSC. First, an increased frequency of PSC in families has been reported (79,80). Moreover, a close association has been noted between the HLA-B8 and HLA-DR3 phenotypes and PSC (81,82). These two haplotypes frequently are found with autoimmune diseases including autoimmune chronic active hepatitis, type I diabetes mellitus, thyrotoxicosis, and myasthenia gravis (83). The increased prevalence of HLA-B8 and HLA-DR3, numerous cellular and humoral immune abnormalities described in PSC, and the association of PSC with IBD and nontropical sprue, two autoimmune diseases, all support an immunologic basis for the pathogenesis of PSC.

Humoral Immunologic Abnormalities

Although PSC is not characterized by a specific serologic marker like the antimitochondrial antibody associated with PBC, numerous humoral abnormalities have been described in PSC (84). For example, PSC patients with and without IBD have elevated circulating immune complexes in the serum (84), a finding seen in various other liver diseases (52). Whether any antigens specific for the hepatobiliary system are contained within these immune complexes has not been determined. Decreased clearance of immune complexes and increased consumption of the classical pathway of the complement system also has been documented (85–88). The serum of patients with PSC also contains antibody that reacts with colonic and biliary epithelium, suggesting the presence of a cross-reactive determinant linking the hepatobiliary disease with the IBD (89). In addition, by an enzyme-linked immunosorbent assay for IgG neutrophil antibody, neutrophil binding by sera from PSC patients is significantly higher than sera from patients with PBC, chronic hepatitis B, and chronic non-A, non-B hepatitis (38). This was noted in PSC patients irrespective of the presence of CUC. A perinuclear pattern of immunofluorescent staining of neutrophils was observed. Others have reported a high prevalence of nuclear neutrophilic antibodies in IBD and PSC (37).

Immune complexes have been detected in the bile of patients with PSC; again, no specific antigens have been characterized (90). Biliary antigens from PSC patients are able to inhibit leukocyte migration *in vitro,* suggesting that these lymphocytes might react with specific biliary antigens (91).

Cellular Immunologic Abnormalities

Reduction in the total number of T cells in the peripheral circulation with a disproportionate decrease in the number of suppresser/cytotoxic (CD8) T cells has been observed in PSC (92–94). This decline is reflected as an increase in the ratio of helper (CD4) to CD8 T cells. Increases in the number and percentage of circulating B cells also have been found and the increased percentage has been correlated with histologic stage on liver biopsy as well as with serum bilirubin, IgG and gamma globulin (92).

Increased numbers of T cells have been noted in liver tissue obtained from PSC patients undergoing liver transplantation (93,94); CD8 T cells were localized to areas of bile duct proliferation and areas of infiltrated ductular epithelium while CD 4 T cells were localized to the lobular side of portal inflammation (93). Others have not observed this T cell subset localization in precirrhotic livers from PSC patients (94).

HLA Antigen Expression

While most nucleated cells express HLA class I antigens, HLA class II antigen expression normally is limited to cells of immune lineage (95). Biliary epithelial cells normally do not express HLA class II antigens; however, most intrahepatic bile duct epithelial cells from patients with PSC do express HLA-DR (class II) antigen at a relatively early stage of the disease (96,97). The ability of bile duct cells to express HLA-DR antigens suggests that these cells may present foreign antigens to T cells, which subsequently undergo activation and enhanced immunoresponsiveness. An alternative explanation for the aberrant expression of HLA-DR antigen on biliary epithelium is that it represents the response of biliary epithelial cells to inflammatory mediators such as interferon gamma, TNFα, or IL-4, which are known to induce HLA class II antigens on a variety of cell types (98,99). The aberrant expression of HLA class II antigen on bile duct cells also has been observed in PBC and with extrahepatic biliary obstruction (96). Thus, it is unclear whether such aberrant expression represents a primary, etiologically important phenomena, or an epiphenomenon secondary to cholestasis. Therefore, what role the aberrant expression of HLA class II antigen plays in the pathogenesis of PSC currently is unclear. However, it is noteworthy that colonic epithelia from patients with active ulcerative colitis also exhibit aberrant HLA class II antigen expression (100).

Table 19–7 summarizes various putative etiologic agents implicated in the pathogenesis of PSC. Based upon current evidence, it seems likely that the pathogenesis of PSC is related to an autoimmune-mediated process. Individuals with a genetic predisposition incur some unknown, possibly viral insult that renders the biliary epithelium susceptible to immune-mediated destruction; however, the mechanism for this process remains unknown.

Animal Models

Several animal models have been developed in an attempt to better understand the pathogenesis of PSC. A rat model of colitis induced by the rectal injection of dilute acetic acid is associated with inflammation in hepatic portal areas (101). Lethal infection with Escherichia coli causes periportal inflammation, increased serum alkaline phos-

Table 19–7
Postulated Etiologic Factors in Primary
Sclerosing Cholangitis

Association with CUC
Infectious Agents
Bacteria/Bacterial products
Viral: Cytomegalovirus
Reovirus
    Hepatitis A, B, C
    Acquired
Copper Toxins:
Bile acids
Chemical irritants (5-FUDR, for-
    malin)
    Vascular: Ischemia
        Genetic
        Familial
        HLA haplotypes
    Immunologic
        Humoral
        Cellular
    HLA-DR expression

---

phatase levels, and Kupffer cell hyperplasia; sublethal doses have no apparent effect (102). Injection into rabbits of heat-inactivated, nonpathogenic E. coli leads to periportal and parenchymal inflammation that resolves after cessation of the injections (103). Last, the surgical creation of self-filling blind loops in the mid-jejunum of rats leads to increased anaerobic bacterial growth and hepatobiliary injury after 2 to 3 weeks (104,105). The periportal inflammation consists of predominantly mononuclear cells and is associated with bile duct injury. These models suggest that bacterial products or possible inflammatory mediators are able to induce periportal inflammation in the liver (106).

Two potential animal models merit further investigation. First, the cotton-topped tamarin develops a spontaneous form of colitis; whether hepatobiliary disease and periportal inflammation accompany this spontaneous colitis is unknown. Second, the injection of peripheral blood lymphocytes from PBC patients into severe combined immunodeficient strains of mice results in lymphocytic infiltration of the portal area as well as the production of human anti-mitochondrial antibody in the serum of these mice (107). Whether a similar observation would be made following the injection of lymphocytes from PSC patients into these mice is unknown. Clearly, the development of better animal models for PSC, particularly those associated with an immune basis, will allow not only a better understanding of PSC, but also permit extension of current therapeutic regimens.

NATURAL HISTORY AND PROGNOSIS

The natural history of primary sclerosing cholangitis is currently in evolution; however, the weight of current evidence suggests that PSC is an unpredictably progressive disease that eventually leads to the complications of chronic cholestasis and hepatic failure (1,2,27,32,44,108). Median survival from the onset of symptoms to death or liver transplantation is approximately 12 years. Prognosis appears to be better in patients who are asymptomatic at the time of their diagnosis, although the survival of asymptomatic patients is significantly decreased compared to a control population (3,44,108,109). During the course of one study, 31% of patients died from underlying liver disease or cholangiocarcinoma; another 10% were referred for orthotopic liver transplantation (44). There may be a subpopulation of PSC patients with a more prolonged, perhaps even benign, course to their disease (110).

The lack of effective medical therapy and the apparent success of orthotopic liver transplantation for the treatment of PSC emphasizes the importance of accurate prognostic indicators in the selection of patients who will most likely benefit from liver transplantation. This has led to the development of mathematical models to provide independent predictors of survival to aid in the selection of patients, both for pharmacologic therapy and for orthotopic liver transplantation. The first report to employ Cox regression analysis for the evaluation of PSC patients found that hepatomegaly and an elevated serum bilirubin were independent predictors of a poor prognosis (27). A similar preliminary model from our institution found that age, serum bilirubin, serum hemoglobin concentration, presence or absence of IBD, and hepatic histologic stage were all independent predictors of survival

(44). The most recent mathematical model to predict survival in PSC patients utilized a geographically heterogeneous patient population from five major medical centers (111). This study found that total serum bilirubin, age, hepatic histologic stage, and splenomegaly were independent predictors of survival with PSC (111).

COMPLICATIONS

Complications secondary to PSC are summarized in Table 19–3, including general complications present in most forms of chronic cholestatic liver diseases. Complications common to most chronic cholestatic liver diseases include hepatic osteodystrophy, steatorrhea, pruritus, and fat-soluble vitamin deficiency. Portal hypertension, gastroesophageal varices, cirrhosis, and hepatic failure generally occur after long-standing disease.

Cholelithiasis and choledocholithiasis also may occur. Chronic cholestasis predisposes to the formation of lithogenic bile and cholesterol gallstones; biliary stasis with or without ascending cholangitis may predispose to pigment stone formation. Thus, cholecystitis must be considered in the appropriate clinical setting in PSC patients. In fact, approximately one third of PSC patients have undergone cholecystectomy during the course of their disease (32).

The development of a dominant stricture or biliary stones is suggested by a sudden clinical and biochemical deterioration such as cholangitis, rising bilirubin, or pruritus. Moreover, distinction between a benign dominant stricture and adenocarcinoma of the bile duct represents a clinical challenge.

Approximately 10 to 15% of PSC patients develop cholangiocarcinoma, the most lethal complication (1,2,29,32,112). This diagnosis may be difficult to establish, and therapy is essentially ineffective. Risk factors for the development of cholangiocarcinoma in PSC include portal hypertension, cirrhosis, and CUC; however, these are not absolute, and cholangiocarcinoma may occur in young patients with early PSC (112,113). Median survival is approximately 5 months after the diagnosis of cholangiocarcinoma in patients with PSC. Preliminary results suggest that CA-19-9 may represent a useful se-

rologic marker for detecting the development of cholangiocarcinoma in PSC (114).

Peristomal varices represent a frequent complication in PSC patients who have had proctocolectomy for CUC with ileostomy (115). These varices are secondary to portal hypertension, are painful, and frequently bleed, sometimes severely, and thus may lead to consideration of the patient for orthotopic liver transplantation as the most effective treatment (115). Reduction of portal hypertension, either medically or by orthotopic liver transplantation, is the treatment of choice. The role of transjugular intrahepatic portosystemic shunting in these patients is unclear.

TREATMENT

Management of Chronic Cholestasis

The progressive nature of PSC provides the clinician with the challenge of both managing the symptoms and complications of this chronic hepatobiliary disease and developing novel approaches to the treatment of the underlying hepatobiliary disease. For the asymptomatic patient with minimal liver function test abnormalities, observation or inclusion in randomized, controlled trials of medical treatment are reasonable approaches. Conversely, patients with complications from long-standing PSC, such as gastroesophageal varices, may require alternative interventions.

The signs and symptoms of chronic cholestasis in PSC include pruritus, steatorrhea, fat-soluble vitamin deficiency, hepatic osteodystrophy, and fatigue. Pruritus is one of the most common complaints of patients with chronic cholestasis. The pruritus usually is worse at night and may lead to insomnia and excoriations. Cholestyramine is an effective treatment for the pruritus, provided that bile flow is sufficient (117). Cholestyramine is initiated at 4 g three times daily taken before or with meals. Once the pruritus has resolved, the dose may be tapered. However, a 2- to 4-day delay is typically seen before the patient observes any benefit from this therapy. If the initial dose fails to alleviate the pruritus, the dose may be increased to 8 g three times a day, but additional increases rarely are beneficial.

Addition of phenobarbital (60 to 90 mg at bedtime) to cholestyramine may provide effective adjunctive therapy by increasing bile flow and providing sedation (116). Colestipol may be substituted for cholestyramine in patients who cannot tolerate the latter (117). Activated charcoal capsules and rifampin also have been effective in the treatment of pruritus (32). In patients refractory to these conventional attempts to control pruritus, large-volume plasmapheresis and ultraviolet B light may be beneficial (117). The presence of intractable pruritus unresponsive to medical management may indicate consideration for orthotopic liver transplantation.

Patients with PSC may have steatorrhea and malabsorption of fat-soluble vitamins (A, D, E, and K). Asymptomatic vitamin A deficiency has been found in almost 50% of PSC patients; a smaller number may develop night blindness (70). Replacement therapy with 25,000 U of vitamin A per day usually is effective in correcting the deficiency. Vitamin K deficiency is unusual and most often observed in patients with chronic jaundice receiving cholestyramine. Coagulation studies usually are normal in PSC patients until end-stage liver disease is present. However, easy bruising or bleeding in a PSC patient merits determination of the prothrombin time and vitamin K therapy if indicated.

Symptomatic bone disease is uncommon in the early stages of PSC, but a significant problem during the advanced stages (32,70,118). When present, osteoporosis rather than osteomalacia is the cause of the associated hepatic osteodystrophy. Determination of bone mineral densitometry is the most sensitive, noninvasive method for establishing the presence of hepatic osteodystrophy. While abnormalities in serum 25-hydroxyvitamin D levels do not correlate with the presence of bone disease, vitamin D should be given if serum levels are low.

Fatigue is a common presenting complaint in PSC patients and one of the most difficult to treat. Organic causes of fatigue, including endocrinopathies, should be evaluated to rule out treatable diseases.

Management of Complications Secondary to Primary Sclerosing Cholangitis

Intermittent episodes of bacterial cholangitis generally are treated with broad-spectrum antibiotics. The role of prophylactic antibiotic therapy, especially for patients with more frequent bouts of cholangitis, based upon anecdotal reports, is unproven, but not unreasonable in selected patients.

Development of a dominant stricture may present as an acute change in a patient's clinical status; after demonstration by cholangiography, this stricture may be relieved by cholangioplasty with or without stent placement (119,120). Biliary stones and debris may cause a similar clinical picture with acute obstruction; patients may be benefited by sphincterotomy, biliary lavage, and/or biliary stent placement. Occult cholangiocarcinoma must be considered when a patient with PSC acutely deteriorates.

Cholangiocarcinoma occurs in approximately 10 to 15% of PSC patients and is often associated with rapid deterioration, progressive jaundice, weight loss, and abdominal discomfort. In many cases, the diagnosis of cholangiocarcinoma complicating PSC is not made until autopsy (112,113). When detected, the tumors usually are found in the advanced stages, precluding any curative resection (112,113). Palliative surgical procedures have little benefit in prolonging survival, and the prognosis for cholangiocarcinoma complicating PSC is uniformly poor. A vigilant awareness for early detection is critical so that more effective therapy might be provided. Clearly, the development of new methods for early detection, localization, and treatment of cholangiocarcinoma in patients with PSC represents a major challenge.

Specific Therapy Directed Toward Primary Sclerosing Cholangitis

Medical Therapy

Various anti-inflammatory, immunosuppressive, and antifibrotic agents have been employed to treat PSC; to date, the results have been disappointing, although assessment of treatment effectiveness is difficult because of the fluctuating, unpredictable clinical course of this disease. The sparsity of controlled clinical trials for most failed therapeutic agents adds to the difficult interpretation of the clinical response.

The first published prospective double-blind clinical trial for the treatment of PSC tested D-penicillamine on the premise that the elevated copper levels present in PSC patients were important in disease progression (71). Unfortunately, penicillamine was not effective therapy for PSC (71). A total of 70 patients were followed for 36 months with no beneficial effects noted for symptoms, liver histology, biochemical serum liver tests, disease progression, or survival (71). Although the treatment did lead to decreased copper levels, the lack of efficacy in disease progression and the drug's toxic side effects indicated that penicillamine is not useful for PSC (71).

Early reports have suggested that corticosteroids may be effective in the treatment of PSC (121,122); others have not observed this favorable response (123). A prospective open-label study from our institution, which evaluated treatment of PSC with prednisone in combination with colchicine, indicated that, after 2 years, no improvement in clinical disease, biochemical serum liver tests, histology, or survival was observed (123). This lack of benefit, coupled with the possibility that corticosteroids might accelerate the associated hepatic osteodystrophy, has dampened enthusiasm for their use in PSC.

Because current views favor an autoimmune mechanism for the etiology of PSC, treatment with cyclosporine has been initiated at our institution (124). Preliminary results from this prospective, double-blind trial indicate that treatment of noncirrhotic PSC patients with cyclosporine has no benefit on clinical symptoms, biochemical liver tests, or survival free of treatment failure (124). While this trial is continuing, the initial results suggest no benefit of cyclosporine for the treatment of PSC.

A case report several years ago suggested that methotrexate improved biochemical liver function tests in a PSC patient with erythroderma (125). Subsequent treatment of a second PSC patient showed similarly promising results (125). This report led to initiation of a prospective, double-blind trial of methotrexate and placebo, the results of which still are pending (117).

Two clinical trials have reported the effects of ursodeoxycholic acid (urso) on patients with PSC (126,127). One study involved 14 patients in a prospective, randomized double-blinded, placebo-controlled trial. Patients treated with urso for 1 year had improvement in serum bilirubin, cholestatic serum enzyme activity, and histologic appearance on liver biopsies compared with the placebo group (126). Expression of the MHC class I molecules on liver cells also was markedly reduced (126). A second open-label pilot study found similar improvement in biochemical markers of cholestasis in PSC patients receiving urso. Improvement in serum enzyme markers and cholesterol was greater after 2 years than after only 6 months of treatment (127). In addition, clinical symptoms of fatigue, pruritus, and diarrhea also were improved by urso (127). Other groups have not observed these improvements with urso therapy for PSC in preliminary reports (128,129). Thus, these results justify larger controlled clinical trials to evaluate the effectiveness of urso as a therapeutic option for PSC.

Interventional Therapy

Radiologic/endoscopic. Radiologic and endoscopic treatment of PSC is designed to alleviate symptoms of cholangitis or pruritus caused by a dominant stricture, biliary debris, or stones (26). Whether by endoscopic or transhepatic approaches, these techniques help to provide relief of symptoms, but do not appear to alter the course of the disease and are unlikely to affect long-term prognosis. Sphincterotomy, cholangioplasty, and stent placement have been used to manage the complications of PSC, but assessment of the long-term benefits of these interventions is difficult in the absence of randomized controlled clinical trials and largely anecdotal reports; however, data from our institution suggest symptomatic benefit for selected patients with PSC who undergo transhepatic balloon dilation for benign dominant strictures (119,120).

Surgical. The purpose of surgical management of PSC generally has been to relieve mechanical biliary tract obstruction caused by dominant strictures. Unfortunately, the associated surgical morbidity, coupled with the lack of convincing data and controlled trials, does not support its efficacy (129). The same goals (i.e., relief of obstruction) generally can be accomplished by nonsurgical approaches, which also do not make subsequent orthotopic liver transplantation more difficult.

The frequent association of PSC with CUC suggested a common etiology and thus a potential role for proctocolectomy. The rationale was that, if some luminal product or infectious agent was being absorbed through a diseased colon, then proctocolectomy would reverse this process. Unfortunately, proctocolectomy for CUC appears to have no role in preventing progression of PSC in patients with both PSC and CUC (47). A retrospective analysis of patients with PSC and CUC demonstrated no difference in the progression of clinical, biochemical, histologic, or cholangiographic features in patients with or without proctocolectomy (47). Moreover, proctocolectomy did not affect overall patient survival. Proctocolectomy may be indicated for colitic symptoms in patients with PSC and CUC, but it has no role in the treatment of PSC.

Orthotopic liver transplantation appears to be the best current treatment for advanced stages of PSC. Although early results of liver transplantation for PSC were not encouraging, improvements in immunosuppressive therapy and surgical expertise have contributed to improved patient survival (130,131). Recent results indicate 5-year survival rates of 74 to 85% for PSC and are not different from other forms of nonmalignant, noninfectious chronic liver disease (131). PSC now represents one of the most frequent indications for adult orthotopic liver transplantation.

Two important issues remain regarding liver transplantation in patients with PSC. First, patients with coexistent CUC who undergo liver transplantation may be at increased risk for the development of colonic malignancy while receiving immunosuppressive therapy. Vigilant screening for colorectal cancer must be continued in these patients. Second, diffuse biliary stricturing occurs more frequently in PSC patients than in patients with other diseases who undergo liver transplantation; this problem probably represents recurrence of the primary disease only in a small number of cases. In the majority, some other pathologic process, such as bacterial or chemical cholangitis or rejection, may be operative.

SUMMARY

Primary sclerosing cholangitis is a chronic, generally progressive cholestatic liver disease of unknown etiology which has become a major focus of attention for gastroenterologists and hepatologists in the last decade. The syndrome occurs in frequent association with chronic ulcerative colitis and most commonly in young men. The disease is characterized by symptoms of fatigue, pruritus, and jaundice with a cholestatic biochemical profile, and evidence of hepatic copper overload. The diagnosis is supported by histologic abnormalities on liver biopsy and generally confirmed by cholangiogram. Although the natural history of the disease is still in evolution, it is generally recognized as a slowly progressive disease that leads to the complications of chronic cholestasis, portal hypertension, and cirrhosis with approximately 10% of patients developing carcinoma of the bile ducts. The etiology of this disease is unknown and is reflected in the lack of effective medical therapy, which is currently directed toward symptomatic treatment, and therapy for complications of PSC. Orthotopic liver transplantation is the treatment of choice for patients with advanced disease. The management of patients with early or asymptomatic disease currently is experimental and directed at prevention of disease progression. A better understanding of the etiology of this disease should allow a more rational approach to current medical therapy.

REFERENCES

1. Wiesner RH, LaRusso NF: Clinicopathologic features of the syndrome of primary sclerosing cholangitis. Gastroenterology *79*:200, 1980.
2. Chapman RWG et al.: Primary sclerosing cholangitis: A review of its clinical features, cholangiography, and hepatic histology. Gut *21*:870, 1980.
3. Hoffman CEE: Verschluss der Gallenwege durch verdickung der Wandungen. Arch Pathol Anat Physiol *49*:206, 1867.
4. Thorpe MEC, Scheuer PJ, Sherlock S: Primary sclerosing cholangitis, the biliary tree, and ulcerative colitis. Gut. *8*:435, 1967.

5. Schrumpf E et al.: Sclerosing cholangitis in ulcerative colitis. A follow up study. Scand J Gastroenterol *17*:33, 1982.

6. MacCarty RL, LaRusso NF, Wiesner RH, Ludwig J: Primary sclerosing cholangitis: Findings of cholangiography and pancreatography. Radiology *149*:39, 1983.

7. Lefkowich JH: Primary sclerosing cholangitis. Arch Intern Med *142*:1157, 1982.

8. Ludwig J: Surgical pathology of the syndrome of primary sclerosing cholangitis. Am J Surg Pathol *13*:43, 1989.

9. Ludwig J: Small-duct primary sclerosing cholangitis. Semin Liver Dis *11*:11, 1991.

10. White TT, Hart MJ: Primary sclerosing cholangitis. Am J Surg *153*:439, 1987.

11. Schwartz SI, Dale WA: Primary sclerosing cholangitis; review and report of six cases. AMA Arch Surg *77*:439, 1958.

12. Wee A, Ludwig J: Pericholangitis in chronic ulcerative colitis: Primary sclerosing cholangitis of the small bile ducts. Ann Intern Med *102*:581, 1985.

13. Thompson HH, Pitt HA, Tomkins RK, Longmire WP: Primary sclerosing cholangitis; a heterogeneous disease. Ann Surg *196*:127, 1982.

14. Pitt HA, Thompson HH, Tomkins RK, Longmire WP: Primary sclerosing cholangitis; results of an aggressive surgical approach. Ann Surg *196*:259, 1982.

15. Vinnik IE, Kern F: Liver disease in ulcerative colitis. Arch Intern Med *112*:87, 1963.

16. Warren KW, Athanassiades S, Monge JI: Primary sclerosing cholangitis. Am J Surg *111*:23, 1966.

17. Shepard HA et al.: Ulcerative colitis and persistent liver dysfunction. Q J Med *208*:503, 1983.

18. Dordal E, Glagov S, Kirsner JB: Hepatic lesions in chronic inflammatory bowel disease; clinical correlations with liver biopsy diagnoses in 103 patients. Gastroenterology *52*:239, 1967.

19. Lupinetti M, Mehigan D, Cameron JL: Hepatobiliary complications of ulcerative colitis. Am J Surg *139*:113, 1980.

20. Eade MN: Liver disease in ulcerative colitis; analysis of operative liver biopsy in 138 consecutive patients having colectomy. Ann Intern Med *72*:475, 1970.

21. Mistilis SP: Pericholangitis and ulcerative colitis. Ann Intern Med *63*:1, 1965.

22. Kreiger J, Seaman WB, Porter MR: The roentgenologic appearance of sclerosing cholangitis. Radiology *95*:369, 1970.

23. Porayko MK, LaRusso NF, Wiesner RH: Primary sclerosing cholangitis: A progressive disease? Semin Liver Dis *11*:18, 1991.

24. Blackstone MO, Nemchausky BA: Cholangiographic abnormalities in ulcerative colitis associated pericholangitis which resemble sclerosing cholangitis. Am J Dig Dis *23*:579, 1978.

25. Brandt DJ et al.: Gallbladder disease in patients with primary sclerosing cholangitis. AJR *150*:571, 1988.

26. MacCarty RL, LaRusso NF, Wiesner RH, Ludwig J: Primary sclerosing cholangitis: Finding on cholangiography and pancreatography. Radiology *149*:39, 1983.

27. Helzberg JH, Peterson JM, Boyer JL: Improved survival with primary sclerosing cholangitis. A review of the clinicopathologic features and comparison of symptomatic and asymptomatic patients. Gastroenterology *79*:200, 1980.

28. Fausa O et al.: Relationship of inflammatory bowel disease and primary sclerosing cholangitis. Semin Liver Dis *11*:31, 1991.

29. LaRusso NF, Wiesner RH, Ludwig J, MacCarty RL: Primary sclerosing cholangitis. N Engl J Med *310*:899, 1984.

30. Lefkowitch JH, Martin EC: Primary sclerosing cholangitis. Prog Liver Dis *8*:557, 1986.

31. Warren KW, Athanassiades S, Monge JI: Primary sclerosing cholangitis. A study of 42 cases. Am J Surg *111*:23, 1966.

32. Wiesner RH, Ludwig J, LaRusso NF, MacCarty RL: Diagnosis and treatment of primary sclerosing cholangitis. Semin Liver Dis *5*:241, 1985.

33. Wiesner RH, LaRusso NF, Ludwig J, Dickson ER: Comparison of the clinicopathologic features of primary sclerosing cholangitis and primary biliary cirrhosis. Gastroenterology *88*:108, 1985.

34. Balasubramanian K, Wiesner RH, LaRusso NF: Primary sclerosing cholangitis with normal serum alkaline phosphatase activity. Gastroenterology *95*:1395, 1988.

35. Gross JB et al.: Abnormalities in tests of copper metabolism in primary sclerosing cholangitis. Gastroenterology *89*:272, 1985.

36. Zauli D et al.: An autoantibody profile in primary sclerosing cholangitis. J Hepatol *5*:14, 1987.

37. Snook JA, Chapman RW, Fleming K, Jewell DP: Anti-neutrophil nuclear antibody in ulcerative colitis, Crohn's disease and primary sclerosing cholangitis. Clin Exp Immunol *76*:30, 1989.

38. Duerr RH, et al.: Neutrophil cytoplasmic antibodies: A link between primary sclerosing cholangitis and ulcerative colitis. Gastroenterology *100*:1385, 1991.

39. MacCarty RL et al.: Cholangiocarcinoma complicating primary sclerosing cholangitis: Cholangiographic appearances. Radiology *156*:43, 1985.

40. Sivak MJ, Farmer RG, Lalli AF: Sclerosing cholangitis: Its increasing frequency of recognition and association with inflammatory bowel disease. J Clin Gastroenterol *3*:261, 1981.

41. Lebovics E, Palmer M, Woo J, Schaffner F: Outcome of primary sclerosing cholangitis. Arch Intern Med *147*:729, 1987.

42. Aadland E et al.: Primary sclerosing cholangitis: A long-term follow-up study. Scand J Gastroenterol *22*:655, 1987.

43. Stockbrugger RW, Olsson R, Jaup B, Jensen J: Forty-six patients with primary sclerosing cholangitis. Radiological bile duct changes in relationship to clinical course and concomitant inflammatory bowel disease. Hepatogastroenterology *35*:289, 1988.

44. Wiesner RH et al.: Primary sclerosing cholangitis: Natural history, prognostic factors and survival analysis. Hepatology *10*:430, 1989.

45. Rabinovitz M et al.: Does primary sclerosing cholangitis occurring in association with inflammatory bowel disease differ from that occurring in the absence of inflammatory bowel disease? A study of sixty-six subjects. Hepatology *11*:7, 1990.

46. Fausa O, Schrumpf E, Elgjo K: Inflammatory bowel disease occurs in almost all patients with primary sclerosing cholangitis. Scand J Gastroenterol *24*(Suppl. 159):53, 1989.

47. Cangemi JR et al.: Effect of proctocolectomy for chronic ulcerative colitis on the natural history of primary sclerosing cholangitis. Gastroenterology *96*:790, 1989.

48. Ludwig J, Wiesner RH, LaRusso NF: Idiopathic adulthood ductopenia: A cause of chronic cholestatic liver disease and biliary cirrhosis. J Hepatology *7*:193, 1988.

49. Whelton MJ: Sclerosing cholangitis. Clin Gastroenterol *2*:163, 1973.

50. Eade MN, Brooke BN: Portal bacteraemia in cases of ulcerative colitis submitted to colectomy. Lancet *1*:1008, 1969.

51. Palmer KR, Duerden BI, Holdsworth CD: Bacteriological and endotoxin studies in cases of ulcerative colitis submitted to surgery. Gut *21*:851, 1980.

52. Ludwig J et al.: Morphologic features of chronic hepatitis associated with primary sclerosing cholangitis and chronic ulcerative colitis. Hepatology *1*:632, 1981.

53. Morecki R et al.: Biliary atresia and reovirus type 3 infection. N Engl J Med *307*:481, 1982.

54. Bangaru B et al.: Comparative studies of biliary atresia in the human newborn and reovirus-induced cholangitis in weanling mice. Lab Invest *43*:452, 1980.

55. Minuk GY, Paul RW, Lee PWK: The prevalence of antibodies to reovirus type 3 in adults with idiopathic cholestatic liver disease. J Med Virol *16*:55, 1985.

56. Finegold MJ, Carpenter RJ: Obliterative cholangitis due to cytomegalovirus: A possible precursor of paucity of intra-hepatic bile ducts. Hum Pathol *13*:662, 1982.

57. Minuk BY et al.: Reovirus type 3 infection in patients with primary biliary cirrhosis and primary sclerosing cholangitis. J Hepatol *5*:8, 1987.

58. Rosser BG et al.: Evidence against a pathogenic role for cytomegalovirus (CMV) in primary sclerosing cholangitis (PSC). Hepatology *16*:193A, 1992.

59. Cello JP: Acquired immunodeficiency syndrome cholangiopathy: Spectrum of disease. Am J Med *86*:539, 1989.

60. Dowsett JF et al.: Sclerosing cholangitis in acquired immunodeficiency syndromes: Case reports and review of the literature. Scand J Gastroenterol *23*:1267, 1988.

61. Record CO et al.: Intra-hepatic sclerosing cholangitis associated with familial immunodeficiency syndrome. Lancet *2*:18, 1973.

62. Thomas IT, Ochs HD, Wedgwood RJ: Liver disease and immunodeficiency syndromes. Lancet *i*:311, 1974.

63. Naveh Y et al.: Primary sclerosing cholangitis associated with immunodeficiency. Am J Dis Child *137*:114, 1983.

64. Di Palma JA, Strobel CT, Farrow JG: Primary sclerosing cholangitis associated with hyperimmunoglobulin M immunodeficiency (dysgammaglobulinemia). Gastroenterology *91*:464, 1986.

65. Pol S et al.: Microsporidia infection in patients with the human immunodeficiency virus and unexplained cholangitis. N Engl J Med *328*:95, 1993.

66. Carey JB: Bile acids, cirrhosis and human evolution. Gastroenterology *46*:490, 1964.

67. Siegel JH, Barnes S, Morris JS: Bile acids in liver disease associated with inflammatory bowel disease. Digestion *15*:469, 1977.

68. Dew MJ, Henegouwen GP, van B Huybregts AWM, Allan RN: Hepatotoxic effect of bile acids in inflammatory bowel disease. Gastroenterology *78*:1393, 1980.

69. Holzbach RT et al.: Portal vein bile acids in patients with severe inflammatory bowel disease. Gut *21*:428, 1980.

70. Lindor KD, Wiesner RH, LaRusso NF: Recent advances in the management of primary sclerosing cholangitis. Semin Liver Dis *7*:322, 1987.

71. LaRusso NF et al.: Prospective trial of penicillamine in primary sclerosing cholangitis. Gastroenterology *95*:1036, 1988.

72. Sherlock S: The syndrome of disappearing bile ducts. Lancet *ii*:493, 1987.

73. Terblanche J, Allison HE, Northover JMA: An ischemic basis for biliary strictures. Surgery *94*:52, 1983.

74. Vierling JM, Fennell RH Jr: Histopathology of early and late human hepatic allograft rejection. Evidence of progressive destruction of interlobular bile ducts. Hepatology *5*:1076, 1985.

75. Kemeny N et al.: Intra-hepatic or systemic infusion of fluorodeoxyuridine in patients with liver metastases from colorectal cancer. A randomized trial. Ann Intern Med *107*:459, 1987.

76. Shea WJ et al.: Sclerosing cholangitis associated with hepatic arterial FUDR chemotherapy: Radiographic-histologic correlation. AJR *146*:717, 1986.

77. Kemeny MM et al.: Sclerosing cholangitis after continuous hepatic artery infusion of FUDR. Ann Surg *202*:176, 1985.

78. Ludwig J et al.: Floxuridine induced sclerosing cholangitis: An ischemic cholangiopathy. Hepatology *9*:215, 1989.

79. Quigley EMM et al.: Familial occurrence of primary sclerosing cholangitis and ulcerative colitis. Gastroenterology *85*:1160, 1983.

80. Jorge AD, Esley C, Ahumada J: Family incidence of primary sclerosing cholangitis associated with immunological diseases. Endoscopy *19*:114, 1987.

81. Chapman RW et al.: Association of primary sclerosing cholangitis with HLA-B8. Gut *24*:38, 1983.

82. Schrumpf E et al.: HLA antigens and immunoregulatory T cells in ulcerative colitis associated with hepatobiliary disease. Scand J Gastroenterol *17*:187, 1982.

83. Eddleson ALWF, Williams R: HLA and liver disease. Br Med Bull *34*:294, 1978.

84. Bodenheimer HC Jr et al.: Elevated circulating immune complexes in primary sclerosing cholangitis. Hepatology *3*:150, 1983.

85. Brinch L, Teisberg P, Schrumpf E, Akesson I: The in vivo metabolism of C3 in hepatobiliary disease associated with ulcerative colitis. Scand J Gastroenterol *17*:523, 1982.

86. Senaldi G et al.: Activation of the complement system in primary sclerosing cholangitis. Gastroenterology *97*:1430, 1989.

87. Minuk GY et al.: Abnormal clearance of immune complexes from the circulation of patients with primary sclerosing cholangitis. Gastroenterology *88*:166, 1985.

88. Minuk GY et al.: Reticuloendothelial system Fc receptor-mediated clearance of IgG-tagged erythrocytes from the circulation of patients with idiopathic colitis and chronic liver disease. Hepatology *6*:1, 1986.

89. Das KM, Vecchi M, Sakamakis S: A shared and unique epitope(s) on human colon, skin and biliary epithelium detected by monoclonal antibody. Gastroenterology *98*:464, 1990.

90. Alberti-Flor JJ, de Medina M, Jeffers L, Schiff ER: Elevated immunoglobulins and immune complexes in the bile of patients with primary sclerosing cholangitis. Hepatology *3*:844, 1983.

91. McFarlane IG et al.: Leukocyte migration inhibition in response to biliary antigens in primary biliary cirrhosis, sclerosing cholangitis and other chronic liver diseases. Gastroenterology *76*:1333, 1979.

92. Lindor KD et al.: Lymphocyte subsets in primary sclerosing cholangitis. Dig Dis Sci *32*:720, 1987.

93. Whiteside RL, Lasky S, Si L, Van Theil DH: Immunologic analysis of mononuclear cells in liver tissues and blood of patients with primary sclerosing cholangitis. Hepatology *5*:468, 1985.

94. Snook JA et al.: Peripheral blood and portal tract lymphocyte populations in primary sclerosing cholangitis. J Hepatol *9*:36, 1989.

95. van de Oord JJ, Sciot R, Desmet VJ: Expression of MHC products by normal and abnormal bile duct epithelium. J Hepatol *3*:310, 1986.

96. Chapman RW et al.: Expression of HLA-DR antigens on bile duct epithelium in primary sclerosing cholangitis. Gut *29*:422, 1988.

97. Broom U, Galumann H, Hulterantz R, Forsum U: Distribution of HLA-DR, HLA-DP, and HLA-DQ antigens in liver tissue from patients with primary sclerosing cholangitis. Scand J Gastroenterol *25*:54, 1990.

98. Wiman K et al.: Occurrence of Ia antigens on tissues of non-lymphoid origin. Nature *276*:711, 1978.

99. Nutali PG et al: Expression of Ia-like antigens in normal human non-lymphoid tissues. Transplantation *31*:75, 1981.

100. Mayer L et al.: Expression of class II molecules on intestinal epithelial cells in humans. Differences between normal and inflammatory bowel disease. Gastroenterology *100*:3, 1991.

101. Hobson CH et al.: Enterohepatic circulation of bacterial chemotactic peptide in rats with experimental colitis. Gastroenterology *94*:1006, 1988.

102. Vinnik IE et al.: Experimental chronic portal vein bacteremia. Proc Soc Exp Biol Med *15*:311, 1964.

103. Kono K et al.: Experimental portal fibrosis produced by intraportal injection of killed nonpathogenic Escherichia coli in rabbits. Gastroenterology *94*:787, 1988.

104. Lichtman SN et al.: Hepatic inflammation in rats with experimental small intestinal bacterial overgrowth. Gastroenterology *98*: 414, 1990.

105. Lichtman SN et al.: Degradation of endogenous bacterial cell wall polymers by the muralytic enzyme mutanolysin prevents hepatobiliary injury in genetically susceptible rats with experimental intestinal bacterial overgrowth. J Clin Invest *90*:1313, 1992.

106. Bjarnason I et al.: Absorption of 51 chromium-labeled ethylcosediaminetetraacetate in inflammatory bowel disease. Gastroenterology *85*:318, 1983.

107. Krams SM, Dorshkind K, Gershwin ME: Generation of biliary lesions after transfer of human lymphocytes into severe combined immunodeficiency (SCID) mice. J Exp Med *170*:1919, 1989.

108. Farrant JM et al.: Natural history and prognostic variables in primary sclerosing cholangitis. Gastroenterology *100*:1710, 1991.

109. Porayko MK et al.: Patients with asymptomatic primary sclerosing cholangitis frequently have a progressive disease. Gastroenterology *98*:1594, 1990.

110. Chapman RWG, Burroughs AK, Bass NM, Sherlock S: Long-standing asymptomatic primary sclerosing cholangitis. Report of three cases. Dig Dis Sci *26*:778, 1981.

111. Dickson ER et al.: Primary sclerosing cholangitis: Refinement and validiation of survival models. Gastroenterology *103*:1893, 1992.

112. Rosen CB et al.: Cholangiocarcinoma complicating primary sclerosing cholangitis. Ann Surg *213*:21, 1991.

113. Rosen CB, Nagorney DM: Cholangiocarcinoma complicating primary sclerosing cholangitis. Semin Liver Dis *11*:26, 1991.

114. Nichols JC et al.: Diagnostic role of CA 19-9 for cholangiocarcinoma in primary sclerosing cholangitis. Hepatology *16*:62A, 1992.

115. Wiesner RH, LaRusso NF, Dozois RR, Beaver SJ: Peristomal varices after proctocolectomy in patients with primary sclerosing cholangitis. Gastroenterology *90*:316, 1986.

116. Redinger RN, Small DM: Primate biliary physiology VIII. The effect of phenobarbital on bile salt synthesis. J Clin Invest *52*: 161, 1987.

117. Kaplan MM: Medical approaches to primary sclerosing cholangitis. Semin Liver Dis *11*:56, 1991.

118. Hay JE et al.: The metabolic bone disease of primary sclerosing cholangitis. Hepatology *14*:257, 1991.

119. May GR, Bender CE, LaRusso NF, Wiesner RH: Nonoperative dilatation of dominant strictures in primary sclerosing cholangitis. Am J Rad *145*:1061, 1985.

120. Bender CE, Wiesner RH, LeRoy AJ, LaRusso NF: Clinical improvement following percutaneous balloon dilatation of dominant bile duct strictures in primary sclerosing cholangitis. Gastroenterology *102*: A780, 1992.

121. Myers RN, Cooper TH, Padis N: Primary sclerosing cholangitis. Complete gross and histologic reversal after long-term steroid therapy. Am J Gastroenterol *53*:527, 1970.

122. Burgert SC, Brown BP, Kirkpatrick RB, LuBrecque DR: Positive corticosteroid response in early primary sclerosing cholangitis. Gastroenterology *86*:1037, 1984.

123. Lindor KD, LaRusso NF, Wiesner RH: Prednisone and colchicine are not of benefit after two years in patients with primary sclerosing cholangitis. Hepatology *10*:638, 1989.

124. Wiesner RH et al.: A controlled clinical trial evaluating cyclosporine in the treatment of primary sclerosing cholangitis. Hepatology *14*:64, 1991.

125. Kaplan MM, Arora S, Pincus SH: Primary sclerosing cholangitis and low-dose oral pulse methotrexate therapy. Clinical and histologic response. Ann Intern Med *106*: 231, 1987.

126. Beuers U et al.: Ursodeoxycholic acid for treatment of primary sclerosing cholangitis: a placebo-controlled trial. Hepatology *16*: 707, 1992.

127. O'Brien CB et al.: Ursodeoxycholic acid for the treatment of primary sclerosing cholangitis: A 30-month pilot study. Hepatology *16*:838, 1992.

128. Van Thiel DH, Wright HI, Gavaler JS: Ursodeoxycholic acid (UDCA) therapy for primary sclerosing cholangitis (PSC): Preliminary report of a randomized controlled trial. Hepatology *16*:71, 1992.

129. Lo SK et al.: Ursodeoxycholic acid in primary sclerosing cholangitis: A double-blind placebo controlled trial. Hepatology *16*: 190, 1992.

130. LaRusso NF, Wiesner RH: Sclerosing cholangitis: Treatment or transplant? *In* Barkin JS, Rogers AI (eds): Difficult Decisions in Digestive Diseases. Chicago, Year Book Medical Publishers, Inc., 1989.

131. Wiesner RH et al.: Selection and timing of liver transplantation in primary biliary cirrhosis and primary sclerosing cholangitis. Hepatology *16*:1290, 1992.

20

Concepts on the Pathogenesis of Cirrhosis

CHARLES S. LIEBER

Over the last century, cirrhosis of the liver has become a major medical concern. Nationwide, cirrhosis of the liver is a major cause of morbidity (3.6 in 1000) and of mortality (ninth cause) (1). It is the fourth cause of all deaths in urban areas in the active age group from 25 to 64 years (2). Common complications of cirrhosis, such as ascites, bleeding, and the other sequelae of portal hypertension, are frequent causes of morbidity and mortality. A recent prospective survey (3) found that, within 48 months, more than half of individuals with cirrhosis and two thirds of patients with cirrhosis plus alcoholic hepatitis had died. This dismal outcome is more severe than that of many cancers, yet is attracting much less concern, both among the public and the medical profession. This may be partly because of the general perception that not much can be done about this major public health issue. Cirrhosis of the liver is the end stage of various hepatic disorders, most commonly alcoholic in the US and other Western countries. At present, except for control of alcohol abuse and liver transplantation for a minority of subjects, there is no effective modality of either prevention or treatment. The purpose of this historical review is to analyze how concepts about cirrhosis have evolved to the present state of knowledge. This chapter will focus primarily on developments over the last century, with only a brief mention of prior contributions extensively reviewed elsewhere (4,5).

BACKGROUND AND PATHOLOGY

Laennec gave the name cirrhosis to the disease in the beginning of the 19th century and provided its first adequate description. The term is derived from the Greek word "kirrhos," meaning orange-colored. Initially and to the end of the 19th century, the disease was considered to represent a diffused inflammatory hyperplasia of the interstitial connective tissue which gradually compressed the liver parenchyma. However, the importance of cell degeneration was recognized eventually, and the concept of the disease was further clarified with the realization that the two types of lesions could coexist. One of the first modern definitions was provided by Mallory: "to the clinician the term cirrhosis usually means a chronic, progressive, destructive lesion of the liver combined with reparative activity and contraction on the part of the connective tissues" (6). Thus he emphasized what has become a key element of the definition of cirrhosis, namely the coexistence of parenchymal destruction and scarring, with some nodular parenchymal regeneration.

Macroscopically, the early cirrhotic liver of the alcoholic is yellow, with small uniform nodules (from 1 to 5 mm) on the surface. Traditionally, this type of cirrhosis is called micronodular or Laennec cirrhosis. The size of the liver varies, depending on the degree of fibrosis, inflammation and steatosis, from a small, shrunken and hard liver to a large organ weighing up to 4 kg. Microscopically, the scar tissue distorts the normal architecture of the liver by forming bands of connective tissue joining portal and central zones. At first, nodules are regular in size and shape. In more advanced cirrhosis, nodules become irregular and frequently larger, with sizes ranging from 5 to

50 mm, and deep scars appear. This macronodular cirrhosis resembles postnecrotic cirrhosis, such as the type that complicates viral hepatitis.

ETIOLOGY, EPIDEMIOLOGY, AND THEIR CONTRIBUTIONS TO PATHOGENETIC CONCEPTS

It was clear from initial recognition of the disease that many causes may be involved, but in Western countries the majority of cases occur in alcoholics. However, the general opinion at the turn of the 20th century held that alcohol had no specific action on the liver except for fatty changes. Interestingly, whereas other much less common causes, such as gallstones, chronic heart failure, and Graves' disease, were readily recognized as "specific underlying causes," the prevailing view, until recently, was that "alcohol cannot be regarded as a specific factor in the etiology of cirrhosis" (4).

Malnutrition Versus Ethanol Toxicity as Causative Agents of Liver Injury in the Alcoholic

Until several decades ago, the concept prevailed that alcoholic liver injury is a deficiency disease correctible with proper dietary management (7) despite abundant epidemiologic evidence of alcohol abuse, the absence of severe nutritional deficiencies, and the failure of dietary management to prevent or control development of cirrhosis. In 1941, Jolliffe and Jellinek pointed out the close correlation between per capita alcohol consumption and cirrhosis mortality (8), an observation subsequently confirmed by Lelbach (9). During the First and Second World Wars in Europe and during the time of Prohibition in the United States, there was a distinct decrease in mortality from cirrhosis (8). In England and Wales, high alcohol taxes were associated with decreased death rates from cirrhosis, from 12 in 100,000 in 1914 to 2 in 100,000 in 1945 (10). Similarly, the termination of alcohol rationing in Sweden in 1955 was followed by an increase in deaths attributable to cirrhosis (11).

Denial of the etiologic role of alcohol persisted, in part, because efforts to reproduce Laennec's cirrhosis in animals by feeding them alcohol had failed. The hypothesis of nutritional deficiencies as the basis of alcoholic fatty liver and cirrhosis was promoted by Klieneberger (12) and Kennedy (13), who maintained that alcohol itself did not act as a direct hepatotoxin and that its ingestion simply contributed to the malnutrition. The dietary origin of cirrhosis received further support from the observation that pancreatectomized dogs given insulin could survive for a year and a half, after which they succumbed with severe fatty livers. The addition of pancreatic enzymes to the diets did not reverse the fatty liver, but replacement with raw pancreas prevented the appearance of hepatic fat (14). Substances, such as choline, casein, cystine, and methionine, which decreased hepatic fat in the depancreatectomized dog, were termed lipotropic agents (15). Connor (16) showed that fatty livers progressed to cirrhosis in depancreatectomized animals maintained on long-term insulin therapy. The same evolution of cirrhosis occurred in normal dogs fed a high-fat diet. The deficiency of lipotropic agents in animals also produced a fatty cirrhosis resembling the human disease (17,18). This choline deficiency model supported the widely held hypothesis that Laennec's cirrhosis was caused by dietary deficiency conditioned by an excessive indulgence in alcohol. High-protein diets then became popular, primarily because they appeared to accelerate recovery from disease (19). In fact, high-protein diets did not accomplish much to improve the condition, but unintentionally helped shed light on the role of high-protein diets in the pathogenesis of hepatic encephalopathy (see subsequent text). In any event, the pathogenic sequence beginning with fatty liver, rupture of fatty cyst, and then development of cirrhosis (20) prevailed in most textbooks until the 1960s.

Weichselbaum (21) reported that rats placed on a low-protein diet died with striking hemorrhages in the liver, and that the lesions could be prevented by sulfur-containing amino acids such as cystine. György and Goldblatt (22) identified the hemorrhages as areas of necrosis. Daft et al. (23) described the evolution of a coarsely nodular cirrhosis following massive hepatic necrosis in rats placed on the cystine-deficient diet. Vitamin E deficiency also was found to cause acute necrosis in the liver of rats (24). In both models—cystine and vitamin E deficiency—the hepatic lesions were enhanced by an excess of unsaturated fatty acids. A role for unsaturated fat also has been shown more recently with alcohol-induced liver injury (25). Finally, Himsworth and Glynn (26) formalized the two nutritional pathways of cirrhogenesis. The first was diffuse fatty liver developing into a finely nodular cirrhosis in the animal model with lipotrope deficiency, a process they considered analogous to alcoholic or Laennec's cirrhosis in humans. The second was massive hepatic necrosis proceeding to coarsely nodular cirrhosis, as produced experimentally by cystine deficiency with, as a proposed human counterpart, acute yellow atrophy progressing into postnecrotic cirrhosis.

The nutritional theories persisted also because they were supported by Best, the prominent codiscoverer of insulin, who wrote that "there is no more evidence of a specific toxic effect of pure ethyl alcohol upon liver cells than there is for one due to sugar" (27). This notion was based largely on experimental work in rats given ethanol in drinking water (27). Under these conditions, no liver lesions developed unless the diet was deficient, and deficiency alone sufficed to produce the liver lesions. However, with the technique of administering alcohol in drinking water, ethanol consumption usually does not exceed 4 to 9 g/kg or about 10 to 25% of the total caloric intake of the animal because rats have an aversion for alcohol. A comparable amount of alcohol, when given with an adequate diet, resulted in negligible ethanol levels in the blood (28). Thus, administration of alcohol in drinking water to rodents was not a suitable model for the human disease. By incorporating ethanol in a totally liquid diet (28–30), the aversion for alcohol was overcome because, to eat or drink, the animals had no choice but to take the alcohol. With this technique, the quantity of ethanol consumed was increased to 36% of total calories, an amount more relevant to alcohol intake in man. The introduction of the liquid diet model represented a turning point in alcohol research, not only by producing substantial blood alcohol levels, but also by allowing better dietary control and strict pair-feeding techniques. Thus, even with nutritionally adequate diets, isocaloric replacement of sucrose or other carbohydrate by ethanol consistently produced a 5- to 10-fold increase in hepatic triglycerides (28–30). Furthermore, isocaloric replacement of carbohydrate by fat instead of ethanol did not produce steatosis (28). More recently, ethanol also was shown to promote accumulation of triacylglycerol in cultured hepatocytes (31).

Volwiler et al. (19) had failed to detect any deleterious effects from alcohol administration in patients recovering from alcoholic fatty liver. However, the amounts of alcohol given were less than the usual intake of alcoholics. With larger amounts of alcohol, Menghini (32) found that the clearance of fat from the alcoholic fatty liver was prevented. Moreover, individuals with a morphologically normal liver (with or without a history of alcoholism) developed a fatty liver when given ethanol in a variety of nondeficient diets as an isocaloric substitution for carbohydrates (28,29). This was evident by both morphologic examination and direct measurement of the lipid content of the liver biopsies, which revealed up to a 25-fold rise in triglyceride concentration. Even with a high protein, vitamin-supplemented diet, there was a significant increase in hepatic triglycerides, as measured in percutaneous biopsies (33). These studies established the fact that, even in the presence of an adequate diet, ethanol can produce the first stage of alcoholic liver injury, namely the fatty liver.

Toxic Factors Other Than Ethanol

The toxicologic era in the study of cirrhosis developed in the 1920s and 1930s. Lichtman (4) summarized the prevailing view at the time when he stated that "it is generally accepted that experimentally, *alcohol alone* will not produce cirrhosis of the liver," and other toxins were implicated. This concept was stimulated by animal studies with the carbon tetrachloride and chloroform models of liver injury. At that time, extensive attention also focused on the toxic contaminants of alcoholic beverages. Tarlike products formed by aging in charred casks (34), and nicotine, manganese, and furfural in wine were incriminated. Mallory (35) also suggested that minute amounts of phosphorus alloyed with iron (which may be present as contaminating traces in liquors) may be an etiologic factor, but later this was not confirmed. Other contaminants have been investigated with negative results. Higher aliphatic aldehydes were found to inhibit mitochondrial acetaldehyde metabolism (36), thereby enhancing the toxicity of acetaldehyde (see subsequent text). Some evidence was presented that prolonged consumption of whiskey might exert more striking undesirable effects on the liver than pure ethanol (37) and that certain alcoholic beverages, particularly brandy, were more toxic to liver cell cultures than pure ethanol (38).

The role of copper contamination dates to 1780, when Ploucquet (cited in 5) believed that copper, derived from copper utensils used for distilling purposes, was an etiologic factor in the pathogenesis of cirrhosis, a hypothesis widely investigated by Mallory (6) and Gerlach (39). Eventually, however, Flinn and Von Glahn (40) excluded copper as a significant factor in the etiology of cirrhosis, except of course for those with a hereditary defect (41). Iron may lead to fibrosis when associated with a hereditary defect in its clearance, namely hemochromatosis, as recognized by Sheldon (42). Iron also can act as a possible toxic congener. Indeed, wine of certain vintages has been shown to contain large amounts of iron (43,44), which accumulated in liver and other organs of experimental animals given the wine over long periods of time (43). This observation explained, at least in part, iron accumulation in various tissues (including the liver) of wine drinkers with cirrhosis of the liver (43,44). By contrast, in non-wine-drinking alcoholics, hepatic iron excess is unusual (45), although increased iron absorption has been attributed to ethanol itself by some observers (46) but not others (47). A unique situation was recognized in South African blacks, who may develop iron overload as a result of drinking home-brewed beer that contains large amounts of iron (48).

The role of toxic xenobiotic agents in the pathogenesis of alcoholic liver injury, popular in the 19th and the beginning of the 20th century, is now coming to the forefront again, but indirectly, because of the discovery (see subsequent text) of an ethanol-inducible cytochrome P4502E1 (49–53) and the realization that it has an unique capacity to activate a variety of xenobiotic agents to highly toxic metabolites. In addition, the hepatic detoxification processes involve glutathione, which is significantly depressed by alcohol in experimental animals and in man (54). This dual jeopardy explains the enhanced vulnerability of the heavy drinker to chemicals in the environment, such as industrial solvents, anesthetic agents, commonly used medications, over-the-counter drugs (such as acetaminophen), carcinogens, and even some vitamins, such as vitamin A (55). It also explains why improving the glutathione level in the liver by providing one of its precursors, namely the activated form of methionine (S-adenosyl-methionine), has beneficial effects, both experimentally (56) and in ongoing clinical studies (57). Glutathione also may promote the detoxification of acetaldehyde (see subsequent text).

Infectious Agents, Immunologic Factors, Endotoxins and Cytokines

Letulle (58) attached special significance to syphilis in the development of a Laennec type of cirrhosis and, at the beginning of this century, the combination of syphilis and alcohol was considered responsible for most cases of Laennec's cirrhosis. Indeed, LeDuc (59) and others found histologic evidence of syphilis in a large percentage of necropsied cases. However, when syphilis was brought under control, there was a significant drop in the incidence of cirrhosis, and it became clear that syphilis played only a contributory role. Similarly, malaria, once considered to be involved (60), was eliminated as a possible etiologic factor in the development of cirrhosis of the liver by the persistence of cirrhosis after the control of malaria. It was recognized that the ova of bilharzia may cause characteristic "pipe-stem" cirrhosis (61) and that Schistosomum japonicum also can produce cirrhosis.

Immune mechanisms have been invoked in the pathogenesis of alcoholic liver injury. Indeed, alcoholic hyaline, when added to lymphocytes from patients with alcoholic hepatitis, causes a significant increase in the production of migration-inhibition factor

(62). Other immune system alterations (e.g., a cell-mediated mechanism) also are present in alcoholic liver disease (63), but there is continuing uncertainty as to whether they are a consequence or a cause of the liver injury. Increased vulnerability of hepatocytes of alcohol-fed baboons to mononuclear cell attack was demonstrated; mononuclear cells of both controls and alcohol-fed animals were more cytotoxic against hepatocytes of alcohol-fed baboons than against those of controls (64).

Because alcoholics have an increased incidence of viral hepatitis, it has been suggested that alcohol-induced liver damage is potentiated by the viral disease. Alcoholism and viral hepatitis can occur in the same patients but, in many subjects with alcoholic cirrhosis, there is no evidence for antecedent viral hepatitis. Furthermore, most current observations do not substantiate a role for hepatitis B virus in alcoholic liver disease (65) or in the associated hepatocellular carcinoma (66). However, hepatitis C is commonly associated and may play a more important role. Parés et al. (67) found an increased prevalence of hepatitis C virus antibodies in alcoholic patients with severe liver injury and concluded that hepatitis C virus is involved in the liver damage of chronic alcoholic patients. Indeed, in alcoholic patients, portal and/or lobular inflammation is strongly associated with HCV antibody, even in the absence of HCV risk factors (68). Thus, as better serologic methods are being developed, there is increasing evidence for the involvement of some viruses in the pathogenesis of chronic hepatitis in alcoholics.

It has been proposed that tumor necrosis factor, a mediator of endotoxic shock and sepsis, plays a role in alcoholic hepatitis. However, circulating tumor necrosis factor and interleukin-1 concentrations remained elevated for up to 6 months after the diagnosis of alcoholic hepatitis, whereas interleukin-6 normalized in parallel with clinical recovery (69). Sheron et al. (70) also found that the cytokine interleukin-6 is activated in severe alcoholic hepatitis and postulated that this may mediate hepatic or extrahepatic tissue damage. Lymphokines, monokines, and other cytokines liberated by activated cells may amplify pre-existing damage in the hepatocytes and thereby con-

tribute to the progression of alcoholic liver disease (71). Concentrations of these cytokines were correlated with biochemical parameters of liver injury. Similarly, cytokines also could modulate fibrogenesis by affecting myofibroblasts, lipocytes, and transitional cells (see subsequent text). The pathogenetic significance of these findings is not known.

Constitutional and Endocrine Factors: Effect of Gender

In earlier years, "constitutional factors" were implicated in diseases with obscure etiology, including cirrhosis. According to Chvostek (72), alcoholic cirrhosis developed only in individuals of a certain constitution, namely males with a scant beard and "feminine" genital hair. It also was recognized that cirrhosis is commonly associated with endocrine disturbances. Barrelet (73), in an anatomic and histologic study, found endocrine gland abnormalities in many instances, including atrophic lesions of the seminiferous tubules of the testes. The thyroid also was atrophic. Thus endocrine changes associated with cirrhosis of the liver have been regarded as consequences of altered hepatic function rather than as etiologic factors (74,75).

Gender also was recognized as an important factor. Cirrhosis of the liver predominates in men over women, 3 to 1. Frerichs (76) found that 20 of 36 cases of cirrhosis were in men. More recently, the male-to-female ratio of mortality was found to be more than 2:1 for all cases of cirrhosis, and it is even greater when restricted to alcoholic cirrhosis (8,11). This male preponderance probably reflects drinking habits. Indeed, until recently, most studies concerning the adverse effects of alcohol focused mainly on men because, on the average, men drink much more than women. However, drinking levels of women have been increasing and soon may approach those of men (77). This trend is particularly significant because it apparently affects selectively young women (78). In fact, some of the evidence accumulated in recent years indicates a greater susceptibility of women to the development of somatic complications of alcoholism, such as liver disease. Lichtman (4) earlier had recognized that "alcohol appeared to be more prone to produce cirrhosis in females," but again he invoked nutritional factors." However, important biologic differences are also involved (79). Women have higher blood ethanol concentrations than men after an equivalent oral dose. This difference has been attributed to a smaller volume of distribution of ethanol because of a lower body water content in women than in men (80). But, according to Frezza et al. (81), the apparent volume of distribution, calculated from intravenous curves, was only 12% larger in normal men than in normal women. Other factors contribute to the higher blood alcohol levels in women, such as lesser gastric alcohol dehydrogenase activity and first-pass metabolism. Indeed, although it is generally recognized that the liver is the main site of ethanol metabolism (82), extrahepatic metabolism occurs: ethanol oxidation in the digestive tract of the rat has been reported (83) and has been related to the alcohol dehydrogenase (ADH) present in this tissue (84). In the rat, the ability of the stomach to oxidize ethanol has been demonstrated (83). However, the magnitude of gastrointestinal ethanol metabolism was assumed to be small (83). The issue was reopened when it was shown that a significant fraction of alcohol ingested in doses in keeping with usual "social drinking" does not enter the systemic circulation in the rat and is oxidized mainly in the stomach (85). This process also was shown to occur in humans, with small (0.15 g/kg), as well as moderate (0.3 g/kg) doses of alcohol (85,86). Moreover, gastrectomy was associated with an abolition of the first-pass metabolism (87). The magnitude of this first-pass metabolism was assessed to amount to about 20% of the ethanol administered when given at a low dose to rats (88) or to humans (89). Thus, it was recognized that the stomach represents some kind of "protective" barrier against the penetration of alcohol into the body by retaining and breaking down part of the alcohol consumed orally; women are less endowed than men in that respect. Gastric alcohol dehydrogenase activities correlated significantly with the magnitude of the first-pass metabolism, and both were found to be lower in women than in men (81). Alcoholism further decreased the ADH activity and first-pass metabolism, with a corresponding rise in blood levels of alcohol. Thus, the effects were most striking in alcoholic women: their blood levels of alcohol were virtually the same, whether the alcohol was given orally or intravenously.

According to some investigators (90) but not to others (91), women have a more rapid elimination of alcohol as compared to men. One explanation of this finding is the fact that the hepatic ADH activity is suppressed by testosterone and its derivatives, both in vivo (91) and in vitro (92), at least at high concentrations. Most importantly, it was observed that the progression to more severe liver injury is accelerated in women (93). In 1932, Meyenburg and Robert (94), in a study of 127 adult cirrhotics, found 72% men and 28% women (2.5 to 1), but the average age for men was 50, and for women 45 years. Wilkinson et al. (95) also found women to be more susceptible than men to the development of alcoholic cirrhosis. Other studies reported the incidence of chronic advanced liver disease to be higher among women than among men for a similar history of alcohol abuse (96). Pequignot et al. (97) observed that a daily intake of alcohol of 40 to 60 g in men but only 20 g in women resulted in a statistically significant increase in the incidence of cirrhosis in a well-nourished population.

The mechanism whereby the female gender potentiates alcohol-induced liver damage is not known. It could obviously relate to the hormonal status since both endogenous and exogenous (i.e. contraceptive) female hormones have been shown to result in some impairment of liver function in a significant number of women (98–101). It is conceivable that an interaction between some of these hormone-related changes and those induced by ethanol may result in more severe liver damage. Other gender-dependent biochemical differences may contribute to the vulnerability to the hepatotoxicity of ethanol. For instance, fatty acid-binding protein (L-FABP) is a major contributor to the ethanol-induced increase in liver cytosolic proteins in the rat (102). This increase in liver FABP may play a role in protecting the liver against the ethanol-induced excess accumulation of free fatty acid by binding them and thereby making them less reactive. It is noteworthy that there is a much smaller increase of cytosolic FABP in females (58%) than in males (161%) (103). Finally, the relative lack of "gastric protective mechanism" in women (see previous text) also may be contributory.

MECHANISMS OF THE HEPATOTOXICITY OF ETHANOL

Perivenular Exacerbation of Injury

A characteristic feature of liver injury in the alcoholic is the predominance of steatosis and other lesions in the perivenular (previously called centrilobular) zone or zone 3 of the hepatic acinus. Several mechanisms for this zonal selectivity have been elucidated over the last three decades.

Role of Hepatic Hypoxia

This hypothesis postulates involvement of a lack of oxygen supply, and propylthiouracil treatment has been proposed to attenuate this deficit. This concept originated from the observation that liver slices from rats fed alcohol chronically consume more oxygen than controls' liver slices (104). It was then postulated that the enhanced consumption of oxygen would increase the gradient of oxygen tensions along the sinusoids to the extent of producing anoxic injury of perivenular hepatocytes. Indeed, in both human alcoholics (105) and animals fed alcohol chronically (105,106), decreases in either hepatic venous oxygen saturation (105) or PO_2 (106) and in tissue oxygen tensions (107) have been found during the withdrawal state. However, these changes disappeared (106,108) or decreased (107) when alcohol was present in the blood. Acute ethanol administration increased splanchnic oxygen consumption in baboons not previously exposed to alcohol, but the consequences of this effect on oxygenation in the perivenular zone were offset by increased blood flow resulting in unchanged hepatic venous oxygen tension (109). Ethanol, in fact, induces an increase in portal hepatic blood flow (106,108–110). In baboons fed alcohol chronically, defective O_2 utilization rather than lack of blood O_2 supply characterized liver injury produced by high concentration of ethanol (109).

Excessive Hepatic NADH Generation

An alternate theory for the perivenular preponderance of liver damage was that the NADH generated from NAD upon oxidation of ethanol to acetaldehyde (by means of alcohol dehydrogenase) and the associated redox shift is exaggerated by the low oxygen tensions normally prevailing in the perivenular zone. This was verified by hepatic vein catheterization and liver biopsies in baboons, in isolated rat hepatocytes, and in the isolated perfused rat liver (106,111). The ethanol-induced redox shift had been the first mechanism invoked to explain, in biochemical terms, the direct hepatic effects of ethanol on lipid metabolism of liver slices (112,113). A number of other metabolic disturbances also were explained on that basis (114), including hypoglycemia (115), hyperlactacidemia, and hyperuricemia (116). Hypoxia increases NADH even further which, in turn, inhibits the activity of NAD^+-dependent xanthine dehydrogenase, thereby favoring that of oxygen-dependent xanthine oxidase (117). Because of the acetate derived from the acetaldehyde, purine metabolites accumulate and are metabolized by means of xanthine oxidase, leading to the production of oxygen radicals which may mediate toxic effects towards liver cells, including lipid peroxidation.

Zonal Distribution of Some Enzymes

Marked heterogeneity was discovered, which also can influence the selective perivenular toxicity. Proliferation of the smooth endoplasmic reticulum after chronic ethanol consumption is maximal in the perivenular zone (118,119), with associated enzyme induction. This proliferation of hepatic microsomal membranes was reminiscent of that produced by other drugs metabolized by liver microsomes and prompted the suggestion that these microsomes are the site for a distinct and adaptive system of ethanol oxidation, named the microsomal ethanol oxidizing system (MEOS) (49,50). The proposal of such an accessory but adaptive pathway of ethanol metabolism (49) was not accepted for more than a decade, but has now gained general acceptance, especially since the demonstration that chronic ethanol consumption results in the induction of a unique cytochrome P-450 (51) purified from rabbit liver microsomes (52), which catalyzed ethanol oxidation at rates much higher than other P-450 isozymes. The purified human protein (now called 2E1) was obtained in a catalytically active form, with a high turnover rate for ethanol and other specific substrates (53). Using antibodies against this 2E1 and the Western blot technique, a 5- to 10-fold induction was found in biopsies of alcoholics (120). Immunohistochemical techniques showed that 2E1 is normally localized within the perivenular region, or zone 3, of the liver lobule, and that induction of 2E1 by prolonged alcohol consumption occurs primarily within the same acinar region. Human ADH was also demonstrated mainly in hepatocytes around the terminal hepatic venule (121). Thus, a presumably higher level of ethanol metabolism in the perivenular zone could contribute to the increased hepatoxicity of ethanol by providing excess free radicals generated by the "induced" microsomal pathway (see previous text), excess NADH by the ADH pathway (see previous text), and an increased amount of the toxic metabolite acetaldehyde (see subsequent text), produced by both pathways.

Mitochondrial Injury and Role of Acetaldehyde

Three decades ago, characteristic ultrastructural changes of early alcoholic liver injury were described, including enlarged and distorted mitochondria, with shortened cristae containing crystalline inclusions. Controlled studies in animals and humans (33,118,119) have shown that these changes are caused by alcohol itself, rather than other factors such as a poor diet. These structural abnormalities are associated with functional impairments, especially decreased oxidation of fatty acids and of a variety of other substrates, including acetaldehyde itself (120). The respiratory capacity of mitochondria was found to be depressed (122). In human volunteers given ethanol, mitochondrial lesions developed even on a high-protein diet (33). Oxidative phosphorylation was found to be altered (123). It is noteworthy that high concentrations of acetaldehyde, the product of ethanol metabolism, mimic the defects produced by chronic ethanol consumption on oxidative phosphorylation (124) and therefore one may wonder to what extent chronic exposure to acetaldehyde is the cause of the defect observed after chronic ethanol consumption.

Acetaldehyde-protein adduct formation is another more recently recognized mechanism of toxicity. Nomura and Lieber (125) reported covalent binding of acetaldehyde to liver proteins. Subsequently, it was shown that acetaldehyde binds covalently to 2E1 (126), other hepatic macromolecules (127), circulating proteins ((serum albumin (128) and hemoglobin (129)), and cytoskeletal proteins such as tubulin. Microtubular alterations lead to swelling of hepatocytes (ballooning) and associated liver injury (130–132). Acetaldehyde adducts may serve as neoantigens, generating an immune response in mice (133) and in humans (134). Niemela et al. (135) found antibodies against acetaldehyde adducts in patients with alcoholic hepatitis, whereas Hoerner et al. detected them in most alcoholics (134,136), including some with simple fatty liver, early fibrosis, or both (136), and in nonalcoholics with liver disease (136). This immune reaction may contribute to the aggravation or perpetuation of liver injury. Acetaldehyde also exerts adverse effects in many other ways, for instance inactivation of nutrients such as pyridoxine (137), or activation of collagen-producing mesenchymal cells in the liver (see subsequent text).

Direct Role of Ethanol in Phospholipid Alterations and in the Production of Cirrhosis

After the demonstration, in both humans and rats, that a fatty liver can be produced by ethanol in the presence of adequate or even enriched diets (see previous text), the experimental debate shifted from the fatty liver to a discussion on the respective etiologic role of alcohol and other factors in the development of fibrosis and the eventual cirrhosis. As for the fatty liver, there was a great reluctance to accept a direct role for alcohol. Other factors were invoked, although epidemiologic evidence indicated otherwise (see previous text). It was again the liquid diet technique that allowed this issue to be settled. Liquid diets were administered by continuous infusion in rodents

(138). This mode of administration allowed control of the rate of diet intake in the various groups of animals and possibly enhanced the overall dose of ethanol metabolized. Using this technique, lesions more severe than simple fatty liver were produced in the rat, including some necrosis and fibrosis (138), but no cirrhosis. In the baboon, however, cirrhosis was successfully produced after consumption of alcohol even in the absence of dietary deficiencies (see subsequent text).

Baboon Model of Alcoholic Cirrhosis

In the aggregate of several studies (139–143), production of cirrhosis was observed in 13 of a total of 63 baboons fed ethanol for 5 years or more, with septal fibrosis developing in an additional 13 animals. No lesions developed in the corresponding pair-fed controls. Ainley et al. (144) challenged the ability of ethanol to produce cirrhosis in the baboon, but it is not known how much alcohol (or diet) was actually consumed by their animals. In addition, only two of these baboons were given ethanol (with the regular diet) for a period exceeding 18 months, whereas the results of other studies (140,143) showed that a longer period of treatment is required to consistently produce septal fibrosis or cirrhosis. Ainley et al. (144), however, confirmed the capacity of alcohol to produce increased circulating transaminase levels, swelling and hydropic degeneration of the hepatocytes with megamitochondria, steatosis, minor inflammatory changes, and pericellular fibrosis. Similar amounts of the same diet (with isocaloric substitution of carbohydrates for ethanol) did not produce any pathology.

Role of Lipotropes

The availability of experimental models of alcoholic fibrosis and cirrhosis allowed reassessment of the lipotrope theories (see previous text). Supplementation with choline failed to prevent the alcohol effect on fibrosis, although very large and even toxic amounts of choline were used (142). By contrast, polyunsaturated lecithin (PUL) was found to be protective in a 10-year study conducted in baboons (143). The mechanism of the protective effect of PUL against fibrosis is not clear at present. A similar question had been raised with regard to the fatty liver of pancreatectomized dogs. The addition of pancreatic enzymes to the diets did not reverse the fatty liver, but replacement with raw pancreas did prevent the appearance of hepatic fat (14). Hershey and Soskin (145) concluded that the preventive precursor in raw pancreas was lecithin. Lecithin has a high choline content, to which some protective effect was ascribed, but such protection was not shown in primates, either baboons (142) or humans. Indeed, clinically, choline treatment of patients suffering from alcoholic liver injury has been found ineffective in the face of continued alcohol abuse (19,146,147). Furthermore, massive supplementation with choline failed to prevent the fatty liver produced by alcohol in volunteer subjects (148). The only situation in humans in which choline may be lacking is among malnourished patients with cirrhosis on severely deficient diets (149).

It is conceivable, of course, that PUL might represent a modality of choline supplementation with less toxicity and/or greater bioavailability than that of native choline. Indeed, it has been shown that in terms of central nervous effects, when choline is provided as lecithin, its biologic activity is significantly increased (150), possibly because of bacterial degradation of free choline in the gut. Whether this also pertains to the alcohol-induced liver injury is uncertain and, in fact, unlikely. Indeed, if this mechanism were operative, it would imply that, in animals fed alcohol, a functional state of choline deficiency exists despite an ample (and even excessive) dietary supply. However, the liver lesions produced by alcohol differ significantly from those resulting from choline deficiency, both chemically (142) and ultrastructurally (118). An alternate hypothesis is that PUL exerts its beneficial effects not simply as a source of choline but by providing some other component. PUL is rich in linoleic acid, but this fatty acid *per se* probably is not responsible for the protective effect because the basic diet was supplemented with linoleate and contained large amounts of corn oil (139) that is rich in linoleic acid. Furthermore, this fatty acid has been incriminated as a permissive rather than as a protective factor in alcoholic liver injury (25). It is possible that the phospholipids themselves might be responsible for some of the protective effects. Indeed, phospholipids rich in essential fatty acids have a high bioavailability. More than 50% of orally administered polyunsaturated phosphatidylcholine is made biologically available for the organism by either intact absorption (lesser extent) or reacylation of absorbed lysophosphatidylcholine (greater extent) (151). Pharmacokinetic studies in humans using $^3H/^{14}C$-labeled phosphatidylcholine showed the absorption to exceed 90% (152). Phosphatidylcholine in the diet is degraded by pancreatic phospholipase A_2, and the products (l-lysophosphatidyl-choline and fatty acids) are absorbed in the jejunum. Polyene phosphatidylcholine is taken up in toto by the liver cells and incorporated into the membrane-containing fractions (153). Thus phosphatidylcholine may directly influence membrane structures and provide a basis for some of the beneficial effects of phospholipids in the treatment of liver disease (154). Indeed, membrane alterations have been described in a variety of liver diseases, and they are particularly prominent in alcoholic liver disease, as shown by scanning electron microscopy of isolated hepatocytes (155).

That ethanol administration alters cellular phospholipids has been shown in various species. In rat hepatic mitochondria, decreases in total phospholipid (156) and in the polyene phospholipid fatty acids have been described (157). In ethanol-fed baboons, the total phospholipid content of the mitochondrial membranes were diminished with a significant decrease in the levels of phosphatidylcholine (158). These alterations in the phospholipid composition of the mitochondrial membranes appeared responsible for some of the depression of cytochrome oxidase activity produced by chronic ethanol consumption (158). This, in turn, may be the cause, at least partly, of the biochemical alterations of baboon hepatic mitochondria after chronic ethanol consumption (159). The ethanol-induced decreases of hepatic phospholipids and phosphatidylcholine (PC) were corrected by PC feeding (160), but the mechanism whereby chronic ethanol consumption alters phospholipids has not been clarified; it may be related to decreased phosphatidylethanolamine-*N*-methyltransferase activity described in cir-

rhotic liver (161). That this abnormality, in fact, is a primary defect related to alcohol is suggested by the observation that the enzyme's activity already is decreased in baboons fed ethanol before the development of cirrhosis (162).

Apart from their structural functions in cell membranes, the polyunsaturated fatty acids of the phospholipids serve as precursors to the prostaglandins and related substances. The prostaglandins can be described generally as a defensive regulatory system, but their postulated role in alcohol-induced liver damage remains largely undefined. It is known, however, that chronic administration of ethanol is associated with abnormalities in essential fatty acid levels in various lipid fractions (163–165). Phospholipids also appear to have a direct effect on fibrous tissue (see subsequent text).

Fibrogenic Cells in the Liver and their Modification by Ethanol, Acetaldehyde and Phospholipids

Fibrous tissue is characterized by excess collagen deposition. In the pathogenesis of liver collagen accumulation, Chojkier (166) incriminated the hepatocyte, whereas a number of other studies suggested a major role for mesenchymal cells. Indeed, the number of the mesenchymal cells increases around the terminal hepatic venules after chronic alcohol consumption. The type of cells involved have been clarified both in patients with alcoholic liver disease and in baboons fed alcohol (167,168). The most common cell around the terminal hepatic venules with fibrosis (in the connective tissue or immediately under the endothelial cells) is the myofibroblast. Gabbiani et al. (169) reported myofibroblasts in granulation tissue. Myofibroblasts also have been described in patients with cirrhosis (170). Nakano et al. (168) first reported myofibroblasts in noncirrhotic human livers. The latter studies also showed that the increase in the number of these cells appears to be one of the earliest detectable events associated with the alcohol-induced fibrotic process. A possible mechanism whereby alcohol consumption may be linked to collagen formation is the increase in tissue lactate and acetaldehyde secondary to alcohol metabolism. Indeed, lactate-stimulated collagen synthesis in myofibroblast cultures and acetaldehyde had a similar effect (171). Processes of myofibroblasts also extend into the Disse space around the sinusoids. However, the most common mesenchymal cell normally encountered there is the lipocyte (fat-storing or Ito cell). Several investigators have examined peri-sinusoidal cells in relation to hepatic fibrogenesis (172,173). After inflammatory stimulation or during the repair process, these cells proliferate in conjunction with collagen deposition; therefore, these cells are considered to play a role in fibrogenesis. After chronic alcohol consumption, most of the lipocytes are replaced by cells transitional between lipocytes and fibroblasts (174). These transitional cells are surrounded by abundant collagen fibers, and they can be seen in the perisinusoidal spaces throughout the lobule associated with a net-like fibrosis, sometimes linking up with the perivenular lesion. A significant correlation was found between the degree of hepatic fibrosis and the percentage of transitional cells (174). Lipocytes, myofibroblasts, and fibroblasts share similarities and may belong to the same cell family. Transformation of Ito cells into myofibroblasts in fact has been suggested.

One of the most potent links between hepatocytes and mesenchymal cells in the pathogenesis of fibrosis is acetaldehyde, the active toxic metabolite produced in abundance from ethanol in the hepatocyte, where it exerts a number of toxic effects (55) (see previous text). It also diffuses out of the hepatocyte and easily reaches the neighboring myofibroblasts and lipocytes, where recent observations revealed striking effects. Acetaldehyde stimulates collagen production in vitro (175) and increases procollagen type I gene transcription in cultured lipocytes (176). PUL selectively prevents the acetaldehyde-induced increase in collagen accumulation in lipocyte cultures, whereas other phospholipids or linoleate (the fatty acids of PUL) have no such effect. PUL did not modify collagen synthesis, but it increased collagenase activity, suggesting that the protective effect exerted by PUL against alcohol-induced fibrosis in vivo (143) is caused at least partly by stimulation of collagen breakdown. The PUL used consisted of several species, mainly dilinoleoyl-phosphatidyl-choline (40–52%), and palmit-

oyl-linoeoyl-phosphatidylcholine (23–24%). Only dilinoleoylphosphatidyl-choline duplicated the effect of the phosphatidylcholine on collagenase and thus dilinoleoyl-phosphatidylcholine may be the active compound and may oppose collagen accumulation partly by promoting its breakdown (160).

Role of Alcoholic Hepatitis

The role of alcoholic hepatitis in the pathogenesis of alcoholic liver fibrosis has been a subject of contention. Traditionally, alcoholic hepatitis is considered the link between fatty liver and cirrhosis and the precursor of the latter, and may contribute to the evolution of cirrhosis. However, it now is recognized that alcoholic hepatitis cannot be regarded as a sine qua non of such progression. Cirrhosis commonly develops in some alcoholics (168,177) without an apparent intermediate stage of florid alcoholic hepatitis and, in experimental animals, alcohol can promote the development of cirrhosis without being preceded by alcoholic hepatitis. Indeed, baboons fed alcohol developed fatty liver, with ballooning of some hepatocytes. The ballooning was associated with some mononuclear inflammation (141) but with very few of the polymorphonuclear cells that are characteristic of human alcoholic hepatitis. By electron microscopy, no alcoholic hyaline was seen. Thus, although the appearance was not that of florid alcoholic hepatitis, septal fibrosis, and/or, typical cirrhosis developed in one third of the animals. Similarly, in some of the patients followed by Nakano et al. (168), cirrhosis developed without an apparent stage of alcoholic hepatitis. Thus, alcoholic hepatitis, as defined by polymorphonuclear inflammation, may not be a necessary intermediate step in the development of alcoholic cirrhosis, but when present, it appears to be a potent stimulus for fibrosis, partly through stimulation of cytokines (see previous text).

HEPATIC ENCEPHALOPATHY

Role of Proteins and Ammonia in the Pathogenesis of the Encephalopathy

Hippocrates (fifth century B.C.) first noted that "those who are mad from bile are vociferous, malignant and will not be quiet" (cited in 5). It may well have been the striking mental changes associated with severe jaundice that influenced Hippocrates to place the site of the soul in the liver. Meat intolerance of the cirrhotic also was noted early, as reflected by Shakespeare in Sir Andrew Aguecheek's (Twelfth Night, 1603) speech about himself: "Methinks sometimes I have no more wit than a Christian or an ordinary man has; but I am a great eater of beef, and I believe that does harm to my wit" (Act I, Sc. iii) (178). In his textbook on liver disease, Frerichs (76) discusses the association of liver disease and nervous system symptoms. The first hint that ammonia, a breakdown product of the amino acids derived from proteins, may be involved in the pathogenesis of hepatic coma was provided by Frerichs' finding that injections of ammonium carbonate caused twitching and convulsions in dogs. The experimental era of the exploration of the liver-brain interactions can be attributed to Hahn, Pavlov, and their associates (179), who produced hepatic coma and other disorders of nervous function in animals with Eck's portacaval fistula when fed large amounts of meat. The liver's role in converting ammonia to urea was appreciated at that time (180) and the importance of protein tolerance ("meat intoxication") arose as a result of several studies, including those of Bollman and Mann (181). Van Caulaert and Deviller (182) even recommended ammonium salts as a test to induce coma in patients with severe liver disease.

Significant progress in the elucidation of the pathogenesis and treatment of hepatic encephalopathy was made when a convenient test for determining blood ammonia became available (183) and was applied clinically (184). Much insight was gained from the observation of complications associated with the surgical performance of portacaval shunts in cirrhotic patients to control variceal hemorrhage (185). Another impetus came from the numerous clinical observations made in patients with liver disease given high protein diets. These diets had become very popular in the 1950s and 1960s as a consequence of the dogma that attributed alcoholic liver disease exclusively to malnutrition. Signs of meat intoxication, previously described in animals, were now com-monly found in these subjects (186). The theory of the toxicity of ammonia derived from bacterial fermentation, particularly the breakdown of proteins, became popular, and its toxicity was explained by a hypothesis formulated by the Bessmans (187), wherein ammonia combines with alpha-ketoglutarte to form glutamic acid and thus removes a link in the brain's Krebs cycle.

A major benefit derived from the theory of ammonia toxicity was the use of low-protein diets (184,188), cleansing of the bowel with antibiotic therapy (189), and administration of lactulose (190). Another form of treatment that was used empirically in patients with severe hepatic coma was steroid administration. The effectiveness of this treatment was finally established in a subgroup of patients with severe alcoholic hepatitis complicated by hepatic encephalopathy (191). One experimental basis for the successful use of steroids had been established three decades before, when it was shown that prednisolone reduced the increased ammonia levels of Eck fistula dogs (192).

The ammonia theory also prompted the search for possible sources of ammonia: the colon was identified as a major site (193,194) and the stomach was also appreciated as an important source. Early in this century, gastric urease emerged as a possibly important enzyme (195), of bacterial or endogenous origin. This question was settled by the observation that gastric urease was not present in germ-free animals (196) and also that, in humans, treatment with a variety of antibiotics suppressed gastric urease activity (197–199). The latter studies clearly showed adverse effects of the ammonia produced by bacterial urease in the stomach, such as decreased gastric acid. These results and their implications were presented at the 1958 World Congress of Gastroenterology in Washington (200), but the role of the spirochetes known to colonize the stomach was virtually ignored until the isolation of the spirochetes from the gastric mucosa (201,202) and their identification as Helicobacter pylori and the recognition of their possible role in the pathogenesis of gastritis and ulcer disease (203–207).

Another area in which the ammonia theory proved to be a productive stimulus was that of inborn errors in the conversion of ammonia to urea. These include carbamyl phosphate synthetase deficiency (208), ornithine carbamyl transferase deficiency (209), argininosuccinate synthetase deficiency (210), and arginase deficiency (211). Reye syndrome (212), with the same endpoint of hepatic encephalopathy, also may belong to this group, especially the variety associated with a defect in the urea cycle (213). The ammonia theory also branched into other areas of hepatology including the hepatorenal syndrome (see subsequent text).

Hepatorenal Syndrome

Austin Flint, Jr. (214) first identified patients with cirrhosis who might succumb to renal failure, but in many patients, the kidneys appeared normal. Charcot (215) also reported the occurrence of uremia in hepatic disorders. The term "hepatorenal syndrome" was introduced by Helwig and Schutz (216). The mechanism by which hepatic disorders may affect renal function has been a subject of continuing controversy (217). In view of the normal anatomic condition of the kidneys and their normal functioning when transplanted to recipients without liver disease, the now prevailing concept is that of a functional abnormality involving blood flow disturbances. Theories in the 1950s centered on plasma-volume depletion (218) or poor cardiac output (219), both of which lead to reduced renal blood flow, or increased sympathetic tone (220), altered renin-angiotensin activity (221), false neurotransmitters (222), endotoxins (223), bradykinin deficiency (224) and, more recently, increased cysteinyl-leukotriene production (225). Excess ammonia derived from urea also may contribute to the clinical disorder of encephalopathy (226), especially in view of the tremendous ammonia generated from endogenous urea in patients with uremia (198). The striking inhibition of this ammonia production by antibiotics, with its therapeutic implications for the encephalopathy, was discussed before.

SUMMARY

During this century, understanding of the pathogenesis of cirrhosis has undergone a progressive evolution. The views that pre-

vailed during the first half of the century were formulated by Jolliffe and Jellinek (8), who stated that "while the association between inebriety and cirrhosis of the liver is definitely established and a *direct* causation through alcohol is ruled out none of the numerous etiological theories of indirect causation can be accepted at present as sufficiently documented." Other toxins, including metals, incriminated at first, were mostly eliminated, except for some hereditary conditions (Wilson's disease, hemochromatosis). Thus, although the investigators could not agree on a specific etiologic agent, they all agreed that "alcohol cannot be regarded as a *specific* cause of cirrhosis" (4). As recently as 1958, Klatskin (227) wrote in the leading medical textbook of the times that "It is generally agreed that alcohol is not a hepatotoxin and that its effects on the liver probably are secondary to an associated nutritional disturbance." Thus, alcohol, because of its high energy content, at first was perceived to act exclusively as "empty calories" displacing other nutrients in the diet and causing primary malnutrition through decreased intake of essential nutrients. More recently, secondary malnutrition was emphasized as a result of a better understanding of maldigestion and malabsorption caused by chronic alcohol consumption and various diseases associated with chronic alcoholism. Dietary therapy alone, however, was not successful in the prevention or treatment of alcoholic liver injury, but it had an unintended result: precipitation and encephalopathy in patients with severe liver disease was recognized as an undesirable side effect of high-protein diets and led to the clarification of the role of protein intolerance and ammonia intoxication in hepatic encephalopathy. Eventually, the dogmatic view that alcoholic liver injury is caused exclusively by dietary deficiencies was rejected by the production of fatty liver with ultrastructural damage in rodents and humans and of liver cirrhosis in subhuman primates with pure ethyl alcohol. Accordingly, the concept of the direct toxicity of alcohol advanced as the primary explanation for injury to the liver. As a consequence, control of alcohol consumption became the basis for the treatment and prevention of cirrhosis. The toxic theory of alcoholic liver disease led to the elucidation of many of the toxic and metabolic effects of alcohol on the basis of the metabolism of ethanol in the liver, first by the alcohol dehydrogenase pathway and later by the microsomal ethanol oxidizing system (MEOS). The discovery of the MEOS explained the increased vulnerability of the alcoholic to the toxicity of many xenobiotic agents. The inducibility of this system also established a basis for enhanced production of acetaldehyde and the associated array of toxic manifestations, including interference with nutrient utilization. Thus, better understanding of the biochemical alterations produced by ethanol in the body also provided insight into processes whereby ethanol alters both the activation and the degradation of key nutrients. In turn, availability of key nutrients and nutritional factors such as S-adenosyl-L-methionine were shown to strikingly affect the detoxification of noxious agents. These nutritional factors, as well as polyunsaturated lecithin, can be viewed as "supernutrients" found to significantly offset some of the toxic manifestations of alcohol. Thus, the original opposition between nutritional and toxic effects of ethanol now has been overcome and, at cellular, biochemical, and molecular levels, nutritional and toxic effects of ethanol now have converged, resulting in better insights into the pathology produced by ethanol and generating prospects for improved therapy. With the recent discovery of hepatitis C, the role of viruses also is emerging, acting either by exacerbating the effects of alcohol or as injurious agents per se.

REFERENCES

1. Dufour MC, Stinson FS, Cases MF: Trends in cirrhosis morbidity and mortality: United States, 1979–1988. Semin Liver Dis *13*:109, 1993.
2. Vital Statistics: New York City: Summary of vital statistics. New York: Department of Health, Bureau of Health Statistics and Analysis, 1986.
3. Chedid A et al.: Prognostic factors in alcoholic liver disease. Am J Gastroenterol *82*: 210, 1991.
4. Lichtman SS: Diseases of Liver, Gallbladder and Bile Duct. Philadelphia, Lea & Febiger, 1942.
5. Chen TS, Chen PS (eds.): Understanding the Liver. A History. Westport, CT; London, Engl, Greenwood Press, 1984.
6. Mallory, FB: Cirrhosis of the liver. Five different types of lesions from which it may arise. Bull Johns Hopkins Hosp *22*:69, 1911.
7. Snell AM: Changing conceptions of portal cirrhosis. J Med *22*:163, 1941.
8. Jolliffe N, Jellinek EM: Vitamin deficiencies and liver cirrhosis in alcoholism. Part VII: Cirrhosis of the liver. Quart J Stud Alcohol *2*:544, 1941.
9. Lelbach WK: Epidemiology of alcoholic liver disease. *In* Popper H, Schaffner E (eds): Progress in Liver Disease. New York, Grune & Stratton, 1976.
10. Stone WD, Islam NRK, Paton A: The natural history of cirrhosis. Quart J Med *37*:119, 1968.
11. Hällen J, Krook H: Follow-up studies on an unselected ten-year material of 360 patients with liver cirrhosis in one community. Acta Med Scand *173*:479, 1963.
12. Klieneberger C: Abdominaltyphus und Lebercirrhose. Zentralb Inn Med *44*:129, 1923.
13. Kennedy JA: Psychosis with alcoholic pellagra. Med Bull Vet Admin (Washington, D.C.) *10*:155, 1933.
14. Allan FN et al.: Behavior of depancreatized dogs kept alive with insulin. Br J Exp Pathol *5*:75, 1924.
15. du Vigneaud V et al.: The transfer of methyl group from methionine to choline and creatine. J Biol Chem *134*:787, 1940.
16. Connor CL: Fatty infiltration of the liver and the development of cirrhosis in diabetes and chronic alcoholism. Am J Pathol *14*: 347, 1938.
17. Rich AR, Hamilton JD: The experimental production of cirrhosis of the liver by means of a deficient diet. Bull Johns Hopkins Hosp *66*:185, 1940.
18. Daft FS et al.: Production and apparent prevention of a dietary liver cirrhosis in rats. Proc Soc Exp Biol Med *48*:228, 1941.
19. Volwiler W, Jones CM, Mallory TB: Criteria for the measurement of result of treatment in fatty cirrhosis. Gastroenterology *11*:164, 1948.
20. Hartroft WS: Diagnostic significance of fatty cysts in cirrhosis. AMA Arch Pathol *55*:63, 1953.
21. Weichselbaum TE: Cystine deficiency in albino rat. Quart J Exp Physiol *25*:363, 1935.
22. György P, Goldblatt H: Hepatic injury on a nutritional basis in rats. J Exp Med *70*: 185, 1939.
23. Daft FS et al.: Prevention by cystine or

methionine of hemorrhage and necrosis of liver in rats. Proc Soc Exp Biol Med *50*:1, 1942.

24. Schwarz K: Tocopherol als Leberschutzstoff. Z Physiol Chem *281*:109, 1944.

25. Nanji AA, French SW: Dietary linoleic acid is required for development of experimentally induced alcoholic liver injury. Life Sci *44*:223, 1989.

26. Himsworth HP, Glynn, LE: Massive hepatic necrosis and diffuse hepatic fibrosis (acute yellow atrophy and portal cirrhosis); their production by means of a diet. Clin Sci *5*:93, 1944.

27. Best CH, Hartroft WS, Lucas CS, Ridout, JH: Liver damage produced by feeding alcohol or sugar and its prevention by choline. Br Med J *II*:1001, 1949.

28. Lieber CS, Jones DP, DeCarli LM: Effects of prolonged ethanol intake: Production of fatty liver despite adequate diets. J Clin Invest *44*:1009, 1965.

29. Lieber CS, Jones DP, Mendelson J, DeCarli LM: Fatty liver, hyperlipemia and hyperuricemia produced by prolonged alcohol consumption, despite adequate dietary intake. Trans Assoc Am Phys *76*:289, 1963.

30. DeCarli LM, Lieber CS: Fatty liver in the rat after prolonged intake of ethanol with a nutritionally adequate new liquid diet. J Nutr *91*:331, 1967.

31. Dich J et al.: Accumulation of triacylglycerol in cultured rat hepatocytes is increased by ethanol and by insulin and dexamethasone. Biochem J *212*:617, 1983.

32. Menghini G: L'Aspect morpho-bioptique du foie de l'alcoolique (non cirrhotique) et son évolution. Bull Acad Suisse Sci Med *16*:36, 1960.

33. Lieber CS, Rubin E: Alcoholic fatty liver in man on a high protein and low fat diet. Am J Med *44*:200, 1968.

34. Moon VH: Experimental cirrhosis in relation to human cirrhosis. Arch Pathol *18*:381, 1934.

35. Mallory FB: Phosphorus and alcoholic cirrhosis. Am J Pathol *9*:557, 1933.

36. Hedlund SG, Kiessling KH: The physiological mechanism involved in hangover. I. The oxidation of some lower aliphatic fusel alcohols and aldehydes in rat liver and their effect on the mitochondrial oxidation of various substrates. Acta Pharmacol Toxicol *27*:381, 1969.

37. Jordo L, Olsson R: Effect of long-term administration of different hard liquors and red wine on the rat liver. Acta Pathol Microbiol Scand *83*:345, 1975.

38. Walker F et al.: Cytotoxic effect of alcohol on liver cells and fibroblast in vitro. Scot Med J *19*:125, 1974.

39. Gerlach W: Alkohol, Kupfer, Leberzirrhose. Schweiz med Wchnschr *65*:194, 1935.

40. Flinn FB, Von Glahn WC: A chemical and pathological study of the effects of copper on the liver. J Exp Med *49*:5, 1929.

41. Wilson SAK: Progressive lenticular degeneration: A familial nervous disease associated with cirrhosis of the liver. Brain *34*:295, 1912.

42. Sheldon JH (ed.): Haemochromatosis. London, Oxford University Press, 1935.

43. Aron E, Paoletti C, Jobard P, Gosse C: Recherches expérimentales sur la cytosidérose au vin. Arch Mal Appar Dig *50*:745, 1961.

44. MacDonald RA, Baumslag N: Iron in alcoholic beverages. Possible significance for hemochromatosis. Am J Med Sci *247*:649, 1964.

45. Jakobovits AW, Morgan MY, Sherlock S: Hepatic siderosis in alcoholics. Dig Dis Sci *24*:305, 1979.

46. Charlton RW, Jacobs P, Sefiel H, Bothwell TH: Effect of alcohol on iron absorption. Br Med J *2*:1427, 1964.

47. Celada A, Rudolf H, Donath A: Effect of a single ingestion of alcohol on iron absorption. Am J Hematol *5*:225, 1978.

48. Bothwell TH, Abrahams C, Bradlow BA, Charlton RW: Idiopathic and banthu hemochromatosis. Comparative histological study. Arch Pathol *79*:163, 1965.

49. Lieber CS, DeCarli LM: Ethanol oxidation by hepatic microsomes: Adapative increase after ethanol feeding. Science *162*:917, 1968.

50. Lieber CS, DeCarli LM: Hepatic microsomal ethanol oxidizing system: In vitro characteristics and adaptive properties in vivo. J Biol Chem *245*:2505, 1970.

51. Ohnishi K, Lieber CS: Reconstitution of the microsomal ethanol-oxidizing system: Qualitative and quantitative changes of cytochrome P-450 after chronic ethanol consumption. J Biol Chem *252*:7124, 1977.

52. Koop DR, Morgan ET, Tarr GE, Coon MJ: Purification and characterization of a unique isozyme of cytochrome P-450 from liver microsomes of ethanol-treated rabbits. J Biol Chem *257*:8472, 1982.

53. Lasker JM et al.: Purification and characterization of human liver cytochrome P-450-ALC. Biochem Biophys Res Commun *148*:232, 1987.

54. Shaw S, Rubin KP, Lieber CS: Depressed hepatic glutathione and increased diene conjugates in alcoholic liver disease: Evidence of lipid peroxidation. Dig Dis Sci *28*:585, 1983.

55. Lieber CS: Biochemical factors in alcoholic liver disease. Semin Liver Dis *13*:136, 1993.

56. Lieber CS et al.: S-adenosyl-L-methionine attenuates alcohol-induced liver injury in the baboon. Hepatology *11*:165, 1990.

57. Lieber CS, Williams R (eds): Recent Advances in the Treatment of Liver Disease. Drugs Vol. 40, Supplement 3. Auckland, New Zealand, Adis International, 1990.

58. Letulle M: La péritonite syphilitique, cause fréquente de l'ascite, dans les cirrhoses du foie. Bull Acad Méd (Paris) *80*:209, 1918.

59. Le Duc DM: A study of atrophic cirrhosis of the liver in relationship to syphilis. Ann Intern Med *2*:932, 1929.

60. Rogers L: Amoebic liver abscess: Its pathology, prevention, and cure. Lancet *i*: 677, 1922.

61. Symmers W St C: Note on a new form of liver cirrhosis due to presence of the ova of bilharzia haematobia. J Pathol Bacteriol *9*:237, 1904.

62. Leevy CM, Chen T, Zetterman R: Alcoholic hepatitis, cirrhosis and immunologic reactivity. Ann NY Acad Sci *252*:106, 1975.

63. Paronetto F: Immunological reactions in alcoholic liver disease. Semin Liver Dis *13*: 183, 1993.

64. Lue SL, Paronetto F, Lieber CS: Cytotoxicity of mononuclear cells and vulnerability of hepatocytes in alcoholic fatty liver of baboons. Liver *1*:264, 1981.

65. Fong TL, Govindarajan S, Valinluck B, Redeker GA: Status of hepatitis B virus DNA in alcoholic disease: A study of a large urban population in the United States. Hepatology *8*:1602, 1988.

66. Walter E et al.: Hepatocellular carcinoma in alcoholic liver disease: No evidence for a pathogenetic role of hepatitis B virus infection. Hepatology *8*:745, 1977.

67. Parés A et al.: Hepatitis C virus antibodies in chronic alcoholic patients: Association with severity of liver injury. Hepatology *12*: 1295, 1990.

68. Rosman AS et al.: Hepatitis C virus antibody in alcoholic patients: Association with the presence of portal and/or lobular hepatitis. Arch Intern Med *153*:965, 1993.

69. Khoruts A et al.: Circulating tumor necrosis factor, interleukin-1 and interleukin-6 concentrations in chronic alcoholic patients. Hepatology *13*:267, 1991.

70. Sheron N et al.: Elevated plasma interleukin-6 and increased severity and mortality in alcoholic hepatitis. Clin Exp Immunol *84*: 449, 1991.

71. McClain C, Hill D, Schmidt J, Diehl AM: Cytokines and alcoholic liver disease. Semin Liver Dis *13*:170, 1993.

72. Chvostek F: Klinische Vorträge. Zur Pathogenese der Leberzirrhose. Wien klin Wchnschr *35*:381, 1922.

73. Barrelet J: Les glandes a sécrétion interne dans la cirrhose hépatique. Ann d'anat Path *9*:385, 1932.

74. Gavaler JS, Van Thiel DH, Lester R: Ethanol: A gonadal toxin in the mature rat of both sexes. Alcoholism: Clin Exp Res *4*: 271, 1980.

75. Gordon GG, Lieber CS: Alcohol, Hormones, and Metabolism. *In* Lieber CS (ed): Medical and Nutritional Complications of Alcoholism. New York, Plenum Medical Book Company, 1992.

76. Frerichs FT: A Clinical Treatise on Diseases of the Liver, Vol II, New York, William Wood & Co., 1879.

77. Mercer PW, Khavari KA: Are women drinking more like men? An empirical examination of the convergence hypothesis. Alcoholism: Clin Exp Res *14*:461, 1990.

78. Corti B, Ibrahim J: Women and alcohol—trends in Australia. Med J Aust *152*: 625, 1990.

79. Van Thiel DH: Gender differences in the susceptibility and severity of alcohol-induced liver disease. Alcohol Alcoholism (Suppl) *1*:9, 1991.

80. Marshall AW, Kingstone D, Boss M, Morgan MY: Ethanol elimination in males and females: Relationship to menstrual cycle and body composition. Hepatology *3*:701, 1983.

81. Frezza M et al.: High blood alcohol levels in women. The role of decreased gastric alcohol dehydrogenase activity and first-pass metabolism. N Engl J Med *322*:95, 1990.

82. Lieber CS: Medical and Nutritional Complications of Alcoholism: Mechanisms and Management. New York, Plenum Medical Book Company, 1992.

83. Lamboeuf Y, La Droitte P, De Saint Blanquat G: The gastrointestinal metabolism of ethanol in the rat. Effect of chronic alcohol intoxication. Arch Int Pharmacodyn Ther *261*:157, 1983.

84. Pestalozzi DM, Buhler R, von Wartburg JP, Hess M: Immunohistochemical localization of alcohol dehydrogenase in the human gastrointestinal tract. Gastroenterology *85*:1011, 1983.

85. Julkunen RJK, Di Padova C, Lieber CS: First pass metabolism of ethanol—a gastrointestinal barrier against the systemic toxicity of ethanol. Life Sci *37*:567, 1985.

86. Di Padova C, Worner TM, Julkunen RJK, Lieber CS: Effects of fasting and chronic alcohol consumption on the first pass metabolism of ethanol. Gastroenterology *92*: 1169, 1987.

87. Caballeria J et al.: The gastric origin of first pass metabolism of ethanol in man: Effect of gastrectomy. Gastroenterology 97:1205, 1989.

88. Caballeria J, Baraona E, Lieber CS: The contribution of the stomach to ethanol oxidation in the rat. Life Sci 41:1021, 1987.

89. Di Padova et al.: Effects of ranitidine on blood alcohol levels after ethanol ingestion: Comparison with other H₂-receptor antagonists. JAMA 267:83, 1992.

90. Mishra L, Sharma S, Potter JJ, and Mezey E: More rapid elimination of alcohol in women as compared to their male siblings. Alcoholism: Clin. Exp. Res. 13:752, 1989.

91. Teschke R, Wiese B: Sex-dependency of hepatic alcohol metabolizing enzymes. J Endocrinol Invest 5:243, 1982.

92. Mezey E, Potter JJ, Diehl AM: Depression of alcohol dehydrogenase activity in rat hepatocyte culture by dihydrotestosterone. Biochem Pharmacol 35:335, 1980.

93. Rankin JG: The natural history and management of the patient with alcoholic liver disease. *In* Fisher MM, Rankin JG (eds): Alcohol and the Liver. New York, Plenum Press, 1977.

94. Meyenburg HV, Robert P: Ueber Leberzirrhose, insbesondere über ihre Häufigkeit und Aetiologie. Schweiz med Wchnschr 62: 1, 1932.

95. Wilkinson P, Santamaria JN, Rankin G: Epidemiology of alcoholic cirrhosis. Austr Ann Med 18:222, 1969.

96. Morgan MY, Sherlock S: Sex-related differences among 100 patients with alcoholic liver disease. Br Med J 1:939, 1977.

97. Pequignot G, Tuyns AJ, Berta JL: Ascitic cirrhosis in relation to alcohol consumption. Int J Epidemiol (London) 7:113, 1978.

98. Allan JS, Tyler ET: Biochemical findings in long-term oral contraceptive usage. I. Liver function studies. Fertil Steril 18:112, 1967.

99. Kappas A: Estrogens and the liver. Gastroenterology 52:113, 1967.

100. Larsson-Cohn U: The 2 hour sulfobromophthalein retention test and the transaminase activity during oral contraceptive therapy. Am J Obstet Gynecol 98:188, 1967.

101. Pihl E, Rais O, Zeuchner E: Functional and morphological liver changes in women taking oral contraceptives. A clinical and ultrastructural study with special reference to the occurrence of cholestasis. Acta Chir Scand 134:639, 1968.

102. Pignon J-P, Bailey NC, Baraona E, Lieber CS: Fatty acid-binding protein: A major contributor to the ethanol-induced increase in liver cytosolic proteins in the rat. Hepatology 7:865, 1987.

103. Shevchuk O et al.: Gender differences in the response of hepatic fatty acids and cytosolic fatty acid-binding capacity to alcohol consumption in rats. Proc Soc Exp Biol Med 198:584, 1991.

104. Videla L, Israel Y: Factors that modify the metabolism of ethanol in rat liver and adaptive changes produced by its chronic administration. Biochem J 118:275, 1970.

105. Kessler BJ, Lieber JB, Bronfin GJ, Sass M: The hepatic blood flow and splanchnic oxygen consumption in alcohol fatty liver. J Clin Invest 33:1338, 1954.

106. Jauhonen P, Baraona E, Miyakawa H, Lieber CS: Mechanism for selective perivenular hepatotoxicity of ethanol. Alcoholism: Clin Exp Res 6:350, 1982.

107. Sato N et al.: Effect of acute and chronic ethanol consumption on hepatic tissue oxygen tension in rats. Pharmacol Biochem Behav 18:443, 1983.

108. Shaw S et al.: Increased hepatic oxygenation following ethanol administration in the baboon. Proc Soc Exp Biol Med 156:509, 1977.

109. Lieber CS et al.: Impaired oxygen utilization: A new mechanism for the hepatotoxicity of ethanol in sub-human primates. J Clin Invest 83:1682, 1989.

110. Stein SW et al.: The effect of ethanol upon systemic hepatic blood flow in man. Am J Clin Nutr 13:68, 1963.

111. Jauhonen P, Baraona E, Lieber CS, Hassinen IE: Dependence of ethanol-induced redox shift on hepatic oxygen tensions prevailing in vivo. Alcohol 2:163, 1985.

112. Lieber CS, DeCarli LM, Schmid R: Effects of ethanol on fatty acid metabolism in liver slices. Biochem Biophys Res Commun 1: 302, 1959.

113. Lieber CS, Schmid R: The effect of ethanol on fatty acid metabolism: Stimulation of hepatic fatty acid synthesis in vitro. J Clin Invest 40:394, 1961.

114. Lieber CS, Davidson CS: Some metabolic effects of ethyl alcohol. Am J Med 33:319, 1962.

115. Freinkel H, Cohen AK, Arky RA, Foster AE: Alcohol hypoglycemia. II. A postulated mechanism of action based on experiments with rat liver slices. J Clin Endocrinol Metab 25:76, 1965.

116. Lieber CS, Jones DP, Losowsky MS, Davidson CS: Inter-relation of uric acid and ethanol metabolism in man. J Clin Invest 41:1863, 1962.

117. Kato S, Kawase T, Alderman J, Lieber CS: Role of xanthine oxidase in ethanol-induced lipid peroxidation in rats. Gastroenterology 98:203, 1990.

118. Iseri OA, Lieber CS, Gottlieb LS: The ultrastructure of fatty liver induced by prolonged ethanol ingestion. Am J Pathol 48: 535, 1966.

119. Lane BP, Lieber CS: Ultrastructural alterations in human hepatocytes following ingestion of ethanol with adequate diets. Am J Pathol 49:593, 1966.

120. Tsutsumi M et al.: The intralobular distribution of ethanol-inducible P450IIE1 in rat and human liver. Hepatology 10:437, 1989.

121. Buhler R, Hess M, von Wartburg JP: Immunohistochemical localization of human liver alcohol dehydrogenase in liver tissue, cultured fibroblasts and hela cells. Am J Pathol 108:89, 1982.

122. Hasumura Y, Teschke R, Lieber CS: Characteristics of acetaldehyde oxidation in rat liver mitochondria. J Biol Chem 251:4908, 1976.

123. Cederbaum AK, Lieber CS, Rubin E: Effects of chronic ethanol treatment on mitochondrial functions. Arch Biochem Biophys 165:560, 1974.

124. Cederbaum AK, Lieber CS, Rubin E: The effect of acetaldehyde on mitochondrial function. Arch Biochem Biophys 165:26, 1974.

125. Nomura F, Lieber CS: Binding of acetaldehyde to rat liver microsomes: Enhancement after chronic alcohol consumption. Biochem Biophys Res Commun 100:131, 1981.

126. Behrens JJ, Hoerner M, Lasker JM, Lieber CS: Formation of acetaldehyde adducts with ethanol-inducible P450IIE1 in vivo. Biochem Biophys Res Commun 154:584, 1988.

127. Lin RC, Smith RS, Lumeng L: Detection of protein-acetaldehyde adduct in the liver of rats fed alcohol chronically. J Clin Invest 81:615, 1988.

128. Donohue TJ, Jr, Tuma DJ, Sorrell MF: Acetaldehyde adducts with proteins: Binding of [$_{14}$C] acetaldehyde to serum albumin. Arch Biochem Biophys 220:239, 1983.

129. Stevens VJ et al.: Acetaldehyde adducts with hemoglobin. J Clin Invest 67:361, 1981.

130. Baraona E, Leo MA, Borowsky SA, Lieber CS: Alcoholic hepatomegaly: Accumulation of protein in the liver. Science 190:794, 1975.

131. Baraona E, Leo MA, Borowsky SA, Lieber CS: Pathogenesis of alcohol-induced accumulation of protein in the liver. J Clin Invest 60:546, 1977.

132. Matsuda Y, Baraona E, Salaspuro M, Lieber CS: Effects of ethanol on liver microtubules and Golgi apparatus possible role in altered hepatic secretion of plasma proteins. Lab Invest 41:455, 1979.

133. Israel Y, Hurwitz E, Niëmelä O, Arnon R: Monoclonal and polyclonal antibodies against acetaldehyde-containing epitopes in acetaldehyde-protein adducts. Proc Natl Acad Sci USA 83:7923, 1986.

134. Hoerner M, Behrens UJ, Worner T, Lieber CS: Humoral immune response to acetaldehyde adducts in alcoholic patients. Res Commun Chem Pathol Pharmacol 54:3, 1986.

135. Niemela O et al.: Antibodies against acetaldehyde-modified protein epitopes in human alcoholics. Hepatology 7:1210, 1987.

136. Hoerner M et al.: The role of alcoholism and liver disease in the appearance of serum antibodies against acetaldehyde adducts. Hepatology 8:569, 1988.

137. Lumeng L, Li TK: Vitamin B$_6$ metabolism in chronic alcohol abuse. Pyridoxal phosphate levels in plasma and the effects of acetaldehyde on pyridoxal phosphate synthesis and degradation in human erythrocytes. J Clin Invest 53:693, 1974.

138. Tsukamoto H et al.: Severe and progressive steatosis and focal necrosis in rat liver induced by continuous intragastric infusion of ethanol and low fat diet. Hepatology 5: 224, 1985.

139. Lieber CS, DeCarli LM: An experimental model of alcohol feeding and liver injury in the baboon. J Med Primatol 3:153, 1974.

140. Lieber CS, DeCarli LM, Rubin E: Sequential production of fatty liver, hepatitis and cirrhosis in sub-human primates fed ethanol with adequate diets. Proc Natl Acad Sci 72: 437, 1975.

141. Popper H, Lieber CS: Histogenesis of alcoholic fibrosis and cirrhosis in the baboon. Am J Pathol 98:695, 1980.

142. Lieber CS et al.: Choline fails to prevent liver fibrosis in ethanol-fed baboons but causes toxicity. Hepatology 5:561, 1985.

143. Lieber CS et al.: Attenuation of alcohol-induced hepatic fibrosis by polyunsaturated lecithin. Hepatology 12:1390, 1990.

144. Ainley CC et al.: Is alcohol hepatotoxic in the baboon? J Hepatol 7:85, 1988.

145. Hershey JM, Soskin S: Substitution of "lecithin" for raw pancreas in the diet of the depancreatized dog. Am J Physiol 98: 74, 1931.

146. Post JJ, Benton H, Breakstone R, Hoffman J: The effects of diet and choline on fatty infiltration of the human liver. Gastroenterology 20:403, 1952.

147. Phillips GR, Davidson CS: Acute hepatic insufficiency of the chronic alcoholic. Arch Intern Med 94:585, 1954.

148. Rubin E, Lieber CS: Alcohol induced hepatic injury in nonalcoholic volunteers. N Engl J Med 278:869, 1968.

149. Chawla RK et al.: Choline may be an essential nutrient in malnourished patients with cirrhosis. Gastroenterology 97:1514, 1989.

150. Wurtman JL: Uses of choline and lecithin in brain disorders. Barbeau A, Growdon J, Wurtman R (eds), Nutrition and the Brain. New York, Raven Press, 1979.

151. Fox JM: Polyene phosphatidylcholine: Pharmacokinetics after oral administration—A review. *In*: Avogaro P et al. (eds): Phospholipids and Atherosclerosis. New York, Raven Press, 1983.

152. Zierenberg O, Grundy SM: Intestinal absorption of polyenephosphatidylcholine in man. J Lipid Res 23:1136, 1982.

153. Lekim D, Graf E: Tierexperimentelle Studien zur Pharmakokinetik der "essentiellen" Phospholipide (EPL). Drug Res 26: 1772, 1976.

154. Kuntz E: Pilotstudie mit Polyenylphosphatidylcholin bei schwerer Leberinsuffizienz. Med Welt 40:1327, 1989.

155. Yamada S, Mak KM, Lieber CS: Chronic ethanol consumption alters rat liver plasma membranes and potentiates release of alkaline phosphatase. Gastroenterology 88: 1799, 1985.

156. French SW, Ihrig TJ, Morin RJ: Lipid composition of RBC ghosts, liver mitochondria and microsomes of ethanol-fed rats. Q J Stud Alcohol 31:801, 1970.

157. Thompson JA, Reitz RC: Effects of ethanol ingestion and dietary fat levels on mitochondrial lipids in male and female rats. Lipids 13:540, 1978.

158. Arai M, Gordon ER, Lieber CS: Decreased cytochrome oxidase activity in hepatic mitochondria after chronic ethanol consumption and the possible role of decreased cytochrome aa_3 content and changes in phospholipids. Biochim Biophys Acta 797: 320, 1984.

159. Arai M et al.: Biochemical and morphological alterations of baboon hepatic mitochondria after chronic ethanol consumption. Hepatology 4:165, 1984.

160. Lieber CS et al.: Dietary dilinoleoylphosphatidylcholine (DLPC) is incorporated into liver phospholipids, protects against alcoholic cirrhosis, enhances collagenase activity and prevents acetaldehyde-induced collagen accumulation in cultured lipocytes. Hepatology 16:87A, 1992.

161. Duce AM, Ortiz P, Cabrero C, Mato JM: S-adenosyl-L-methionine synthetase and phospholipid methyltransferase are inhibited in human cirrhosis. Hepatology 8:65, 1988.

162. Lieber CS, Leo MA, Robins S, DeCarli LM: Ethanol decreases hepatic phosphati-

dyl methyltransferase activity whereas phosphatidylcholine increases it, with protection against cirrhosis. FASEB 7:A842, 1993 (abstract).

163. Alling C, Aspenstrom G, Dencker S: Essential fatty acids in chronic alcoholism. Acta Med Scand (Suppl) 63:1, 1979.

164. Rouach H et al.: Fatty acid composition of rat liver mitochondrial phospholipids during ethanol inhalation. Biochim Biophys Acta 795:125, 1984.

165. Horrobin DF: Essential fatty acids, prostaglandins, and alcoholism: An overview. Alcoholism: Clin Exp Res 11:2, 1987.

166. Chojkier M: Hepatocyte collagen production in vivo in normal rats. J Clin Invest 78: 333, 1986.

167. Nakano M, Lieber CS: Ultrastructure of initial stages of perivenular fibrosis in alcohol-fed baboons. Am J Pathol 106:145, 1982.

168. Nakano M, Worner T, Lieber CS: Perivenular fibrosis in alcoholic liver injury: Ultrastructure of histologic progression. Gastroenterology 83:777, 1982.

169. Gabbiani G, Ryan GB, Majno G: Presence of modified fibroblasts in granulation tissue and their possible role in wound contraction. Experientia (Basel) 17:549, 1971.

170. Bhathal PS: Presence of modified fibroblasts in cirrhotic livers in man. Pathology 4:139, 1972.

171. Savolainen ER, Leo MA, Timpl R, Lieber CS: Acetaldehyde and lactate stimulate collagen synthesis of cultured baboon liver myofibroblasts. Gastroenterology 87:777, 1984.

172. McGee JO, Patrick RS: The role of perisinusoidal cells in hepatic fibrogenesis: An electron microscopic study of acute carbon tetrachloride liver injury. Lab Invest 26: 429, 1972.

173. Kent G, Inouye T, Minick OT, Bahu RJ: Role of lipocytes (perisinusoidal cells) in fibrogenesis. *In* Eisse W, Knook DL (eds): Kupffer Cells and Other Liver Sinusoidal Cells. Amsterdam, Elsevier/North Holland Biomedical Press, 1977.

174. Mak KM, Leo MA, Lieber CS: Alcoholic liver injury in baboons: Transformation of lipocytes to transitional cells. Gastroenterology 87:188, 1984.

175. Moshage H, Casini A, Lieber CS: Acetaldehyde selectively stimulates collagen production in cultured rat liver fat-storing cells but not in hepatocytes. Hepatology 12:511, 1990.

176. Casini A, Cunningham M, Rojkind M, Lieber CS: Acetaldehyde increased procollagen type 1 and fibronectin gene transcrip-

tion in cultured rat fat-storing cells through a protein synthesis-dependent mechanism. Hepatology *13*:758, 1991.

177. Karasawa T et al.: Morphologic spectrum of liver diseases among chronic alcoholics. Acta Pathol Jpn *30*:505, 1980.

178. Summerskill WHJ: Aguecheeks' disease. Lancet *ii*:288, 1955.

179. Hahn M et al.: Die Eck'sche Fistel zwischen der unteren Hohlvene und der Pfortader und ihre Folgen für den Organismus. Arch Exp Pathol Pharmakol *32*:161, 1893.

180. Salaskin S: Über das Ammoniak in physiologischer und pathologischer Hinsicht und die Rolle der Leber im Stoffwechsel stickstoffhaltiger Substanzen. Z Physiol Chem *25*:449, 1898.

181. Bollman JL, Mann FC: Physiology of impaired liver. Ergeb Physiol *38*:445, 1936.

182. van Caulaert C, Deviller C: Ammoniémie expérimentale après ingestion de chlorure d'ammonium chez l'homme à l'état normal et pathologique. Compt. Rend. Soc. Biol. *11*:50, 1932.

183. Conway EJ: Micro-diffusion, Analysis and Volumetric Error, 3d Ed. New York, Van Nostrand, 1950.

184. Lieber CS, Lefevre A: Ammonia and intermediary metabolism in hepatic coma: Value of the determination of blood ammonia in the diagnosis and management of cirrhosis. Acta Clin Belg *13*:328, 1958.

185. McDermott Jr, WV, Adams RD: Episodic stupor associated with an Eck fistula in the human, with particular reference to metabolism of ammonia. J Clin Invest *33*:1, 1954.

186. Phillips GB, Schwartz R, Gabuzda GJ, Davidson CS: The syndrome of impeding hepatic coma in patients with cirrhosis of the liver given certain nitrogenous substances. N Engl J Med *247*:239, 1952.

187. Bessman SP, Bessman AN: The cerebral and peripheral uptake of ammonia in liver disease with an hypothesis for the mechanism of hepatic coma. J Clin Invest *34*:622, 1955.

188. Chalmers TC: An evaluation of dietary protein in the treatment of liver disease. Ann Intern Med *48*:320, 1958.

189. Silen W et al.: Effect of antibacterial agents on ammonia production within intestine. Proc Soc Exp Biol Med *88*:138, 1955.

190. Bircher J et al.: Treatment of chronic portal-systemic encephalopathy with lactulose. Lancet *i*:890, 1966.

191. Imperiale TF, McCullough AJ: Do corticosteroids reduce mortality from alcoholic hepatitis? A meta-analysis of the randomized trials. Ann Intern Med *113*:299, 1990.

192. Lieber CS, Lefevre A, Lustman F: Effect of prednisolone on the increased ammonia blood level in Eck fistula dogs. Rev Belg Pathol *26*:414, 1958.

193. Folin O, Denis W: Protein metabolism from the standpoint of blood and tissue analysis. 2. The origin and significance of the ammonia in the portal blood. J Biol Chem *11*:161, 1912.

194. Martini GA et al.: The bacterial content of the small intestine normal and cirrhotic subjects: Relation to methionine toxicity. Clin Sci *16*:35, 1957.

195. Luck JM, Seth TN: The physiology of gastric urease. Biochem J *19*:357, 1925.

196. Delluva AM, Markley K, Davies RE: The absence of gastric urease in germ-free animals. Biochim Biophys Acta *151*:646, 1968.

197. Lieber CS, Lefevre A: Effect of oxytetracycline on acidity, ammonia and urea in gastric juice in normal and uremic subjects. CR Soc Biol (Paris) *151*:1038, 1957.

198. Lieber CS, Lefevre A: Ammonia as source of gastric hypoacidity in patients with uremia. J Clin Invest *38*:1271, 1959.

199. Meyers S, Lieber CS: Reduction of gastric ammonia by ampicillin in normal and azotemic subjects. Gastroenterology *70*:244, 1976.

200. Lieber CS, Lefevre A: Effects of antibiotics on gastric juice in normal and uremic subjects: Ammonia as source of hypoacidity in uremic patients. *In* Proceedings of World Congress Gastroenterology. Baltimore, Williams & Wilkins Publishing Company, 1959.

201. Warren JR: Unidentified curved bacilli on gastric epithelium in active chronic gastritis. Lancet *i*:1273, 1983.

202. Marshall B: Unidentified curved bacilli on gastric epithelium in active chronic gastritis. Lancet *i*:1273, 1983.

203. Kawano S et al.: Chronic effect of intragastric ammonia on gastric mucosal structures in rats. Dig Dis Sci *36*:33, 1991.

204. Triebling AT et al.: Severity of helicobacter-induced injury correlates with gastric juice ammonia. Dig Dis Sci *36*:1089, 1991.

205. Uppal R et al.: Chronic alcoholic gastritis: Roles of ethanol and helicobacter pylori. Arch Intern Med *151*:760, 1991.

206. Graham DY, Go MF, Evans DJ Jr: Review article: urease, gastric ammonium/ammonia, and helicobacter pylori—the past, the present, and recommendations for future research. Aliment Pharmacol Ther *6*:659, 1992.

207. Leung KM, Hul PK, Chan WY, Thomas TMM: Helicobacter pylori-related gastritis and gastric ulcer. A continuum of progres-

sive epithelial degeneration. Am J Clin Pathol *98*:569, 1992.

208. Freeman JM et al.: Ammonia intoxication due to a congenital defect in urea synthesis. J Pediat *65*:1039, 1964.

209. Russell A et al.: Hyperammonaemia. A new instance of an inborn enzymatic defect of the biosynthesis of urea. Lancet *ii*:699, 1962.

210. McMurray et al.: Citrullinuria: A new aminoaciduria associated with mental retardation. Lancet *i*:138, 1962.

211. Terheggen HE et al.: Arginnaemia with arginase deficiency. Lancet *ii*:748, 1969.

212. Reye RD et al.: Encephalopathy and fatty degeneration of the viscera. A disease entity in childhood. Lancet *ii*:749, 1963.

213. Thaler MM et al.: Reye's syndrome due to novel protein-tolerant variant of ornithine-transcarbamylase deficiency. Lancet *ii*:438, 1974.

214. Flint Jr A: Clinical report on hydroperitoneum, based on an analysis of 46 cases. Am J Med Sci *45*:306, 1863.

215. Charcot JM: L'abaissement de l'excrétion urinaire d'urée au cours de la fièvre intermittente hépatique, *In* leçons sur les maladies du foie, 1877.

216. Helwig FC, Schutz CB: Liver kidney syndrome; Clinical, pathological, and experimental studies. Surg Gynec Obstet *55*:570, 1932.

217. Epstein M: Alcohol and kidney. *In* Lieber CS (ed): Medical and Nutritional Complications of Alcoholism. New York-London, Plenum Medical Book Company, 1992.

218. Bradley SE, Bradley GP: The effect of increased intra-abdominal pressure on renal

219. Lancestremere RG et al.: Renal failure in Laennec's cirrhosis. 2. Simultaneous determination of cardiac output and renal hemodynamics. J Clin Invest *41*:1922, 1962.

220. Baldus WP et al.: Renal circulation in cirrhosis: Observations based on catheterization of the renal vein. J Clin Invest *43*:1090, 1964.

221. Haynes FW, Dexter L: Renal humoral pressor mechanism in man; hypertensinogen content of plasma of normal patients and patients with various diseases. J Clin Invest *24*:78, 1945.

222. Fischer JE, Baldessarini RJ: False neurotransmitters and hepatic failure. Lancet *ii*: 75, 1971.

223. Wilkinson SP et al.: Endotoxaemia and renal failure in cirrhosis and obstructive jaundice. Br Med J *2*:1415, 1976.

224. Wong PY et al.: Kallikrein-kinin and renin-angiotensin systems in functional renal failure of cirrhosis of the liver. Gastroenterology *73*:1114, 1977.

225. Huber M et al.: Analysis of cysteinyl leukotrienes in human urine: enhanced excretion in patients with liver cirrhosis and hepatorenal syndrome. Eur J Clin Invest *19*:53, 1989.

226. Lieber CS, Davidson CS: Complications resulting from renal failure in patients with liver disease. Arch Intern Med *106*:749, 1960.

227. Klatskin G: Jaundice and other manifestations of liver disease, *In* Harrison TR (Ed.): Principles of Internal Medicine, New York: McGraw Publishing Co. 1958.

function in man. J Clin Invest *26*:1010, 1947.

21

The Contribution of Transplantation to Gastroenterologic Knowledge

THOMAS E. STARZL

How whole-organ transplantation came to be a clinical discipline has been told elsewhere by many of the persons directly involved (1). Although the history of the field through 1959 was dominated by the kidney (2), the extrarenal vacuum rapidly filled in the late 1950s with the development in several laboratories of canine transplant models with which to study all of the intraabdominal (Fig. 21–1) and thoracic organs.

EARLY ANIMAL MODELS

The Liver

Auxiliary Transplantation

In 1955, C. Stuart Welch of Albany, New York, described the insertion of an extra (auxiliary) canine liver into the pelvis or right paravertebral gutter of nonimmunosuppressed recipients (3). The allograft hepatic artery was revascularized from the aorta or iliac artery, and the portal flow was restored by rerouting the high volume systemic venous return of the host inferior vena cava into the graft portal vein (Fig. 21–2). It was not discovered until a decade later that factors other than rejection were involved in the rapid destruction of the auxiliary transplant (see subsequent section on hepatotrophic physiology).

Orthotopic Liver Transplantation

The first mention of liver replacement (orthotopic transplantation) (Fig. 21–3) was by Dr. Jack Cannon of the University of California, Los Angeles, who cited Welch's article as the stimulus for his own "several successful" operations in dogs "without survival of the patient" (4). Assuming that the liver played an important role in rejection, Cannon speculated that the graft would not contribute to its own repudiation. No details were given about the operation, which remained virtually unknown until its independent investigation in dogs beginning in the summer of 1958 at the Peter Bent Brigham Hospital (Boston) (5–7) and at Northwestern University (Chicago) (8,9). The Boston effort under the direction of Francis D. Moore was part of an immunologically oriented institutional commitment to organ transplantation that initially was preoccupied with the kidney (10).

In contrast, the Northwestern initiative stemmed from a conviction that the liver was a modulator of endogenous insulin, or instead was governed by this hormone (11–13). Such metabolic questions and their investigation ultimately led to the development of a new field called "hepatotrophic physiology" (14,15). To pursue them, a new technique of total hepatectomy (the first half of a transplant operation) was developed (16). The second step of inserting an allograft into the vacated hepatic fossa soon followed; from the outset, the superior liver-supporting qualities of portal versus systemic venous blood were obvious (8).

Although there was no effective way to prevent rejection, an astonishing amount of

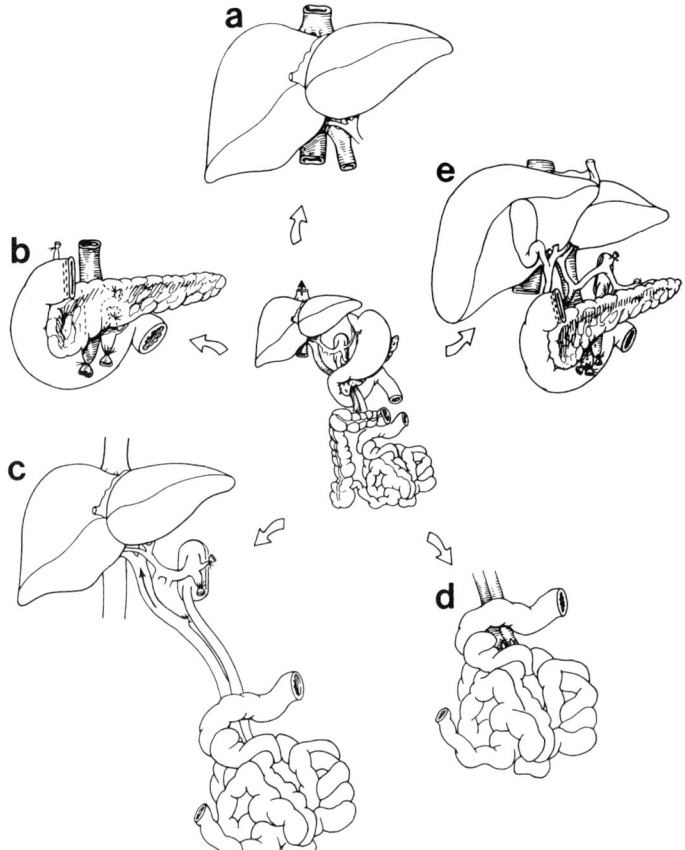

Fig. 21–1. The complex of intra-abdominal viscera which has been transplanted as a unit (center) or as separate components. Counterclockwise: *a,* liver; *b,* pancreas; *c,* liver-intestine; *d,* intestine; *e,* liver-pancreas.

information about orthotopic liver transplantation was compiled in 1958 and 1959. At the April 1960 meeting of the American Surgical Association, Moore reported on 31 canine experiments with 7 survivors of 4 to 12 days. In discussing his paper (17), I described an experience that was in press elsewhere (8) with more than 80 dogs, of which 18 had lived for 4 to 20-1/2 days. Rejection was always present after 5 or 6 days and usually was the cause of death thereafter.

Beyond demonstrating the need to revascularize the hepatic graft with splanchnic venous blood, the work in Boston and Chicago clarified the other requirements for successful liver replacement. Preservation of the transplanted liver was accomplished with intraportal infusion of chilled electrolyte solutions in much the same way as practiced clinically today (8). Improved infusates in the succeeding years (18,19)

eventually replaced the originally used lactated Ringer's and saline solutions. Until 1987, the safe preservation time was only 5 or 6 hours, but since then, the University of Wisconsin (UW) solution (20) has permitted reliable safe refrigeration of human livers for 18 to 24 hours (21,22).

The final requirement for success in dogs was the use of plastic external venous bypasses that passively redirected blood from the occluded splanchnic and systemic venous beds to the superior vena cava during the so-called anhepatic stage while recipient hepatectomy was performed and the new liver was installed (6,8). Such venous decompression was later shown to be expendable in dogs submitted several weeks in advance of transplantation to common bile duct ligation, because of the development in the interim of decompressing venous collaterals (23). Similarly, venous bypasses

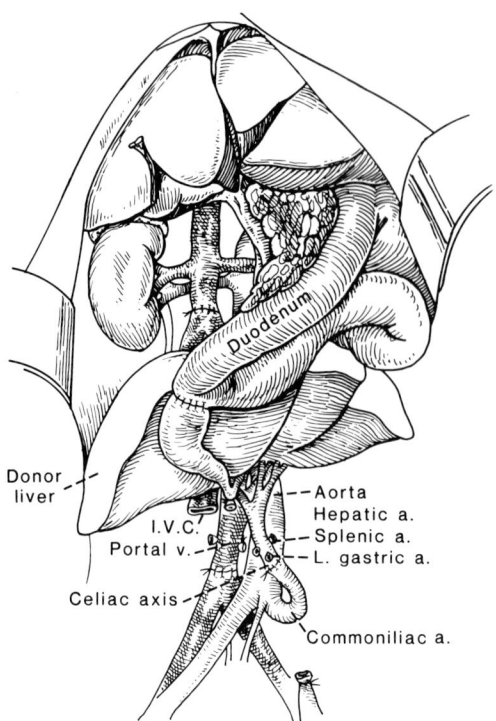

Fig. 21–2. Auxiliary liver transplantation in a dog by a modification of Welch's original technique. Note that the reconstituted portal blood supply is from the distal inferior vena cava. Redrawn with permission from Starzl TE, et al.: Immunosuppression after experimental and clinical homotransplantation of the liver. Ann Surg *160*:411, 1964.

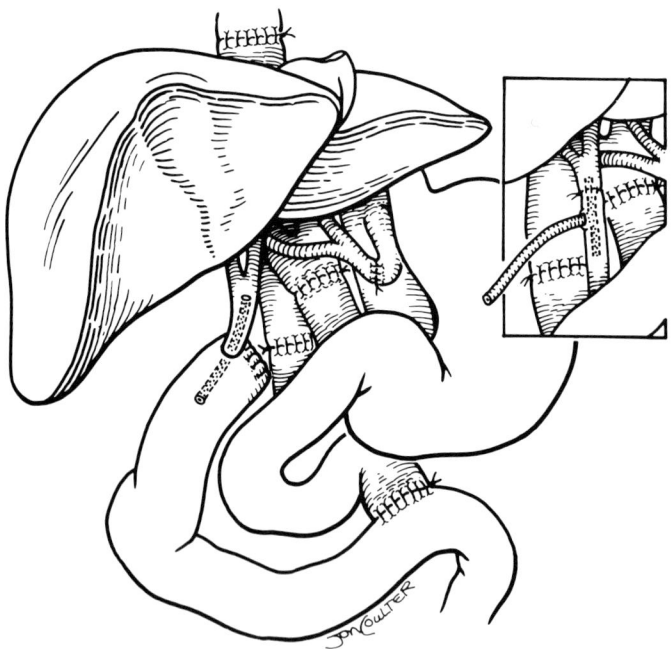

Fig. 21–3. Orthotopic liver transplantation (liver replacement). Biliary tract reconstruction is usually with choledochojejunostomy (to a Roux limb) or (inset) with a choledochocholedochostomy, which is stented with a T tube. Reproduced with permission from Starzl TE et al.: Medical progress: Liver transplantation. N Engl J Med *321*:1014, 1989.

were shown to be nonessential in most clinical cases if the operation was performed by highly experienced surgeons (24,25). Nevertheless, the introduction of pump-driven venovenous bypasses in the 1980s, first with (25) and then without anticoagulation (26–28), made the operation less stressful in humans, placed it well within the grasp of most competent general and vascular surgeons, and allowed the systematic training of a new generation of liver transplant surgeons.

Multivisceral and Intestinal Transplantation

Isolated Intestine

Nearly 90 years ago, Alexis Carrel and C.C. Gunthrie performed canine intestinal transplantations. Little more was added until the similar studies of small bowel transplantation in dogs by Richard Lillehei of the University of Minnesota (29), who replaced the entire small intestine in unmodified recipients except for short segments of jejunum and ileum. The graft was preserved by immersing it in iced saline, and the blood vessels were anastomosed to companion recipient structures in an anatomically normal way. Although it was later demonstrated in Toronto (30), London (Ontario) (31), Pittsburgh (32), Kiel (33), and Paris (34) that the gut could be successfully replaced with long survival in large animals under immunosuppression, the clinical application of this procedure languished. The first clinical successes did not come until the late 1980s (35,36).

Multivisceral Transplantation

The multiple organ allograft in this versatile operation (37) was envisioned as a grape cluster with a double central stem consisting of the celiac axis and superior mesenteric artery (Fig. 21–1, center). In variations of the operation used clinically nearly 30 years later, the grapes, or individual organs, could be removed or retained according to the surgical objectives (Fig. 21–1, periphery), but both arterial stem structures were preserved (38). The venous outflow was kept intact up to or beyond the liver.

Two observations were made in the unmodified canine multivisceral recipients of

1959 that have dominated the field of gastroenterologic transplantation since then. First, rejection of the organs making up the composite graft was less severe than that seen when the organs were transplanted individually (39). This finding was confirmed and greatly extended in 1969 by Calne et al. (40), who described in pig liver recipients the protection of kidney and skin grafts from the hepatic donor; these experiments identified the liver as the "protective" organ. Calne's conclusion about hepatic tolerogenicity has been confirmed by the Japanese surgeon Naoshi Kamada, whose experiments were performed in rats (41), and by many others. Most recently, Valdivia et al. (42) demonstrated the similar protection of hamster heart and skin xenografts in rats by simultaneous or prior xenotransplantation of a hamster liver.

The second fundamental issue raised at the outset was the specter of graft-versus-host disease (GVHD) with the multivisceral procedure. GVHD was well known in 1960 from the prior work of Billingham and Brent (43) and Trentin (44), but this was associated almost exclusively with bone marrow or splenocyte (not whole organ) transplantation. Histopathologic evidence of GVHD was found in recipient tissues of our multivisceral canine recipients (39), who quickly developed multiple organ failure. Later experiments by Monchik and Russell (45) confirmed the potential threat of GVHD, using the F_1 hybrid model in which the parent and F_1 hybrid offspring were donor and recipient respectively. However, these studies vastly overestimated the GVHD threat after splanchnic organ transplantation for reasons explained in the subsequent section on "Mechanisms of Graft Acceptance."

The multivisceral operation is not often indicated clinically, but it has spawned many variations (38) and was itself the procedure with which the first long survival (>6 months) of a functioning human intestinal graft was accomplished (46).

Pancreas Transplantation

Transplantation of the pancreas alone has not been considered in these historical notes because this procedure is done only for endocrine objectives. However, the effect of pancreatic insulin secretion on the liver is a vital concern with all gastroenterologic transplant procedures (see next section). Furthermore, even the transplantation of the whole pancreas "alone" implies the concomitant engraftment of a segment of duodenum which receives exocrine pancreatic secretions and with which the pancreas shares its blood supply in humans and animals (Fig. 21–1b). Thus, it was not surprising that pancreaticoduodenal grafts were used in the first reported acute experiments on pancreas transplantation (47,48). When immunosuppression became available, essentially the same pancreaticoduodenal graft was used in dogs (49) and eventually in humans (50).

HEPATOTROPHIC PHYSIOLOGY: LIVER ATROPHY AND REGENERATION

The Eck Fistula and Liver Transplantation

C. S. Welch's conclusion that rejection was solely responsible for the rapid destruction of the auxiliary liver graft (3,51) was based on an erroneous concept about liver physiology that had evolved from nearly 80 years of research with the experimental procedure of Eck's fistula (portacaval shunt) in dogs. The operation of canine Eck fistula is well known to gastroenterologists. When it is performed, blood returning from the pancreas, intestines, and other splanchnic viscera by way of the portal vein is diverted around the liver instead of through it. Thus, the liver, which now is supplied only by the hepatic artery, loses much of its total blood flow. The liver shrinkage that occurs in dogs (and also in rats, baboons, and humans [15,52]) and the wasting, hair loss, and brain damage that follow were ascribed until the mid 1960s to the diminution of flow rather than the loss of exposure to the liver of any specific substance(s) in the portal blood (53–56). This became known as the flow hypothesis of portal physiology.

Although Welch accepted this false dogma and attributed auxiliary graft destruction to rejection alone, he unwittingly had created an experimental model of great power. The principle of the model was the coexistence of two livers in the same animal

with similar conditions except for the content of the blood delivered to the graft and native portal veins. When we repeated Welch's experiments in 1963 under immunosuppression, auxiliary livers protected from rejection by azathioprine but deprived of splanchnic venous inflow shrank within a few days to a fraction of their original size (57). This acute atrophy was not seen in normally vascularized orthotopic livers. The atrophy could be prevented in auxiliary livers if they were nourished with normal portal blood; then, it afflicted the native liver that was deprived of its portal supply (58).

Soon, nontransplant models were developed in which the animal's own liver was divided into two parts, each of which could be given the venous blood that came from different organs or different parts of the body (59,60) (Fig. 21–4). It was apparent that the healthy and hypertrophic liver fragment with first access to the portal blood, particularly that returning from the upper abdominal viscera, was able to remove substance(s) so completely that little was left for the competing fragment which shriveled up (Fig. 21–5). From the outset, it was postulated that insulin was the most important, although not the only, liver-supporting substance (60–63). This conclusion was supported by later experiments in which the effect on the liver of removing the nonhepatic visceral organs was tested (64,65).

Meanwhile, infusion experiments had been performed showing that insulin, when injected alone into the tied-off central vein after portacaval shunt (Fig. 21–6), could prevent most of the consequences to the liver that were caused by the Eck fistula (66). As other liver growth factors of pancreatic, enteric, and nonsplanchnic origin have become available in recent years, they have been screened and evaluated for potency with the Eck fistula model (67,68). In this preparation, an active test substance prevents in the infused liver lobes the expected acute hepatocyte atrophy, organelle disruption, and fatty infiltration caused by depriving the liver of portal venous blood—the comparison of protected versus nonprotected hepatic tissue being similar to that in Figure 21–5.

In addition to affecting the size of hepatocytes, the most potent factors tested in the model shown in Figure 21–6 also promote

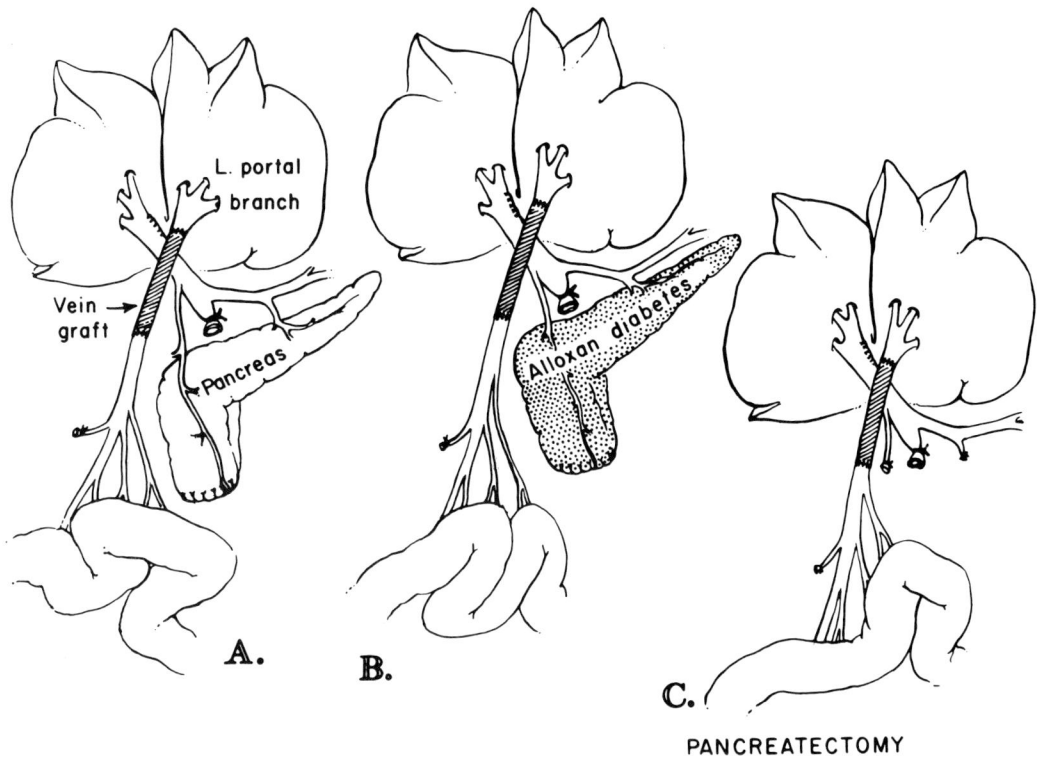

Splanchnic division

Fig. 21–4. Splanchnic division experiments. In these dogs, the right liver lobes received venous return from the pancreaticogastroduodenosplenic region, and the left liver lobes received venous blood from the intestines. *A,* nondiabetic dogs; *B,* alloxan-induced diabetic dogs; *C,* dogs with total pancreatectomy. Reproduced with permission from Starzl TE et al.: The effect of diabetes mellitus on portal blood hepatotrophic factors in dogs. Surg Gynecol Obstet *140*:549, 1975.

proliferation—beginning with insulin (66) but also including the immunosuppressive agents cyclosporine (69) and FK 506 (70) and the growth factors, insulin-like growth factor (IGF-II), transforming growth factor-alpha (TGFα) and hepatocyte growth factor (HGF) (68). By virtue of these developments, hepatotrophic physiology has become a consistent countertheme of all research on the transplantation of splanchnic organs as well as a common ground shared by liver transplantation, clinical portal shunt operations (all are variations of Eck's fistula), and the regeneration that follows hepatic resection (15,71). In the portal shunt field, the new insight into portal hepatotrophic physiology provided an incentive to use portal flow-sparing procedures such as the Warren shunt in reference to complete portal diversion for the treatment of portal hypertension (15).

In contrast, the completely diverting portacaval shunt has been used preferentially to palliate several inborn errors of metabolism (15). The principle was to create with complete portal diversion a subtle kind of liver disease that inhibited the synthesis and accumulation of abnormal glycogen in patients with certain glycogen storage diseases (72), or alpha-1-antitrypsin in patients with alpha-1-antitrypsin deficiency (73,74). Because portal diversion reduces the production of cholesterol that cannot be normally catabolized in the disease of familial hypercholesterolemia, portacaval shunt lowered serum cholesterol in patients with this diagnosis (75,76). The manufacture in the liver of many other substances also is

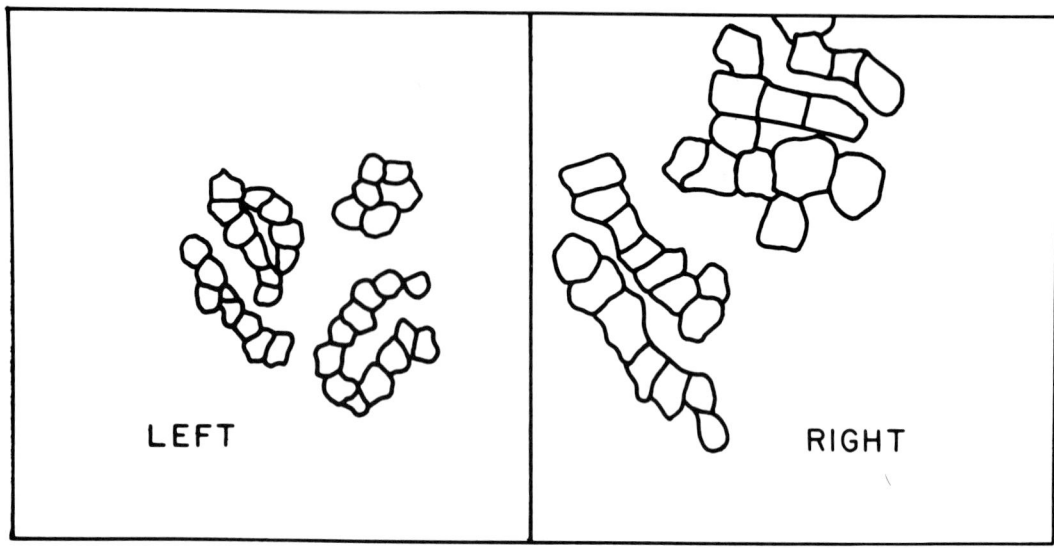

Fig. 21–5. Hepatocyte shadows traced during histopathologic examination of liver biopsies from experiments shown in Figure 21–4A. These were later cut out on standard paper and weighed as an index of hepatocyte size. The right lobes with the large hepatic cells received venous blood from the pancreas, stomach, duodenum, and spleen. The relatively shrunken left lobes with the small hepatocytes received intestinal blood. Reproduced with permission from Starzl TE et al.: Surg Gynecol Obstet *137*:179, 1973. The origin, hormonal nature, and action of hepatotrophic substances in portal venous blood.

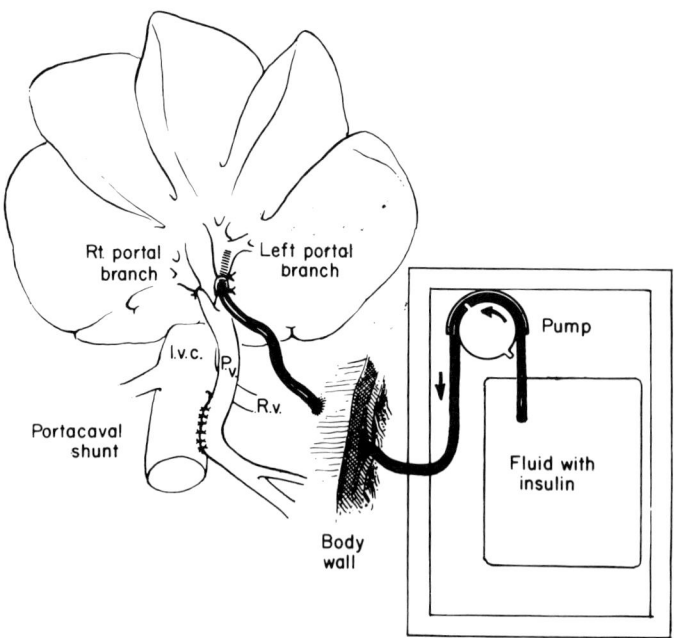

Fig. 21–6. Experiments in which postoperative infusions of hormones are made into the left portal vein after performance of Eck fistula. Reproduced with permission from Starzl TE et al.: Lancet *1*:821, 1976. Effects of insulin, glucagon, and insulin/glucagon infusions on liver morphology and cell division after complete portacaval shunt in dogs.

curtailed by portal diversion, but the consequent adverse effects in patients with the metabolic diseases were superseded in significance by the gain in control of the abnormal or runaway metabolites. Eventually, it was shown that all three of the cited inborn errors, as well as many others, could be corrected definitively by liver replacement (see subsequent section). When this occurred, the use of portal diversion for metabolic purposes became obsolete.

An additional ripple effect of research in transplantation was stimulated by the referral for liver replacement of patients with large but still localized liver neoplasms that were thought to be unresectable. As an alternative to transplantation, we standardized and popularized the previously dangerous operation of right trisegmentectomy (77) and introduced the new operation of left trisegmentectomy (extended left hepatic lobectomy) (78).

IMMUNOSUPPRESSION

While the gastroenterologic transplant operations were being perfected, other developments had raised hopes of their potential clinical application. The literature on these developments, which has been summarized elsewhere (79), began with the demonstration by Medawar in 1944 that rejection is an immunologic event (80,81). The deliberate weakening of the immune system with total body irradiation (82), and corticosteroid therapy (83,84), and (much later) the thiopurine compounds, 6-mercaptopurine and azathioprine (85–89) ameliorated the rejection of skin grafts in rodents and renal grafts in dogs. However, complete control of rejection with a single agent was rarely

achieved in animals without lethal side effects. This same thing was seen in discouraging clinical trials of renal transplantation (90–95). In the numerous clinical trials of *kidney* transplantation from January 1959 through the autumn of 1962, there were only 8 examples of survival for at least 5 months—2 in Boston (90–92) and 6 in Paris (96,97). All except the last of these patients were treated primarily with total body irradiation; the final patient was the first to have long survival with azathioprine (92).

This discouraging picture changed dramatically during 1962 and 1963 in Colorado, where the synergism of azathioprine and prednisone was known from animal investigations (98). When these two drugs were used together from the outset in human kidney transplant recipients, the results exceeded everyone's expectations (99,100) and precipitated a revolution in clinical transplantation. Success hinged, first, on the fact that acute rejection usually could be reversed with prednisone and, second, that the amount of drug treatment required to achieve stability of graft function often became less in time (99–102).

The reversibility of rejection and change in host-graft relationship were eventually verified with all other transplanted organs, beginning with the liver (103,104). Although immunosuppression has improved, the central therapeutic dogma for whole organ transplantation that had emerged by 1963 (99,100) has changed little in nearly 30 years. The dogma calls for daily treatment with one or two baseline drugs with further immune modulation by the highly dose-maneuverable adrenal cortical steroids to whatever level is required to maintain stable graft function (Table 21–1). This means that every organ recipient goes through a trial

Table 21–1
Central Therapeutic Dogma

Strategy	Baseline Agents	Sites of Action
1. Baseline therapy with one or two drugs	1. Azathioprine	DNA synthesis
2. Secondary adjustments with steroids or antilymphoid agents	2. Cyclophosphamide	DNA synthesis
	3. Cyclosporine	IL-2 production
3. Case-to-case trial (and potential error) of weaning	4. FK 506	IL-2 production

Table 21–2
Principal Immunosuppressive Drug Regimens and Adjuncts* Used Clinically

Agents	Year Described and Reported (Ref.)	Place	Deficiencies	Used for GI Organs
Total body irradiation	1960 (90)	Boston	Ineffective, dangerous	No
Azathioprine	1962 (91)	Boston	Ineffective, dangerous	No
Azathioprine-steroids	1963 (99)	Denver	Suboptimal	Yes, liver
Thoracic duct drainage as adjunct	1963 (105)	Stockholm	Nuisance: requires 20 to 30 days pretreatment	Yes†, liver
Thymectomy as adjunct	1963 (106)	Denver	Unproven value	Yes, rarely in 1963
Splenectomy as adjunct	1963 (106)	Denver	No longer necessary	Yes, once commonly for liver
ALG as adjunct	1966 (107)	Denver	Suboptimal	Yes
Cyclophosphamide substitute for azathioprine	1970 (108)	Denver	No advantage except for patients with azathioprine toxicity	Yes‡, liver
Total lymphoid irradiation	1979 (109, 110)	Palo Alto, Minneapolis	Dangerous, extensive preparation, not quickly reversible	Yes§, for liver
Cyclosporine	1978–1979 (111)	Cambridge	Suboptimal	Yes
Cyclosporine-steroids	1980 (112)	Denver	Nephrotoxicity; rejection not always controlled	Yes
FK506-steroids	1989 (114)	Pittsburgh	Nephrotoxicity; rejection not always controlled	Yes

* Until 1966, these were developed with kidney transplantation and applied for livers. From 1966 onward, the liver increasingly became the dominant test organ.

† It was not realized until much later that pretreatment for 3 to 4 weeks before transplantation was a necessary condition for effective use of TDD (113).

‡ These trials were summarized many years later with at least 10 years follow-up for surviving patients (25).

§ By Professor J. A. Myburgh of Johannesburg.

and potential error experience as drugs are weaned to maintenance levels.

The principal regimens used clinically within this format over the ensuing 30 years are summarized in Table 21–2. Aside from the simplicity and the consequent ease with which the therapeutic formula could be taught, it proved applicable to each new drug regimen or immune modulating technique used clinically over the next 30 years (105–114) and to each new organ, of which the liver was the first after the kidney and the intestine the most recent.

The history of this remarkable phase in transplantation has been told elsewhere (79). Even at the end of 1962, transplantation still seemed like a mirage. One year later, a wild proliferation of kidney transplant centers had begun on both sides of the Atlantic, driven by knowledge of the efficacy of the "drug cocktail" approach, of which the first example was the azathioprine-prednisone combination. Trials with the liver, the next vital organ beyond the kidney, had started (115) and clinical kidney xenotransplantation with chimpanzee (116) and baboon (117) donors had been systematically tried with encouraging, although ultimately unsatisfactory, results.

CLINICAL TRIALS OF LIVER TRANSPLANTATION

Phase I: The Failed First Cases

The prospect of establishing a forerunner kidney program in Denver in preparation for liver transplantation was the reason for my move from Northwestern to the University of Colorado in late 1961 (118). Now, the effectiveness of azathioprine-prednisone cocktail for kidney grafting having been proved, a decision was taken to move on to the liver (115,119). The first recipient was a 3-year-old boy with biliary atresia who had had multiple previous operations. The transplantation could not be completed because of a fatal hemorrhage from venous collaterals and an uncontrollable coagulopathy. Even for a team that had been fully prepared for technical vicissitudes by hundreds of animal operations, the exsanguination of this child was a terrible shock.

Two more liver transplantations were carried out in the next 4 months. In both, the procedures seemed satisfactory, but the recipients died after 22 and 7-1/2 days, respectively (115,119). The strategy of coagulation control introduced after the death of the first patient had a delayed backfire in all of the liver transplant recipients in whom it was used. During the time when the livers were sewn in, the plastic external bypasses were used to reroute venous blood around the area of the liver in the same way as had been worked out in dogs. In the humans who were being given drugs and blood products to promote clots, these clots formed in the bypass tubing and passed on to the lungs. There, they caused abscesses and other lung damage which contributed to or caused delayed death of all four of the patients who survived the intraoperative period (57,115). A pall settled over the liver

program, with a self-imposed moratorium that lasted more than 3 years. By this time, isolated attempts also were unsuccessful at the Brigham (120) and in France (121).

When these first seven liver transplantations failed in three different centers (Table 21–3), pessimism settled in worldwide. The operation seemed too difficult to allow practical application, the methods of preservation were thought inadequate for an organ so seemingly sensitive to ischemic damage, and it began to be asked if immunosuppression available was considered too primitive to permit success. This last reservation was reinforced by the fact that truly chronic survival after liver replacement had never been achieved to this time in experimental animals.

Phase 2: Feasible But Impractical Therapy

By the summer of 1967, these deficiencies had been at least partially rectified by 3 more years of laboratory effort. Many long-term canine survivors had been obtained (103), some dogs having passed the 3-year postoperative mark. Better immunosuppression with the so-called triple drug therapy was now available, following the development and first clinical trials in the world of antilymphocyte globulin (ALG) prepared from sensitized horses (107) and used to supplement azathioprine and prednisone. Finally, improved techniques of organ preservation had been developed (122,123).

On July 23, 1967, a 1-1/2 year old child with a huge hepatoma was restored almost immediately from a moribund state to seemingly good health after liver replacement. More cases followed. The ripple effect of successfully transplanting a vital organ other than the kidney was far-reaching (124). If the liver, the most difficult of all organs, could be transplanted, anything seemed possible. The smoldering embers in other specialty centers burst into flames: first, with the heart transplantation in Capetown by Christiaan Barnard (December 1967), then with attempts at intestinal transplantation by Richard Lillehei and William Kelly (University of Minnesota, 1967), and finally with the first successful lung transplantation on November 14, 1968 (by F. Derom of Louvain, Belgium).

Table 21–3
The First 7 Attempts of Clinical Orthotopic Liver Transplantation

No.	Location (Ref.)	Age (Yr)	Disease	Survival (Days)	Main Cause of Death
1	Denver (115)	3	Extrahepatic biliary atresia	0	Hemorrhage
2	Denver (115)	48	Hepatocellular cancer, cirrhosis	22	Pulmonary emboli, sepsis
3	Denver (115)	68	Duct cell carcinoma	7½	Sepsis, pulmonary emboli, gastrointestinal bleeding
4	Denver (57)	52	Hepatocellular cancer, cirrhosis	6½	Pulmonary emboli, hepatic failure, pulmonary edema
5	Boston (120)	58	Metastatic colon carcinoma	11	Pneumonitis, liver abscesses, hepatic failure
6	Denver (57)	29	Hepatocellular cancer, cirrhosis	23	Sepsis, bile peritonitis, hepatic failure
7	Paris (121)	75	Metastatic colon carcinoma	0	Hemorrhage

Most of these attempts failed early, and all of the patients eventually died. For the liver also, it was not a time of triumph. The child who became the first long-term survivor after hepatic replacement died of recurrent cancer after 400 days. The maximum survival of the other six liver recipients treated between July 1967 and March 1968 was 2-1/2 years (25,124). For the next 12 years, the 1-year mortality after liver transplantation never fell below 50% in cases that were accrued at the University of Colorado at the rate of about one per month. The terrible losses were concentrated in the first postoperative months. After this, the life survival curve flattened, leaving a residual group of stable and remarkably well survivors. Thirty (18%) of the first 170 patients in the consecutive series that started 1 March 1963 and ended in December 1979 lived more than a decade; 23 are still alive after 13 to 23 years. All were treated with azathioprine (or cyclophosphamide), prednisone, and polyclonal ALG (25).

In the meanwhile, Professor Roy Calne at Cambridge University (England) began clinical trials of liver transplantation on May 23, 1967. As in our earlier experience, his first patient exsanguinated (125). A few

months later, Calne formed a collaboration that endured for more than two decades with the hepatologist, Professor Roger Williams, at Kings College Hospital in London. The Colorado and Cambridge-London teams continued their clinical efforts through the years, in spite of frequent disappointments and many tragic failures. The long survival of patients in both series was a testimonial for liver transplantation, but it was asked increasingly on both sides of the Atlantic if such a small dividend could justify the prodigious effort that had brought liver transplantation this far (126). Other teams established subsequently in Hannover (Rudolf Pichlmayr, 1972) and Paris (Henri Bismuth, 1974) also reported the nearly miraculous benefits of liver transplantation when this treatment was successful, but always with the notation that the mortality was too great to allow its practical use. Liver transplantation was a feasible but impractical operation.

Phase 3: The Cyclosporine/FK 506 Era

The frustration ended when cyclosporine became available clinically in 1979 (111), but only after this drug was combined with prednisone or lymphoid depletion in the first of the cyclosporine-based cocktails (112). Of our first 12 liver recipients treated with cyclosporine and prednisone in the first 8 months of 1980, 11 lived for more than a year (127) and 7 are still alive more than 12 years later. As the news was confirmed that 1-year patient survival of at least 70% was readily achievable, new liver programs proliferated worldwide. When FK 506 was substituted for cyclosporine in 1989 (114), the 1-year patient and liver graft survival rose another 15% in the Pittsburgh experience (128). An improvement also was recorded in a multicenter European trial. By now, liver transplantation had become the accepted court of last appeal for almost all non-neoplastic liver diseases, and even for selected patients with otherwise nonresectable hepatic malignancies. The principal limitation of the technology quickly became the supply of organs to meet the burgeoning needs.

Although the ascension of liver transplantation was dominated by improvements in immunosuppression, other significant improvements occurred, including modified details of the operation itself. The incidence of biliary duct complications (obstruction, fistula, and cholangitis), which had been more than 30% (129), was reduced by the use of choledochocholedochostomy with a T-tube stent, or if this was not feasible, by choledochojejunostomy to a Roux limb (25). Management of coagulopathies was facilitated by the use of the thromboelastagram to follow the minute-to-minute clotting changes in the operating room (115,130). The systematic use of veno-venous bypasses without anticoagulation also greatly diminished the hemorrhages of nightmare proportions that were common at one time (131).

ORGAN PROCUREMENT

Hypothermia and Core Cooling

Steps in the development of liver graft procurement and preservation have been few. However, these steps have had an importance far beyond their application for liver replacement, because the principles were applied equally to other whole organs. The first step was core cooling by infusion of chilled lactated Ringer's solution into the portal vein (8) a laboratory technique promptly modified for use in clinical kidney transplantation (132).

Today, core cooling is the first step in the preservation of all whole organ grafts, but in contrast to the original method, this is most often done by some variant of the in-situ technique originally developed at the University of Colorado to cool and continuously perfuse cadaveric liver and kidney donors before the acceptance of brain death conditions (133,134). Ackerman and Snell (135) and Merkel and colleagues (136) simplified the in-situ cooling of cadaveric kidneys with cold electrolyte solutions infused into the distal aorta. Finally, in-situ cold infusion techniques were perfected that allowed removal of all thoracic and abdominal organs, including the liver, without jeopardizing any of the individual organs (137). Modifications of this procedure have been made for unstable donors and even for donors whose hearts have ceased to beat (138). In less than 5 years, multiple-organ procurement, using techniques that are interchangeable not only from city to city but from country to country, had become standardized in all parts of the world.

The technique is versatile. A complete midline abdominal and thoracic incision is made. The aorta at the diaphragm is encircled so that it can be crossclamped when the core cooling is begun. The distal aorta is used as an entry site for the fluid infusion. By coordination of the fluid infusion and the crossclamping of the great vessels and by dissection and ligation of appropriate arterial branches, the cold infusate can be made to go selectively to the organs (including the liver) that are to be transplanted. The portal vein of the liver also is infused after a catheter is placed into it through the splenic vein or other major tributary. Core cooling of the thoracic organs is accomplished with the same principles (137). After the chilled organs have been removed, subsequent preservation may be by simple refrigeration, or by sophisticated methods of continuous perfusion.

INDICATIONS FOR LIVER TRANSPLANTATION

Because the potentially suitable candidates for liver transplantation outnumber

Table 21–4
Generic Listing of Liver Diseases
Treatable by Hepatic Transplantation

Disease

Parenchymal
  Postnecrotic cirrhosis
  Alcoholic cirrhosis
  Acute liver failure
  Budd-Chiari syndrome
  Congenital hepatic fibrosis
  Cystic fibrosis
  Neonatal hepatitis
  Hepatic trauma
Cholestatic
  Biliary atresia
  Primary biliary cirrhosis
  Sclerosing cholangitis
  Secondary biliary cirrhosis
  Familial cholestasis
Inborn errors of metabolism
Tumors
  Benign
  Primary malignant
  Metastatic

the available organs by 3 to 1, the selection of appropriate recipients from such a large pool requires highly individualized assessment. By 1989, the list of benign diseases treatable by transplantation had become so long that it was increasingly given in broad categories such as cholestatic or parenchymal disease (Table 21–4). The simplification made it easy to lose sight of the fact that nearly 100 distinct diseases have been treated with liver transplantation, including more than 20 in the broad category of cholestatic disorders. Because products of hepatic synthesis permanently retain the original metabolic specificity of the donor after transplantation (139,140), liver transplantation is a decisive way to treat many liver-based or liver-influenced inborn errors of metabolism (Table 21–5).

Diseases that precluded transplantation 5 or 10 years ago, such as alcoholic cirrhosis, are no longer absolute contraindications. In addition, scarring from multiple upper abdominal operations and prior portal-systemic shunts that at one time would have ruled out liver transplantation are no longer overriding deterrents in any major center. Extensive thrombosis of the portal and superior mesenteric veins which previously made liver transplantation difficult or impossible has been almost eliminated as a contraindication to attempted liver transplantation by the use of vein grafts (141–145).

Inflexible age proscriptions at either the upper or lower range have been dropped. The shortage of appropriate-sized donors for very small pediatric recipients was greatly ameliorated by the use of liver fragments. The first known reduced liver graft operation was performed in Denver in 1975 (146) but was not reported until long after the landmark descriptions of this technique by Henri Bismuth and Didier Houssin of Paris (147) and the team of Rudolf Pichlmayr and Christoph Broelsch of Hannover (148).

The use of conventional liver transplantation to treat otherwise nonresectable primary or metastatic hepatic cancers has resulted in a very high rate of recurrence (139). Nevertheless, the use of liver transplantation to treat cancer is still being investigated by many transplantation teams, almost invariably in combination with adjuvant chemotherapy or other experimental treatment protocols. Certain kinds of neoplasms have a better prognosis than others. A crucial condition of candidacy involves ruling out the possibility that the tumor has spread beyond the liver.

A radical extension of this concept is the removal of organ clusters to en bloc (liver, pancreas, spleen, stomach, duodenum, proximal jejunum, and right colon) to treat extensive sarcomas and carcinoid tumors of the pancreas or duodenum with liver metastases, bile duct carcinomas with liver metastases, and hepatomas that had invaded the duodenum and colon (149). The excised organs have been replaced with hepatopancreaticoduodenal grafts (see Fig. 21–1e), or in some cases by the liver alone.

CLINICAL TRIALS OF INTESTINAL TRANSPLANTATION IN COMPOSITE VISCERAL GRAFTS OR ALONE

Composite Grafts

Function for more than a half year of a cadaveric intestine was not accomplished until 1987 (150,151). In November of that

Table 21–5
Inborn Errors of Metabolism Treated with Liver Transplantation—Most of the Patients Were in University of Colorado—University of Pittsburgh Series. Follow-up to January 1989 (139).

Disease	Explanation of Disease	Longest Survival	Associated Liver Disease
α_1Antitrypsin deficiency	Structural abnormality of the protease inhibitor synthesized in liver	13 yr	Cirrhosis
Wilson's disease	Abnormal biliary copper excretion, decreased copper binding to ceruloplasmin, and copper accumulation in tissues; autosomal recessive gene mapped to chromosome 13	16.5 yr	Cirrhosis
Tyrosinemia	Fumaroylacetoacetate hydrolase deficiency	7.5 yr	Cirrhosis, hepatoma
Type I glycogen storage disease	Glucose-6-phosphatase deficiency	7 yr	Glycogen storage, fibrosis, tumors
Type IV glycogen storage disease	Amylo-1:4,1:6-transglucosidase (branching enzyme) defect	4.5 yr	Cirrhosis
Cystic fibrosis	Unknown; pancellular disease, liver often affected	4.5 yr	Cirrhosis
Niemann-Pick disease	Sphingomyelinase deficiency, sphingomyelin storage	2 yr (died)	None
Sea-blue histiocyte syndrome	Unknown, neurovisceral lipochrome storage	7 yr	Cirrhosis
Erythropoietic protoporphyria	Hepatic ferrochelatase deficiency, ?overproductive of protoporphyrin by erythropoietic tissues	1.5 yr	Cirrhosis
Crigler-Najjar syndrome	Glucuronyl transferase deficiency	4 yr	None
Type 1 hyperoxaluria	Peroxisomal alanine:glyoxylate aminotransferase deficiency	8 mo.	None
Urea cycle enzyme deficiency (3 types)	Ornithine carbamoyltransferase deficiency	8 mo.	None
C protein deficiency	Defective C protein synthesis	2.25 yr	None
Familial hypercholesterolemia	Low-density lipoprotein receptor deficiency, low-density lipoprotein overproduction	6 yr	None
Hemophilia A	Factor VIII deficiency	4 yr	Cirrhosis, a complication of blood component therapy
Hemophilia B	Factor IX deficiency	6 mo.	Cirrhosis, a complication of blood component therapy

year, the recipient of a multivisceral graft who was treated with cyclosporine, prednisone, and the antilymphoid agent, OKT3, survived for 192 days before dying of a B cell lymphoma (46). Several subsequent recipients of the full multivisceral graft (see Fig. 21–1, center) are alive after as long as 17 months under treatment with FK 506 (36,152).

A variant procedure in which only the liver and small bowel are retained (see Fig. 21–1c) was described by Grant et al. (153) of London, Ontario. This operation has been particularly useful in patients with the short gut syndrome who developed liver failure after prolonged hyperalimentation (36). Using FK 506, 13 (76.5%) of 17 patients in the Pittsburgh series of liver-intestinal grafts are alive after 5 to 31 months—all but one liberated from total parenteral hyperalimentation (TPN) (36,152).

Intestinal Transplantation Alone

As recently as late 1991, some workers in the field believed that the protection to the intestine afforded by the concomitant transplantation of the liver from the same donor (see previous text) was sufficiently great to justify combined liver and intestinal transplantation even when only a technically simpler intestinal transplant was needed. Enthusiasm for this draconian strategy began to fade with the successful transplantation in March 1989 of a cadaveric small intestine by Goulet et al. (35) of Paris, and of an ileal segment from a living related donor by Deltz of Kiel, Germany (154).

These were isolated straws in the wind. The routine survival of cadaveric intestinal recipients then became possible in Pittsburgh under immunosuppression with FK 506, where the results have been better with isolated intestinal transplantation than with either the multivisceral operation or its liver-intestine variant (36,152). Eight of 9 such recipients are alive, several after 1 to 2 years—all but one being TPN-free. The expected release of FK 506 for general use in the near future is certain to stimulate rapid further development of the intestinal transplantation field.

Metabolic Interactions

Nonimmunologic factors can influence the success or failure of abdominal organ grafts. Normally, the venous effluent from all of the nonhepatic splanchnic organs contributes to the portal blood supply, ensuring the liver of first-pass exposure to the intestinal nutrients, and the so-called portal hepatotrophic substances, of which insulin is the most important.

When partial multivisceral grafts such as the liver-intestine are used in recipients whose pancreas and other upper abdominal organs are retained, it is preferable to direct the venous effluent from the residual host organs into the portal circulation of the new liver. Otherwise, subtle injury of the liver typical of, although less severe than, that caused by Eck fistula, can be produced. Similarly, when the intestine is transplanted alone, the ideal route of venous return is through the liver. However, the inability for technical reasons to drain intestinal return into the host liver has not caused severe hepatic complications in a small number of our human recipients (36).

MECHANISM OF GRAFT ACCEPTANCE

Throughout the modern history of transplantation, it has not been known how grafts were able, with the aid of immunosuppression, to weather the initial attack by the recipient immune system, and later to merge half-forgotten into the host. Study of the gastrointestinal organs and their recipients has provided unique insights into this process (155,156). In 1969, the liver became the first transplanted organ to be recognized as having a composite (chimeric) structure. It was noted that the Kupffer cells and other tissue leukocytes became predominantly recipient-phenotype within 100 days after transplantation while the hepatocytes permanently retained their donor specificity. At the time and long afterward, this transformation was assumed to be unique to the hepatic allograft.

However, 22 years later, first in rat models (157), and then in humans (158), it was realized that the same process occurred in all successfully transplanted intestines. The epithelium of the bowel remained that of the donor, whereas the lymphoid, dendritic and other leukocytes of recipient origin quickly became the dominant cells in the lamina propria, Peyer's patches, and mesenteric nodes. Subsequent studies of the kidney and thoracic organs made it obvious that all whole-organ grafts underwent a similar transformation that differed only quantitatively from organ to organ. The number of substituted tissue leukocytes ranged from large in the case of the liver to small in organs like the kidney and heart.

What remained to be determined was the fate of the leukocytes vacating the grafts. The answers were provided in the spring and summer of 1992 by the longest survivors of kidney and liver transplantation (155,156,159,160). Samples were taken from the transplanted organ as well as from the patient's own skin, lymph nodes, and other tissues. After special staining procedures (immunostaining or sex identification after fluorescence in-situ hybridization), the tissues were examined under the microscope to see if the individual cells that made them up had come from the organ donor, the recipient's own body, or both. Alternatively, the donor and recipient contributions to any specimen could be separated by polymerase chain reactions ("DNA fingerprinting") techniques.

Within minutes after restoring the blood supply of any whole organ transplant, myriads of sessile but potentially migratory leukocytes that are part of the normal structure of all organs left the graft and migrated all over the recipient while similar recipient cells took their place in the transplant without disturbing the highly specialized donor parenchymal cells (Fig. 21–7). The relocated donor and recipient leukocytes learned to live in harmony, provided they were given sufficient protection during their nesting by immunosuppressive drugs. The same process applied to the intestine and all whole organs. In this new context, the drugs could be viewed as traffic directors, allowing movement of the white cells in both directions (to and from the graft) but preventing the immune destruction that is the normal purpose of this traffic.

It is not known yet how the two sets of white cells—a small population of predomi-

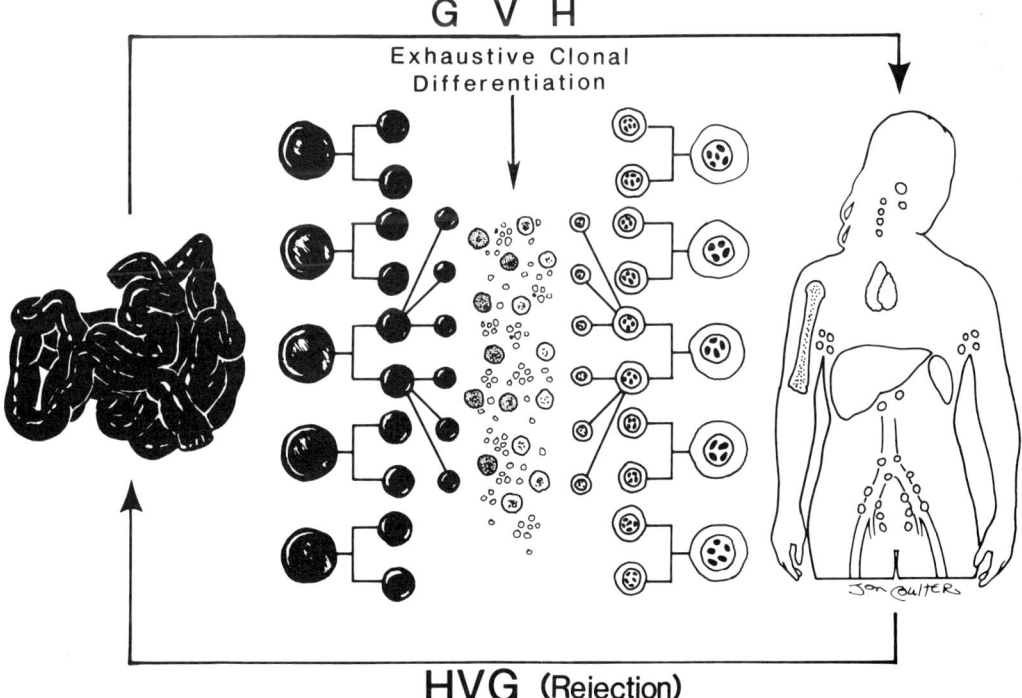

Fig. 21–7. Current understanding of the graft and systemic chimerism that occurs after transplantation, in this case of the intestine. Evolution of this concept has explained how grafts are accepted (see text).

nantly dendritic cells from the donated organ and a large one that is in essence the entire recipient immune system of the patient—reach a "truce." This is so complete in some cases that immunosuppression can be stopped, particularly after liver transplantation and less constantly with other organs. Such a stable biologic state can be induced more easily by the liver than by other transplanted organs because of the liver's higher content of the critical missionary leukocytes. This was thought to be the explanation for the protection afforded the intestine by a concomitantly transplanted liver (38,39).

While still incomplete, this much information already provides a tool with which to shape future strategies (156,159). The migratory cells can be purified from the bone marrow or spleen of a donor and then infused to improve the "acceptability" of various organs from that specific donor including those taken from an animal for use in humans as xenografts. The cell migration and mixed chimerism phenomena make comprehensible the unexpected inability of donor-recipient HLA matching to accurately predict the outcome of whole organ transplantation (161). As a result of the mutual cell engagement, neither the new organ nor its new host remains the same as at the time of the matching tests.

WHOLE-ORGAN XENOTRANSPLANTATION

When organs are transplanted from a significantly disparate species, the first immunologic hurdle is that of preformed xenospecific antibodies, which quickly devascularize the graft and exclude it from recipient circulation by damaging its blood vessels (162). If this barrier can be surmounted, the process of xenograft acceptance involves the same bidirectional cell migration and consequent systemic chimerism as with allotransplantation (163). This means that successful clinical xenotransplantation must be visualized along the same lines of donor-recipient cellular migration and repopulation as with allograft acceptance.

SUMMARY

Over a period of 38 years, it has become possible to successfully transplant individual intra-abdominal viscera or combinations of these organs. The consequences have been, first, the acquisition of new information about the metabolic interrelations that the visceral organs have in disease or health; second, the addition of several transplant and nontransplant procedures to the treatment armamentarium for GI diseases; and third, the development of a more profound understanding of the means by which all whole organ grafts are "accepted."

REFERENCES

1. Terasaki PI: History of Transplantation: Thirty-Five Recollections. UCLA Tissue Typing Laboratory, Los Angeles, CA, 1991, pp. 1–691.
2. Woodruff WMA: The Transplantation of Tissues and Organs. Springfield, Charles C Thomas, 1960.
3. Welch CS: A note on transplantation of the whole liver in dogs. Transplant Bull 2:54, 1955.
4. Cannon JA: Brief Report. Transplant Bull 3:7, 1956.
5. Moore FD et al.: One-stage homotransplantation of the liver following total hepatectomy in dogs. Transplant Bull 6:103, 1959.
6. Moore FD et al.: Experimental whole organ transplantation of the liver and of the spleen. Ann Surg 152:374, 1960.
7. McBride RA et al.: Homotransplantation of the canine liver as an orthotopic vascularized graft. Histologic and functional correlations during residence in the new host. Am J Pathol 41:501, 1962.
8. Starzl TE et al.: Reconstructive problems in canine liver homotransplantation with special reference to the postoperative role of hepatic venous flow. Surg Gynecol Obstet 111:733, 1960.
9. Starzl TE, Kaupp HA Jr, Brock DR, Linman JW: Studies on the rejection of the transplanted homologous dog liver. Surg Gynecol Obstet 112:135, 1961.
10. Moore FD: Give and Take. The Development of Tissue Transplantation. Philadelphia, WB Saunders Company and Garden City, New York, Doubleday and Company, 1964, pp. 1–182.

11. Meyer WH Jr, Starzl TE: The reverse portacaval shunt. Surgery *45*:531, 1959.

12. Meyer WH Jr, Starzl TE: The effect of Eck and reverse Eck fistula in dogs with experimental diabetes mellitus. Surgery *45*:760, 1959.

13. Starzl TE: A trip south. *In The Puzzle People*. Pittsburgh, University of Pittsburgh Press, 1992. pp. 47–58.

14. Porter R, Whelan J (eds): Hepatotrophic Factors Ciba Foundation Symposium No. 55. Amsterdam, Excerpta Medica (Elsevier North-Holland), 1978, pp. 1–396.

15. Starzl TE, Porter KA, Francavilla A: The Eck fistula in animals and humans. Curr Probl Surg *20*:687, 1983.

16. Starzl TE, Bernhard VM, Benvenuto R, Cortes N: A new method for one-stage hepatectomy in dogs. Surgery *46*:880, 1959.

17. Starzl TE: *In*: Moore FP et al. (Reference 6): Discussion. Ann Surg *152*:386, 1960.

18. Wall WJ et al.: Simple hypothermic preservation for transporting human livers long distance for transplantation. Transplantation *23*:210, 1977.

19. Benichou J et al.: Canine and human liver preservation for 6 to 18 hours by cold infusion. Transplantation *24*:407, 1977.

20. Jamieson NV et al.: Successful 24- to 30-hour preservation of the canine liver: A preliminary report. Transplantation Proceedings *20*(Suppl. 1):945, 1988.

21. Kalayoglu M et al.: Extended preservation of the liver for clinical transplantation. Lancet *i*:617, 1988.

22. Todo S et al.: Extended preservation of human liver grafts with UW solution. JAMA *261*:711, 1989.

23. Picache RS, Kapur BML, Starzl TE: The effect of liver disease on the need for venous decompression during the anhepatic phase of canine orthotopic liver transplantation. Surgery *67*:319, 1970.

24. Starzl TE et al.: Orthotopic homotransplantation of the human liver. Ann Surg *168*: 392, 1968.

25. Starzl TE et al.: Evolution of liver transplantation. Hepatology *2*:614, 1982.

26. Denmark SW, Shaw BW, Starzl TE, Griffith BP: Veno-venous bypass without systemic anticoagulation in canine and human liver transplantation. Surg Forum *34*:380, 1983.

27. Shaw BW et al.: Venous bypass in clinical liver transplantation. Ann Surg *200*:524, 1984.

28. Griffith BP et al.: Veno-venous bypass without systemic anticoagulation for transplantation of the human liver. Surg Gynecol Obstet *160*:270, 1985.

29. Lillehei RC, Goott B, Miller FA: The physiologic response of the small bowel of the dog to ischemia including prolonged in vitro preservation of the bowel with successful replacement and survival. Ann Surg *150*: 543, 1959.

30. Craddock GN et al.: Small bowel transplantation in the dog using cyclosporine. Transplantation *35*:284, 1983.

31. Grant D et al.: Successful intestinal transplantation in pigs treated with cyclosporine. Transplantation *45*:279, 1988.

32. Diliz-Perez HS et al.: Successful small bowel allotransplantation in dogs with cyclosporine and prednisone. Transplantation *37*:126, 1984.

33. Deltz E et al.: Graft-versus-host reaction in small bowel transplantation and possibilities for its circumvention. Am J Surg *151*: 379, 1986.

34. Ricour C et al.: Successful small bowel allografts in piglets using cyclosporine. Transplant Proc *15*:3019, 1983.

35. Goulet O et al.: Successful small bowel transplantation in an infant. Transplantation *53*:940, 1992.

36. Todo S et al.: Intestinal transplantation in composite visceral grafts or alone. Ann Surg *216*:223, 1992.

37. Starzl TE, Kaupp HA Jr: Mass homotransplantation of abdominal organs in dogs. Surg Forum *11*:28, 1960.

38. Starzl TE et al.: The many faces of multivisceral transplantation. Surg Gynecol Obstet *172*:335, 1991.

39. Starzl TE et al.: Homotransplantation of multiple visceral organs. Am J Surg *103*: 219, 1962.

40. Calne RY et al.: Induction of immunological tolerance by porcine liver allografts. Nature *223*:472, 1969.

41. Kamada N: The immunology of experimental liver transplantation in the rat. Immunology *55*:369, 1985.

42. Valdivia LA et al.: Successful hamster to rat liver xenotransplantation under FK506 immunosuppression induces unresponsiveness to hamster heart and skin. Transplantation *56*:2:489, 1993.

43. Billingham R, Brent L: Quantitative studies on transplantation immunity. IV. Induction of tolerance in newborn mice and studies on the phenomenon of runt disease. Philos Trans R Soc Lond (Biol) *242*:439, 1956.

44. Trentin JJ: Mortality and skin transplantibility in X-irradiated mice receiving isologous or heterologous bone marrow. Proc Soc Exper Biol Med *92*:688, 1956.

45. Monchik GJ, Russell PS: Transplantation of the small bowel in the rat: Technical and

immunologic considerations. Surgery *70*: 693, 1971.

46. Starzl TE et al.: Transplantation of multiple abdominal viscera. JAMA *26*:1449, 1989.

47. Houssay BA: Technique de la greffe pancreaticoduodenal au cou. CR Soc Biol *100*: 138, 1929.

48. DeJode LR, Howard JM: Studies in pancreaticoduodenal homotransplantation. Surg Gynecol Obstet *114*:553, 1962.

49. Idezuki Y, Feemster JA, Dietzman RH, Lillehei RC: Experimental pancreaticoduodenal preservation and transplantation. Surg Gynecol Obstet *126*:1002, 1968.

50. Kelly WD et al.: Allotransplantation of the pancreas and duodenum along with the kidney in diabetic nephropathy. Surgery *61*: 827, 1967.

51. Goodrich EO Jr et al.: Homotransplantation of the canine liver. Surgery *39*:244, 1956.

52. Putnam CW, Porter KA, Starzl TE: Hepatic encephalopathy and light and electron micrographic changes of the baboon liver after portal diversion. Ann Surg *184*:155, 1976.

53. Mann FC: The William Henry Welch Lectures: II. Restoration and pathologic reactions of the liver. J Mt Sinai Hosp *11*:65, 1944.

54. Child CG, Barr D, Holswade GR, Harrison CS: Liver regeneration following portacaval transposition in dogs. Ann Surg *138*: 600, 1953.

55. Fisher B, Russ C, Updegraff H, Fisher ER: Effect of increased hepatic blood flow upon liver regeneration. Arch Surg *69*:263, 1954.

56. Bollman JL: The animal with an Eck fistula. Physiol Rev *41*:607, 1961.

57. Starzl TE et al.: Immunosuppression after experimental and clinical homotransplantation of the liver. Ann Surg *160*:411, 1964.

58. Marchioro TL et al.: Physiologic requirements for auxiliary liver homotransplantation. Surg Gynecol Obstet *121*:17, 1965.

59. Marchioro TL et al.: The effect of partial portacaval transposition on the canine liver. Surgery *61*:723, 1967.

60. Starzl TE et al.: The origin, hormonal nature, and action of hepatotrophic substances in portal venous blood. Surg Gynecol Obstet *137*:179, 1973.

61. Starzl TE et al.: The effect of diabetes mellitus on portal blood hepatotrophic factors in dogs. Surg Gynecol Obstet *140*:549, 1975.

62. Starzl TE, Porter KA, Kashiwagi N, Putnam CW: Portal hepatotrophic factors, diabetes mellitus and acute liver atrophy, hypertrophy and regeneration. Surg Gynecol Obstet *141*:843, 1975.

63. Starzl TE, Lee IY, Porter KA, Putnam CW: The influence of portal blood upon lipid metabolism in normal and diabetic dogs and baboons. Surg Gynecol Obstet *140*:381, 1975.

64. Starzl TE, Francavilla A, Porter KA, Benichou J: The effect upon the liver of evisceration with or without hormone replacement. Surg Gynecol Obstet *146*:524, 1978.

65. Starzl TE et al.: The effect of splanchnic viscera removal upon canine liver regeneration. Surg Gynecol Obstet *147*:193, 1978.

66. Starzl TE, Watanabe K, Porter KA, Putnam CW: Effects of insulin, glucagon, and insulin/glucagon infusions on liver morphology and cell division after complete portacaval shunt in dogs. Lancet *i*:821, 1976.

67. Starzl TE et al.: Growth-stimulating factor in regenerating canine liver. Lancet *i*:127, 1979.

68. Francavilla A et al.: Screening for candidate hepatic growth factors by selective portal infusion after canine Eck fistula. Hepatology *14*:665, 1991.

69. Mazzaferro V et al.: The hepatotrophic influence of cyclosporine. Surgery *107*:533, 1990.

70. Starzl TE et al.: Hepatotrophic effects of FK 506 in dogs. Transplantation *51*:67, 1991.

71. Starzl TE, Terblanche J: Hepatotrophic substances. *In* Popper H, Schaffner F (eds): Progress in Liver Diseases, Volume 6 New York, Grune and Stratton, 1979, pp. 135–152.

72. Starzl TE et al.: Portal diversion for the treatment of glycogen storage disease in humans. Ann Surg *178*:525, 1973.

73. Starzl TE, Porter KA, Francavilla A, Iwatsuki S: Reversal of hepatic alpha-1-antitrypsin deposition after portacaval shunt. Lancet *ii*:424, 1983.

74. Starzl TE, Porter KA, Busuttil RW, Pichlmayr R: Portacaval shunt in 3 children with alpha-1-antitrypsin deficiency: 9 to 12–1/3 years later. Hepatology *11*:152, 1990.

75. Starzl TE, Chase HP, Putnam CW, Porter KA: Portacaval shunt in hyperlipoproteinemia. Lancet *ii*:940, 1973.

76. Starzl TE et al.: Portacaval shunt in patients with familial hypercholesterolemia. Ann Surg *198*:273, 1983.

77. Starzl TE, Bell RH, Beart RW, Putnam CW: Hepatic trisegmentectomy and other liver resections. Surg Gynecol Obstet *141*: 429, 1975.

78. Starzl TE et al.: Left hepatic trisegmentectomy. Surg Gynecol Obstet *155*:21, 1982.

79. Starzl TE: The French heritage in clinical

kidney transplantation. Transplantation Reviews *7*:65, 1993.

80. Medawar PB: The behavior and fate of skin autografts and skin homografts in rabbits. J Anat *78*:176, 1944.

81. Medawar PB: Second study of behavior and fate of skin homografts in rabbits. J Anat *79*:157, 1945.

82. Dempster WJ, Lennox B, Boag JW: Prolongation of survival of skin homotransplants in the rabbit by irradiation of the host. Br J Exp Pathol *31*:670, 1950.

83. Billingham RE, Krohn PL, Medawar PB: Effect of cortisone on survival of skin homografts in rabbits. Br Med J *1*:1157, 1951.

84. Morgan JA: The influence of cortisone on the survival of homografts of skin in the rabbit. Surgery *30*:506, 1951.

85. Meeker WR et al.: Prolongation of skin homograft survival in rabbits by 6-mercaptopurine. Proc Soc Exp Biol *102*:459, 1959.

86. Schwartz R, Dameshek W: The effects of 6-mercaptopurine on homograft reactions. J Clin Invest *39*:952, 1960.

87. Calne RY: The rejection of renal homografts: Inhibition in dogs by 6-mercaptopurine. Lancet *i*:417, 1960.

88. Zukoski CF, Lee HM, Hume DM: The prolongation of functional survival of canine renal homografts by 6-mercaptopurine. Surg Forum *11*:470, 1960.

89. Calne RY, Murray JE: Inhibition of the rejection of renal homografts in dogs by Burroughs Wellcome 57–322, Surg Forum *12*:118, 1961.

90. Murray JE et al.: Study of transplantation immunity after total body irradiation: Clinical and experimental investigation. Surgery *48*:272, 1960.

91. Murray JE et al.: Kidney transplantation in modified recipients. Ann Surg *156*:337, 1962.

92. Murray JE et al.: Prolonged survival of human-kidney homografts by immunosuppressive drug therapy. New Engl J Med *268*:1315, 1963.

93. Woodruff MFA et al.: Homotransplantation of kidney in patients treated with preoperative administration of antimetabolite (Imuran). Lancet *ii*:675, 1963.

94. Goodwin WE, Martin DC: Transplantation of the kidney. Urol Survey *13*:229, 1963.

95. Groth CG: Landmarks in clinical renal transplantation. Surg Gynecol Obstet *134*:323, 1972.

96. Hamburger J et al.: Renal homotransplantation in man after radiation of the recipient. Am J Med *32*:854, 1962.

97. Kuss R et al.: Homologous human kidney transplantation. Experience with six patients. Postgrad Med J *38*:528, 1962.

98. Marchioro TL et al.: The role of adrenocortical steroids in reversing established homograft rejection. Surgery *55*:412, 1964.

99. Starzl TE, Marchioro TL, Waddell WR: The reversal of rejection in human renal homografts with subsequent development of homograft tolerance. Surg Gynecol Obstet *117*:385, 1963.

100. Starzl TE: Experience in Renal Transplantation. Philadelphia, WB Saunders Company, 1964, pp. 1–383.

101. Starzl TE et al.: Long term (25 year) survival after renal homotransplantation—the world experience. Transplant Proc *22*:2361, 1990.

102. Hume DM et al.: Renal transplantation in man in modified recipients. Ann Surg *158*:608, 1963.

103. Starzl TE et al.: Factors determining short- and long-term survival after orthotopic liver homotransplantation in the dog. Surgery *58*:131, 1965.

104. Starzl TE: Early liver rejection in patients without hepatic gangrene. *In* Experience in Hepatic Transplantation Philadelphia, WB Saunders Company, 1969, pp. 277–307.

105. Franksson C: Survival of homografts of skin in rats depleted of lymphocytes by chronic drainage from the thoracic duct. Lancet *i*:1331, 1984.

106. Starzl TE, Marchioro TL, Talmage DW, Waddel WR: Splenectomy and thymectomy in human renal transplantation. Proc Soc Exp Biol Med *113*:929, 1963.

107. Starzl TE et al.: The use of heterologous antilymphoid agents in canine renal and liver homotransplantation and in human renal homotransplantation. Surg Gynecol Obstet *124*:301, 1967.

108. Starzl TE et al.: Cyclophosphamide and whole organ transplantation in humans. Surg Gynecol Obstet *133*:981, 1971.

109. Strober S et al.: Transplantation tolerance after total lymphoid irradiation. Transplant Proc *11*:1032, 1979.

110. Najarian JS et al.: Fractional total lymphoid irradiation (TL1) as preparative immunosuppression on high risk renal transplantation. Ann Surg *196*:442, 1982.

111. Calne RY et al.: Cyclosporin A initially as the only immunosuppressant in 34 recipients of cadaveric organs: 32 kidneys, 2 pancreases, and 2 livers. Lancet *ii*:1033, 1979.

112. Starzl TE et al.: The use of cyclosporin A and prednisone in cadaver kidney transplantation. Surg Gynecol Obstet *151*:17, 1980.

113. Starzl TE et al.: Thoracic duct drainage before and after cadaveric kidney transplantation. Surg Gynecol Obstet *149*:815, 1979.

114. Starzl TE et al.: FK 506 for human liver, kidney and pancreas transplantation. Lancet *ii*:1000, 1989.

115. Starzl TE et al.: Homotransplantation of the liver in humans. Surg Gynecol Obstet *117*:659, 1963.

116. Reemtsma K et al.: Renal heterotransplantation in man. Ann Surg *160*:384, 1964.

117. Starzl TE et al.: Renal homotransplantation from baboon to man: Experience with 6 cases. Transplantation 2:752, 1964.

118. Starzl TE: Substance or Stunts? In The Puzzle People. Pittsburgh, University of Pittsburgh Press, 1992, pp. 70–82.

119. Starzl TE: The Failed Liver Transplant Trials. In: The Puzzle People. Pittsburgh, University of Pittsburgh Press, Pennsylvania, 1992, pp. 96–105.

120. Moore FD et al.: Immunosuppression and vascular insufficiency in liver transplantation. Ann NY Acad Sci *102*:729, 1964.

121. Demirleau NN et al.: Tentative d'homogreffe hepatique (Attempted hepatic homograft). Mem Acad Chir (Paris) *90*:177, 1964.

122. Starzl TE: The Donors and the Organs. In The Puzzle People. Pittsburgh, University of Pittsburgh Press, 1992.

123. Brettschneider L et al.: The use of combined preservation techniques for extended storage of orthotopic liver homografts. Surg Gynecol Obstet *126*:263, 1968.

124. Starzl TE: A pyrrhic victory. In The Puzzle People. Pittsburgh, University of Pittsburgh Press, 1992, pp. 162–172.

125. Calne RY, Williams R: Liver transplantation in man. I. Observations on technique and organization in five cases. Br Med J *4*: 535, 1968.

126. Starzl TE: Icebergs and hammer blows. In The Puzzle People. Pittsburgh, University of Pittsburgh Press, 1992, pp. 173–196.

127. Starzl TE et al.: Liver transplantation with the use of cyclosporin A and prednisone. N Engl J Med *305*:266, 1981.

128. Todo S et al.: Liver, kidney, and thoracic organ transplantation under FK 506. Ann Surg *212*:295, 1990.

129. Starzl TE et al.: Biliary complications after liver transplantation: With special reference to the biliary cast syndrome and techniques of secondary duct repair. Surgery *81*:212, 1977.

130. Groth CG: Changes in coagulation. In Starzl TE: Experience in Hepatic Transplantation. Philadelphia, WB Saunders Company, 1969, pp. 159–192.

131. Starzl TE, Groth CG, Makowka L: Liver transplantation: In Clio Chirurgica. Austin, Texas, Silvergirl, Inc. 1988, pp. 1–363.

132. Starzl TE: Experience in Renal Transplantation. Philadelphia, WB Saunders Company, 1964, pp. 68–71.

133. Marchioro TL, Huntley RT, Waddell WR, Starzl TE: Extracorporeal perfusion for obtaining postmortem homografts. Surgery *54*:900, 1963.

134. Starzl TE: Experience in Hepatic Transplantation. Philadelphia, WB Saunders Company, 1969, pp. 45–48.

135. Ackerman JR, Snell ME: Cadaveric renal transplantation. Br J Urol *40*:515, 1968.

136. Merkel FK, Jonasson O, Bergan JJ: Procurement of cadaver donor organs. Evisceration technique. Transplant Proc *4*:585, 1972.

137. Starzl TE et al.: A flexible procedure for multiple cadaveric organ procurement. Surg Gynecol Obstet *158*:223, 1984.

138. Starzl TE, Miller C, Broznick B, Makowka L: An improved technique for multiple organ harvesting. Surg Gynecol Obstet *165*: 343, 1987.

139. Starzl TE, Demetris AJ, Van Thiel DH: Medical progress: Liver transplantation. N Engl J Med Part I *321*:1014, 1989; Part II *321*:1092, 1989.

140. Starzl TE: The Little Drummer Girls. In The Puzzle People. Pittsburgh, University of Pittsburgh Press, 1992, pp. 318–333.

141. Starzl TE et al.: Vascular homografts from cadaveric organ donors. Surg Gynecol Obstet *149*:737, 1979.

142. Shaw BW Jr, Iwatsuki S, Bron K, Starzl TE: Portal vein grafts in hepatic transplantation. Surg Gynecol Obstet *161*:66, 1985.

143. Sheil AGR et al.: Mesoportal graft for thrombosed portal vein in liver transplantation. Clin Transplant *1*:18, 1987.

144. Tzakis A, Todo S, Stieber A, Starzl TE: Venous jump grafts for liver transplantation in patients with portal vein thrombosis. Transplantation *48*:530, 1989.

145. Stieber AC et al.: The spectrum of portal vein thrombosis. Ann Surg *213*:199, 1991.

146. Starzl TE, Demetris AJ. Liver Transplantation: A 31-Year Perspective. Chicago, Year Book Medical Publishers, Inc. 1990, pp. 38–41.

147. Bismuth H, Houssin D: Reduced-size orthotopic liver graft in hepatic transplantation in children. Surgery *95*:367, 1984.

148. Broelsch CE et al.: Orthotope transplantation von Lebesegmenten bei mit gallengangsatresien. (Orthotopic transplantation of hepatic segments in infants with biliary atresia). In Kolsowski L (ed): Chirurgisches Forum 1984, F. Experim U. Klimische Forschung Hrsga. New York, Springer-Verlag, 1984, pp. 105–109.

149. Starzl TE, Todo S, Tzakis A: Abdominal

organ cluster transplantation for the treatment of upper abdominal malignancies. Ann Surg *210*:374, 1989.

150. Pritchard TJ, Kirkman RL: Small bowel transplantation. World J Surg *9*:860, 1985.

151. Schroeder P, Goulet O, Lear P: Small bowel transplantation: European experience. Lancet *336*:110, 1990.

152. Starzl TE, Todo S, Tzakis A, Fung J: The transplantation of gastrointestinal organs. Gastroenterology *104*:673, 1993.

153. Grant D et al.: Successful small bowel/liver transplantation. Lancet *335*:181, 1990.

154. Deltz E et al.: Successful clinical small-bowel transplantation. Transplant Proc *22*: 2501, 1990.

155. Starzl TE et al.: Cell migration, chimerism, and graft acceptance. Lancet *339*:1579, 1992.

156. Starzl TE et al.: Cell migration and chimerism after whole organ transplantation: The basis of graft acceptance. Hepatology *17*: 1127, 1993.

157. Murase N et al.: Long survival in rats after multivisceral versus isolated small bowel allotransplantation under FK 506. Surgery *110*:87, 1991.

158. Iwaki Y et al.: Replacement of donor lymphoid tissue in human small bowel transplants under FK 506 immunosuppression. Lancet *337*:818, 1991.

159. Starzl TE et al.: Cell chimerism permitted by immunosuppressive drugs is the basis of organ transplant acceptance and tolerance. Immunology Today *14*:326, 1993.

160. Starzl TE et al.: Chimerism after liver transplantation for type IV glycogen storage disease and Type I Gaucher's disease. N Engl J Med *328*:745, 1993.

161. Starzl TE, Demetris AJ, Trucco M: HLA matching and the point system. Clinical Transplant *7*:4:Pt1:353, 1993.

162. Starzl TE: The future of xenotransplantation. Ann Surg *216(4)*:supplemental article, October, 1992.

163. Starzl TE et al.: Baboon to human liver transplantation. Lancet *341*:65, 1993.

Gallbladder

22

Developments in Cholelithiasis During the 20th Century*

LESLIE J. SCHOENFIELD

Cholelithiasis is the most common disorder of the biliary system. Gallstones are found in 10 to 20% of adults worldwide. They are classified as either cholesterol or pigment gallstones. Cholesterol gallstones are categorized as either pure, which contain over 90% cholesterol, or mixed, which contain 50 to 90% cholesterol. Pigment gallstones, which contain principally calcium bilirubinate and less than 20% cholesterol, are either black or brown (1).

In the United States and Europe, about 80% of gallstones are the cholesterol type (mostly mixed) and 20% are the pigment type (mostly black). In Asia, brown pigment gallstones predominated in the early part of this century; subsequently, however, fewer brown pigment gallstones and more cholesterol and black pigment gallstones were found, a pattern increasingly resembling the pattern in the Western world (2).

Gallstones are a major medical problem, even though most do not cause symptoms. When gallstones migrate from the gallbladder to obstruct the cystic duct, however, they cause biliary colic or acute cholecystitis; when they block the common bile duct, they cause biliary colic, cholangitis, jaundice, or acute pancreatitis. Accordingly, each year in the United States alone, one million new cases of gallstones are diagnosed and 600,000 cholecystectomies are done.

* Supported in part by the National Institute of Diabetes and Digestive and Kidney Diseases, Grant No. AM 37080.

Cholecystectomy has remained the treatment of choice since the early part of this century for most patients with symptomatic gallstones. In the past two decades, however, based on advances in understanding the physiochemistry involved in the formation of cholesterol gallstones, medical dissolution of gallstones by orally administered bile acids has provided an alternative therapy for some patients. Then, in the past few years, laparoscopic cholecystectomy, in whirlwind fashion, has virtually supplanted conventional cholecystectomy.

The early history of gallstones—that is, before the 20th century—has been the subject of scholarly publications by, among others, Donald C. Balfour (3), John M. Beal (4), Frank Glenn (5), Gordon Gordon-Taylor (6), William P. Longmire (7), and A. J. Harding Rains (8). Gallstones have been known for centuries. In fact, the first documentation of gallstones was in an Egyptian mummy, a priestess of Amen in the 21st Dynasty, around 1500 BC. The purpose of this chapter is to review developments in the field of cholelithiasis during the 20th century to highlight current areas of research and envision future areas.

PATHOGENESIS OF GALLSTONES

The pathogenesis differs between pigment gallstones and cholesterol gallstones, and more attention has been directed to the formation of cholesterol gallstones. The major issues in the pathogenesis of gall-stones that were addressed during the 20th century were the roles of infection, meta-bolic abnormalities, and the gallbladder.

Infection

According to A. J. Harding Rains (8), Bernard Naunyn in 1892 in Strassburg (Germany, at the time) believed that infection of the gallbladder was a cause rather than a result of gallstones (9). Naunyn determined that the desquamated, inflamed mucosal cells that he found in the gallbladder-bile of patients with gallstones were rich in cholesterol. Furthermore, he observed the formation of crystals of cholesterol in this bile. He believed that the crystals originated from the cholesterol in the inflamed cells.

By the start of the 20th century, coliform and typhoid organisms had been isolated from inflamed gallbladders (10). Also, Salmonella typhi had been injected into the gallbladders of rabbits and produced gallstones. In 1916, Rosenow injected streptococci parenterally into rabbits, simulating a blood-borne infection that caused cholecystitis and then gallstones (11). Wilkie, in 1927, extended Rosenow's observations. He injected streptococci cultured from cystic duct nodes of patients with cholecystitis directly into rabbits' gallbladders (12). The results were acute cholecystitis and gallstones in the rabbits.

Investigators continued to pursue an infectious cause of gallstones by culturing bile, gallbladder-tissue, or gallstones in patients with cholecystitis and by injecting organisms into animals (13). Coliform organisms were cultured most often, although in 1962, Rains cultured Actinomyces from about 50% of gallstones (14). The idea behind these lines of research was that infection of the gallbladder led to the production by the inflamed mucosa of abnormal proteins and excess cholesterol. The proteins, the exfoliated cells, or even the clumps of bacteria then could serve as a center or nidus for the growth of pigment or cholesterol gallstones.

In 1966, Maki from Japan showed that the enzyme beta-glucuronidase, found in the bacteria in bile, deconjugates the bilirubin glucuronides in bile (15). Escherichia coli, a source of this enzyme, was the most frequently cultured organism in bile in the Orient (16). The resulting unconjugated bilirubin precipitates with calcium. Maki proposed that the calcium bilirubinate then goes on to form pigment gallstones or becomes the nidus of cholesterol gallstones.

Contemporary thinking, however, holds that infection is involved in the pathogenesis of only brown pigment gallstones (17). The formation of cholesterol gallstones or of black pigment gallstones, by contrast, is based on metabolic and physicochemical abnormalities. Of course, secondary inflammation or infection of the gallbladder can result from each type of gallstone. During the past 20 years or more, Ostrow and his colleagues (18) and Soloway and his colleagues (19) have contributed substantially to our understanding of the chemistry and physiology involved in the formation of pigment gallstones.

Metabolic Abnormality

A. J. Harding Rains described the concept, as understood at about the turn of the last century, of a metabolic abnormality as the basis for formation of gallstones (8). He related that J. L. W. Thudichum of London, in the latter part of the 19th century, studied the solubilization of cholesterol by bile salts and the crystallization of cholesterol in bile. Thudichum proposed that, as an initial step in the formation of gallstones, both cholesterol and bile pigment somehow were decomposed chemically and precipitated in the bile ductules of the liver; then, most gallstones grew in the gallbladder (20).

In 1900, J. Boysen developed novel sectioning techniques to study the microscopic appearance of the centers of gallstones (21). From his observations, he extended Thudichum's theory and suggested that granules of calcium bilirubinate were transported from the ducts of the liver by the flow of bile to the lumen of the gallbladder. There, according to Boysen, the granules either grow to form pigment gallstones or are infiltrated with cholesterol from the bile to form cholesterol gallstones.

Ludwig Aschoff and A. Bacmeister in Freiburg, Germany in 1909 observed the frequent occurrence of gallstones without antecedent infection or inflammation of the gallbladder (22). They had examined the bile and gallstones from more than 200 gallbladders removed by operation. Based on their data, they postulated that both a metabolic increase of biliary cholesterol and stasis of bile in the gallbladder were responsible for precipitation of cholesterol crystals and formation of gallstones. In 1925, Thorkild Rovsing from Copenhagen, studying the structure, composition, and bacteriology of gallstones, likewise favored a metabolic etiology for cholesterol gallstones (23). The concept was that the liver secreted bile that was saturated with cholesterol which then precipitated (that is, nucleated) from the saturated bile in the gallbladder.

Saturation

The detergent properties of bile salts, which are responsible in large part for maintaining cholesterol in solution in bile, have been recognized for almost 200 years. As already mentioned, Thudichum in the late 1800s investigated the solubilization of cholesterol by bile salts as a factor in the formation of gallstones. In 1913, McBain elaborated on the physicochemical properties of micelles of bile salts (24). He demonstrated that the ability of these ionic aggregates to lower the surface tension of solutions was responsible for their detergent or dissolving properties. In 1931, Andrews and colleagues showed that most of the cholesterol in human bile was present in water-soluble complexes with bile salts (25).

In 1954, Isaksson, extending the earlier work of several investigators, found that lecithin, the major phospholipid in bile, associates with the micelles of bile salts (26). The resultant mixed micelles of bile salts and lecithin are swollen and therefore have an augmented capacity to dissolve cholesterol. Isaksson showed in vitro that, if the weight ratio of bile salt plus lecithin to cholesterol were above 11:1, cholesterol precipitated out of solution. In the clinical situation, he found that more than 75% of patients with cholesterol gallstones had a ratio above 11:1. His ratio was somewhat flawed, however, in that it was an imprecise representation of the micellar solubilization of cholesterol.

In the early 1960s, Rains demonstrated that with increasing biliary concentration of bile salts and, therefore, increasing formation of micelles, the amount of cholesterol solubilized in bile increased steadily (14). On the other hand, he suggested that, as a result of an increase of cholesterol or a decrease of bile salts in bile, cholesterol would come out of solution. Accordingly, an excess of cholesterol beyond the capacity of bile to hold cholesterol in solution would provide the solid, crystalline cholesterol for the formation and growth of gallstones.

Alan Hofmann's contributions in the 1960s and 1970s to understanding the metabolism of bile acids, the enterohepatic circulation, and the solubilization of lipids, are legion (27). Also, during these two decades, the physicochemical studies carried out by Donald Small with Dervichian at the Institut Pasteur in Paris and then with Admirand and Carey in Boston validated the importance of saturation of bile with cholesterol in the formation of cholesterol gallstones (28–30). In landmark studies, Small and his colleagues used triangular coordinates to plot the relative molar concentrations of bile salts, lecithin, and cholesterol in model solutions and in bile (Fig. 22–1). Thus, any single point on the graph would fall into a zone representing saturated or unsaturated solutions.

Admirand and Small showed that the bile from patients with cholesterol gallstones virtually always was saturated or supersaturated with cholesterol. As a consequence, most investigators in cholelithiasis in the 1970s focused their research on saturation of biliary lipids. Also, a resurgence of interest in medical dissolution of gallstones during those years was attributable largely to this research. The results of analyses of biliary lipids can be presented on triangular coordinate graphs, as demonstrated by Admirand and Small, or alternatively as saturation indices or percentages; a value of 1 or 100% indicates saturated bile; higher values, supersaturated; and lower values, unsaturated (31). Because the saturation index or percentage was quantitative and easy to calculate, it became the usual way to present data on saturation of bile with cholesterol.

The most recently described vehicles for solubilization of cholesterol in bile are vesicles of lecithin, as reported in 1983 by Somjen and Gilat from Israel (32). The vesicles were characterized by quasi-elastic light scattering as large 700 Angstrom particles.

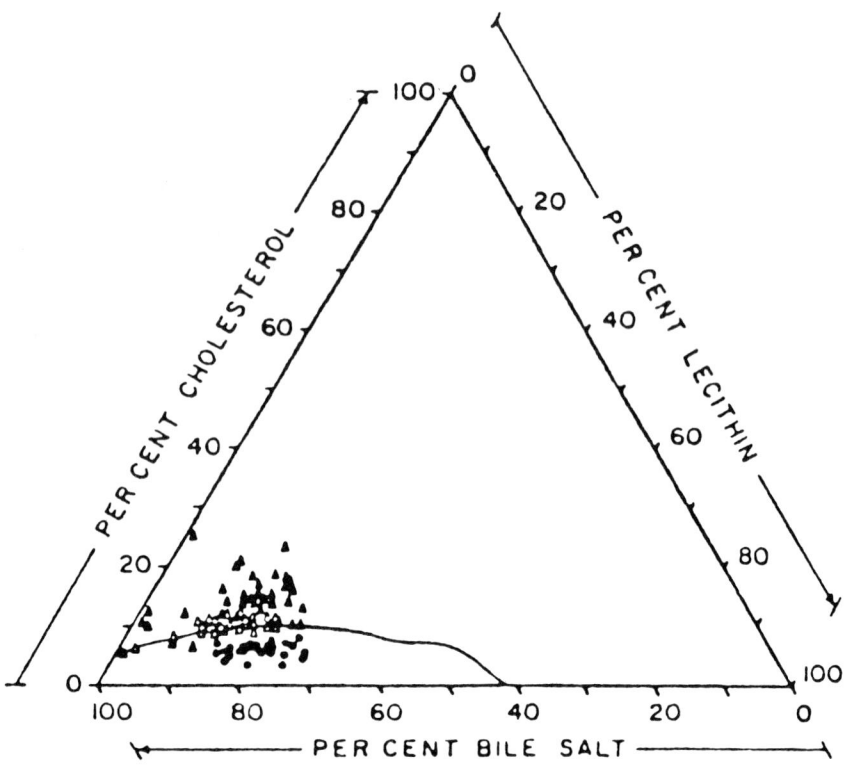

Fig. 22–1. The composition of gallbladder bile from normal subjects and patients with gallstones compared with the limits of cholesterol solubility as determined from a model system. The line representing maximal cholesterol solubilization has been superimposed on the triangle. The composition of bile from normal subjects (represented by closed circles) is such that all circles fall within the micellar zone. The bile samples from patients with cholesterol or mixed gallstones in which no microcrystals were present (open triangles) fall on or very near the line, indicating maximum cholesterol solubilization. The bile samples from gallstone patients, which contain microcrystals of cholesterol (closed triangle), fall well above the line of maximum saturation. Reproduced with permission from Admirand WH and Small DM: The physicochemical basis of cholesterol gallstone formation in man. J Clin Invest 47:1043, 1968, by copyright permission of the American Society for Clinical Investigation.

When the capacity of mixed micelles (20 to 60 Angstroms) to solubilize cholesterol is surpassed, the excess cholesterol is solubilized by the vesicles. Bile becomes saturated when the hepatic secretion of cholesterol is increased relative to that of the solubilizing agents, bile salts and lecithin. Indeed, most investigators have found that an increased secretion of cholesterol is the main secretory defect in most patients with cholesterol gallstones (33).

Today, we recognize several possible sources for the increased biliary cholesterol (34). For example, increased hepatic uptake of cholesterol can result from increased dietary or other extrahepatic cholesterol or from increased hepatic receptors. In fact,

animal models for formation of gallstones that depend on dietary alterations, used at least since the 1950s, have made important contributions to our understanding of the pathogenesis of gallstones (35,36). Other possible reasons for increased biliary secretion of cholesterol include increased hepatic synthesis of free cholesterol, decreased hepatic esterification of cholesterol, or decreased synthesis of bile acids from cholesterol. Research in the future will address the molecular basis for enzymatic or other cellular abnormalities.

Nucleation

Holzbach and his colleagues in 1973 observed that saturated bile often is found in individuals without cholesterol gallstones (37). Accordingly, although saturation of bile is prerequisite for the formation of cholesterol crystals and gallstones, it is not sufficient. These investigators, in 1979, then made a major discovery. They found that a short nucleation time in the bile of patients with gallstones distinguished these patients from control subjects without gallstones (Fig. 22–2) (38). (The nucleation time is the time it takes for saturated bile that is incubated in a test tube to nucleate its first crystal of cholesterol.) Accordingly, since then, nucleation has been the subject of most research on the pathogenesis of cholelithiasis.

For example, Harvey and colleagues, in 1987, observed that nucleation of cholesterol crystals from saturated solutions occurred from the vesicles of lecithin rather than from the mixed micelles (39). At about the same time, Halpern and colleagues, using time-lapse microscopy, depicted the sequence of events leading to nucleation (40). First, the vesicles, which are unilamellar, aggregate. Next, they fuse to form multilamellar vesicles or liquid crystals from which the solid crystals of cholesterol monohydrate emerge. In the meantime, the temporal sequence of events in bile—from biochemical changes to shortening of the nucleation time to formation of cholesterol crystals—was documented in patients who

are prone to form gallstones because of rapid weight loss (41).

As recently summarized by Afdahl and Smith, an increase in promoters of nucleation or a decrease in inhibitors of nucleation in bile favors nucleation (42). The putative promoters include, for example, mucous glycoproteins, immunoglobulins, and calcium. The putative inhibitors include apolipoproteins, low molecular weight proteins, and the vesicles of lecithin. Moreover, prostaglandins (perhaps coming from arachidonyl lecithin), by stimulating the gallbladder to produce mucous glycoproteins or by inhibiting contractility of smooth muscle, may be involved in formation of gallstones (34). One other important area for future research on the pathogenesis of gallstones will be the growth of individual cholesterol crystals and the growth of microscopic gallstones by aggregation of the crystals.

Role of the Gallbladder

The functions of the gallbladder were described elegantly by J. E. Sweet from Philadelphia in 1924 (43). He recognized that the primary purpose of the gallbladder is to store and concentrate bile between meals and then to deliver the bile to the intestine during meals to aid in digestion. To accom-

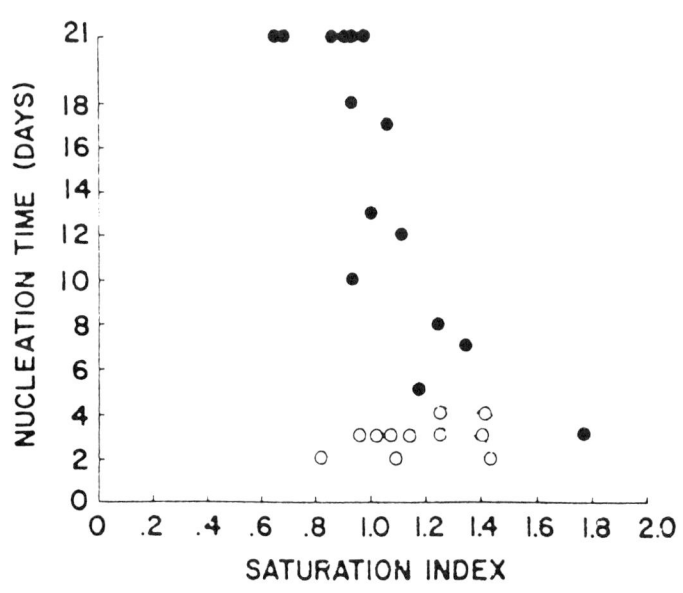

Fig. 22–2. The nucleation time of bile from patients with gallstones (open circles) was more rapid than that from controls without gallstones (closed circles), even when the saturation indices were similar. Modified from Holan KR, et al.: Nucleation time: A key factor in the pathogenesis of cholesterol gallstone disease. Gastroenterology 77: 611, 1979. Reproduced with permission.

plish this purpose, the crucial functions of the gallbladder are absorption to concentrate the bile and regulated emptying to discharge the concentrated bile in a timely manner. The gallbladder empties in response to the intestinal hormone, cholecystokinin. The concentrating process in the gallbladder was reviewed in detail by Henry Wheeler in 1971 (44).

The concept of stasis of bile or incomplete emptying of the gallbladder contributing to the formation of gallstones, as proposed by Aschoff and Bacmeister in 1909, was supported by the observations of Tera in 1960 (45). He described stratification of bile within the gallbladder sampled at the time of abdominal operations. The idea was that the stratification of the components of bile into layers was evidence of stasis of the gallbladder. Moreover, the interface between layers of proteinacious solutions of different specific gravities would provide a mileau for the precipitation of cholesterol.

More recent studies have shown that emptying of the gallbladder is abnormal, at least in some patients with gallstones. For example, Fisher and colleagues in 1982 (46), using the technique of cholescintigraphy developed by Spellman and colleagues (47), demonstrated significantly delayed emptying of the gallbladder in patients with gallstones compared to controls without gallstones. Accordingly, the concept of stasis of bile contributing to the formation of gallstones currently is in vogue. Furthermore, modern studies at the molecular level have found that receptors for cholecystokinin are decreased in the smooth muscle of gallbladders that empty poorly (48). Whether impaired emptying of the gallbladder is a cause or an effect of the gallstones, however, remains to be determined.

Nevertheless, an essential role for the gallbladder in the pathogenesis of cholesterol gallstones is well accepted (49). Clearly, the gallbladder is important because gallstones virtually always form in the gallbladder and rarely recur after cholecystectomy. In fact, the absorptive, secretory, and motor activities of the gallbladder each are thought to be involved in the formation of gallstones. Thus, concentration of bile promotes nucleation, insufficient acidification of bile hampers solubilization of calcium compounds, and impaired motility

provides the time for nucleation and growth. Moore and his colleagues recently have published extensively on the physicochemistry and solubilization of calcium bilirubinate and calcium channels in bile (50).

CLINICAL ASPECTS

Advances in the clinical area in the 20th century have been primarily in defining the natural history of gallstones, understanding their symptoms, and developing the technology for diagnostic imaging.

Epidemiology and Clinical Course

The most reliable epidemiologic information on gallstones in the 20th century has been acquired in the last 25 years or so. Before then, the data were apt to be biased because they were obtained from symptomatic patients (51) or autopsy studies (52). Then, in 1970, Sampliner and colleagues in Phoenix determined the true prevalence and the epidemiology of cholelithiasis in the Pima Indians, a well-defined population at high risk for developing gallstones (53). The overall prevalence of gallbladder disease, based on chart review, symptoms, cholecystography, and autopsy was strikingly high—50%. Most of these patients were asymptomatic at the time of diagnosis.

All epidemiologic studies have revealed that women have perhaps twice as many cholesterol gallstones as men, although the prevalence of cholesterol and pigment gallstones increases with age in both genders (54). Still, the prevalence of gallstones differs widely among various racial groups. For example, among women in the United States, the prevalence was 14.7% in Mexican-Americans, 9% in whites, and 4.5% in blacks (55).

Many other clinical associations with gallstones have been debated over the years; a few correlations have been established. For example, obesity clearly has been identified as a risk factor for the formation of gallstones (56). Furthermore, as originally noted by Burrill Crohn in 1958 (57), obese patients develop gallstones during rapid loss of weight (58). Also, significant associations of gallstones with female sex hormones have been made in several collaborative studies, as in young women on oral contraceptives (59), older women taking estrogens (60), and even men treated with estrogens to lower serum lipids (61). Finally, rather solid data obtained by Gilat and colleagues in 1983 using oral cholecystography demonstrated the familial nature of gallstones (62). In the future, even larger studies using ultrasonography and biochemical markers or molecular probes will establish the genetics of cholelithiasis.

Two extensive, ongoing, prospective epidemiologic surveys in Italy, using ultrasonography to detect gallstones, began in the mid-1980s and already have provided much information. The Sirmioni Study found an 11% prevalence of gallstones, more than three quarters of which were in asymptomatic patients (63). The GREPCO Study in Rome observed that older women have only a slightly higher incidence than men but that the gallstones are symptomatic more often in these women (64). Neither study thus far has been able to identify characteristics of the patients or their stones that predispose to the development of biliary symptoms.

The conclusion by W. J. Mayo in 1911 that innocent gallstones are a "myth" was based on the clinical diagnosis of cholelithiasis without the aid of imaging techniques (65). Decades later, in 1982, Gracie and Ransohoff reported on the natural history of gallstones detected by routine cholecystography in asymptomatic faculty at the University of Michigan (66). The investigators found that only 18% of the patients developed biliary symptoms during 10 to 20 years of follow-up. These data established the concept that asymptomatic gallstones, with few exceptions, should be managed by observation alone (67). Perhaps an earlier study in 1948 by Comfort and colleagues at the Mayo Clinic had suggested as much (68). Certainly, subsequent studies of asymptomatic gallstones, including those detected by routine ultrasonography (69), confirmed the innocuous clinical course.

Modern data on the natural history of symptomatic gallstones also has been obtained. In these patients, in accordance with the earlier reports (70), recurrent biliary symptoms or complications develop during follow-up far more often than in asymptomatic patients (71). Accordingly, symptomatic gallstones usually require treatment.

Still, data from the placebo group of the National Cooperative Gallstone Study indicated that the longer the symptom-free interval, the less the chance of developing future biliary pain (72).

Biliary Pain

Remarkably, considering that no specific diagnostic methods were available at the time, physicians as early as the 16th and 17th centuries recorded certain manifestations of gallstones, notably jaundice, abdominal pain, adhesions, fistulas, and fever. In 1925, within a year after the introduction of contrast cholecystography, Sir Humphrey Rolleston of London provided a comprehensive description of the clinical manifestations of gallstones (73). He classified the manifestations as mechanical or infectious, emphasizing their dependence on the location of the gallstones or of the inflammation. Still, the mechanism of biliary pain was not yet well understood.

In 1933, Zollinger performed experiments in humans to elucidate biliary pain (74). After completing a cholecystostomy for gallstones in six patients, he distended the gallbladder and common bile duct with a balloon during the surgery. The distension consistently produced epigastric pain.

The mechanism of biliary pain was studied further by Schein and Beneventano in 1968 (75). They induced choledochal hypertension by instillation of radiopaque material through a T-tube into the common bile duct 10 to 14 days after cholecystectomy. A manometer was attached to the T-tube. They found that the infusion led sequentially to increased intraductal pressure, dilation of the duct, and finally biliary pain when the distension was maximal. More recently, prostaglandins have been implicated as mediators of biliary pain while inhibitors of prostaglandins—specifically, nonsteroidal anti-inflammatory drugs—were shown to alleviate the pain (76).

The clinical characteristics of biliary colic, described by Littler and Ellis in 1952 (77) and French and Robb in 1963 (78), and the patterns of referral of biliary pain detailed by Doran in 1967 (79) were substantiated for the most part by Gunn and Keddie in 1972 (80). Colic actually is a misnomer because biliary colic is a steady pain rather than a colicky pain. It is of sudden onset, severe, often requires a narcotic for relief, and lasts up to 6 hours. The pain is usually in the epigastrium or right upper quadrant and may radiate to the interscapular area, tip of the right scapula, or right shoulder. The patient often is nauseated and moves about with the pain, seeking but failing to find a position of relief.

Does spasm of the sphincter of Oddi also cause biliary pain? In the 1940s and 1950s, Boyden provided a definitive description of the musculature of the sphincter of Oddi (81). But it was not until 1977 that Geenen and his colleagues developed a perfusion system to provide accurate manometric pressure recordings from the sphincter (82). Since then, dysfunction (including spasm) of the sphincter of Oddi has been documented by these investigators as a cause of biliary pain (83). Furthermore, the pain in these patients could be relieved by endoscopic sphincterotomy.

Koch and Donaldson in 1964 dispelled the notion, held even by Rolleston in 1925, that dyspepsia or fried and fatty food intolerance is caused by gallstones (84). They found no characteristic patterns of food intolerance among patients with specific gastrointestinal diseases, including gallstones. Rather, as subsequently suggested by Johnson, patients with nonspecific dyspepsia may have increased reflux of duodenal contents into the stomach causing mucosal injury (85). The underlying mechanism of the nonspecific dyspepsia, then, is thought to be an abnormality of antroduodenal motility.

All of the foregoing discussion of biliary pain notwithstanding, the established definition of biliary pain is being reevaluated currently and in fact, questioned. For example, in one contemporary epidemiologic study, the sensitivity and specificity of acute pain in the upper abdomen for the diagnosis of gallstones were very low (86). Still another study, extending the definition of biliary pain somewhat, demonstrated better sensitivity and a high specificity (87). Furthermore, a circadian rhythm recently has been recognized wherein biliary pain, in contrast to renal colic, occurs most often at about 1 a.m. (88). So, we have not heard the last of this debate on the nature of biliary pain.

Diagnosis

The diagnosis of gallstones is suspected clinically based on the patient's symptoms, but is established usually by biliary imaging and occasionally by biliary drainage.

Biliary Imaging

The developments in imaging of the biliary system for the diagnosis of gallstones are reviewed in more detail in another chapter. From the time of the discovery of x-rays by William Conrad Roentgen in 1895 until 1924, only plain films to detect radiopaque gallstones were available. Then, the development of intravenous and oral cholecystography, introduced by Everts Graham and Warren Cole, was a major advance for the diagnosis of gallstones (89). The contrast techniques reigned until the technologic advances of the 1960s and 1970s. Then, ultrasonography, which obviated exposure to x-rays and was much quicker than oral cholecystography, became the technique of choice to detect gallstones in the gallbladder (90).

CAT scan and MRI are important for abdominal imaging but have little applicability for the diagnosis of gallstones. During the technologic era, however, endoscopic retrograde cholangiography (91) and the skinny needle technique for transhepatic cholangiography (92) were developed and perfected to visualize the bile ducts. At about the same time, hepatobiliary scanning with technicium labeled compounds was shown to be useful for the diagnosis of acute calculous cholecystitis (93).

Biliary Drainage

Meltzer in 1917 developed the hypothesis of contrary innervation, whereby relaxation of the sphincter of Oddi triggers reflex contraction of the gallbladder which consequently discharges bile into the duodenum (94). Then, in 1919, biliary drainage was introduced by Lyon for the diagnosis of gallstones (95). In this so-called Meltzer-Lyon test, bile is aspirated through a duodenal tube after inducing contraction of the gallbladder by magnesium sulfate (later replaced by cholecystokinin or its octapeptide). The bile then is examined microscopically for cholesterol crystals which, if found, indicate the presence of cholesterol gallstones in the gallbladder. (The clinical significance of finding bilirubinate granules in the drainage is not certain.) With the advent of oral cholecystography for the diagnosis of gallstones, however, diagnostic biliary drainage largely was abandoned.

Approximately 30 years later, biliary drainage was resurrected, stimulated by the detailed studies of Kerrison Juniper in 1957 (96). Today, the test is useful in patients who have biliary-type pain and a normal cholecystogram and ultrasonogram (97). If these patients have tiny cholesterol gallstones, microscopic examination of the biliary drainage usually reveals cholesterol crystals. (Gallstones less than 1 or 2 mm in diameter are too small to visualize by cholecystography or ultrasonography.) In contrast, the ultrasonographic finding of sludge in the gallbladder cannot be used to suggest the diagnosis of gallstones. Although sludge purportedly comprises cholesterol crystals, calcium bilirubinate granules, and mucin (98), and provides an appropriate milieu for the formation of gallstones, the relevance of ultrasonographic sludge in the diagnosis or, for that matter, pathogenesis of gallstones has not been established.

TREATMENT

Cholecystectomy is the treatment of choice for most patients with symptomatic gallstones. Medical dissolution, however, provides an alternative for some of these patients.

Cholecystectomy

According to Longmire (7), the first well-documented cholecystostomy (to incise and close the gallbladder), although described and possibly done earlier by Thudichum, was performed by John Bobbs in Indianapolis in 1868 (99). The first cholecystostomy (to maintain a stoma in the gallbladder) was accomplished by James Marion Sims in New York in 1878 (100). Then, Carl Langenbuch performed the first planned cholecystectomy for gallstones in Berlin in 1882 (101). Langenbuch believed that cholecystostomy to remove gallstones was not

adequate treatment. He recommended removal of the gallbladder, not just because it contained gallstones, but because it formed them (102).

The first cholecystectomy in America was done in 1886 by Justus Ohage in St. Paul, Minnesota (103). He echoed Langenbuch's opinion that the gallbladder is not essential for life. Some species actually lack a gallbladder, yet their digestion is not impaired. Years later, Wakim and Mahour evaluated the pathophysiologic consequences of cholecystectomy (104). They acknowledged that the operation deprives the patient of such functions of the gallbladder as storage, concentration, and pressure regulation. They concluded, however, that postoperative functional and structural adaptations are sufficient to compensate the digestive process for the loss of the gallbladder.

From the late 19th century to the early 20th century, the increasing application of several major advances in science greatly facilitated the performance of abdominal surgery. These advances included antiseptic techniques, general anesthesia, and parenteral nutrition. Subsequently, antibiotics, transfusions of blood, and vitamin K for hypoprothrombinemia furthered the safety of biliary surgery.

In the first two decades of the 20th century, however, cholecystectomy still was hazardous, carrying a mortality of about 20%. During those years, the relative merits of cholecystostomy and cholecystectomy were debated hotly (105). The main problem with cholecystostomy was recurrence of gallstones. So, by 1926, when W. J. Mayo reported that cholecystectomy was accomplished with a very low (<2%, then <1%) mortality rate, cholecystectomy became the operation of choice (106).

Along the way, Mirizzi and Losada of Argentina in 1932 introduced operative cholangiography to visualize ductal gallstones (107). More recently, for the same purpose, Berci and colleagues in the United States refined operative choledochoscopy (108). Accordingly, these intraoperative techniques seem to have substantially reduced the incidence of retained ductal gallstones.

Phillip Mouret from Lyons, France, is said to have performed the first laparoscopic cholecystectomy in 1987. Then, within just a few years, stimulated largely by the experience of Reddick in the United States (109) and Dubois (110) and Perissat (111) in France, an estimated 80% of cholecystectomies were done by this technique. Laparoscopic cholecystectomy offers distinct advantages over open cholecystectomy. It decreases postoperative pain and disability because of the small incisions, without increasing mortality or overall morbidity. However, the frequency of injury to the common bile duct appears to be increased, and a longer follow-up of its safety still is needed.

Medical Dissolution

At the end of the 19th century, Naunyn reported, as had other investigators, that human gallstones placed in the gallbladder of dogs dissolved in a few months (9). The gallstones disappeared because the cholesterol from the gallstones was solubilized in the bile of the dogs, which normally has a relatively low concentration of cholesterol. As the gallstones dissolved, the bile of the dogs became saturated with the cholesterol. This canine model and an increasing understanding of the mechanisms for solubilization of cholesterol provided the scientific basis for the use of bile acids to dissolve cholesterol gallstones.

Oral Bile Acids

In 1876, William C. Dabney of Charlottesville, Virginia reported the oral administration of choleate of soda to four patients who had attacks of "gallstone colic" (112). Dabney credits Moritz Schiff in Florence, Italy with proposing, about 3 years earlier, this treatment to prevent gallstones (113). The rationale was that the choleate of soda would solubilize the cholesterol in bile before the cholesterol could form the gallstones that cause the colic. In Dabney's case reports, three of the four patients remained free of the colic for some months during the treatment.

Then, it was not until 1937 that Allan Rewbridge at the University of Minnesota administered bile salts (the chemical type was not specified) and olive oil orally to five patients with gallstones in the gallbladder (114). The bile salts were given because they were known to be choleretic and to solubi-

lize cholesterol, and were thought to be deficient in patients with cholesterol gallstones. After 9 months of this treatment, the gallstones disappeared on the oral cholecystograms in two of the five patients. Whether the gallstones passed into the intestine or were dissolved, however, was not determined. Among the three patients with unchanged gallstones, the gallbladder had failed to visualize in one, the gallstones were calcified in another, and no explanation was given in the third.

Rewbridge's promising results were not to be reproduced soon, although 20 years later, two groups of investigators administered oral bile salts to patients with gallstones in the bile ducts. Thus, Johnston and Nakayama from Detroit administered lecithin-fortified ox bile in unspecified amounts orally or through a T-tube to 26 patients, 5 of whom had retained gallstones in the common bile duct (115). The lecithin was added to increase the solubilizing capacity of the bile salts for cholesterol in the ox bile. As anticipated, the biliary concentrations of bile salts and lecithin increased, even after administration of the bile acids orally; however, the biliary cholesterol also increased, the solubilizing capacity of bile for cholesterol did not increase, and the gallstones were not dissolved. These investigators also administered sitosterol (to block absorption of cholesterol) or alpha-phenyl-n-butylamide (to inhibit synthesis of cholesterol) but biliary cholesterol was not affected. Noting that ox bile contains mostly cholic acid, they presciently suggested trying the other primary bile acid, chenodeoxycholic acid, to dissolve the gallstones.

In the very same year (1957), Cole and Harridge from Chicago reported administration of bile salts of unspecified type to nine patients who had residual ductal gallstones after cholecystectomy (116). They gave 3 to 4 g orally of the bile salts daily. Unlike Johnston and Nakayama, they appeared to have success. After 8 to 31 weeks of treatment, the shadows (presumed to be gallstones) on the T-tube cholangiograms disappeared in 7 of the 9 patients. The investigators reasoned that the gallstones dissolved, disintegrated, or passed into the intestine, and they believed that the bile salts were responsible.

In 1966, Grundy and colleagues at the Rockefeller Institute published an abstract indicating that administration of cholic acid orally to humans decreased the endogenous synthesis of cholesterol (117). Then, another seemingly solid rationale for the use of oral bile acids to dissolve gallstones was discovered by Vhlacevic and colleagues in 1970 (118). These investigators found a small bile acid pool in patients with gallstones. Soon thereafter, in 1971, investigators from the Mayo Clinic administered several pure bile acids individually to patients with radiolucent gallstones in the gallbladder (119). Only chenodeoxycholic acid (chenodiol) unsaturated the bile and dissolved the gallstones (120); cholic acid did not.

Stimulated by these and other promising reports on dissolution of gallstones by chenodiol (121), The National Cooperative Gallstone Study (NCGS) was initiated in 1971 (122). This randomized controlled trial documented the efficacy and safety of chenodiol and led to approval of this bile acid by the Food and Drug Administration (FDA) in 1983. Because of chenodiol's low efficacy relative to its side-effects, however, it was received by clinicians with little enthusiasm.

Moreover, another bile acid, ursodeoxycholic acid, the 7-beta epimer of chenodeoxycholic acid had just been shown by Japanese investigators to dissolve gallstones, virtually without side-effects (123). Ursodeoxycholic acid, a major bile acid in the bile of the bear, is found in low concentrations in the bile of humans. Actually, bear bile had been used as a virtual panacea in Japan since ancient times. Ursodiol was approved by the FDA in 1988 and, since then, has supplanted chenodiol for dissolution of gallstones (124). In Europe, however, the two bile acids often are used in combination (125). Although each of these bile acids repletes the pool of bile acids (126), their major mechanism of action turns out to be to decrease the biliary secretion of cholesterol (127). At present, bile acids are indicated for symptomatic radiolucent gallstones in patients who are too ill to undergo cholecystectomy or who prefer to avoid the risk of general anesthesia (128).

Extracorporeal Lithotripsy

Oral bile acids also are being used as adjuvant therapy for extracorporeal shock wave lithotripsy (ESWL). Researchers in Munich in 1986 introduced ESWL to shatter gallstones in the gallbladder so that the tiny fragments pass through the bile ducts into the intestine. In addition, because of an increased surface area of the fragments, the gallstones are dissolved more rapidly by the bile acids (129). Adapted from ESWL treatment of renal stones, ESWL for gallstones requires no general anesthesia or hospitalization, takes 1 to 2 hours, and appears to be safe (130). Whereas bile acids alone usually are administered for an average of 18 months, bile acids after ESWL are given for only about half that time to dissolve gallstones that were originally of comparable size.

ESWL still is an investigational technique in the United States and has not yet been approved by the FDA. In fact, in contrast to the situation in Europe, enthusiasm for ESWL has been only lukewarm in the United States, partly at least because of the concurrent phenomenal popularity of laparoscopic cholecystectomy. The ideal candidate for ESWL plus bile acids has a solitary radiolucent gallstone 10 to 20 mm in diameter. Multiple, calcified, or larger gallstones are less responsive to ESWL. Patients having smaller or floating multiple gallstones can be treated by bile acids alone.

Contact Dissolution

As early as 1891 and soon after the first cholecystectomy had been performed, Walker in London perfused ethyl ether through a cholecystostomy tube to dissolve gallstones in the gallbladder (131). The ethyl ether and some other organic solvents that were tried subsequently, however, proved too toxic to perfuse into the gallbladder or bile ducts. Then, in 1972, Way and colleagues perfused micellar solutions of sodium cholate through T-tubes to dissolve gallstones in the common bile duct (132).

More recently, infusions of other compounds such as heparin, mono-octanoin, or other bile acids with or without lecithin were tried to dissolve ductal gallstones (133). These likewise were essentially abandoned because they dissolved cholesterol gallstones too slowly and pigment gallstones not at all, and produced some adverse effects. Moreover, by this time, endoscopic sphincterotomy, introduced by Classen and Demling in 1974 (134), had been shown to be a safe and effective treatment for most patients with gallstones in the bile ducts.

Then, in the late 1980s, at about the same time as ESWL was introduced, Thistle and colleagues at the Mayo Clinic developed the technique of percutaneous perfusion of methyl tert-butyl ether (MTBE) into the gallbladder for contact dissolution of gallstones (135). MTBE, with a boiling point of 57°C, in contrast to ethyl ether, remains liquid at body temperature. This investigational technique, not yet approved by the FDA, is applicable to any size and number of CAT scan-radiolucent gallstones. The treatment takes a few days to complete, although bile acids usually then are administered for 6 months to a year. As with ESWL, percutaneous contact dissolution with MTBE needs no general anesthesia or hospitalization and is reasonably safe.

Catheterization of the gallbladder for contact dissolution, however, requires the expertise of an interventional radiologist. Solvents that are even more suitable than MTBE for contact dissolution, such as ethyl propionate, and pumps for rapid transfer of the solvents are currently being evaluated (136). Alternatively, as Forrsher has shown recently, the solvents can be delivered through a catheter placed endoscopically through the ampulla of Vater into the gallbladder (137).

Interventional radiology already had made other important contributions to the treatment of gallstones, starting in the 1970s and 1980s. For example, Burhenne championed a procedure whereby gallstones in the bile ducts were extracted with basket forceps through a sinus tract that had matured after removal of a T-tube (138). Also, percutaneous catheterization of the gallbladder or bile ducts, in competition again with endoscopic techniques for access, allows intracorporeal fragmenting of gallstones (by laser or electrohydraulic techniques) or stenting or dilating of the bile ducts (139,140).

In the future, bile acids or other compounds may be used to prevent recurrence of gallstones after dissolution (141). Even more exciting would be prevention of the initial formation of gallstones in patients who are at high risk for developing them. In fact, the first example of primary prophylaxis already has been reported (58). Ursodiol prevented gallstones from developing in patients during rapid loss of weight. In the coming years, look for research in molecular biology and genetics to unravel the fundamental basis for the formation of gallstones and to pave the way for the discovery of novel agents for prophylaxis or treatment.

ACKNOWLEDGMENT

We thank Ms. Patsy Johnson for her superb help in preparing this manuscript.

REFERENCES

1. Malet PF et al.: Black and brown pigment gallstones differ in microstructure and microcomposition. Hepatology *4*:227, 1984.
2. Hikasa Y et al.: Epidemiology and etiology of gallstones. Arch Jap Chir *49*:555, 1980.
3. Balfour DC: Gallstones. *In* Bett WR (ed): The History of Common Diseases. Norman, University of Oklahoma Press, 1954, pp. 220–23.
4. Beal JM: Historical perspective of gallstone disease. Surg Gyn Obstet *158*:181, 1984.
5. Glenn F: Biliary tract disease since antiquity. Bull NY Acad Med *47*:329, 1971.
6. Gordon-Taylor G: On gallstones and their sufferers. Br J Surg *25*:241, 1937.
7. Longmire WP Jr: Historic landmarks in biliary surgery. South Med J *75*:1548, 1982.
8. Rains AJH: Gallstones. Causes and Treatment. Springfield, Illinois, Charles C Thomas, 1964.
9. Naunyn B: A Treatise on Cholelithiasis, translated by AE Garrod. London, New Sydenham Society, 1896.
10. Richardson MW: On the role of bacteria in the formation of gallstones. J Boston Soc Med Sci *3*:79, 1898.
11. Rosenow EC: The etiology of cholecystitis and gallstones and their production by the intravenous injection of bacteria. J Infect dis *19*:527, 1916.
12. Wilkie AL: The bacteriology of cholecystitis: Clinical and experimental study. Br J Surg *15*:450, 1927.
13. Brown RO: A study on the etiology of cholecystitis and its production by the injection of streptococci. Arch Intern Med *23*:185, 1919.

14. Rains AJH: Researches concerning the formation of gallstones. Br J Med 2:685, 1962.
15. Maki T: Pathogenesis of calcium bilirubinate gallstones: Role of E. Coli, beta-glucuronidase and coagulation by inorganic ions, polyelectrolytes and agitation. Ann Surg 164:90, 1966.
16. Tabata M, Nakayama F: Bacteria and gallstones, etiological significance. Dig Dis Sci 26:218, 1981.
17. Cetta FM: Bile infection documented as initial event in the pathogenesis of brown pigment biliary stones. Hepatology 6:482, 1986.
18. Ostrow JD: The etiology of pigment gallstones. Hepatology 4:215 (Supplement), 1984.
19. Soloway RD, Trotman BW, Ostrow JD: Pigment gallstones. Gastroenterology 72:167, 1977.
20. Thudichum JLW: Treatise on gallstones: Their chemistry, pathology and treatment. London, Churchill, 1863, p. 323.
21. Boysen J: Galdestenenes struktur og pathogenese, Kjobenhavn, Doktorafhandling, 1900.
22. Aschoff L, Bacmeister A: Die cholelithiasis. Jena, Gustav Fischer, 1909.
23. Rovsing T: Weitere Beitrage zur pathogenese der gallensteinkrankheit. Acta Chir Scand 56:207, 1924.
24. McBain JW: Mobility of highly-charged molecules. Trans Faraday Soc 9:99, 1913.
25. Andrews E, Schoenheimer R, Hrdina L: Etiology of gallstones. III Bile salt-cholesterol ratio in human gallstone disease. Proc Soc Exper Biol Med 28:947, 1931.
26. Isaksson B: On the dissolving power of lecithin and bile salts for cholesterol in human bladder bile. Acta Soc Med Upsalein 59:296, 1954.
27. Hofmann AF: The medical treatment of gallstones: A clinical application of the new biology of bile acids. The Harvey Lectures, Series 74, 1978, pp. 23–48.
28. Small DM, Bourges M, Dervichian DG: Ternary and quaternary aqueous systems containing bile salt, lecithin, and cholesterol. Nature 211:816, 1966.
29. Admirand WH, Small DM: The physicochemical basis of cholesterol gallstone formation in man. J Clin Invest 47:1043, 1968.
30. Carey MC, Small DM: The physical chemistry of cholesterol solubility in bile. Relationship to gallstone formation and dissolution in man. J Clin Invest 61:998, 1978.
31. Metzger AL, Heymsfield S, Grundy SM: The lithogenic index—a numerical expression for the relative lithogenicity of bile. Gastroenterology 62:499, 1972.
32. Somjen GJ, Gilat T: A non-micellar mode of cholesterol transport in human bile. FEBS 156:265, 1983.
33. Key PH et al.: Biliary lipid synthesis and secretion in gallstone patients during treatment with chenodeoxycholic acid. J Lab Clin Med 95:816, 1980.
34. Hay DW, Carey MC: Pathophysiology and pathogenesis of cholesterol gallstone formation. Semin Liver Dis 10:159, 1990.
35. Dam H: Nutritional aspects of gallstone formation with particular reference to alimentary production of gallstones in laboratory animals. World Rev Nutr and Dietetics 11:199, 1969.
36. Brenneman DE, Connor WE, Forker EL, DenBesten L: The formation of abnormal bile and cholesterol gallstones from dietary cholesterol in the prairie dog. J Clin Invest 51:1495, 1972.
37. Holzbach RT: Cholesterol solubility in bile: Evidence that supersaturated bile is frequent in healthy man. J Clin Invest 52:1467, 1973.
38. Holan KR et al.: Nucleation time: A key factor in the pathogenesis of cholesterol gallstone disease. Gastroenterology 77:611, 1979.
39. Harvey PR et al.: Nucleation of cholesterol from vesicles isolated from bile of patients with and without cholesterol gallstones. Biochem et Biophys Acta 921:198, 1987.
40. Halpern Z et al.: Rapid vesicle formation and aggregation in abnormal human biles. Gastroenterology 90:875, 1986.
41. Marks JW, Bonorris GG, Albers G, Schoenfield LJ: The sequence of biliary events preceding the formation of gallstones in man. Gastroenterology 103:566, 1992.
42. Afdahl NH, Smith BF: Cholesterol crystal nucleation: A decade-long search for the missing link in gallstone pathogenesis. Hepatology 11:699, 1990.
43. Sweet JE: The gallbladder: Its past, present, and future (Mutter Lecture). Internat Clin 1:187, 1924.
44. Wheeler HO: Concentrating function of the gallbladder. Am J Med 51:588, 1971.
45. Tera H: Stratification of human gallbladder bile in vivo. Acta Chir Scand (Suppl) 256:1, 1961.
46. Fisher RS, Stelzer F, Rock E, Malmud LS: Abnormal gallbladder emptying in patients with gallstones. Dig Dis Sci 27:1019, 1982.
47. Spellman SJ, Shaffer EA, Rosenthal L: Gallbladder emptying in response to cholecystokinin, Gastroenterology 77:115, 1979.
48. Pearson RK, Hadac EM, Miller LJ: Preparation and characterization of a new chole-

cystokinin receptor probe that can be oxidatively radioiodinated. Gastroenterology *90*:1985, 1986.

49. LaMorte WW, Schoetz DJ Jr, Birkett DH, Williams LF Jr: The role of the gallbladder in the pathogenesis of cholesterol gallstones. Gastroenterology *77*:580, 1979.

50. Moore EW: Biliary calcium and gallstone formation. Hepatology *12*:206 (Supplement), 1990.

51. Lund J: Surgical indication in cholelithiasis; prophylactic cholecystectomy elucidated on the basis of long-term follow-up on 526 non-operated cases. Ann Surg *151*: 153, 1960.

52. Torvik A, Hoivik B: Gallstones in an autopsy series. Incidence, complications, and correlations with carcinoma of the gallbladder. Acta Chir Scand *120*:168, 1960.

53. Sampliner RE et al.: Gallbladder disease in Pima Indians: demonstration of high prevalence and early onset by cholecystography. N Engl J Med *283*:1358, 1970.

54. Heaton KW et al.: Symptomatic and silent gallstones in the community. Gut *32*:316, 1991.

55. Diehl AK, Stern MP, Ostrower VS, Freidman PC: Prevalence of clinical gallbladder disease in Mexican-American, Anglo, and Black women. South Med J *73*:438, 1980.

56. Bennion LJ, Grundy SM: Effects of obesity and caloric intake on biliary lipid metabolism in man. J Clin Invest *56*:996, 1975.

57. Crohn BB: Some effects of too rapid reduction in weight. Proceedings of the World Congress of Gastroenterology, Washington, D.C. (Abstract), 1958, pp. 106–107.

58. Broomfield PH et al.: Formation and prevention of lithogenic bile and gallstones during loss of weight. N Engl J Med *319*: 1567, 1988.

59. Boston Collaborative Drug Surveillance Program: Oral contraceptives and venous thromboembolic disease, surgically confirmed gallbladder disease, and breast tumors. Lancet *i*:1399, 1973.

60. Boston Collaborative Drug Surveillance Program, Boston University Medical Center: Surgically confirmed gallbladder disease, venous thromboembolism, and breast tumors in relation to post-menopausal estrogen therapy. N Engl J Med *290*:15, 1974.

61. Coronary Drug Project Research Group: Gallbladder disease as a side effect of drugs influencing lipid metabolism. N Engl J Med *296*:1185, 1977.

62. Gilat T et al.: An increased familial frequency of gallstones. Gastroenterology *84*: 242, 1983.

63. Barbara L et al.: A population study on the prevalence of gallstone disease: The Sirmione study. Hepatology *7*:913, 1987.

64. GREPCO (The Rome group for epidemiology and prevention of cholelithiasis). The epidemiology of gallstone disease in Rome, Italy. Part II. Factors associated with the disease. Hepatology *8*:907, 1988.

65. Mayo WJ: 'Innocent' gallstones a myth. JAMA *61*:1021, 911.

66. Gracie WA, Ransohoff DF: The natural history of silent gallstones. N Engl J Med *307*: 798, 1982.

67. Schoenfield LJ et al.: Asymptomatic gallstones: Definition and treatment. Gastroenterol Internat *1*:25, 1989.

68. Comfort MW, Gray HK, Wilson JM: The silent gallstone: A ten to twenty year follow-up study of 112 cases. Ann Surg *128*: 931, 1948.

69. Cucchiaro G et al.: Clinical significance of ultrasonographically detected coincidental gallstones. Dig Dis Sci *35*:417, 1990.

70. Friedman GD, Kannel WB, Dawber TR: The epidemiology of gallbladder disease: observations in the Framingham study. J Chronic Dis *19*:273, 1966.

71. McSherry CK et al.: The natural history of diagnosed gallstone disease in symptomatic and asymptomatic patients. Ann Surg *202*: 59, 1985.

72. Thistle LJ et al.: The natural history of cholelithiasis: The National Cooperative Gallstone Study. Ann Intern Med *101*:171, 1984.

73. Rolleston H: Medical aspects of gallstones. Postgrad Med J *1*:4, 1925.

74. Zollinger R: Observations following distension of the gallbladder and common duct in man. Proc Soc Exp Biol Med *30*:1260, 1933.

75. Schein CJ, Benneventano TC: Choledochal dynamics in man. Surg Gynecol Obstet *126*: 591, 1968.

76. Thornell E, Jansson R, Kral JG, Svanvik J: Inhibition of prostaglandin synthesis as a treatment for biliary pain. Lancet *i*:584, 1979.

77. Littler TR, Ellis GR: Gallstones: A clinical survey. Br Med J *i*:842, 1952.

78. French EB, Robb WAT. Biliary and renal colic. Br Med J *2*:135, 1963.

79. Doran FSA: The sites of which pain is referred from the common bile duct in man and its implications for the theory of referred pain. Br J Surg *54*:599, 1967.

80. Gunn A, Keddie N: Some clinical observations on patients with gallstones. Lancet *ii*: 239, 1972.

81. Boyden EA: The anatomy of the choledochoduodenal junction in man. Surg Gyn Obstet *104*:641, 1957.

82. Geenen JE et al.: Endoscopic electrosurgical papillotomy and manometry in biliary tract disease. JAMA *237*:2075, 1977.

83. Geenen JE et al.: The efficacy of endoscopic sphincterotomy in post-cholecystectomy patients with sphincter of Oddi dysfunction. N Engl J Med *320*:82, 1989.

84. Koch JP, Donaldson RM Jr: A survey of food intolerances in hospitalized patients. N Engl J Med *271*:657, 1964.

85. Johnson AG: Pyloric function and gallstone dyspepsia. Br J Surg *59*:449, 1972.

86. Jorgensen T: Abdominal symptoms and gallstone disease. An epidemiological investigation. Hepatology *9*:856, 1989.

87. Diehl AK, Sugarek NJ, Todd KH: Clinical evaluation for gallstone disease: Usefulness of symptoms and signs in diagnosis. Am J Med *89*:29, 1980.

88. Rigas B et al.: The circadian rhythm of biliary colic. J Clin Gastroenterol *12*:409, 1990.

89. Graham EA, Cole W: Roentgenologic examination of the gallbladder; preliminary report of a new method utilizing the intravenous injection of tetrabromphenolphthalein. JAMA *82*:613, 1924.

90. Leopold GR, Amberg J, Gosink BB, Mittelstaedt C: Gray scale ultrasonic cholecystography: A comparison with conventional radiographic techniques. Radiology *121*:445, 1976.

91. Rabinov KR, Simon M: Peroral cannulation of the ampulla of Vater for direct cholangiography and pancreatography: Preliminary report of a new method. Radiology *85*:693, 1965.

92. Okuda K et al.: Nonsurgical percutaneous transhepatic cholangiography: Diagnostic significance in medical problems of the liver. Dig Dis Sci *19*:21, 1974.

93. Fonseca C et al.: 99m Tc-IDA imaging in the differential diagnosis of acute cholecystitis and acute pancreatitis. Radiology *130*:525, 1979.

94. Meltzer SJ: The disturbance of the law of contrary innervation as a pathogenic factor in the disease of the bile ducts and gallbladder. Am J Med Sci *153*:469, 1917.

95. Lyon BBV: Diagnosis and treatment of diseases of the gallbladder and bile ducts: Preliminary report on a new method. JAMA *73*:980, 1919.

96. Juniper K Jr, Burson EN Jr: Biliary tract studies. II. The significance of biliary crystals. Gastroenterology *32*:175, 1957.

97. Marks JW, Bonorris GG: Intermittency of cholesterol crystals in duodenal bile from gallstone patients. Gastroenterology *87*:622, 1984.

98. Lee SP, Nichols JF: Nature and composition of biliary sludge. Gastroenterology *90*:677, 1988.

99. Bobbs JS: Case of lithotomy of the gallbladder. Trans Indiana Med Soc *18*:68, 1868.

100. Sims JM: Remarks on cholecystostomy in dropsy of the gallbladder. Br Med J *i*:811, 1878.

101. Langenbuch C: Ein fall von exstirpation der gallenblase wegen chronischer cholelithiasis. Heilung. Berliner Klinische Wochenschrift *19*:725, 1882.

102. Ammon HV, Hofmann AF: The Langenbuch paper. I. An historical perspective and comments of the translators. Gastroenterology *85*:1426, 1983.

103. Ohage J: The surgical treatment of diseases of the gallbladder. Med News *50*:233, 1887.

104. Wakim KG, Mahour GH: Pathophysiologic consequences of cholecystectomy. Surg Gyn Obstet *133*:113, 1971.

105. Mayo CH: The relative merits of cholecystostomy and cholecystectomy. Surg Gynecol Obstet *24*:281, 1917.

106. Mayo WJA: Short discourse on surgery of the gallbladder. Surg Gynecol Obstet *43*:46, 1926.

107. Mirizzi PL, Losada CQ: Die untersuchung der gallenwege wahrend der operation. Deut Ztschr Chir *236*:755, 1932.

108. Berci G: Endoscopy. New York, Appleton-Century-Crofts, 1976.

109. Reddick EJ et al.: Laparoscopic laser cholecystectomy. Laser Med Surg News Adv *7*:38, 1989.

110. DuBois F et al.: Coelioscopic cholecystectomy: Preliminary report of 36 cases. Ann Surg *211*:60, 1990.

111. Perissat J, Collet D, Belliard R: Gallstones: Laparoscopic treatment-cholecystectomy, cholecystostomy and lithotripsy. Surg Endosc *4*:1, 1990.

112. Dabney WC: The use of choleate of soda to prevent the formation of gallstones. Am J Med Sci *71*:410, 1876.

113. Schiff M: Il coleinato di soda nella cura dei calcoli biliari. L'Imparziale *13*:97, 1873.

114. Rewbridge AG: The disappearance of gallstone shadows following the prolonged administration of bile salts. Surgery *1*:395, 1937.

115. Johnston CG, Nakayama F: Solubility of cholesterol and gallstones in metabolic material. Arch Surg *75*:436, 1957.

116. Cole WH, Harridge WH: Disappearance of "stone" shadows in postoperative cholangiograms. JAMA *164*:238, 1957.

117. Grundy SM, Hofmann AF, Davignon J, Ahrens EH Jr: Human cholesterol synthesis is regulated by bile acids. J Clin Invest *45*:1018, 1966.

118. Vlahcevic ZR et al.: Diminished bile acid pool size in patient with gallstones. Gastroenterology *59*:165, 1970.

119. Thistle JL, Schoenfield LJ: Induced alterations in composition of bile of persons having cholelithiasis. Gastroenterology *61*:488, 1971.

120. Danzinger RG, Hofmann AF, Schoenfield LJ, Thistle JL: Dissolution of cholesterol gallstones by chenodeoxycholic acid. N Engl J Med *286*:1, 1972.

121. Bell GD, Whitney B, Dowling RH: Gallstone dissolution in man using chenodeoxycholic acid. Lancet *ii*:1213, 1972.

122. Schoenfield LJ, Lachin JM, Steering Committee: Chenodiol (chenodeoxycholic acid) for dissolution of gallstones: The National Cooperative Gallstone Study. A controlled trial of the efficacy and safety of chenodiol for dissolution of gallstones. Ann Intern Med *95*:257, 1981.

123. Nakagawa S, Makino I, Ishizaki T, Dohi I: Dissolution of cholesterol gallstones by ursodeoxycholic acid. Lancet *ii*:367, 1977.

124. Salen G: Clinical perspective in the treatment of gallstones with ursodeoxycholic acid. J Clin Gastroenterol *10*:12 (Suppl), 1988.

125. Podda M et al.: Efficacy and safety of a combination of chenodeoxycholic and ursodeoxycholic for gallstone dissolution: A comparison with ursodeoxycholic acid alone. Gastroenterology *96*:222, 1989.

126. Danzinger RG et al.: Effect of oral chenodeoxycholic acid on bile acid kinetics and biliary lipid composition in women with cholelithiasis. J Clin Invest *52*:2809, 1973.

127. Nilsell K, Angelin B, Leijd B, Einarsson K: Comparative effects of ursodeoxycholic acid and chenodeoxycholic acid on bile acid kinetics and biliary lipid secretion in man. Evidence for different modes of action on bile acid synthesis. Gastroenterology *85*:1248, 1983.

128. Schoenfield LJ, Marks JW: Oral contact dissolution of gallstones. NIH Consensus Development Conference. Am J Surg *165*: 427, 1993.

129. Sauerbruch T et al.: Fragmentation of gallstones by extracorporeal shock waves. N Engl J Med *314*:818, 1986.

130. Schoenfield LJ, investigators of the Dornier National Biliary Lithotripsy Study: The effect of ursodiol on the efficacy and safety of extracorporeal shock-wave lithotripsy of gallstones. N Engl J Med *323*:1239, 1990.

131. Walker JW: The removal of gallstones by ether solution. Lancet *i*:874, 1891.

132. Way LW: Retained common duct stones. Surg Clin North Am *53*:1139, 1973.

133. Toouli J, Jablowski P, Watts JM: Dissolution of human gallstones. The efficacy of bile salt, bile salt plus lecithin, and heparin solutions. J Surg Res *19*:47, 1975.

134. Classen M, Demling L: Endoskopische sphinkterotomie der papilla vateri und steinextraktion aus dem ductus choledochus. Dtsch Med Wschr *99*:496, 1974.

135. Allen MJ et al.: Rapid dissolution of gallstones by methyl tert-butyl ether. N Engl Med *312*:217, 1985.

136. Hofman AF, Schteingart CD, vanSonnenberg E: Contact dissolution of cholesterol gallstones with organic solvents. Gastroenterol Clin Am *20*:183, 1991.

137. Foerster ECH, Buhler H, Domschke W: Direct dissolution of gallbladder gallstones. Lancet *i*:954, 1989.

138. Burhenne HJ: Nonoperative roentgenologic instrumentation technics of the postoperative biliary tract: Treatment of biliary stricture and retained stones. Am J Surg *128*:111, 1974.

139. van Sonnenberg E et al.: Diagnostic and therapeutic percutaneous gallbladder procedures. Radiology *160*:23, 1986.

140. Ferrucci JT: Biliary lithotripsy. Am J Radiol *153*:15, 1989.

141. Villanova N et al.: Gallstone recurrence after successful oral bile acid treatment. Gastroenterology *97*:726, 1989.

Pancreas

23

An Eclectic History of the Anatomy, Physiology, and Some Diseases of the Exocrine Pancreas*

EUGENE P. DIMAGNO

Information about the pancreas began with anatomic descriptions in the 17th and 18th centuries (1). Sporadic descriptions of acute and chronic pancreatitis appeared during the 18th and early 19th centuries. Definite recognition of acute and chronic pancreatitis, however, occurred only after Bernard determined that pancreatic secretion was important for digestion (2). Now, important progress is being made in the application of molecular biology to the study of pancreatitis. Another outstanding accomplishment has been the rapid advance in knowledge of cystic fibrosis since its recognition 60 years ago.

The purpose of this chapter is to present a chronologic perspective of some important aspects of the exocrine pancreas. The topics selected for review are: (1) pancreatic anatomy; (2) the critical importance of pancreatic secretion to normal digestive processes; (3) the imperfect understanding of mechanisms that control pancreatic secretion; and (4) present knowledge of acute pancreatitis. The treatment of pancreatic insufficiency, the history of chronic pan-

creatitis, the endocrine pancreas, cancer of the pancreas, and surgery of the pancreas are not included. The first two of these latter topics are considered in a recent publication (3).

ANATOMY OF THE PANCREAS

As with most medical disciplines, anatomists were the first to investigate the pancreas, e.g., the ducts of Wirsung and Santorini, the ampulla of Vater, and the sphincter of Oddi. In Padua, in 1643, Wirsung described a single pancreatic duct. Santorini, who studied medicine at Bologna, Padua and Pisa and was an anatomist in Venice, described two pancreatic ducts, a smaller one emptying two fingerbreadths below the major duct, which emptied with the bile duct (according to Bernard (2)). He also described the communication between the two ducts. The ampulla of Vater was named after Abraham Vater, who described the structure in 1720. According to Luigi Belloni (4), while Ruggero Oddi was a fourth-year medical student at Perugia (1886–1887), he observed marked dilatation of the bile ducts in a a dog that had had a previous cholecystectomy. He surmised "that at the outlet of the choledochus into the duodenum there was a special device which allowed the flow of the bile only at certain times, preventing it at others, so that

---

* This chapter utilized an eclectic approach to select "what appears to be best from various doctrines methods or styles" (1) rather than establishing primacy of discovery, and is based chiefly on secondary sources or translations. Secondary sources are identified in the text and secondary sources or references quoted by others and unavailable for review are bracketed in the references.

391

the bile, no longer accumulating in the gall-bladder, but compelled to create a space in the larger bile ducts, caused their enormous dilation."

Debate about the ductal anatomy of the pancreas, which started in the mid-19th century, continues today. According to Bernard, the original description of the accessory pancreatic duct was made by Regnier de Graf who, in 1671, published an illustration of a single pancreatic duct, a century before Santorini. However, Bernard comments that de Graf ". . . later described two quite distinct ducts that anastomosed with each other . . . the larger of the two had a common opening with the bile duct. . ." Bernard also credits Meckel (1835) with suggesting that the two ducts "represented an anomalous state, or perhaps the persistence of a foetal condition." Indeed, later investigators showed that the presence of two ductal systems was due to fusion of two anlage of the pancreas, each having its own duct.

Later in this century, Odgers (5) recognized His (His W: Mitteilungen zur Embryologie der Saugetiere und des Menschen. Arch. f. Anat. und Phys., 1881) as originally describing the dorsal pancreas and Phisalix (Phisalix: Etude d'un embryon humain de 10 mm. Arc. Zool. experim. et generale. T. 6, 1888) as describing the ventral pancreas in 1888. Stern (6) recently reviewed the history of the pancreatic ducts and the ampulla of Vater and concluded that these structures should be called only by their proper anatomic names because of the difficulty of establishing primacy for their original discovery.

Stern points out that descriptions of the accessory pancreatic duct had been made by Johan Rhode in 1646 and 1647, Thomas Wharton in 1656, and Regnier de Graff and Niels Stensen in 1664. Stern also notes that Samuel Collins in 1685 gave an "unambiguous description of pancreas divisum." According to Stern, Andrea Vesalius "had already given an obscure account of this region in 1543, Collins gave a clear description of the ampulla in 1685, and Velasco-Suarez credited Santorini with describing the area and suggested that the ampulla of Vater should be named Santorini's valves." (Stern references: Velasco-Suarez C. The

Santorini valves. Mt. Sinai J Med (NY) *48*: 149, 1981).

It is not well known that the ventral pancreatic bud also consists of two parts. Avery, in his classical textbook of developmental anatomy (7) identifies Odgers as noting that the ventral pancreas is originally a paired structure that fuses. Odgers stated that W. Felix in 1892 (Arch. f. Anat. u. Phys.) first noted that the ventral pancreas came from two outgrowths that blended together; the right outgrowth was larger, the left rudimentary: this observation was confirmed by others, including S. A. Siews in 1926 (8). Odgers examined a series of embryos 5 to 23 mm long and showed that the ventral pancreas arose from two separate proliferations from the hepatic diverticulum, which fuse early and share in the formation of the adult gland.

Several clinical entities continue to sustain interest in the embryology of the exocrine pancreas. Two conditions, annular pancreas and pancreatic heterotopia, may arise from abnormal fusion of the two ventral anlage. Nonfusion of the ventral and dorsal anlage produces pancreas divisum.

Annular pancreas was described by Tiedemann in 1818 (9), and the name was given by Ecker in 1862 (10). The two hypotheses about the cause of the anomaly date to 1910 and they have not been resolved. Leco (11) believed that the tip of the ventral pancreas adhered to the duodenum as the ventral pancreas rotates posteriorly around the duodenum on its way to join the dorsal pancreas. Baldwin (12) postulated that the annular pancreas occurred because either the small left bud of the ventral pancreas (see previous text) did not disappear and continued to grow and envelop the duodenum or resulted from excessive growth of the right bud of the ventral anlage. This anomaly continues to be important because there is an association with peptic ulcer disease or pancreatitis in up to one half of the patients. There also is an increased incidence of Down's syndrome, congenital cardiac abnormalities, intestinal malrotation, and duodenal atresia. Obstruction of the bile ducts is common, and many patients may be jaundiced. Moreover, the appropriate treatment is a bypass operation rather than a transection or resection of the pancreas.

Heterotopia of the pancreas is present in

1 to 2% of autopsies. According to De Castro Barbosa et al. (13), Horgan (1921) hypothesized that during the rotation of the dorsal pancreas, the anlage comes into contact with other parts of the gastrointestinal tract that are growing in the opposite direction; pieces of the pancreas are pulled away and eventually grafted into the foreign location. Warthin (1904) had a similar concept, but he believed that accessory pancreatic tissue was formed from lateral budding of the pancreatic ducts which were snared off by the longitudinally growing intestine. Lordy (1930), on the other hand, attributed the accessory pancreas to persistence or incomplete regression of the left ventral anlage.

The most controversial concept, erroneous in my opinion, is that the persistence of the non-fused dorsal and ventral ducts, pancreas divisum, predisposes to pancreatitis. Episodes of acute pancreatitis in patients with pancreas divisum were noted by Rosch et al. in 1976 (14). Soon afterward, an etiologic relationship between the two conditions was suggested by Gregg (15), Heiss and Shea (16), and Cotton (17).

Essential in solving this controversy is the study of Delhaye et al. (18), who showed that in patients undergoing ERCP, pancreas divisum was present in the same proportion of patients with and without pancreatitis. These data suggest that pancreas divisum is a normal variant and has no relationship to the etiopathogenesis of pancreatitis, but reports to the contrary continue to appear (19). Consequently, sphincterotomy and stent placement are not indicated.

PANCREATIC SECRETION

Early History of Pancreatic Enzyme Secretion

In 1856, Bernard (2) demonstrated that pancreatic juice contained substances that digested fat. But it was not until 1890 that Abelman (20), working under the direction of Minkowski, demonstrated that pancreatic secretion was necessary for protein absorption by showing that extirpation of the pancreas in dogs caused both fat and protein malabsorption. Confusion about the necessity of pancreatic secretion from the absorption of carbohydrate continued almost to the present. Nearly a century after Bernard, Lagerlof (21) stated that "starch hydrolysis . . . (is) practically normal even in the absence of pancreatic juice. This has been proved experimentally and clinically." Only recently, by using breath hydrogen tests (22) in patients with pancreatic insufficiency and using amylase inhibitors (23) in normal individuals and in patients with diabetes mellitus (24) has it been shown that lack of intraluminal amylase activity causes carbohydrate malabsorption.

Bernard (2) correlated clinical observations in the literature with his findings in dogs in which the pancreas had been destroyed. One of the seven dogs survived more than 2 days after the pancreatic ducts were injected with a variety of materials (air, blood, fat, candle wax), with and without tying the ducts. The pancreatic duct of this one dog had been injected with mutton fat. After recovering from the operation, the dog's appetite became voracious and the dog passed undigested food (trips) in pale, clay-like, greasy, foul-smelling stools. At autopsy 24 days later, the pancreas was partly atrophied. Bernard noted that the stools of this dog resembled the stools of eight patients reported in the literature who had an abnormal pancreas at autopsy. Accurate diagnoses on all the patients were not possible, but four appear to have had a cancer of the pancreas, distal bile duct, ampulla, or duodenum; and one patient had chronic pancreatitis (stones in the pancreatic duct).

Bernard concluded that the ". . . pancreas plays a unique role in the digestion of fat; interference with the normal working of the gland prevents, or seriously impedes, the absorption of fat from the intestine in such a way as to cause fat to appear along with otherwise normal excreta. The presence of fat is pathognomonic of the failure of pancreatic juice to reach the intestine. This can occur through disease of the organ itself, through blockage of the duct(s), or through a fistula."

Quantification of Human Pancreatic Enzyme Secretion

One hundred seventeen years after Bernard's studies, we showed that fat and protein malabsorption did not occur until lipolytic and proteolytic activity decreased by more than 90% (25). Previously, Kalser et al. (26) had demonstrated that patients with chronic pancreatitis and a 75% distal resection of the pancreas had no steatorrhea. By contrast, similar patients with a 95% resection had only mild steatorrhea (69 to 91, coefficient of absorption). Earlier, Whipple and Bauman in 1941 (27) and Wollaeger et al. in 1948 (28) demonstrated that patients with pancreaticoduodenectomies had moderately severe fat and protein malabsorption. Sarles' data suggested that steatorrhea did not occur until pancreatic secretion was reduced by 75% (29).

We also found that, in chronic pancreatitis, lipolytic activity decreased much faster than trypsin (30). This finding explains why steatorrhea occurs sooner than azotorrhea, why malabsorption is a late sequelum of chronic pancreatitis and why it is necessary to increase the intraluminal concentration of pancreatic enzymes to 5 to 10% of normal before malabsorption is abolished (31).

CONTROL OF PANCREATIC SECRETION

After Bernard, Pavlov was the next outstanding physiologist to profoundly influence the direction of pancreatic research. The first edition of his work published in 1897 comprised his lectures at the Imperial Institute for Experimental Medicine in St. Petersburg. In this edition, Pavlov asserted that exocrine pancreatic secretion was regulated by neural reflex mechanisms. By the time of the second English edition, published in 1910 (32), Bayliss and Starling (33) had discovered secretin and described its release from the proximal small intestine in response to acid.

In the 1910 edition, Pavlov postulated that acid exerted its effect by one of three mechanisms: (1) a neural reflex by acting on an "end apparatus of centripetal nerves in the mucous membrane" or "locally through a peripheral nervous mechanism;" (2) it may be absorbed into the blood and stimulate the pancreatic cells directly; or (3) by its action on the duodenal mucous membrane, it may produce an excitant which circulates through the bloodstream to the pancreas.

Interestingly, observations made before Bayliss and Starling should have led investigators to their conclusions. Popielski found that acid in the duodenum stimulated pancreatic secretion after section of both vagi, splanchnic nerves, extirpation of the solar plexus, and destruction of the spinal cord. Wertheimer and Lepage confirmed these results. In addition, they showed that the effects were not abolished by atropine and that the effect of acid diminished in the distal small intestine. These investigators, influenced by Pavlov, interpreted their findings as demonstrating that pancreatic secretion occurred secondary to a peripheral nerve reflex.

Bayliss and Starling confirmed the experiments of the foregoing investigators, but then proceeded to demonstrate that acid instilled into a denervated loop of jejunum stimulated pancreatic secretion. Because they knew from the work of Wertheim and Lepage that acid introduced into the circulation did not stimulate pancreatic secretion, they surmised that acid in the duodenum caused a substance to be secreted into the blood stream that stimulated pancreatic secretion. This hypothesis was tested by preparing an acid extract of jejunal mucosa and demonstrating the increased volume of pancreatic secretion. Bayliss and Starling named this substance secretin and proposed the term hormone, after the Greek word meaning "I set in motion." According to Babkin (34), these observations were rapidly confirmed by others, including Enriques and Hallion, who performed cross-circulation experiments.

Investigators continue to study the stimuli involved in the release of secretin and the secretion of pancreatic bicarbonate, electrolytes, and water by the pancreas. By using bicarbonate secretion as a bioassay of secretion, Thomas and Crider in 1940 (35) and Meyer, Way, and Grossman in 1970 (36) showed that the threshold pH for secretin release was 4.5. Chey, in 1982 (37), confirmed these findings using a secretin radioimmunoassay. Secretin also is released by long-chain triglycerides (38) and bile (39). Many investigators subsequently have studied pancreatic secretion, including Babkin (34), Melanby (40), Ivy (41), Lagerlof (21),

Hollander (42), and Dreiling and Janowitz (43).

Years after the discovery of secretin, Harper and Raper found in 1943 (44) another hormone, pancreozymin, that influenced pancreatic secretion. In the interval between the discoveries of secretin and pancreozymin, the prevailing opinion regarding the control of pancreatic enzyme secretion was as stated by Lagerlof (21) in 1942: "... pancreatic secretion is regulated by both the hormone secretin and by nervous impulses which reach the gland through vagal and sympathetic fibers. Secretin regulates the fluid and bicarbonate secretion. The nerves are mainly concerned in the regulation of the enzyme secretion, but they also act indirectly upon the secretion of fluid by giving impulses to the blood vessels and glandular ducts."

Melanby in 1925 (40) found that secretin had no effect on the secretion of enzymes and postulated that pancreatic enzyme secretion was under a "dual hormonal and nervous control: Secretin controlling the amount and bicarbonate content of the juice, the vagus nerve controlling its enzyme content." However, several investigators had found that intravenous secretin increased pancreatic enzyme secretion, and Harper and Vass earlier observed an increased enzyme content of pancreatic juice when food was introduced into the denervated intestine of cats. Harper and Raper (44) concluded that these discrepancies "could be explained if there were present in the intestinal epithelium a hormone capable of stimulating the production of enzymes by the pancreas." Harper and Raper then demonstrated that an extract of small intestinal mucosa, separate from secretin, had such an effect, despite section of the vagi and uninfluenced by atropine.

At that time it appeared that there were three hormones in the duodenal mucosa, secretin, cholecystokinin and pancreozymin. Earlier, Ivy and Oldberg (45) had demonstrated that crude secretin preparations caused gallbladder contraction and called the hormone cholecystokinin. Later, Ivy and coworkers demonstrated that cholecystokinin also relaxed the sphincter of Oddi (46). In 1966, Jorpes and Mutt (47) proved that pancreozymin and cholecystokinin

were the same substance; since then the hormone has been called cholecystokinin.

The release of cholecystokinin from the duodenal mucosa is not a simple process. Cholecystokinin is released from the duodenal mucosa in response to fat and protein, but release probably is regulated by a protease-dependent negative feedback mechanism, at least in animals. Small amounts of "free" proteolytic activity within the duodenal lumen, either as a result of diminished pancreatic secretion or postprandially when proteolytic activity is bound to food, cause hypercholecystokininemia. By contrast, large amounts of "free" proteolytic activity reduce cholecystokinin levels. In rats, two peptides exist that stimulate CCK release and both are digested by proteolytic enzymes. One peptide is secreted from the duodenal mucosa by a cholinergic mechanism (CCK-releasing factor, CCK-RF) (48) and another is secreted by the pancreas (monitor peptide) (49). In the absence of ingested protein, proteolytic enzymes hydrolyze CCK-RF or the monitor peptide and enzyme output declines.

These experiments suggest that the amount of "free enzymes" may be an important regulatory mechanism. In turn, the amount of free enzymes depends on the stability of enzymes in the gastrointestinal tract and the rate of food absorption. Layer, working in my laboratory (50), showed that lipase is extremely fragile and loses its activity rapidly, particularly after the absorption of food in the proximal gut. Earlier, Borgstom (51) in 1957 used gastrointestinal intubation techniques and nonabsorbable markers to show that most carbohydrate, fat, and proteins were absorbed by the time chyme reached the proximal to mid-jejunum. Currently, work is under way in several laboratories to identify the mechanisms underlying these relationships. These studies may provide new insights as to the dietary and enzyme treatment of patients with pancreatic insufficiency.

The role of food in pancreatic secretion was investigated in Pavlov's laboratory by Kuvshinskii, who, by performing sham feeding experiments, demonstrated a cephalic (psychic) stimulation of the pancreas (32). By timing the beginning of pancreatic secretion after the onset of sham feeding, he determined that rapidity of secretion had to result from neural stimulation. Acid was the most powerful stimulus for volume secretion; starch did not increase the volume of pancreatic secretion, but exerted a "trophic influence" by increasing the amylolytic quantity of the juice.

Pavlov and his coworkers showed that fat increased the flow of pancreatic juice, and Babkin (34) found that sodium oleate introduced into the stomach increased pancreatic secretion. According to Fleig, soap extracts of the duodenal and jejunal mucosa injected intravenously also increased pancreatic secretion; an effect inhibited by atropine (Savitsch).

At the end of the Pavlovian era, the effect of food in the digestive tract on pancreatic secretion remained poorly understood. A cephalic phase of pancreatic secretion was recognized as the result of neural impulses arising from the oral cavity, but it was believed that food in the stomach had no effect on pancreatic secretion except for causing gastric acid secretion which increased pancreatic secretion by releasing secretin when it entered the duodenum. Later, Babkin (34) postulated, as did Pavlov before him, that the effects of food stimulated enzyme secretion through neural mechanisms, specifically the vagus nerve, because the effects of fat in the duodenum could be inhibited by atropine.

In 1950, Wang and Grossman transplanted the distal denervated pancreas to the breast of lactating dogs and anastomosed the pancreatic duct to the mammary duct (52). When they infused nutrients into the duodenum, they observed maximal enzyme secretion from both the in situ and transplanted organs. The enzyme response was maximal for fat, intermediate for protein, and low for carbohydrate. These data proved conclusively that pancreatic secretion in response to food is at least partly caused by a hormone(s). Twenty-one years later, after pancreatic transplantation was pioneered at the University of Minnesota as a treatment of end-stage diabetes mellitus, we tried to mimic these experiments in a human (53) and demonstrated that, in a diabetic patient with a pancreatoduodenal allotransplant, the transplanted pancreas responded to essential amino acids infused into the transplanted duodenum.

The effects of individual amino acids, triolein, fatty acids, and carbohydrates and the interaction among these foods and bile on human pancreatic enzyme secretion were elucidated by Go and colleagues in the late 1960s and 1970s. They showed that essential amino acids (methionine, phenylalanine, valine and perhaps tryptophan) caused a submaximal enzyme output and infusing a 78 mM mixture of all eight essential acids increased enzyme output to 50% of maximum (54). Triglycerides or fatty acids induced a maximal enzyme output; long-chained fatty acids were more potent than short- and medium-chained fatty acids (55). The effect of bile acids is complex: they are probably an intraluminal modulator of pancreatic enzyme secretion (56). They delay absorption of amino acids, which reduces postprandial hyperglucagonemia and inhibition of pancreatic secretion. Therefore, bile acids prevent the premature inhibition of postprandial pancreatic enzymes secretion (57). Paradoxically, bile acids modulate pancreatic secretion stimulated by fat by enhancing the absorption of fat, thereby reducing the length of intestine exposed to fat and presumably decreasing the release of hormones that stimulate pancreatic secretion.

Originally, through the work and influence of Pavlov, the neural hypothesis dominated. In the middle of this century, most work was devoted to hormones and in a series of experiments, Grossman and others refined the concepts of additive and potentiating effects of hormones. What is intriguing is that current data suggest that, at least in the case of cholecystokinin, the neural and hormonal mechanisms are co-mingled. There is increasing evidence that CCK acts primarily through cholinergic pathways and not directly on pancreatic acinar cells (58). Thus, Pavlov and Bayliss and Starling both were correct.

At the end of his chapter on pancreatic secretion, Pavlov stated that his laboratory was interested in organ physiology and such questions as what is the "peripheral-end apparatus of the centripetal nerve, how does it perceive excitation, and what are the phenomena by which reactions and molecular changes in the secretory cell leads to the formation of this or that ferment, or to the preparation of this or that reagent." These comments, of course, heralded modern studies of the molecular biology of pancreatic secretion.

In the past 25 years, much work has been devoted to identifying secretagogues of pancreatic secretion other than secretin and cholecystokinin and their mode of action. The secretagogues have been classed as those that increase intracellular calcium (acetylcholine, cholecystokinin, substance P, gastrin-releasing peptide); and those that activate adenylate cyclase and increase cyclic AMP (secretin and vasoactive intestinal polypeptide). In the United States, much of this knowledge has arisen from work done in the laboratories of J. D. Gardner and R. T. Jensen at the National Institutes of Health, J. Williams at the University of Michigan, L. J. Miller at the Mayo Clinic, J. D. Jamieson and F. Gorelick at Yale, and G. A. Scheele and M. Steer at Harvard.

Major work in progress is concerned with acinar cell physiology and function, including receptor function and regulation, intracellular mediators of secretagogues, intracellular calcium, intracellular ionic currents, lysosomal function, exocytosis and aggregation of pancreatic secretory proteins, and their precipitation in pancreatic ducts.

For example, it appears that CCK binds to a receptor that assumes two or more affinity states depending on its association with a guanine-binding nucleotide-binding receptor protein (G-protein) (59). Presumably, assumption of a particular affinity state changes the activity of G proteins leading to cellular events such as the activation of phospholipase C or adenylate cyclase (60). By using patch clamping to measure calcium wave propagation in acinar cells, Jamieson and his group showed that the initial calcium wave signal originates at the apex of the cell and migrates to the basolateral region (61), and Peterson showed that muscarinic and CCK stimulation cause different patterns of calcium fluctuation (62).

Much work has been devoted to the control of stimulated pancreatic secretion, but the control of unstimulated pancreatic secretion is receiving increased attention because of its relationship to the pathogenesis of pancreatic diseases. The patterns of fasting, "interdigestive pancreatic secretion" were described by Boldyreff (63), a pupil of Pavlov, in 1911, but were ignored until rediscovered in 1978 by us (64) and by Vantrappen (65). Cycles of interdigestive pancreatic enzyme secretion are accompanied by cycles of hormones (66,67) and are influenced by autonomic neural input (68–72), but the controlling mechanisms are not completely understood.

Interdigestive pancreatic secretion is present overnight when the upper gastrointestinal tract contains no food. Loss of normal cycling of pancreatic juice through the ducts, particularly if there is a high protein concentration, favors precipitation of protein within the ducts (see subsequent text). Thus, this phenomenon may be important in the pathogenesis of pancreatic diseases, particularly chronic pancreatitis if the prevailing hypothesis that intraductal precipitation of protein is central to inducing pancreatitis proves correct.

ACUTE PANCREATITIS

In 1889, Reginald Fitz (73) divided acute pancreatitis into hemorrhagic, suppurative, and gangrenous types. In a remarkable paper, he described 16, 22, and 15 patients, respectively, with these conditions. The patients were mostly culled from the literature but also included patients from his personal experience.

According to Fitz, Classen (Die Krankh. d. Bauchspeicheidr., 1842) elevated acute pancreatitis from a theoretic belief to a clinical reality. Classen collected six patients from the literature, but Fitz dismissed all but two, one patient described by Morgagni in 1765 (De Sedibus et Caus. Morb, 1765, iii., Epist., xxx., art. 10) and one by Lieutaud (His. anat. Med., 1767, i, obs. 1021).

Fitz described 16 patients with hemorrhagic pancreatitis, which today would probably be classified as fatal necrotizing pancreatitis. On section of the pancreas at autopsy, "the color may be dark-red, reddish-brown, violet, reddish-black or even black." He noted that "nearly one-sixth of patients were addicted to the abuse of alcohol" and that "nearly one-half were abundantly or superabundantly provided with fat tissue." They were usually in good health at the time of the attack. "The pain was violent, intense, or severe, either constant or paroxysmal . . . located in the upper abdomen . . . and in one-fifth of the cases, the abdominal pain became general." Vomiting was frequent, fever inconstant, and constipation obstinate. Generalized or upper abdominal "tympanitic swelling" was common, and death occurred between the second and sixth day after onset of the attack. A better clinical description of severe acute pancreatitis has not been written! The 15 patients that Fitz classified as having gangrenous pancreatitis had a clinical presentation similar to the patients with hemorrhagic pancreatitis except that they succumbed within several weeks instead of days.

Fitz also credits Lieutaud in citing Bartholinus, Tulpius, Aubert, and Patin in the 18th century as describing patients with suppurative pancreatitis. Fitz believed the suppuration arose from sites other than the pancreas; and his description of the clinical course of suppurative pancreatitis is remarkably accurate. Although death could occur at the end of the first week and with acute abdominal pain, the usual course was chronic, the patients had mild symptoms and death from cachexia occurred from 1 to 11 months.

Many patients had gallstones, and alcohol abuse was present in some, but Fitz did not correlate gallstones or alcohol with pancreatitis. Rather, Fitz wrote, "acute pancreatitis commonly arises by extension of a gastroduodenal inflammation along the pancreatic duct. It may also be induced by occurrence of hemorrhage in the pancreas. This may be traumatic in origin, although usually arising from unknown causes. The pancreatic hemorrhage may likewise be secondary to inflammation of the pancreas." Interestingly, Fitz also noted that two patients had worms; one patient had a lumbricus half in a vein and half in the abscess, and a second patient had a roundworm in the pancreatic duct. In this patient, the worm might have caused the pancreatitis, but Fitz decided that the worm entered the duct after establishment of inflammation.

Fitz considered treatment as palliative, but with the "formation of pus in the omental cavity comes the opportunity for the surgeon. The possibility of the removal of the gangrenous pancreas is suggested by the healthy condition of a patient seventeen years after he had discharged this organ

from his bowels!" Although, Fitz clearly suspected that infection had a significant role in necrotizing and in suppurative pancreatitis, it has taken a century to make significant advances in detecting necrotizing and infected pancreatitis and improve its treatment.

A breakthrough in this area was the use of contrast-enhanced computed tomography to detect necrotizing pancreatitis (74). In 1986, the Ulm surgical group headed by Hans Beger clearly showed that 39% of patients with necrotizing pancreatitis submitted to necrosectomy had bacterial infection (75). One year later Gerzof, et al. (76) popularized the technique of percutaneous computed tomography-guided aspiration of the pancreas to determine if microbial infection was present. Lastly, in 1992, the Ulm group (77) showed that, among the antibiotics tested, bactericidal concentration in pancreatic infections could be achieved with ciprofloxacin, ofloxacin, and metronidazadole. Thus, in a few short years, we acquired the ability to diagnose pancreatic necrosis and infection of the pancreas without resorting to surgery. In the near future, randomized control trials may reveal if antibiotics that penetrate the pancreas should be used to prevent and treat pancreatic infection.

Eugene L. Opie was another important investigator in the area of acute pancreatitis. In 1901, he wrote three papers describing the association of biliary colic and gallstones with acute pancreatitis (78–80). In what I believe were the first two papers, Opie actually hypothesized that obstruction of the pancreatic duct causes the pancreatitis and the subsequent fat necrosis (79,80). He stated that "a gallstone lodged near the orifice of the common duct might compress the pancreatic duct." He also commented on experiments in cats in which he ligated the pancreatic duct and caused fat necrosis. He concluded (78), "A small stone impacted in the diverticulum of Vater may occlude the common orifice of the bile duct and the duct of Wirsung and convert them into a closed continuous channel. Bile enters the pancreas by way of the pancreatic duct and the pancreas becomes the seat of inflammatory changes characterized by necrosis of the parenchymatous cells, hemorrhage and the accumulation of inflammatory products. Anatomical peculiarities of the diverticulum of Vater do not permit this sequence of events in all individuals." By this he meant that complete obstruction by gallstones at the ampulla could occur only when the dorsal duct (if it communicated with the ventral duct) did not open into the duodenum. He noted that this anatomic arrangement occurred in only 34 of 104 autopsies performed by Schirmer. This may be another explanation of why gallstones may pass and not cause acute pancreatitis in many patients.

Opie also found that bile injected into the pancreatic ducts of dogs caused hemorrhagic pancreatitis accompanied by fat necrosis. He concluded by declaring that "the frequent association of cholelithiasis with hemorrhagic and gangrenous pancreatitis is the result of impaction of gallstones at the orifice of the diverticulum of Vater and penetration of bile into the pancreas."

Opie additionally noted that the patient with a stone impacted in the ampulla was "a large framed muscular man with abundant subcutaneous fat (78,79). He died following an operation to relieve suppurative pancreatitis and autopsy revealed a stone in the bile duct 1.5 cm from the diverticulum of Vater, fat necrosis, and a black necrotic pancreas." This description of necrosis of fat and the pancreas in a fat person was observed also by Fitz and is of interest in relation to recent studies linking the mortality of acute pancreatitis to obesity (Imrie and Banks noted that body weight is linked to severity of disease). Most of my patients who have necrotizing pancreatitis, abscess, or resolving pseudocyst are fat.

These experiments of Opie and his bile reflux hypothesis continue to arouse controversy. Currently, Steer (81) and Moody (82) are investigating "biliary pancreatitis" in the American opossum. The difference in these models is that Moody's animals are infected with salmonella but Steer's animals are not. Moody showed that necrotizing pancreatitis occurred with ligation of the bile duct below the entrance of the pancreatic duct as well as when the pancreatic and bile ducts were ligated separately so that bile could not reflux into the pancreatic duct. Moody's animals, however, did not develop severe pancreatitis when only the pancreatic duct was ligated, and death was not prevented by decompressing the biliary tree. Steer's group, in contrast, showed that pancreatic duct ligation alone produced necrotizing pancreatitis similar to ligation of the bile duct below the entry of the pancreatic duct. Even more interestingly, Steer showed that releasing the ligature prevented death (83).

These studies may have important therapeutic implications. Since the description of endoscopic papillotomy, the extraction of gallstones from the papilla has been used to treat patients with biliary pancreatitis. These data suggest that relief of obstruction early in the course of gallstone pancreatitis may prevent necrotizing pancreatitis.

MOLECULAR BASIS FOR PANCREATITIS

The molecular basis of pancreatic disease arose from the pioneering work of Claude, deDuve, Palade and Porter (84–87), who used molecular biologic techniques to study the process of cellular protein synthesis. To enhance these investigations, James Jamieson developed an in vitro lobule system for further investigation (64–67). From these workers one can trace most of the current investigation of the molecular basis of acute and chronic pancreatitis. The hypothesis generated by this approach is that disordered synthesis and trafficking of intracellular proteins and subsequent intracellular activation of enzyme are the basis of acute pancreatitis (deDuve and Palade).

Most workers credit Chiari (88) as first suggesting that activation of pancreatic enzymes was the initial event in acute pancreatitis. However, it was not until relatively recently that active proteolytic enzymes were demonstrated within acinar cells of the pancreas (89). Current efforts in several laboratories are directed to unraveling the mechanisms of intracellular proteolytic enzyme activation. Steer and colleagues (90,91) have postulated that all causes of pancreatitis begin as an inhibition of pancreatic secretion (a block of exocytosis) followed by colocalization of lysosomal and digestive enzymes within vacuoles in the acinar cell. With colocalization, trypsinogen is activated by cathepsin B, leading to damage of the acinar cells when the activated enzymes leak into the cytoplasm of the acinar cell. Other investigators confirmed that lysosomal hydrolases colocalize with zymogen granules (92) and that activation of proteases occurs within isolated acinar cells (93), but the mechanisms of activation remain controversial.

CYSTIC FIBROSIS

There has been extraordinary progress from the recognition of cystic fibrosis 60 years ago to the present time. In the 1930s, cystic fibrosis was separated from celiac disease and labeled as a disease having pancreatic fibrosis and bronchiectasis (94,95), and in 1938 received its name (96).

An important early finding was that cystic fibrosis was inherited in an autosomal recessive pattern (97). Most of the initial efforts were devoted to understanding the underlying pathophysiologic abnormalities including the abnormal electrolyte composition of sweat (98) and identification of the chloride transport defect (99,100).

Beginning in the 1980s, rapid progress ensued toward identifying and characterizing the cystic fibrosis gene. Finally, through the collaboration of several laboratories, this goal was realized in 1989 (101). The mutated cystic fibrosis gene is on the long arm of chromosome 7 and is a 3-base pair deletion resulting in a loss of phenylalanine at position 508. Since this work, other mutations have been discovered, but approximately 70% of mutant genes have this change.

The normal gene encodes a 1480-amino acid protein termed the cystic fibrosis transmembrane conductance regulator (CFTR) (102) that most believe is a cAMP-activated chloride channel. The abnormal gene produces a significantly altered protein that does not conduct chloride. In several tissues, including the pancreas (103), CFTR is present in the apical region of epithelial cells. It is presumed that, in this location, the abnormal CFTR reduces chloride excretion by the pancreatic ducts and diminishes the hydration of pancreatic juice. In time, the viscous juice obstructs pancreatic ductules causing destruction of acinar cells, fibrosis and subsequent pancreatic insufficiency. The genetic advances encourage the possibility of reversing the cystic fibrosis

abnormality by delivering to epithelial cells normal genes by means of viral vectors or liposomes.

CONCLUSION

During the 17th and 18th centuries, the advances in the area of the exocrine pancreas were primarily to define its anatomy. After the important contribution of Bernard in the mid-19th century, interest in the organ increased as more was understood about its physiology. Beginning in the late 19th century and extending to the middle of the 20th century, diseases of the exocrine pancreas became recognized as significant clinical entities. During the last half of this century, there has been an outpouring of knowledge concerning the cellular mechanisms of exocrine pancreatic secretion, concomitantly with clinical studies, developments that promise to lead to the prevention and cure of the diseases of the exocrine pancreas.

REFERENCES

1. Websters New Twentieth Century Dictionary Unabridged. Second edition. New York, Simon and Schuster, 1979.
2. Bernard C: Memoir on the pancreas and on the role of pancreatic juice in digestive processes, particularly in the digestion of neutral fat (1856). (Translated by Henderson J). London, Academic Press, Inc., 1985.
3. DiMagno EP: A short eclectic history of exocrine pancreatic insufficiency and chronic pancreatitis. Gastroenterology *104*:5:1255, 1993.
4. Belloni L: Oddi, Ruggero. *In* Dictionary of Scientific Biography, volume 11. New York, Charles Scribner's Sons, 1975, pp 175–176 [from Luigi Belloni, "Sulla vita e sull'opera di Ruggero Oddi (1864–1913)," in Rendiconti dell'Instituto lombardo di scienze e lettere, Classe di scienze (B), *99*:35, 1965.]
5. Odgers PNB: Some observations on the development of the ventral pancreas in man. J Anat *65*:1, 1930.
6. Stern CD: A historical perspective on the discovery of the accessory duct of the pancreas, the ampulla 'of Vater' and pancreas divisum. Gut *27*:203, 1986.
7. Avery LB: Developmental Anatomy. 6th

Edition. Philadelphia, WB Saunders Company, 1954.

8. Siewe SA: Pankreasstudien. Morph Jahrb *57*:84, 1926.

9. [Tiedemann F: Über die Verschiedenheiten des Ausführungsganges der Bauchspeicheldruse bei den Menschen und Säugetieren. Dtsch Arch Physiol *4*:403, 1818.]

10. [Ecker A: Bildungsfehler des Pankreas und des Herzens. Z Art Med *14*:354, 1862.]

11. [Leco TM: Zur Morphologie des pankreas annulare. Sitzungsb Akad Wissensch *119*: 391, 1910.]

12. Baldwin WM: A specimen of annular pancreas. Anat Rec *4*:299, 1910.

13. Barbosa J deC, Dockerty MB, Waugh JM: Pancreatic heterotopia. Review of the literature and report of 41 authenticated surgical cases of which 25 were clinically significant. Surg Gynecol Obstet *82*:527, 1946.

14. Rösch W, Koch H, Schaffner O, Demling L: The clinical significance of the pancreas divisum. Gastrointest Endosc *22*:206, 1976.

15. Gregg JA: Pancreas divisum: Its association with pancreatitis. Am J Surg *134*:539, 1977.

16. Heiss FW, Shea JA: Association of pancreatitis and variant ductal anatomy. Am J Gastroenterol *70*:158, 1978.

17. Cotton PB: Congenital anomaly of pancreas divisum as a cause of obstructive pain and pancreatitis. Gut *21*:105, 1980.

18. Delhaye M, Engleholm L, Cremer M: Pancreas divisum: Congenital anatomic variant or anomaly? Gastroenterology *89*:951, 1985.

19. Bernard JP, Sahel J, Giovannini M, Sarles H: Pancreas divisum is a probable cause of pancreatitis: A report of 137 cases. Pancreas *5*:248, 1990.

20. [Abelman.: Über die Ausnützung der Nahrungsstoffe nach Pankreasextirpation, Dissert. Dopat, 1890.] (quoted by Tileston W: The diagnosis of complete absence of pancreatic secretion from the intestine with the results of digestion and absorption experiments. Trans A Am Phys *26*:511, 1911).

21. Lagerlof HO: Pancreatic function and pancreatic disease. Acta Medica Scandinavica, supplentum CXXVIII. Stockholm, P.A. Norstedt & Söner, 1942.

22. Mackie RD, Levine AS, Levitt MD: Malabsorption of starch in pancreatic insufficiency. (Abstr) Gastroenterology *80*:1220, 1981.

23. Layer P, Zinsmeister AR, DiMagno EP: Effects of decreasing intraluminal amylase activity on starch digestion and postprandial function in humans. Gastroenterology *91*: 41, 1986.

24. Boivin M, et al.: Gastrointestinal and metabolic effects of amylase inhibition in diabetes. Gastroenterology *94*:387, 1988.

25. DiMagno EP, Go VLW, Summerskill WHJ: Relations between pancreatic enzyme outputs and malabsorption in severe pancreatic insufficiency. N Engl J Med *288*: 813, 1973.

26. Kalser MH, Leite CA, Warren WD: Fat assimilation after massive distal pancreatectomy. N Engl J Med *279*:570, 1968.

27. Whipple AO, Bauman L: Observations on pathologic physiology of insular and external secretion of human pancreas. Am J Med Sci *201*:629, 1941.

28. Wollaeger EE, Comfort MW, Clagett OT, and Osterberg AE: Efficiency of gastrointestinal tract after resection of head of pancreas. JAMA *137*:838, 1948.

29. Sarles H: Comment in Symposium on the Exocrine Pancreas Normal and Abnormal Function (Ciba Foundation). London, J and A Churchill, Ltd., 1962.

30. DiMagno EP, Malagelada J-R, Go VLW: Relationship between alcoholism and pancreatic insufficiency. Ann NY Acad Sci *252*:200, 1975.

31. Regan PT et al.: Comparative effects of antacids, cimetidine, and enteric coating on the therapeutic response to oral enzymes in severe pancreatic insufficiency. N Engl J Med *297*:854, 1977.

32. Pavlov IP: The work of the digestive glands. (Translated by Thompson WH). London, Charles Griffin & Company, Limited, 1910.

33. Bayliss WM, Starling EH: The mechanism of pancreatic secretion. J Physiol *28*:325, 1902.

34. Babkin BP: The secretory mechanism of the digestive glands. Second Edition. New York, Paul B. Hoeber, Inc. (Medical book department of Harper & Brothers), 1950.

35. Thomas JE, Crider J: A qualitative study of acid in the intestine as a stimulus of the pancreas. Am J Physiol *131*:394, 1940.

36. Meyer JH, Way LW, Grossman MI: Pancreatic bicarbonate response to various acids in the duodenum. Am J Physiol *219*: 964, 1971.

37. Chey WY, Konturek SJ: Plasma secretin and pancreatic secretion in response to liver extract with varied pH and exogenous secretin in the dog. J Physiol *324*:263, 1982.

38. Watanabe S, Chey WY, Lee KY, Chang TM: Fat release secretin in dogs. Gastroenterology *86*:1293, 1984.

39. Osnes M, Hanssen LE, Flaten O, Myren J: Exocrine pancreatic secretion and immunoreactive secretin (IRS) release after in-

traduodenal instillation of bile in man. Gut *19*:180, 1978.

40. Mellanby J: The mechanism of pancreatic digestion—the function of secretin. J Physiol *60*:85, 1925.

41. Voegtlin WL, Greengard H, Ivy AC: The response of the canine and human pancreas to secretin. Am J Physiol *110*:198, 1934.

42. Hollander F, Birnbaum D: The role of carbonic anhydrase in pancreatic secretion. Trans NY Acad Sci *15*:56, 1952.

43. Dreiling DA, Janowitz HD: The secretion of electrolytes by the human pancreas. Gastroenterology *30*:382, 1956.

44. Harper AA, Raper HS: Pancreozymin, a stimulant of the secretion of pancreatic enzymes in extracts of small intestine. J Physiol *102*:115, 1943.

45. Ivy AC, Oldberg E: A hormone mechanism for gallbladder contraction and evacuation. Am J Physiol *86*:599, 1928.

46. Sandblom P, Voegtlin WL, Ivy AC: The effect of cholecystokinin on the choledochal mechanism (sphincter of Oddi). Am J Physiol *113*:175, 1935.

47. Jorpes E, Mutt V: Cholecystokinin and pancreozymin, one single hormone? Acta Physiol Scand *66*:196, 1966.

48. Lu L, Louie D, Owyang C: A cholecystokinin releasing peptide mediates feedback regulation of pancreatic secretion. Am J Physiol *256*:G430, 1989.

49. Iwai K et al.: Purification and sequencing of a trypsin-sensitive cholecystokinin-releasing peptide from rat pancreatic juice. J Biol Chem *262*:8956, 1987.

50. Layer P, Go VLW, DiMagno EP: Fate of pancreatic enzymes during small intestinal aboral transit in humans. Am J Physiol *251* (Gastrointest. Liver Physiol *14*):G475, 1986.

51. Borgstrom B, Dahlqvist A, Lundh G, Sjovall J: Studies of intestinal digestion and absorption in the human. J Clin Invest *36*: 1521, 1957.

52. Wang CC, Grossman MI: Physiological determination of the release of secretin and pancreozymin from intestine of dogs with transplanted pancreas. Am J Physiol *164*: 527, 1951.

53. DiMagno EP et al.: Functions of a pancreaticoduodenal allograft in man. Gastroenterology *61*:363, 1971.

54. Go VLW, Hofmann AF, Summerskill WHJ: Pancreozymin bioassay in man based on pancreatic enzyme secretion: Potency of specific amino acids and other digestive products. J Clin Invest *49*:1558, 1970.

55. Malagelada J-R, DiMagno EP, Summerskill WHJ, Go VLW: Regulation of pancreatic and gallbladder function by intraluminal fatty acid and bile acids in man. J Clin Invest *58*:493, 1976.

56. Malagelada J-R, Go VLW, DiMagno EP, Summerskill WHJ: Interactions between intraluminal bile acids and digestive products on pancreatic and gallbladder function. J Clin Invest *52*:2160, 1973.

57. DiMagno EP, Go VLW, Summerskill WHJ: Intraluminal and post-absorptive effects of amino acids on pancreatic enzyme secretion. J Lab Clin Med *82*:241, 1973.

58. Adler G et al.: Interaction of the cholinergic system and cholecystokinin in the regulation of endogenous and exogenous stimulation of the pancreatic secretion in humans. Gastroenterology *100*:537, 1991.

59. Molero X, Miller LJ: The gallbladder cholecystokinin receptor exists in two guanine nucleotide-binding protein-regulated affinity states. Molec Pharmacol *39*:150, 1991.

60. Matozaki T, Zhu W-Y, Goke B, Williams JA: Intracellular mediators of bombesin action on rat pancreatic acinar cells. Am J Physiol (Gastroint Liver Physiol) *260*: G858, 1991.

61. Nathason MH et al.: Mechanism of Ca^{2+} wave propagation in pancreatic acinar cells. J Biol Chem *267*:18118, 1992.

62. Wakumi M, Kase H, Petersen OH: Cytoplasmic Ca (2+) signals evoked by an activation of cholecystokinin receptors. Ca (2+) dependent recording in internally perfused pancreatic acinar cells. J Membr Biol *267*:3569, 1991.

63. Boldyreff W: Einige neue Seiten der Tatigheit des Pankreas. Der Übertritt des Pankreassaftes und anderer Darmsekrete in den Magen. Die physiologische und klinische Bedeutung dieser Erscheinung. Ergebn Physiol *11*:185, 1911.

64. DiMagno EP, Hendricks JC, Dozois RR, Go VLW: Relations among canine fasting pancreatic and biliary secretions, pancreatic duct pressure and duodenal phase III motor activity-Boldyreff revisited. Dig Dis Sci *24*:689, 1979.

65. Vantrappen GR, Peeters TL, Janssens J: The secretory component of the interdigestive component in man. Scand J Gastroenterol *14*:663, 1979.

66. Keane FB, DiMagno EP, Dozois RR, Go VLW: Relationships among canine interdigestive exocrine pancreatic and biliary flow, duodenal motor activity, plasma pancreatic polypeptide, and motilin. Gastroenterology *78*:310, 1981.

67. Lee KY et al.: A hormonal mechanism for the interdigestive pancreatic secretion in dogs. Am J Physiol *251*:G759, 1986.

68. Layer P, Chan ATH, Go VLW, DiMagno EP: Human pancreatic secretion during phase II antral motility of the interdigestive cycle. Am J Physiol *154*:G249, 1988.

69. Layer PH et al.: Andrenergic modulation of interdigestive pancreatic secretion in humans. Gastroenterology *103*:990, 1992.

70. Layer P et al.: Cholinergic modulation of interdigestive pancreatic secretion in humans. Pancreas *8*:181, 1993.

71. Zimerman DW et al.: Cyclical interdigestive pancreatic exocrine secretion: Is it mediated by neural or hormonal mechanisms? Gastroenterology *102*:1378, 1992.

72. Magee DF, Naruse S: The neural control of periodic secretion of the pancreas stomach in fasting dogs. J Physiol *344*:153, 1983.

73. Fitz RH: Acute pancreatitis. A consideration of pancreatic hemorrhagic, suppurative, and gangrenous pancreatitis, and of disseminated fat-necrosis. Med Rec *35*:187, 225, 253, 1889.

74. Kivisaari L et al.: Early detection of acute fulminant pancreatitis by contrast enhanced computed tomography. Scand J Gastroenterol *187*:39, 1983.

75. Beger HG, Bittner R, Block S, Buchler M: Bacterial contamination of pancreatic necrosis. A prospective clinical study. Gastroenterology *91*:433, 1986.

76. Gerzof GG et al.: Early diagnosis of pancreatic infection by computed tomography-guided aspiration. Gastroenterology *93*:1315, 1987.

77. Büchler M et al.: Human pancreatic tissue concentration of bactericidal antibiotics. Gastroenterology *103*:1902, 1992.

78. Opie EL: The relation of cholelithiasis to disease of the pancreas and fat necrosis. Am J Med Sci *121*:27, 1901.

79. Opie EL: The relation of cholelithiasis to disease of the pancreas and to fat-necrosis. Johns Hopkins Hosp Bull *118*:19, 1901.

80. Opie EL: The etiology of acute hemorrhagic pancreatitis. Johns Hopkins Hosp Bull *121*:27, 1901.

81. Lerch MM et al.: Pancreatic duct obstruction triggers acute necrotizing pancreatitis in the oppossum. Gastroenterology *104*:853, 1993.

82. Senninger N, Moody FG, Coehlo JCU, Van Buren DH: The role of biliary obstruction in the pathogenesis of acute pancreatitis in the opossum. Surgery *99*:688, 1986.

83. Runzi M et al.: Early ductal decompression prevents the progression of biliary pancreatitis: An experimental study in the opossum. Gastroenterology *104*:3:853, 1993.

84. Claude A: Fractionation of mammalian liver cells by differential centrifugation I. Problems, Methods, and Preparation of Extract. II. Experimental Procedures and Results. J Exp Med *85*:51, 61, 1946.

85. deDuve C: Exploring cells with a centrifuge. Science *189*:186, 1975.

86. Palade G: Intracellular aspects of the process of protein synthesis. Science *189*:347, 1975.

87. Porter KR, Claude A, Fullam EF: A study of tissue culture cells by electron microscopy. J Exp Med *81*:233, 1945.

88. [Chiari H: Ueber Selbstverdauung des menschlichen Pankreas. Z Helik *17*:69, 1896.]

89. Yamaguchi H, Kimura T, Mimura K, Nawata H: Activation of proteases in caerulein induced pancreatitis. Pancreas *4*:565, 1989.

90. Steer ML, Meldolesi J, Figarella C: Pancreatitis: The role of lysosomes. Dig Dis Sci *29*:934, 1984.

91. Steer ML, Meldolesi J: The cell biology of experimental pancreatitis. N Engl J Med *326*:144, 1987.

92. Willemer S, Bialedk R, Adler G: Localization of lysosomal and digestive enzymes in cytoplasmic vacuoles in caerulein pancreatitis. Histochemistry *94*:161, 1990.

93. Leach SD, Modlin IM, Scheele GA, Gorelick FS: Intracellular activation of digestive zymogens in rat pancreatic acini. J Clin Invest *87*:362, 1991.

94. Fanconi G, Uehlinger E, Knauer C: Das Coeliakiesyndrom bei angeborener zystischer Pankreasfibromatose und Bronchiektasien. Wien Med Wochenschr *86*:753, 1936.

95. Hess JH, Saphir O: Celiac disease (chronic intestinal digestion). A report of three cases with autopsy findings. J Pediatr *6*:1, 1935.

96. Anderson DH: Cystic fibrosis of the pancreas and its relation to celiac disease: A clinical and pathological study. Am J Dis Child *56*:344, 1938.

97. Anderson DH, Hodges RG: Celiac syndrome. V. Genetics of cystic fibrosis of the pancreas with a consideration of etiology. Am J Dis Child *72*:62, 1946.

98. de Sant'Agnese PA, Darling RC, Perea GA, Shea E: Abnormal electrolyte composition of sweat in cystic fibrosis of the pancreas. Clinical significance and relationship to disease. Pediatrics *12*:549, 1953.

99. Quinton PM: Chloride impermeability in cystic fibrosis. Nature *301*:421, 1983.

100. Knowles M, Gatzy J, Boucher R: Relative

ion permeability of normal and cystic fibrosis epithelium. J Clin Invest *71*:1410, 1983.

101. Rommens JM et al.: Identification of the cystic fibrosis gene: Chromosome walking and jumping. Science *245*:1059, 1989.

102. Riordan JR et al.: Identification of the cystic fibrosis gene: Cloning and characterization of complementary DNA. Science *245*: 1066, 1989.

103. Marino CR, Matovick LM, Gorelick FS, Cohn JA: Localization of the cystic fibrosis transmembrane conductance regulator in pancreas. J Clin Invest *88*:712, 1991.

General

24

Nutrition

MICHAEL D. SITRIN

Although concern with hunting and food gathering has been a major preoccupation of humans since primitive times, the science of nutrition is principally a 20th-century development (1). The ancient Greek physicians considered selection of an appropriate diet the cornerstone of scientific medicine, and frequently prescribed dietary treatments for various diseases (1,2). The Hippocratic school, however, believed that foods contained only one "aliment" and various poisons or drugs (1,2). Thus, although elegant descriptions of classic nutritional deficiency diseases can be found in ancient writings, their relationships to specific dietary practices were not appreciated. The concept that food contained only a single "aliment" persisted until well into the 19th century (1).

Many authorities date the beginning of modern nutritional science with the demonstration by Lavoisier in the late 18th century that utilization of food in the human body was equivalent to combustion (3). Lavoisier's student, the great French physiologist Magendie, demonstrated in the early 1800s the requirement for nitrogen in the form of protein (4), and William Prout is credited with proposing in about 1834 that food contained three important nutrients, carbohydrate, fats, and protein (5). Shortly thereafter, the importance of dietary salt and bone minerals became appreciated (1). In the second half of the 19th century, nutrition science progressed mainly in two areas. The chemical compositions of various foods were defined by Liebig and his disciples using the newly developed methods of or-

ganic chemistry (1,6). Most of the amino acids in dietary protein were isolated and chemically characterized. In 1896, Atwater and colleagues published the famous Bulletin No. 28 of the U.S. Office of Experimental Stations, entitled "The Chemical Composition of American Food Materials," which remained the standard reference in the field for almost 50 years (7,8). During the same period, a group of physiologists, mainly from Germany and the Untied States, including Voit, Rubner, Atwater, Lusk, Benedict and others, developed calorimetric and metabolic balance methods to study the effects of diet, physical activity, and disease on energy metabolism (1,7,8). The "Atwater units" of 9, 4, and 4 calories per gram for fat, carbohydrate, and protein, respectively, were determined (7,8).

Thus, at the beginning of the 20th century, nutritional knowledge was confined to a rudimentary knowledge of food chemistry and basic energy and protein metabolism, and nutritional therapeutics continued to be based primarily on folklore rather than on science. This century has seen an explosion of knowledge in basic nutrition science and in its application to health maintenance and disease prevention and treatment. Nutrition is an integrative science, and advancements have come through the combined efforts of chemists and their descendants, the biochemists, physiologists, and clinical practitioners and scientists (1). It would be impossible in this short chapter to do justice to all the remarkable scientific achievements in this diverse area. Instead, representative examples have been chosen to illustrate contributions that have had a major impact on the course of nutrition research or practice, emphasizing areas of particular relevance to the field of gastroenterology.

STUDIES OF AMINO ACID REQUIREMENTS

In the early part of the 20th century, most of the amino acids that are components of dietary protein had been identified, and it was recognized that different food proteins varied considerably in their amino acid compositions (9,10). Willock and Hopkins (9,11) had demonstrated that the corn-derived protein zein, used as the only source of nitrogen, was unable to maintain growth in young mice, and that addition of tryptophan improved animal survival, but did not normalize growth. The great nutrition scientists Thomas B. Osborne and Lafayette B. Mendel, working at Yale, reported in 1915 that zein plus tryptophan permitted survival of growing rats, and that zein plus tryptophan and lysine supported growth (12–14). This was the first convincing evidence that certain specific amino acids were required in the diet to prevent nutritional deficiency. Osborne and Mendel developed a protein-free milk containing the sugar and salts of milk, yellow-green pigments, and small amounts of other unidentified substances (9,15). Using this milk as a base, it was then possible to compound a nearly purified diet for rats, permitting the systematic investigation of the nutritional value of different dietary proteins and amino acids. For example, studies by these investigators showed that addition of cystine greatly improved the growth of rats fed casein as a protein source (12). The discoveries of methionine in 1922 and threonine in 1935 as amino acid constituents of protein set the stage for the critical studies which determined essential amino acid requirements in man (10).

William Rose and colleagues pioneered the method of using defined diets in which single amino acids were eliminated from the food one at a time, which permitted the identification of the essential dietary amino acids (10). In their initial rat studies, they found that 10 of the amino acids ordinarily found in food proteins were necessary in the diet for maximal weight gain, whereas the others could be synthesized in vivo in adequate amounts and were not required in food (10). Similarly, using amino acid-based defined experimental diets, they demonstrated that 8 amino acids were essential for adult humans, using nitrogen balance as the criterion for adequacy of the diet (10,16). In a further refinement of this method, diets were developed in which the composition of seven of the essential amino acids was kept constant, while the amount of the eighth was progressively lowered, maintaining total nitrogen contents by the addition of glycine or urea (10). The minimal requirement was defined as the amount needed to maintain nitrogen balance. It is now recognized that the essential amino acid requirements are altered during growth and with various disease states, and new tracer methodologies have suggested that the amounts of various essential amino acids needed to maintain normal amino acid homeostasis may differ from Rose's original estimates (17). Nevertheless, Rose's values for the requirements of essential amino acids have served as an important basis for dietary recommendations for the public and for the design of products for enteral and parenteral nutrition support.

NUTRITIONAL BIOCHEMISTRY: THE DISCOVERY OF THE VITAMINS

In the first half of the 20th century, the discovery of essential micronutrients, particularly the vitamins, was one of the most exciting developments in all of chemistry and biology, and numerous Nobel prizes were awarded for these research achievements. The most important pioneer in this area of research was Elmer V. McCollum, who worked at the University of Wisconsin and subsequently at Johns Hopkins University (18–20). After completing his graduate studies in organic and biologic chemistry at Yale, McCollum took a position in Agricultural Chemistry in the College of Agriculture at the University of Wisconsin. He was assigned to work on a project to determine the causes of malnutrition in dairy cows fed certain single grain sources. Because McCollum had never analyzed a food or conducted an animal study during his graduate work in chemistry, he performed an extensive literature search related to the chemistry of living substances and nutrition. He found several reports of studies using diets containing "purified" constituents, and noted that animals, mostly mice, grew poorly on these diets. He concluded that "the most important problem in nutrition was to discover what was lacking in diets containing only 'purified constituents' (18)." McCollum also reasoned that it would be best to conduct experiments using small animals, which would grow and reproduce more rapidly than dairy cows, and which consume little food so that one could afford to perform the necessary chemical analyses of the diets (18).

McCollum presented these ideas to Professor E. Hart, director of the cow research project. Hart was offended that McCollum was proposing abandoning the research effort on cows, and was contemptuous of the rat experiments. Emeritus Professor Steven M. Babcock, however, was extremely impressed by McCollum's proposal and took him to Dean H. L. Russell. Dean Russell was steadfastly opposed to the concept of using state and federal funding to do studies of the nutritional requirements of a farm pest. Because of the support of Dr. Babcock, the most distinguished member of the College of Agriculture, McCollum was finally allowed to establish his rat colony, but was not given any financial support for the project (18–20).

Using home-made cages and beginning with 12 albino rats purchased from a pet store (early attempts to use captured wild rats were abandoned because of the ferociousness of the animals), McCollum and his coworker Marguerite Davis began their studies. They found a certain diet, containing only "purified" substances, which was able to sustain growth for several weeks when supplemented with either butter or egg yolk fat. Substitution of lard or olive oil caused decreased growth and an eye disease, with swollen lids, corneal ulceration, and ultimately destruction of the eye (18). McCollum called this lipid factor nutrient fat-soluble A, now known as vitamin A. The discovery of this essential nutrient in butter fat more than justified McCollum's experimental approach as relevant to the Wisconsin dairy industry. Further studies demonstrated that there was a factor or factors

presented in the water-soluble fraction of milk which also supported the nutrition of rats fed purified diets (18).

McCollum's work established what he termed the "Biological method for analysis of a foodstuff," but which today would be called a bioassay (18,19,21). This revolutionary technique permitted the assessment in various foodstuffs of micronutrients that could not be measured by the conventional chemical techniques of the day. Returning to his initial project to determine why cows fed wheat fared so poorly, McCollum recognized that the wheat rations did not contain the leaf of the plant, which was a better source of essential micronutrients than the seed. Ultimately, it was found that deficiencies of vitamin A and calcium were the most important in the wheat-fed dairy cows (18).

McCollum moved to Johns Hopkins University in 1917, and continued to use the bioassay method to identify more essential nutrients. Cod-liver oil could prevent or treat both rickets and the eye disease associated with vitamin A deficiency. McCollum and colleagues demonstrated that, by passing heated air bubbles through the cod liver oil, it was possible to destroy the vitamin A activity, but that the treated oil was still active in treating or preventing rickets (18). A second fat-soluble vitamin was therefore established, which they named vitamin D. McCollum's later work demonstrated the need for various inorganic elements in the diet of animals, including some required in very small quantities which are today termed essential trace minerals (18).

McCollum's contributions to nutrition extended well beyond his laboratory research. He served as an important advisor to the United States government on nutrition, and devoted much effort to better public education concerning good nutrition practices. He frequently spoke and wrote articles in the lay press encouraging the public to diversify its diet and in particular to include leafy green vegetables, fruits, meat, milk, eggs, and whole-grain cereals as "protective foods" (19,20).

Many other distinguished investigators contributed to the characterization and chemical identification of vitamins. In the late 1920s, only two components of the water-soluble vitamin B complex were recognized: vitamin B_1, the antineuritic factor ultimately identified as thiamine, and vitamin B_2, the antipellagra factor (22). Studies by Paul Gyorgy and colleagues observed the green-yellow fluorescence of the vitamin B_2 complex, and riboflavin was the first component of the vitamin B_2 complex that was isolated and identified (22,23). It was, however, not the pellagra-preventive factor, and it was some years later before niacin was clearly identified as the antipellagra vitamin (see subsequent text). Riboflavin was the first vitamin that was appreciated as functioning as part of an enzyme system, and thus linking nutrition with cellular metabolism (24). Over the next two decades, many laboratories identified other essential nutrients as components of the original vitamin D complex (22,25), including the studies by Lepkovsky, Keresztesy, and Gyorgy on pyridoxine (26–28); Williams and associates on thiamine (29); Lepkovsky, Jukes, and Krause on pantothenic acid (30); Goldberger and Elvehjem on niacin (see subsequent text), Mitchell, Snell, Williams, Stokstad, Pfiffner, Angier, and others on folate (31–33); and Rickes et al. and Smith and Parker on vitamin B_{12} (34,35). Ascorbic acid was identified as the anti-scurvy vitamin by the work of Szent-Gyorgy, King, Waugh, Haworth, and others (36–38). The ability to chemically synthesize large amounts of these vitamins not only provided vitamin preparations for therapeutic purposes, but also made possible large-scale food fortification, an approach to public health nutrition which has certainly had many benefits, but continues to spark much discussion and controversy.

CONTRIBUTIONS OF CLINICAL INVESTIGATORS: THE LEGACY OF JOSEPH GOLDBERGER

The contributions of physicians/clinical investigators to the advancement of nutrition science and clinical nutrition in the 20th century can perhaps best be illustrated by the remarkable work of Dr. Joseph Goldberger to discover the cause of pellagra (39–41). These classic studies have led many to consider Dr. Goldberger the father of clinical nutrition in the United States, and they continue to serve as a model for careful epidemiologic and clinical research.

In the early 1900s, pellagra was recognized as a prevalent endemic disease in the southern United States. A national conference was held in Columbia, South Carolina in 1908, at which time thousands of cases were identified (39). The medical authorities of the day considered pellagra to be an infectious disease, probably spread by an insect vector, and thus there was great concern that the disease would rapidly spread. In 1914, the Surgeon General assigned one of his young researchers, Dr. Joseph Goldberger, to investigate this major public health problem.

Goldberger began to observe the cases of pellagra that occurred in orphanages and other institutions in the South, and noted that, although the disease was prevalent among the inmates, it never affected the staff (42). Previously, Dr. Goldberger had investigated various infectious diseases, and knew that if pellagra were an infectious disease, it would affect some of the staff. Indeed, he himself had contracted various infectious diseases, including yellow fever, dengue, and typhus, during his research on them. Goldberger, therefore, decided to examine the diets of patients and staff in these institutions. He observed that, although the inmates had an ample quantity of food, they consumed little of the more expensive animal products like eggs, milk, and meat. The most telling observations were made in the Methodist orphanage in Jackson, Mississippi, where about one third of the children contracted pellagra (43). He noted that the affected children were almost all between the ages of 6 and 12 years. Goldberger found that older children, who were rarely affected, were able to scavenge for other food sources to supplement their institutional diet, and that the youngest children below age 6 years, who also rarely developed pellagra, were given all of the available milk. It was the children in the age group 6 to 12 who consumed very little meat and milk.

Goldberger subsequently performed an intervention trial in this orphanage (43). He secured funds to add milk, meat, and eggs to the diet of children at risk, and no new cases of pellagra appeared. When the money ran out and the children reverted to their previous institutional diet, pellagra reappeared. Goldberger proceeded to use convict volunteers to demonstrate that pellagra could be induced by a deficient diet, but was not transmitted as an infectious disease (44). In his subsequent work, using black tongue disease in the dog as an experimental model, Goldberger and colleagues tested various foods for the antipellagra factor, and demonstrated that yeast was a rich source (45).

Elvehjem and colleagues at the University of Wisconsin identified nicotinamide as the antipellagra nutrient in food (46). In fact, nicotinic acid had been available as a chemical since 1867, and could be easily synthesized. In 1929, the year Goldberger died of carcinoma, and with the onset of the Depression, pellagra was at its peak, with some 7000 deaths recorded and an estimated 200,000 cases (39). With the introduction of nicotinic acid as a treatment, deaths from pellagra almost disappeared.

Dr. Joseph Goldberger's legacy of careful clinical observations and controlled therapeutic trials greatly influenced the work of other physicians/clinical investigators, including William Sebrell Jr.'s studies of riboflavin deficiency (39,47), the investigations by Minot, Murphy, and Castle of pernicious anemia and the roles of "intrinsic factor" and "extrinsic factor" (vitamin B_{12}) (25,48), and others. The combination of epidemiologic observations with controlled clinical studies, which are refined as advances in biochemistry occur, continues to be the mainstay of research in clinical nutrition until this day.

SPECIALIZED NUTRITION SUPPORT

Parenteral Nutrition

For centuries, astute clinicians have noted the association between malnutrition and poor recovery from injury or illness, and have been interested in the possibility of parenteral administration of nutrients to patients who could not consume an adequate dietary intake. Other than the early experiments with blood transfusion, alcohol was the first nutrient administered intravenously, beginning in the 1600s (49,50). Atwater and Benedict (51), using calorimeteric techniques, demonstrated that oral ethanol was used as a caloric source, providing 7 kcal/g, and was protein sparing. These findings were demonstrated by Rice and Stricker (52) for intravenous alcohol, and for many years ethanol was used in a commercial intravenous nutrition preparation. As described in a review by Levenson et al. (49), milk was the first complete nutrient mixture to be administered intravenously to patients by Hodder in 1873 (53). This therapy was not designed as nutritional therapy, but as a method for treating acute dehydration caused by cholera (53).

. . . a stout build farmer, who had come to Toronto on business, was admitted. He was in a state of collapse, cold, pulseless, blue, and shriveled; the secretion of urine was arrested, there were vomiting and purging of rice-water fluid; —in fact, he seemed dying. [Hodder has assembled his colleagues to observe this novel treatment.]*. . . "Then, gentlemen" I said, "I am about to try the experiment of transfusing milk into his veins."—"If you do, you will kill him," was the reply. Thereupon I invited them to be present at the operation, but three out of the four left the building; the fourth remained, but would not assist. Everything being ready, I ordered a cow to be driven up the shed; and, while she was being milked into a bowl (the temperature of which was raised to about 100° Fahr.) through gauze, I opened a vein in the arm and inserted a tube and then filled my syringe (also previously warmed) and injected slowly therewith. No perceptible change, either for the better or for worse, took place, so after waiting two or three minutes, I again filled the syringe, and injected seven ounces more. The effect was magical: in a few moments the patient expressed himself as feeling better; the vomiting and purging ceased, the pulse returned at the wrist; the surface of the body became warm; —in fact, the man rallied, and speedily recovered without a bad symptom.*

Two more patients were similarly treated, with one recovering and one dying, in Hodder's view because he was not given a sufficient infusion of milk. In an attempt to further investigate this therapeutic modality,

Dr. Bovell and myself then applied to the Corporation for a good cow, and a few articles indispensably necessary for the comfort and well-being of the patients; they were refused, and we thereupon sent in our resignations. (53)

Thomas continued to enthusiastically support milk infusions because of the similarities it had to chyle, and in 1878 reported the results on treatment of seven patients (54), concluding:

> *. . . I would be false to my own convictions if I did not predict for intravenous lacteal injection a brilliant and useful future.*

Although milk infusion continued to be used often over the next 5 years, the practice was eventually abandoned, undoubtedly because of fat embolization and other complications, and attention in the 20th century turned to other types of nutrient infusions.

Beginning in the 1930s, various investigators (including Whipple, Yuilie, Albright, and others) examined the intravenous infusion of plasma proteins (49). They demonstrated that, in protein-fasted adult dogs, intravenous infusion of homologous plasma protein could meet the animals' protein requirements (49). Studies performed using radiolabeled plasma protein demonstrated a gradual decline in plasma radioactivity and a gradual increase in tissue radioactivity (49,55,56). In contrast, when similarly radiolabeled protein was given by mouth, there was rapid incorporation into tissue and loss of radioactivity in the urine. Albright et al. found that, although the nitrogen from intravenously administered plasma was retained in the body, the nitrogen from an intravenous protein hydrolysate was promptly excreted, similar to the fate of the same protein taken orally (57). Albright et al. concluded (57):

> *. . . there are three fates of i.v. administered plasma protein: (1) to be burned, which can be measured by the increased excretion of nitrogen; (2) to be converted into protoplasm, which can be measured by the decreased excretion of phosphorus or potassium; (3) to remain unchanged.*

To further demonstrate that intravenous plasma protein could be metabolically utilized, Allen et al. compared puppies maintained for 99 days on intravenous plasma with littermates fed protein by mouth (58). These studies demonstrated that the animals receiving intravenous plasma proteins were in positive nitrogen balance, and grew and gained weight comparably to their orally fed littermates.

The discovery that dietary protein was digested in the gastrointestinal tract to amino acids and small peptides and released into the portal venous system as amino acids stimulated research into the use of intravenous protein hydrolysates and amino acids that provides the basis for modern parenteral nutrition. In the early 1900s, studies demonstrated that intravenously administered amino acids were rapidly cleared from the plasma, with only a small amount appearing in the urine, and the remainder being taken up in tissues (49,59). Henriques and Anderson (60) achieved positive nitrogen balance by intravenous infusion of a meat hydrolysate, glucose, and salt into a goat for 16 days. As discussed, Rose et al. performed classic studies of amino acid requirements in experimental animals and man, defining the essential amino acids. Rose stated:

> *Indeed, it is not wholly improbable that methods may be devised whereby this ideal mixture (of amino acids) may be employed for parenteral administration to human subjects when the prevention of undue loss of body structure is an important consideration (49,61)*

A series of important experimental animal and clinical studies by Elman and others clearly demonstrated the efficacy of parenteral nutrition support regimens containing protein hydrolysates or amino acids in improving the nutritional status of patients with various injuries or illnesses that prevented adequate food consumption by way of the gastrointestinal tract (49,62,63). With the development of methods for mass production of individual L-amino acids, crystalline amino acid formulations became the mainstay of modern parenteral nutrition support because they avoided the problems of nonuniformity of hydrolysis and incomplete utilization of peptides that plagued the use of protein hydrolysates. Special amino acid formulations to meet the altered requirements of patients with renal disease, hepatic failure, and severe stress and trauma have been developed. Although the clinical use of these specialized amino acid mixtures remains controversial, the availability of crystalline amino acids for intravenous administration continued to stimulate new research into the design of special formulations suitable for optimizing the nutritional, metabolic, and immunologic status of patients with specific disease states.

The great French physiologist Claude Bernard is credited with being the first to infuse sugars into experimental animals, and demonstrated that intravenous glucose was not excreted into urine, and, therefore, was presumably utilized (64). Subsequent studies in the early 1900s defined the amount of glucose that could be infused without producing glycosuria (65). In 1945, Zimmerman (66) showed that catheters in the superior vena cava could be used for intravenous infusions of hypertonic solutions, and Dennis reported beneficial effects of treatment of malnutrition in seriously ill patients, including many with chronic ulcerative colitis, with a constant infusion of hypertonic glucose, vitamins, electrolytes, and plasma (67,68).

In the late 17th century, Courten administered olive oil intravenously to dogs, and observed that the animals died of severe respiratory distress, probably caused by pulmonary fat emboli (49,69,70). In the 19th century, subcutaneous administration of fat was studied in experimental animals and humans, but this approach was greatly limited by the severe pain associated with the infusions (69,71). In the early 20th century, many laboratories investigated methods for preparing stable fat emulsions that could be used for parenteral nutrition. Building on the work of Stare, Geyer, and others (72,73), fairly stable cottonseed oil emulsions were developed and produced commercially by the Upjohn Company. These early products, however, tended to produce fever and sometimes more severe problems such as shortness of breath, hypoxia, tachycardia, hypotension, hemolysis, thrombocytopenia, and back pain (68). Wretlind and colleagues (69,74,75) in Sweden developed a lipid emulsion based on soybean oil and egg yolk phospholipids that was the first to be well tolerated by humans. This emulsion made it possible to supply intravenously a high-density source of calories and to provide essential fatty acids.

Much of the methodology for modern parenteral nutrition had its origin in the laboratories of the Department of Surgery at the University of Pennsylvania (76–79). Previous research by Cuthbertson, Whipple, and others (80) had emphasized the marked negative nitrogen balance that accompanied trauma or sepsis, and studies by investigators in the Pennsylvania surgical group had demonstrated that the calories and amino acids that could be given by peripheral vein were generally insufficient to achieve nitrogen equilibrium in these patients. Rhoads and colleagues (77,78) developed an approach that used diuretics to permit an increased rate of fluid administration by way of the peripheral vein (the 5 liter program). Although this method allowed delivery of increased amounts of nutrients, meticulous care was required to replace diuretic-induced electrolyte losses and to avoid fluid overload and pulmonary edema (77,78). This research group devoted itself to developing techniques for long-term central venous catheterization that would allow administration of concentrated nutrient solutions that could meet the patient's nutritional requirements (76,78). Using small-bore plastic tubing that was initially developed as electrical insulation, these investigators established methods for prolonged central venous catheterization, and in a classic study reported by Dudrick et al. in 1968 (81) demonstrated that six beagle puppies fed intravenously for 72 to 256 days achieved growth, development, and weight gain comparable to those of their littermates that were orally fed isocaloric diets. Subsequent studies in patients with chronic complicated gastrointestinal disease demonstrated efficacy in the clinical setting. Over the past 25 years, total parenteral nutrition has become a mainstay of the hospital management of patients with a wide variety of surgical and medical diseases, contributing significantly to decreases in morbidity and mortality in patients with inflammatory bowel disease, fistulas, burns, short bowel syndrome, cancer, etc. Techniques rapidly developed for safe total parenteral nutrition in the home setting, permitting medical and social rehabilitation of many patients previously confined permanently to the hospital. The thousands of patients who have been successfully supported by total parenteral nutrition are a testimony to the many advances in nutrition science in the 20th century, and demonstrate that physicians have learned much about nutritional requirements in various diseases states. Of equal importance, however, are the many observations of nutritional deficiencies and metabolic complications in patients receiving total parenteral nutrition. Evaluation of these patients has greatly increased our understanding of gastrointestinal physiology, metabolism, and requirements for trace elements and vitamins, and continue to stimulate new research into methods for optimizing the nutritional and metabolic status of patients.

Enteral Nutritional Support

The use of feeding by placing a tube in the gastrointestinal tract was described in ancient Egypt and Greece, where nutrient enemas (clysters) were a commonly prescribed therapy. Various materials including wine, milk, barley broth, and fatty or gummy substances were used to treat diarrheal diseases and to preserve health (82). In 1882, Bliss (83) reported over 400 cases in the literature of rectal feeding, including that of President Garfield, who had developed acute parotitis after his injury that severely limited oral intake. As the processes of digestion and intestinal absorption became understood, it was apparent that absorption of nutrients administered by way of the colon or rectum was limited, and attention focused on tube feeding into the upper gastrointestinal tract.

Tubes for feeding into the stomach developed from devices used for dilation of esophageal strictures or for extraction of foreign bodies, and many intriguing feeding tubes were described. For example, the famous surgeon John Hunter reported a patient who had suffered a stroke and was unable to swallow (84). He used a tube made of eel skin that was introduced over a flexible whalebone probe, and the patient was fed through it twice daily for 5 weeks until his ability to swallow returned. Stomach tubes that were large in diameter and inflexible were widely used in asylums for the insane in England, and Reeve (85) noted the many

complications that occurred. Commenting on the expertise and patience required for tube feedings, Reeve noted that tube feeding, "if confined to ignorant keepers, was perilous" (82,85). In his review of the techniques and instruments available for tube feeding, Nesbitt noted that:

> . . . a demonstration or sighting of the apparatus will often produce the happiest results; and that food will be voluntarily taken by the patient when the alternative of not doing so is fairly placed before him (82,86).

Fortunately, improved nasogastric tubes were developed, and by the end of the 19th century, tube feeding into the esophagus or stomach using common foods was well established (82). In the first half of the 20th century, tubes for feeding into the small intestine were developed (82), and several surgeons devised tubes for combined gastric decompression and intrajejunal feeding of the post-operative patient. In the 1950s, Pareira et al. (87) and Barron (88) published reviews of hundreds of patients who had received tube feedings, including some who had fed themselves by tube at home.

Techniques for surgical placement of a gastrostomy or jejunostomy were developed in the early 20th century, principally for palliation in patients with carcinoma of the upper digestive tract (82,89). More recently, endoscopic and radiologic approaches for placing gastrostomies and jejunostomies have been popularized, avoiding much of the postsurgical morbidity and mortality while still permitting long-term access to the gastrointestinal tract and avoiding uncomfortable chronic nagogastric or nasointestinal tubes (90,91).

The studies by Rose that established the essential amino acid requirements for humans previously described provided the scientific basis for the development of "elemental" diets in which mixtures of essential and nonessential amino acids serve as the protein source. Greenstein and colleagues investigated these "elemental" diets in experimental animals and subsequently in cancer patients, achieving positive nitrogen balance in some (92,93). Research funded by the National Aeronautics and Space Administration (NASA) further developed these formulas because they were found to cause a dramatic reduction in stool weight, which made them attractive for feeding in space (82). Subsequent studies by many laboratories have demonstrated the utility of "elemental" diets in the treatment of patients with malabsorptive disorders and other chronic gastroenterologic diseases (83,94).

Although both total parenteral nutrition and enteral alimentation by tube feeding are now well-accepted treatment modalities, considerable controversy remains concerning the optimal use of these therapies. In the 1970s and 1980s, patients with various chronic gastrointestinal diseases, particularly inflammatory bowel disease, were often treated with total parenteral nutrition and nothing by mouth ("bowel rest"), with a goal of achieving nutritional repletion and disease remission. More recently, the important role of enteral nutrition in maintaining the metabolic, immunologic, and barrier functions of the gastrointestinal tract has received greater emphasis (95,96). Several clinical studies have found lower complication rates and better outcomes in postoperative patients receiving enteral nutrition than in those on total parenteral nutrition (97,98), and patients with Crohn's disease generally respond equally well to elemental diets or to total parenteral nutrition (96,99,100). Much current research is being directed toward better understanding of the effects of specific nutrients on the structure and function of the gastrointestinal tract.

REFERENCES

1. Harper AE: Nutrition: Where are we? Where are we going? Am J Clin Nutr 22: 87, 1969.
2. Ackerknecht EH: The end of the Greek diet. Bull Hist Med 42:242, 1971.
3. Rappaport R: Antoine-Laurent Lavoisier—a biographical sketch. J Nutr 79:1, 1963.
4. Fenton PF: Francois Magendie. J Nutr 43: 3, 1951.
5. Ahrens R: William Prout (1785–1850). A biographical sketch. J Nutr 107:17, 1977.
6. Thomas K: Justus von Liebig. J Nutr 7:3, 1934.
7. Darby WJ: Nutrition science: An overview of American genius. Nutr Rev 34:1, 1976.
8. Hegsted DM: Nutrition: The changing scene. Nutr Rev 43:357, 1985.
9. Leverton R: Building blocks and stepping stones in protein nutrition. J Nutr 91(Suppl 1):39, 1967.
10. Rose WC: The sequence of events leading to the establishment of the amino acid needs of a man. AJPH 58:2020, 1968.
11. Willock EG, Hopkins FG: The importance of individual amino acids in metabolism. Observations on the effect of adding tryptophane to a diet in which zein is the sole nitrogenous constituent. J Physiol 35:88, 1906–7.
12. Mendel LB: Nutrition and growth. JAMA 64:1539, 1915.
13. Smith AH: Lafayette Benedict Mendel. J Nutr 60:3, 1956.
14. Vickery HB: Thomas Burr Osborne. In Darby WJ, Jukes TH (eds): Founders of Nutrition Science. Bethesda, MD, American Institute of Nutrition, 1992.
15. Osborne TB, Mendel LB: Feeding experiments with isolated food substances. Carnegie Institution of Washington. Publ. 156: 53, 1915.
16. Rose WC, Haines WJ, Warner DT: The amino acid requirements of man. V. The role of lysine, arginine, and tryptophan. J Biol Chem 206:421, 1954.
17. Young VR, Bier DM: Amino acid requirements in the adult human: How well do we know them? J Nutr 117:1484, 1987.
18. McCollum EV: The paths to the discovery of vitamins A and D. J Nutr 91(Suppl 1): 11, 1967.
19. Herriott RM: Life and contributions of Elmer V. McCollum. Fed Proc 39:2713, 1980.
20. Rider AA: Elmer Verner McCollum—a biographical sketch. J Nutr 100:3, 1970.
21. Schneider HA: Rats, fats, and history. Perspect Biol Med 29:392, 1986.
22. Gyorgy P: Reminiscences on the discovery and significance of some of the B vitamins. J Nutr 91(Suppl 1):5, 1967.
23. Gyorgy P, Kuhn R, Wagner-Jauregg T: Vitamin B_2. A review. Klin Wochenschr 12: 1241, 1933.
24. Gyorgy P, Kuhn R, Wagner-Jauregg T: Flavins and flavoproteins as vitamin B_2. Z Physiol Chem 223:241, 1934.
25. Todhunter EN: Chronology of some events in the development and application of the science of nutrition. Nutr Rev 34:353, 1976.
26. Gyorgy P: Crystaline vitamin B_6. J Am Chem Soc 60:983, 1938.
27. Lepkovsky S: Crystalline factor 1. Science 87:169, 1938.
28. Keresztesy JC, Stevens JR: Vitamin B_6. J Am Chem Soc 60:1267, 1938.

29. Williams RR, Cline JK: Synthesis of vitamin B_1. J Am Chem Soc *58*:1504, 1936.

30. Lepkovsky S, Jukes TH, Krause ME: The multiple nature of the third factor of the vitamin B complex. J Biol Chem *115*:557, 1936.

31. Pfiffner JJ, et al.: Isolation of the antianemia factor (vitamin B_c) in crystalline form from liver. Science *97*:404, 1943.

32. Stokstad ELR: Some properties of a growth factor for lactobacillus casei. J Biol Chem *149*:573, 1943.

33. Angier RB et al.: Synthesis of a compound identical with the L. Casei factor isolated from liver. Science *102*:227, 1945.

34. Rickes EL et al.: Crystalline vitamin B_{12}. Science *107*:396, 1948.

35. Smith EL, Parker LFJ: Purification of antipernicious anaemia factor. Biochem J *43*: viii, 1948.

36. Widdowson EM: Nutrition research in Britain. J Am Dietetic Assn *55*:233, 1969.

37. King CG: The discovery and chemistry of vitamin C. Proc Nutr Soc *12*:219, 1953.

38. Ault RG et al.: Synthesis of d- and l-ascorbic acid and of analogous substances. J Chem Soc *2*:1419, 1933.

39. Sebrell WH: Clinical nutrition in the United States. AJPH *58*:2035, 1968.

40. Sebrell WH: Joseph Goldberger. J Nutr *55*: 3, 1955.

41. Bollet AJ: Politics and pellagra: The epidemic of pellagra in the U.S. in the early twentieth century. Yale J Biol Med *65*:211, 1992.

42. Goldberger J: The etiology of pellagra: The significance of certain epidemiological observations with respect thereto. Pub Health Rep *29*:1683, 1914.

43. Goldberger J, Waring CH, Willets DG: The prevention of pellagra: A test of diet among institutional inmates. Pub Health Rep *30*: 3117, 1915.

44. Goldberger J, Wheeler GA: The experimental production of pellagra in human subjects by means of diet. Hyg Lab Bull *120*:7, 1920.

45. Goldberger J, Wheeler GA, Lillie RD, Rogers LM: A further study of butter, fresh beef, and yeast as pellagra preventives, with consideration of the relation of factor P-P of pellagra (and black tongue of dogs) to vitamin B. Pub Health Rep *41*:297, 1926.

46. Elvehjem CA, Madden RJ, Strong FM, Wooley DW: Relation of nicotinic acid and nicotinic acid amide to canine black tongue. J Am Chem Soc *59*:1767, 1937.

47. Sebrell WH, Butler RE: Riboflavin deficiency in man. (ariboflavinosis). Pub Health Rep *54*:2121, 1939.

48. Castle WB, Health CW, Strauss MB, Heinle RW: Observations of the etiologic relationship of achylia gastrica to pernicious anemia. VI. The site of the interaction of food (extrinsic) and gastric (intrinsic) factors; failure of in vitro incubation to produce a thermostable hematopoietic principle. Am J Med Sci *194*:618, 1937.

49. Levenson SM, et al.: Early history of parenteral nutrition. Fed Proc *43*:1391, 1984.

50. Wren C: An account of the method of conveying liquors immediately into mass of blood. As reported by Henry Oldenburn. Philos Trans R Soc London, 1665. Cited by Annan GL: An exhibition of books on the growth of our knowledge of blood transfusions. Bull NY Acad Med *15*:623, 1939.

51. Atwater WO, Benedict FC: An experimental inquiry regarding the nutritive value of alcohol. Mem Natl Acad Sci *8*:235, 1897.

52. Rice CO, Stricker JL: Parenteral nutrition in elderly surgical patients. Geriatrics *7*: 232, 1952.

53. Hodder EM: Transfusion of milk in cholera. Practioner *10*:14, 1873.

54. Thomas TG: Intravenous injection of milk as a substitute for transfusion of blood. NY State J Med *27*:449, 1878.

55. Yuilie CL, Lamson BG, Miller LL, Whipple GH: Conversion of plasma protein to tissue protein without evidence of protein breakdown. Results of giving plasma proteins labelled with carbon[14] parenterally to dogs. J Exp Med *93*:539, 1951.

56. Yuilie CL, O'Dea AE, Lucas FV, Whipple GH: Plasma protein labelled with lysine C^{14}, its oral feeding and related protein metabolism in the dog. J Exp Med *95*:247, 1952.

57. Albright F, Forbes AP, Reifenstein EC: The fate of plasma proteins administered intravenously. Trans Assoc Am Phys *59*: 221, 1946.

58. Allen JG, Stemmer EM, Head LR: Similar growth rates of litter puppies maintained on oral protein with those on the same quantity of protein as daily intravenous plasma for 99 days as the only protein source. Ann Surg *144*:349, 1956.

59. Van Slyke DD, Meyer GM: The fate of protein digestion products in the body. J Biol Chem *16*:197, 1913.

60. Henriques V, Anderson AC: Uber parentaler Ernahrung durch intravenose Injektion. Z Physiol Chem *88*:357, 1913.

61. Rose WC: The significance of amino acids in nutrition. Harvey Lect *30*:49, 1934–5.

62. Elman R, Lischer CE: Amino acids, serum and plasma in the replacement therapy of fatal shock due to repeated hemorrhage, an

experimental study. Ann Surg *118*:225, 1943.

63. Elman R, Weiner DO: Intravenous alimentation with special reference to protein (amino acid) metabolism. JAMA *112*:796, 1939.

64. Bernard C: Leçons sur les propriétés physiologiques et les altérations pathologiques des liquides de l'organisme. Paris *2*:459, 1859.

65. Woodyatt RT, Sansum WD, Wilder RM: Prolonged and accurately timed injection of sugar. JAMA *65*:2067, 1915.

66. Zimmerman B: Intravenous tubing for parenteral therapy. Science *101*:567, 1945.

67. Dennis C: Preoperative and postoperative care for the bad risk patient. Minn Med *27*: 538, 1944.

68. Dennis C, Karlson KE: Surgical measures as supplements to the management of idiopathic ulcerative colitis; cancer, cirrhosis, and arthritis as frequent complications. Surgery *32*:892, 1952.

69. Wretlind A: Recollections of pioneers in nutrition: Landmarks in the development of parenteral nutrition. J Am Coll Nutr *11*: 366, 1992.

70. Courten W: Experiments and observations of the effects of several sorts of poisons upon animals made at Montpelier in the years 1678 and 1679 by the late William Courten. Philos Trans R Soc London *27*: 485, 1710.

71. Friedrich PL: Die kunstliche subkutane Ernahrung in der praktischen Chirurgie. Arch Klin Chirurgie *73*:507, 1904.

72. Geyer RP: Parenteral nutrition. Physiol Rev *40*:150, 1960.

73. Stare FJ: Recollections of pioneers in nutrition: Establishment of the first department of nutrition in a medical center. J Am Coll Nutr *8*:248, 1989.

74. Schuberth O, Wretlind A: Intravenous infusion of fat emulsions, phosphatides and emulsifying agents. Acta Chir Scand *278(Suppl)*:1, 1961.

75. Wretlind A: Development of fat emulsions. JPEN *5*:230, 1983.

76. Vars HM: Early research in parenteral nutrition. JPEN *4*:467, 1980.

77. Rhoads JE: The evolution of intravenous hyperalimentation. World J Surg *6*:144, 1982.

78. Rhoads JE, Vars HM, Dudrick SJ: The development of intravenous hyperalimentation. Surg Clin North Am *61*:429, 1981.

79. Dudrick SJ: The genesis of intravenous hyperalimentation. JPEN *1*:23, 1977.

80. Cuthbertson DP: The metabolic response to injury and its nutritional implications. *In* Cuthbertson DP (ed). Progress in Nutrition and Allied Sciences. Edinburgh and London, Oliver and Boyd, 1963.

81. Dudrick SJ, Wilmore DW, Vars HM, Rhoads JE: Long-term total parenteral nutrition with growth, development, and positive nitrogen balance. Surgery *64*:134, 1968.

82. Randall HT: Enteral nutrition: Tube feeding in acute and chronic illness. JPEN *8*: 113, 1984.

83. Bliss DW: Feeding per rectum. As illustrated in the case of the late President Garfield and others. Med Rec *22*:64, 1882.

84. Hunter J: A case of paralysis of the muscles of deglutition cured by an artificial mode of conveying food and medicines in the stomach. Trans Soc Improv Med Chir Know *1*: 182, 1793.

85. Reeve J: Apparatus for administering nourishment to insane persons who refused food. Lancet *i*:520, 1851.

86. Nesbitt PR: Forced alimentation. Br Med J *11*:587, 1859.

87. Pareira MD et al.: Therapeutic nutrition with tube feeding. JAMA *156*:810, 1954.

88. Barron J: Tube feeding of postoperative patients. Surg Clin North Am *39*:1481, 1959.

89. Torosian MH, Rombeau JL: Feeding by tube enterostomy. Surg Gynecol Obstet *150*:918, 1980.

90. Mamel JJ: Percutaneous endoscopic gastrostomy. Am J Gastroenterol *84*:703, 1989.

91. Gray RR, St Louis EL, Grosman H: Percutaneous gastrostomy and gastro-jejunostomy. Br J Radiol *60*:1067, 1987.

92. Greenstein JP, et al.: Quantitative nutritional studies with water-soluble, chemically defined diets. I. Growth, reproduction, and lactation in rats. Arch Biochem *72*:396, 1957.

93. Greenstein JP, et al.: Quantitative nutritional studies with water-soluble, chemically defined diets. X. Formulation of a nutritionally complete liquid diet. J Nat Cancer Inst *24*:211, 1960.

94. Heymsfield SB, et al.: Enteral hyperalimentation: An alternative to central venous hyperalimentation. Ann Intern Med *90*:63, 1979.

95. Wilmore DW, et al.: The gut: A central organ after surgical stress. Surgery *104*:917, 1988.

96. Sitrin MD: Nutrition support in inflammatory bowel disease. Nutr Clin Pract *7*:53, 1992.

97. Kudsk KA, et al.: Enteral versus parenteral feeding. Effects on septic morbidity after

blunt and penetrating abdominal trauma. Ann Surg *215*:503, 1992.

98. Moore FA, et al.: TEN versus TPN following major abdominal trauma—reduced septic morbidity. J Trauma *29*:916, 1989.

99. Greenberg GR, et al.: Controlled trial of bowel rest and nutritional support in the management of Crohn's disease. Gut *29*: 1309, 1988.

100. Wright RA, Adler EC: Peripheral parenteral nutrition is no better than enteral nutrition in acute exacerbation of Crohn's disease: A prospective trial. J Clin Gastroenterol *12*:396, 1990.

25

Psychosocial and Psychophysiologic Mechanisms in GI Illness

DOUGLAS A. DROSSMAN

Our understanding of how psychosocial factors relate to GI illness depends partly on the changing belief systems or explanatory ("folk") models of the time. For example, the popularity of searching for psychogenic causes of GI diseases in the 1940s related more to the influence of established psycho-analytically oriented theorists than to research findings specific for these diseases. This psychosomatic model arose after some failure in finding infectious etiologies (the previous "folk" model) for many chronic diseases. By the 1960s, the psychosomatic model was refuted. With improved techniques to measure intestinal motility, a parallel movement of psychophysiologic investigation became more popular, but with little appreciation of intervening psychosocial influences. The fact that neither model was sufficient to explain symptoms, health behaviors, or other clinical paradoxes, has led to interest in a more integrated explanatory model.

Although explanatory models arise in response to new technologies and the need for clinical solutions, they have their roots in theories that have existed for centuries. In this chapter, I will trace the evolution of theory and research relating psychosocial factors with GI illness and will then discuss current knowledge in the context of the existing (biopsychosocial) model.

ANTIQUITY THROUGH THE LATE 19TH CENTURY

Beliefs about the interaction between mind and body in western civilization re-

lates historically to two competing concepts: *dualism*, which separates, and *holism*, which unifies these two entities. The most widely recognized proponent of dualism was the philosopher Rene Descartes, who in 1637 proposed the separation of the thinking mind (res cognitans) from the machine-like body (res extensa) (1). Consistent with dualism is the concept of psychogenesis: if mind and body are separate, then psychologic processes (as an external factor) can cause (rather than be a part of) medical disease. The possibility that "passions" or emotions could lead to the development of medical disease was first proposed by Galen (2), and has been upheld by medical writers into the 20th century. This supposition is not surprising, since it is easy to observe the effects of intense emotion on autonomic arousal, the production of chest or abdominal pain or even sudden death (3). Even today, when the pathophysiology of a disease is unknown, it is common to attribute it to a psychogenic etiology.

The concept of holism, from the Greek holos, or whole, was first proposed by Plato, Aristotle, and Hippocrates in ancient Greece (1). It postulates that mind and body are integrated and inseparable, and the study of medical disease must take into account the whole person rather than merely the diseased part. By the 17th century, these ideas were eclipsed by the strong influence of Cartesian duality on western medicine. Nevertheless, holistic theory was occasionally defended by some authors, such as Claude Bernard, who promoted the concept of a homeostatic relationship involving mind and body. In the United States, the most notable proponent of holism was Dr. Benjamin Rush, who stated; "He [man] is, in the eye of a physician, a single and indivisible being, for so intimately united are his soul and body, that one cannot be moved, without the other" (4). Rush sought to integrate psychologic and medical knowledge in the diagnosis and treatment of medical illness. However, after his death in 1813, psychiatry was separated from medical practice and relegated to the asylums. In addition, and unintentionally (5), Pasteur's discovery of microorganisms and Koch's development of the germ theory of disease further moved medicine in the direction of duality and biologic reductionism. Only in recent years (for example, with tuberculosis and AIDS) have we learned that infectious agents are conditional factors in disease etiology; host resistance and the social environment also contribute.

Because of limited technology, explanatory models through the 19th century developed from natural observations, which were then interpreted in terms of etiology. However, an important advancement occurred in 1833 with William Beaumont's studies of Alexis St. Martin, a voyageur who developed a traumatic gastric fistula. Beaumont's studies systematically reported the association of emotions such as anger and fear on gastric mucosal morphology and function (6), and are probably the first psychophysiologic investigations of the human GI tract.

OBSERVATIONAL STUDIES IN THE EARLY TO MID-20TH CENTURY (1900–1959)

Studies of Gastrointestinal Function

Beaumont set the stage for further investigations of the effects of emotion on gastrointestinal function. Cannon noted a cessation in bowel activity among cats reacting to a growling dog (7). Pavlov (8) studied surgically produced fistulas in dogs, which led to an understanding of the role of the vagus nerve in mediating the cephalic phase of acid secretion. Selye (9) observed gastric erosions and adrenal enlargement in rats exposed to a variety of noxious stimuli, and

this led to the concept of a generalized bodily response to stress, the "general adaptation syndrome." Later studies of Tom (10) and Monica (11), two people with gastric fistulas, demonstrated that different emotional configurations are associated with distinct changes in gastric function. Gastric hyperemia and increased motility and secretion occurred with feelings of anger, intense pleasure, or aggressive behavior patterns related to the subject's active engagement with the environment. Conversely, mucosal pallor and decreased secretion and motor activity occurred with fear or depression: states of withdrawal ("giving-up" behavior) or disengagement from others.

Other investigators reported that esophageal spasm occurred in response to strong emotion (12), and a series of experiments by Almy et al. indicated that physical and psychologic stimuli led to increased sigmoid motility and vascular engorgement in healthy subjects (13) and in subjects with irritable bowel syndrome (IBS) (14). Almy's later studies with IBS patients using an emotive ("stress") interview attempted to correlate mood with symptoms and motility. He reported increased motility concurrent with states of aggression (particularly in those with constipation), and decreased motility associated with feelings of helplessness (and diarrhea) (15). These patterns were not associated with fixed personality features, but varied with the patient's mood.

The medical investigators of the time are to be credited for their careful observation and documentation of psychologic and physiologic variables. The data provide scientific evidence that the gut is physiologically responsive to emotion and environmental (stressful) stimuli. However, the studies were limited in two ways: (1) the measurement techniques were rudimentary, and (2) the studies were unidirectional; for example, no effort was made to evaluate the reciprocal effects of changes in gut physiology on mental functioning.

Psychosomatic Investigation of GI Disorders

A parallel line of investigation in the U.S. occurred during the psychoanalytically dominated era of psychosomatic medicine.

Freud set the stage for psychiatric investigators to consider the unconscious mind as a stimulus for the development of medical disease. The most rigid hypothesis was proposed by Groddeck, who believed that physical diseases were caused by symbolic inner conflicts, and these diseases existed to prevent these conflicts from becoming conscious (16). The more moderate (and more popular) view was developed by Franz Alexander (17) and other academic psychoanalysts who emigrated from Western Europe in the early part of the century. Alexander and his coworkers emphasized that psychodynamic conflicts and specific personality features, in addition to a biologic predisposition (Factor X), contributed to the development of a disease. Therefore, the proper environmental stimulus could activate the psychologic conflict, and the biologically predisposed individual would develop or exacerbate the disease. Ulcerative colitis, duodenal ulcer, and five non-GI disorders (asthma, rheumatoid arthritis, hypertension, neurodermatitis, and thyrotoxicosis) were identified as psychosomatic.

Using peptic ulcer as an example, it was proposed that acid hypersecretion in the infant might lead to a greater requirement for feeding to neutralize excess secretion and relieve internal tension. If this need were not met by a gratifying environment (mother), then a chronic or repetitive state of tension would develop. The child might generalize this experience and later have difficulty gaining confidence in the environment as a source of support. A psychodynamic pattern (oral-dependent) for securing gratification would develop to satisfy the increased needs. Thus, a person with this personality pattern would be more likely to view the real or threatened loss of a source of support as distressing. This hypothesis was tested in a study of 2073 Army recruits in basic training because leaving home provided an appropriate stressful environment. Among 63 acid hypersecretors, psychiatrists were able to blindly identify seven of nine men who had ulcers based on the psychologic features of an "ulcer-prone" personality (18). The "core" conflict for ulcerative colitis was less developed. It related to the development of over-dependency on certain key persons (e.g., a controlling or dominant mother), leading to a sensitivity to rejection, and difficulty in forming trusting relationships. Disruption of a key relationship, such as by death or separation, would lead to activation of disease through changes in bowel vascularity or intestinal microflora (17).

Aside from the Weiner study (18), the psychosomatic literature consisted of numerous retrospective case reports that were flawed because of small sample sizes, skewed sampling of psychiatric patients, uncontrolled psychologic assessment, and limited disease validation (19,20). In retrospect, the psychosomatic theory is too simplistic because it proposed that emotional factors were etiologic rather than a part of the illness. Furthermore, attention was directed solely at intrapsychic factors; life stress, the social environment, and the patient's coping style were not considered. The results that were reported probably relate more to a general effect of psychologic distress on illness exacerbation than to findings specific for any disease. By the 1960s, this theory became unpopular among patients and physicians because of its stigmatizing features. Nevertheless, these investigators contributed to the first systematic study of psychodynamic processes, and supported an association between psychologic factors and the clinical expression of medical disease.

THE BIOMEDICAL ERA (1960–1979)

With the explosion of medical technology after 1960, and perhaps as a result of the somewhat unfounded "bad press" of the psychosomatic research, social and political forces moved scientists into an era of biomedical (dualistic and reductionistic) research. The search for the etiology and pathophysiology of disease took precedence over the study of the patient. Psychosocial processes were considered important, but only as secondary phenomena: if the cause of a disease could be found, then certainly any psychosocial difficulties would disappear.

Physiologic Investigation of the GI Tract

By the early 1970s, notable GI physiologists such as Horace Davenport, Charles

Code, Sidney Cohen, James Christensen, and Sidney Phillips were developing and testing physiologic systems to better evaluate the motor and electrical activity of the gastrointestinal system. Investigators systematically studied most areas of the GI tract (21–23), and were able to delineate mechanisms for many of the esophageal motor disorders (e.g., achalasia, scleroderma, diffuse esophageal spasm), and to determine the somewhat paradoxic mechanism of constipation (increased sigmoid pressures) and diarrhea (decreased pressures) (24,25).

A logical extension of this research effort was to explore the pathophysiology of the functional GI disorders. These disorders, represented primarily by the IBS, were heretofore unexplained, but the symptoms were presumed to arise from intestinal dysmotility. These studies showed that when patients with IBS were compared to normals, they had an enhanced motor response to various environmental stimuli such as psychological stress (14), peptide hormones (26) and fatty meals (27), and it also was reported that the increased motility was associated with symptoms of pain (28).

In the late 1970s, interest focused on finding a specific physiologic marker for IBS, and little attention was paid to evaluation of the patient's psychologic state. Some authors reported a unique myoelectrical pattern: although the predominant basic electrical rhythm (BER) or pacesetter potential of the colon is six to nine cycles per min (comprising 90% of an observation period), patients with IBS had an increased frequency (up to 40% of the time) of three cycles per minute electrical activity (29,30). Furthermore, stimulation of the bowel also led to increased contractile activity at the same frequency (31). Later work using more sophisticated techniques had difficulty in reproducing these findings, and the concept of physiologic specificity was further challenged when Latimer et al. (32) reported the same electrical pattern in patients with psychiatric disturbance who did not have bowel symptoms. Investigators also began to recognize that the correlation between altered motility and painful symptoms was poor: experimentally induced motility in IBS did not usually produce pain, and many patients with functional GI disorders did not have abnormal motility when having pain. It took another 10 years for investigators to begin to consider alternative explanations for the symptoms of IBS.

Psychosocial Investigation of GI Disorders

For the most part, psychosocial investigation during this period remained out of the mainstream of medical research, and was limited to mental health scientists and a few medical investigators. Despite efforts to promote an integrated understanding of mind and body (or gut), their research was undertaken separately from physiologic investigations, and the findings were not generally known to the medical community.

Psychologic Factors in Functional GI Illness

The notion of a physiologic etiology for the functional GI disorders was challenged by reports that patients with IBS had a very high frequency of psychologic distress or disturbance (33–35). For example, in one study, 72% of patients with IBS met research criteria for psychiatric illness (36). Some then argued that IBS was a psychiatric disorder, and refuted the prevailing notion that the psychologic disturbance resulted from chronic GI symptoms. However, the patients having other chronic GI diseases who served as controls in these studies were psychologically normal. The ongoing argument as to whether IBS was "medical or psychiatric" was later clarified by epidemiologic studies in the 1980s.

Life Events Research

Meanwhile, psychiatric investigators were shifting the direction of their research from case reports about intrapsychic processes to larger studies linking stressful life events with the incidence and prevalence of disease. Also, the investigators studied the general effects of stress on disease susceptibility, rather than searching for disease-specific psychologic markers. In one study of thousands of subjects, the authors found that persons working in a more high-pressure job (air traffic controllers compared to airmen) were more likely to have stress-induced illnesses such as peptic ulcer and hypertension (37). It was hypothesized that chronic frustration from this job produced physiologic effects that increased the likelihood for these diseases to develop.

To standardize this type of research, Holmes and Rahe developed a 43-item questionnaire that included experiences (e.g., divorce, death of a spouse, financial difficulties) that would be considered distressing to most persons. Using this scale, they reported that the greater the number of such life events, the greater the likelihood of a change in health status (38). The life events research during this period, although narrow in scope, was an improvement over the previous psychosomatic studies because of: (1) the emphasis on hypothesis testing, (2) the use of standardized questionnaires to gather psychosocial data, (3) the focus on interactional rather than just intraindividual processes, and (4) the affirmation of the multifactorial nature of illness.

Behavioral Medicine

By the 1960s, research psychologists were aware that autonomic or other physiological functioning such as GI secretion and motility could be modified through operant or classical conditioning (39,40). Conditioning experiences might also lead to a psychophysiologic disorder, as demonstrated in the following hypothetic example (41):

A young child wakes up on the day of a dreaded examination at school with anxiety and "fight-or-flight" symptoms of tachycardia, diaphoresis, abdominal cramps, and diarrhea. The parent keeps the child home because of a "tummyache," and allows him to stay in bed and watch TV. Several days later, as the child is about to go to school, the symptoms recur.

This hypothetic case demonstrates how attention to the abdominal discomfort through "rewards" such as absence from school can produce relief by avoiding the feared situation. Repetition of this behavior could then condition the development of future GI symptoms when the person experiences similar distressing circumstances (39).

The awareness that such behavioral conditioning could affect physiologic dysfunction and illness behavior set the stage in 1977 for the development of the new psychologic field of behavioral medicine. This psychologic discipline differed from its contemporaries through the use of behavioral psychology to develop therapeutic techniques (42). If GI dysfunction can be learned, then it may be unlearned through behavioral techniques such as biofeedback.

Early efforts to improve disordered GI function (43,44) through biofeedback were generally unsuccessful, the exception being treatment of fecal incontinence (45). Although biofeedback could modify GI motility, it did not lead to improved symptoms, and this further challenged the belief that functional GI symptoms resulted from disturbed motility. The currently accepted role for biofeedback and other relaxation techniques in medical illness is to reduce stress and improve the patient's sense of control over pain and other symptoms (46).

THE REEMERGENCE OF HOLISM (1980–?)

The 1980s saw the beginning of a period of major changes in the psychosocial understanding of GI disease and illness. Until this point, the biomedical model maintained dominance in modern theory and research. Particularly in the 1960s and 1970s, it was believed that technologic advances would lead to finding the cause (and cure of) many GI disorders. However, by the end of this period, clinicians and scientists were confronted with the inefficiencies of this model: (1) diagnostic imaging and physiologic assessment did not fully explain the symptoms of many, if not most patients presenting with functional complaints; (2) the prominence of psychosocial disturbances and illness behaviors, particularly among those seen at referral centers, did not correlate well with the observed physiologic disturbance or disease pathology; (3) social and political forces led to increased interest in understanding psychosocial issues of the aged and chronically ill; (4) newer psychosocial methods of assessment shifted interests away from disease activity and toward the patient; and (5) advances in brain-gut physiology yielded findings that could not fit with the reductionistic biomedical concept.

Biopsychosocial (Systems) Model

Although many psychiatrists wrote about the importance of psychosocial factors in medical illness, the pivotal event that changed the thinking of most medical physicians began in 1977 with Engel's series of publications on the biopsychosocial model (47–49). Engel, an internist and psychoanalyst, offered the first modern exposition of holistic (now called systems) theory by proposing that illness is the product of biologic, psychologic, and social subsystems interacting at multiple levels (Fig. 25–1). Consider a man with Crohn's disease recently suffering from the loss of a spouse, who develops increased disease activity with worsening inflammation, abdominal pain, and diarrhea. The spouse's death could affect the person's appraisal of his symptoms (e.g., as life threatening), the pain threshold, his psychologic state (acute grief), and even the degree of inflammation, through its association with immune or inflammatory mediators. Similarly, exacerbation of disease can affect the patient's daily functional status and capacity to cope with the loss. Rather than consider any one factor as etiologic, Engel proposed that it is the interaction of the conditions that determines the illness. The subsystems cannot be separated, because they simultaneously explain the person's illness experience, which in turn reciprocates with its contributors.

The biopsychosocial or systems model offers certain advantages for modern patient care and research: (1) an understanding of human illness that reconciles the discrepancies between biomedical thought and clinical observation, (2) a clinical framework for the physician to integrate the broad range of biomedical and psychosocial that explain the illness experience, and (3) a unifying structure for the new multidisciplinary research methodology and findings in GI illness that emerged over the next decade: enhancements in psychosocial assessment and analysis.

Major advances in psychosocial assessment evolved with: (1) improved research questionnaires having better reliability and validity, (2) the development of new scales to assess broader psychosocial domains, (3) a shift in research focus from measurement of disease to that of patient perceptions and behaviors, (4) inclusion of both psychosocial and physiological assessments in study protocols, (5) evaluation of "softer" outcomes (e.g., health care use, daily function, symptom severity, general well-being) than death or disease complications, and (6) use of multivariate statistical methods to simultaneously control for interacting variables.

Psychiatric Diagnosis

The need for standardization in psychiatric diagnosis in research led to the development of questionnaires (50,51) based on the American Psychiatric Association's Diag-

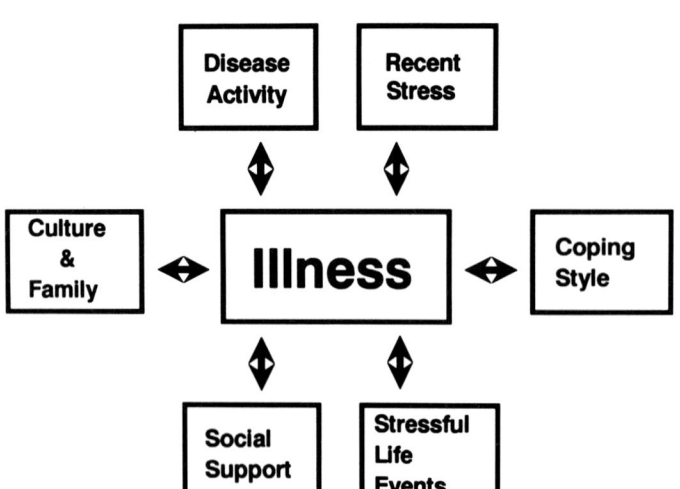

Fig. 25-1. Biopsychosocial model of illness. Illness is shown to result from, and in turn influence, multiple interacting biologic and psychosocial subsystems. Reproduced with permission from Drossman DA: Psychosocial Considerations in Gastroenterology. *In* Gastrointestinal Disease, Fifth Edition. Philadelphia, W.B. Saunders Co., 1993.

nostic and Statistical Manual (currently in its third revision) (52). Using these questionnaires, investigators confirmed that patients with IBS (53) and functional dyspepsia (54) had higher frequencies of psychiatric diagnoses than patients with other GI problems, and the psychiatric diagnosis antedated the onset of the bowel disorder (53). For inflammatory bowel disease, psychiatric illness was associated primarily with patients having more severe physical illness (55).

Improvements in Life Events Research

Criticisms of the Holmes and Rahe life events scale led to two improvements. The Life Experiences Survey (56) evaluated not only the presence of an event, but also how it was appraised, either as positive or negative, and its intensity. For example, a divorce or job change might be viewed as positive by one individual and negative by another, and these interpretations might have different psychosocial impact. Using this scale (57), patients with IBS were found to have lower positive life event scores than persons with IBS who had not seen physicians (nonpatients) or normals. But surprisingly, IBS patients had *lower* negative life event scores than IBS nonpatients and normals. Further analysis showed no group differences in the number of events, but the IBS patients played down their severity. Stated another way, this new scale showed that IBS patients are more likely to deny or minimize their appraisal or reporting of negatively perceived life experiences.

Another concern was that persons experiencing psychologic distress might overreport life events. For this reason, the Life Events and Difficulties Schedule (LEDS) was designed to validate these events by having raters independently determine the degree to which an event is threatening to an average person (58). Using this scale, Creed found that, although the frequency of life events was similar in patients with functional and organic GI illness, severe life events were more frequent in the functional GI group, and these events preceded the onset of pain (59). These findings were independent of the degree of the patient's psychologic disturbance, and existed even when the patients denied this association.

Study of Newer Psychosocial Domains

The newly developed field of health psychology produced scientists who were vested in simultaneously studying a broad range of psychosocial domains. They recognized that simple analyses of medical and psychiatric diagnoses, personality, and even life stress were not sufficient to explain the multiplicity of factors affecting the illness experience. This led to the development of new standardized questionnaires to assess psychologic distress (60), social support (61), coping style (62), and functional status (63).

Health-Related Quality of Life

The growing scientific interest in the patient's psychosocial responses to chronic illness influenced the development of research in health related quality of life (64). This method uses standardized scales to assess patient perceptions, the illness experience, and functional status in response to a particular medical disorder. In gastroenterology, most of the studies involve inflammatory bowel disease, and several scales specific for this disorder have been developed (65–67). The studies have shown that: (1) IBD patients generally have a good quality of life compared to patients with other chronic illness (e.g., rheumatoid arthritis, chronic pain, obstructive lung disease) (68,69), but worse than the general population or HMO patients (67,68); (2) their illness impact occurs more in terms of psychosocial (e.g., functional, recreational, social, economic, emotional) than physical dysfunction (70,71); (3) patient's with Crohn's disease have greater emotional distress and disability than those with ulcerative colitis (71,72), but this relates primarily to disease severity (71); (4) disease-related worries and concerns have independent impact on quality of life, which may be ameliorated through physician counseling and education (66); (5) certain coping strategies such as education and social support are adaptive in improving quality of life (71); and (6) for ulcerative colitis, colectomy improves quality of life (73,74), but (7) ileoanal and Koch pouches are preferred over Brooke ileostomies for sports and sexual activities (74).

Epidemiologic Psychosocial Assessment

The previous dilemma relating to the role of psychosocial factors in the functional GI disorders was clarified by applying a unique epidemiologic study design. Following the development of questionnaires to identify IBS by survey (75,76), it was possible to compare the psychosocial profiles of those in the community (IBS nonpatients) with those of patients seen by physicians. If psychosocial disturbance were linked to the GI disorder, then the findings would be similar in the two groups. Conversely, if the psychosocial disturbances in IBS patients were not seen in the community, then they were not related to the disorder per se, but influenced the decision to seek health care. The latter (self-selection) hypothesis was confirmed by finding that nonpatients with IBS were not psychologically different from normal persons (57,77,78). This finding contributed to the understanding of psychosocial factors as modulators of illness behaviors, and set the stage for the health outcome research to follow.

Health Outcome Research

Health outcome research is new to gastroenterology. It exemplifies the research application of the biopsychosocial model since, through statistical techniques, it permits simultaneous analysis of multiple interacting variables.

This research model is illustrated in Figure 25–2, which depicts the relationship of biologic and psychosocial factors on health outcome. Genetic, biologic, and environmental factors early in life determine one's susceptibility to developing a medical disorder. Following this, psychosocial modifiers, along with the biologic nature of the disease, determine whether or when the disease is experienced as an illness, subsequent illness behaviors, and ultimately, the clinical outcome. Outcome is understood in broad terms: the patient's general well-being and daily function, symptom severity, health care use (including physician visits, hospitalizations, and surgeries) and finally, the clinical course of the disease, its complications, and possibly death. The clinical outcome will, in turn, have reciprocal effects on its precedents.

As an example, the assumption that the biologic nature of the disorder determines outcome has been challenged for chronic GI disorders with new evidence that psychosocial factors also have effects (57,77–79). It is then clinically relevant to determine which factors are more important, and this has implications for treatment. Using multiple regression techniques, the anticipated medical and psychosocial variables are put into an analytic model where their relative contribution (while controlling for each other) in predicting a selected outcome, is determined.

This approach has been used to determine the effects of physical and sexual abuse on health outcome in a GI referral practice (80). All women attending the University of North Carolina GI clinic were surveyed with regard to demographic factors, medical diagnosis, medical symptoms, health care use, and abuse history. It was found that an abuse history (independent of demographic factors and medical disease) predicted:

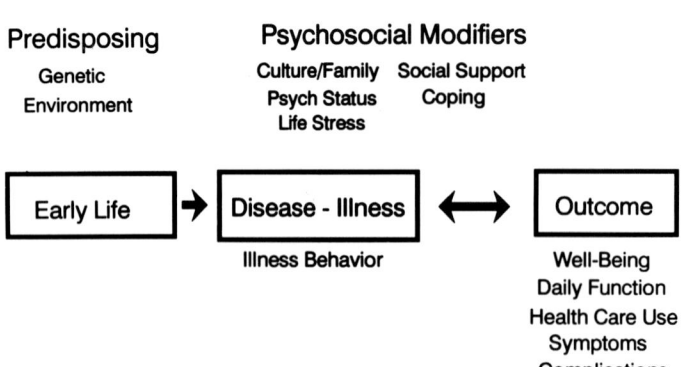

Fig. 25-2. Relationship of predisposing factors and psychosocial modifiers on disease susceptibility, illness and its outcome. Reproduced with permission from Drossman DA: Psychosocial Considerations in Gastroenterology. *In* Gastrointestinal Disease, Fifth Edition. Philadelphia, W.B. Saunders Co., 1993.

(1) more frequent GI and non-GI painful symptoms, (2) more lifetime surgeries (2.8 vs. 2.0 surgeries; p < 0.009), and (3) more frequent physician visits (4.2 versus 3.3 visits in 6 months; p < 0.09). The findings suggest that efforts directed at treating the psychosocial concomitants of abuse may improve the clinical outcome over and above treatment of the disease.

Physiologic Investigations Relating to GI Disease

Since the 1980s, the focus of physiologic research has shifted from etiology to understanding the mediating effects of physiologic systems on brain-gut interactions.

Neuroenteric Physiologic Research—The Brain-Gut Axis

Previous psychophysiologic studies assumed a unidirectional relationship between CNS (e.g., "stress") and GI function. In the 1980s, this was revised with the description of a "hard-wired" system that permitted multidimensional interactions among the brain, the enteric nervous system, and its neuroendocrine and immune connections (41). Figure 25-3 shows how extrinsic or enteroceptive (including mental) information has the capability to affect GI function, and GI function can reciprocally affect CNS activity (81). Disturbances in any of the subsystems resonate throughout the brain-gut axis, leading to possible effects on pain sensation, motility, and mood.

Further modulation of this system occurs by way of brain-gut neurotransmitters, which include: VIP, TRH, 5HT and its congeners, Substance P, CCK, and the enkephalins. These substances have integrated activities on gastrointestinal function and human behavior depending upon their location. The heterotopic locations of the enkephalins lead to varied and potent integrated effects on pain control (82), GI motility (83), feeding activity (84), emotional behavior, and immunity (85).

New findings over the last decade provide an understanding of how abnormalities in afferent sensation, motor function, and psychologic status can interact to explain functional GI symptoms. Psychologic states affect intestinal motor function (86,87), and intestinal motor disturbance reciprocally af-

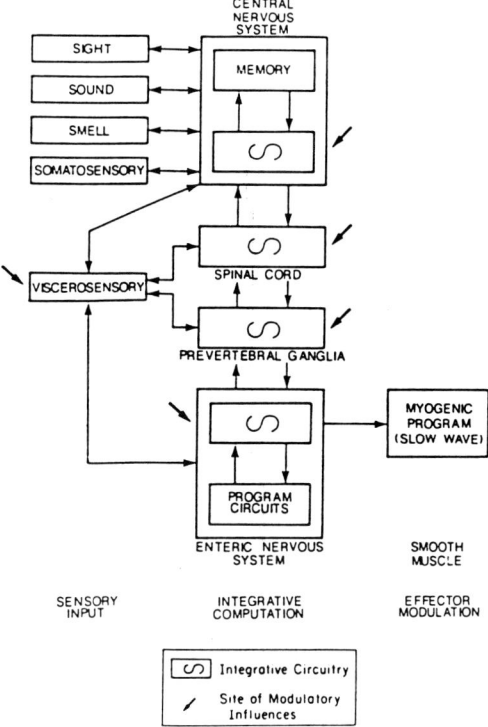

Fig. 25-3. Processing of information within the brain-gut axis. External and internal sensory information are integrated within neural circuits in the central nervous system, spinal cord, prevertebral ganglia, and enteric nervous system. This multidirectional system allows resonating circuits, which explain potential relationships between altered pain sensation, gut dysmotility, and mood disturbance. Reproduced with permission from Mayer EA, Raybould HE: Role of visceral afferent mechanisms in functional bowel disorders. Gastroenterology 99:1692, 1990.

fects emotional centers in the brain (88). But clinicians know that altered motility is not enough to explain symptoms. Recent studies also indicate the existence of abnormalities in pain perception and pain threshold in patients with functional esophageal (89), gastroduodenal (90) and bowel (91) disorders. These pain thresholds are modified by CNS/psychosocial processes including psychologic distress and coping (92), and abuse history (93). These new findings provide the basis for future treatment trials to improve pain symptoms by means of peripheral (e.g., visceral neurotransmitter blocking agents) and central (e.g., psychopharmacologic or behavioral) techniques.

Psychoneuroimmunology and Psychoneuroendocrinology

One of the more exciting new research areas relates to studying effects of natural and experimentally induced stressors on cognitive and emotional centers, and their subsequent alteration of immune function and disease susceptibility (94). It is now clear that the CNS, through the hypothalamic-pituitary (through the corticotropic releasing hormone) and neuroadrenergic (through the locus ceruleus) systems coordinate both behavioral and immunologic adaptation to stressful situations. These systems reciprocate with the interleukin-cytokine system of immune-inflammatory cells and can modulate inflammatory activity in disorders such as rheumatoid arthritis (95) and possibly inflammatory bowel disease.

Clinically, studies also have shown that medical students under stress from examinations decrease their interferon production and have an increased incidence of infectious diseases (96), and these effects appear to be dose-related (97). Animal studies show that the immune and emotional response to stress are associated with increased neural activity in the amygdala and hippocampus, and lesions in the limbic system reduce negative emotion and produce immune enhancement (98).

These psychoimmune processes are amenable to behavioral interventions. In one study, mucosal mast cells were classically conditioned to secrete an immune mediator (Protease II) in response to an audiovisual cue (99). The same conditioning model also has been shown to delay the development of murine lupus erythematosus and prolong survival in NZB-NZW hybrid mice (100).

Although future studies are needed to clarify the degree of effect these relationships will have in human gastrointestinal disease, the pathophysiologic framework exists, and the implications are significant. Studies over the next decade are likely to elaborate on the mediating mechanisms for the clinically observed association of psychosocial stress with exacerbation of peptic and inflammatory bowel disease, and for the benefits of supportive interpersonal care in ameliorating chronic illness and improving health (101).

THE FUTURE

The biopsychosocial model has provided the framework for future studies that will increase our knowledge of the relationships among psychosocial processes, GI function, disease susceptibility, and clinical outcomes. Greater integration among the basic sciences (e.g., molecular biology, neuroenteric physiology, immunity) and its clinical concomitants (symptoms, disease activity and its complications, health related quality of life) will occur through interdisciplinary collaborations and sophisticated research models. The knowledge obtained is likely to bring on a new era of therapeutics using biologic and behavioral interventions.

APPENDIX—GLOSSARY OF TERMS

1. *Disease/Illness.* For this discussion, a distinction is made between *disease,* externally measurable abnormalities in the structure and function of organs and tissues, and *illness,* the person's experience of ill health and bodily dysfunction (102).
2. *Psychogenic.* Refers to the belief that psychologic factors lead to the development of illness and disease. It implies a linear or reductionistic (i.e., cause → effect) association.
3. *Holism.* An ancient concept which proposes that mind and body are inseparably linked. Although the term has been promulgated by proponents of alternative medicine, it is more appropriately understood as having evolved into the biopsychosocial model.
4. *Psychophysiologic reaction.* A psychologically induced alteration in function of a target organ without structural change. The persistence of an altered physiologic state or an enhanced physiologic response to psychologic stimuli is considered by some a *psychophysiologic disorder.*
5. *Psychosomatic disease.* An overused term considered by some synonymous with psychogenically induced disease or illness. The traditional definition relates to a disease that results both from preexistent biologic susceptibility and specific psychologic characteristics (17). Ul-

cerative colitis and peptic ulcer were considered as two of the seven "classic" psychosomatic diseases. This term should be ignored when discussing current psychosocial theory.

6. *Biopsychosocial.* An explanatory model which proposes that health, illness, and disease are the result of multiple interacting systems at the cellular, tissue, organismal, interpersonal and environmental level. As the term implies, it incorporates biologic, psychologic, and sociocultural dimensions.

7. *Health status/Health-related quality of life.* A composite measure used in research of an individual's perceptions, concerns, illness experience, and functional status. It incorporates social, cultural, psychologic, and disease-related factors.

8. *Outcome.* The predicted effect or result of the illness/disease or any interventions. Outcome variables may include "hard" measures (e.g., death, disease complications), or "soft" measures (e.g., general well-being, physical or psychologic function, health care use), as used in health status and outcome research.

9. *Stress.* Any influence on the person's steady state that requires adjustment or adaptation can be considered stress. The term is nonspecific and encompasses both the stimulus and its effects. The stimulus can be a biologic event such as infection, a social event such as a change in residence, or a disturbing thought. Stress can be desirable or undesirable, although some stimuli, such as pain, sex, or threat of injury elicit predictable responses. In contrast, certain life events can have more varied effects (e.g., a change in job). The effects may vary among people, or within the same person at different times. There may be no effect, physiologic changes (e.g., diarrhea), a psychologic response (e.g., anxiety, depression), disease onset (e.g., asthma, colitis), or any combination. An individual's appraisal of a stimulus as stressful or not, and his or her response, depend on prior experience, attitudes, coping mechanisms, personality, culture, and biologic factors, including susceptibility to disease.

REFERENCES

1. Lipowski ZJ: Psychosomatic medicine: Past and present Part 1, historical background. Can J Psychiatry *31*:2, 1986.
2. Ackerknecht EH: The history of psychosomatic medicine. Psychol Med *12*:17, 1982.
3. Engel GL: Psychologic stress, vasodepressor (vasovagal) syncope, and sudden death. Ann Intern Med *89*:403, 1978.
4. Rush B: Sixteen introductory lectures, Philadelphia, Bradford and Inns-keep, 1811.
5. Dubos R, Escande JP: Reflections on Medicine, Science and Humanity, New York, Harcourt Brace Jovanovich, 1979.
6. Beaumont W: Experiments and Observations on the Gastric Juice and the Physiology of Digestion, Plattsburg, FP Allen, 1833.
7. Cannon WB: The movements of the intestine studied by means of roentgen rays. Am J Physiol *6*:251, 1902.
8. Pavlov I: The Work of the Digestive Glands. London, C Griffen and Company, 1910.
9. Selye H: The general adaptation syndrome and the diseases of adaptation. J Clin Endocrinol Metab *6*:117, 1946.
10. Wolf S, Wolff HG: Human Gastric Function, New York, Oxford University Press, 1943.
11. Engel GL, Reichsman F, Segal HL: A study of an infant with gastric fistula. I. Behavior and the rate of total hydrochloric acid secretion. Psychosom Med *18*:374, 1956.
12. Jacobson E: Spastic esophagus and mucous colitis. Arch Intern Med *37*:443, 1927.
13. Almy TP, Kern F Jr, Tulin M: Alteration in colonic function in man under stress: II. Experimental production of sigmoid spasm in healthy persons. Gastroenterology *12*:425, 1949.
14. Almy TP, Hinkle LE Jr, Berle B, Kern F Jr: Alterations in colonic function in man under stress. III. Experimental production of sigmoid spasm in patients with spastic constipation. Gastroenterology *12*:437, 1949.
15. Almy TP: Experimental studies on the irritable colon. Am J Med *10*:60, 1951.
16. Groddeck G: The Book of the It. New York, Vintage Books, 1961.
17. Alexander F: Psychosomatic Medicine: Its Principles and Applications. New York, WW Norton, 1950.
18. Weiner H, Thaler M, Reiser M, Mirsky IA: Etiology of duodenal ulcer—I. Relation of specific psychological characteristics to

rate of gastric secretion. Psychosom Med *19*:1, 1957.

19. Drossman DA: Psychosocial aspects of ulcerative colitis and Crohn's disease. *In* JB Kirsner, RG Shorter (eds): Inflammatory Bowel Disease. Philadelphia, Lea & Febiger, 1988, p. 209–26.

20. Aronowitz R, Spiro HM: The rise and fall of the psychosomatic hypothesis in ulcerative colitis. J Clin Gastroenterol *10*:298, 1988.

21. Watson WC, Sullivan SN: Hypertonicity of the cricopharyngeal sphincter: A cause of globus sensation. Lancet *ii:2*:1417, 1974.

22. Bar-meir S et al.: Biliary and pancreatic duct pressures measured by ERCP manometry in patients with suspected papillary stenosis. Dig Dis Sci *24*:209, 1979.

23. Schuster MM, Hendrix TR, Mendeloff AI: The internal sphincter response. Manometric studies on its normal physiology, normal pathways and alteration in bowel disease. J Clin Invest *42*:196, 1963.

24. Connell AM: The motility of the pelvic colon. Part II: Paradoxical motility in diarrhoea and constipation. Gut *3*:342, 1962.

25. Wangel AG, Deller DJ: Intestinal motility in man. III. Mechanisms of constipation and diarrhea with particular reference to the irritable colon syndrome. Gastroenterology *48*:69, 1965.

26. Harvey RF, Read AE: Effect of cholecystokinin on colon motility and symptoms in patients with the irritable bowel syndrome. Lancet *i*:1, 1973.

27. Sullivan MA, Cohen S, Snape WJ: Colonic myoelectrical activity in irritable-bowel syndrome. New Engl J Med *298*:878, 1978.

28. Connell AM, Jones FA, Rowlands EN: Motility of the pelvic colon. IV. Abdominal pain associated with colonic hypermotility after meals. Gut *6*:105, 1965.

29. Snape WJ, Carlson GM, Cohen S: Colonic myoelectric activity in the irritable bowel syndrome. Gastroenterology *70*:326, 1976.

30. Taylor I, Duthie DL, Smallwood R: The effect of stimulation on the myoelectrical activity of the rectosigmoid of man. Gut *15*:599, 1974.

31. Snape WJ, Carlson GM, Matarazzo SA: Evidence that abnormal myoelectrical activity produces colonic motor dysfunction in the irritable bowel syndrome. Gastroenterology *72*:326, 1977.

32. Latimer PR et al.: Colonic motor and myoelectrical activity: A comparative study of normal patients, psychoneurotic patients and patients with irritable bowel syndrome (IBS). Gastroenterology *80*:893, 1981.

33. Mendeloff AI, Monk M, Siegel CI, Lilienfeld A: Illness experience and life stresses in patients with irritable colon and with ulcerative colitis. An epidemiologic study of ulcerative colitis and regional enteritis in Baltimore, 1960–1964. N Engl J Med *282*:14, 1970.

34. Esler MD, Goulston KJ: Levels of anxiety in colonic disorders. N Engl J Med *288*:16, 1973.

35. Palmer RL et al.: Psychological characteristics of patients with the irritable bowel syndrome. Postgrad Med J *50*:416, 1974.

36. Young SJ, Alpers DH, Norland CC, Woodruff RA: Psychiatric illness and the irritable bowel syndrome. Practical implications for the primary physician. Gastroenterology *70*:162, 1976.

37. Cobb S, Rose RM: Hypertension, peptic ulcer and diabetes in air traffic controllers. JAMA *224*:489, 1973.

38. Holmes TH, Rahe RH: The social readjustment rating scale. J Psychosom Res *11*:213, 1967.

39. Miller NE: Learning of visceral and glandular responses. Science *163*:434, 1969.

40. Miller NE: Effect of learning on gastrointestinal functions. Clin Gastroenterol *6*:533, 1977.

41. Drossman DA: Psychosocial considerations in gastroenterology. *In* Sleisenger MH et al. (eds): Gastrointestinal Disease: Pathophysiology, Diagnosis, Management. Philadelphia, WB Saunders Co., 1993.

42. Miller NE, Dworkin BR: Effects of learning on visceral functions—biofeedback. N Engl J Med *296*:1274, 1977.

43. Bueno-Miranda F, Cerulli M, Schuster MM: Operant conditioning of colonic motility in irritable bowel syndrome. Gastroenterology *70*:867, 1976 (Abstract).

44. Schuster MM, Nikoomanesh P, Welles D: Biofeedback control of lower esophageal sphincter contraction. Clin Res *21*:521, 1973.

45. Marzuk PM: Biofeedback for gastrointestinal disorders: A review of the literature. Ann Intern Med *103*:240, 1985.

46. Drossman DA: Psychosocial factors in the care of patients with gastrointestinal diseases. *In* Yamada T (ed.): Textbook of Gastroenterology. Philadelphia, JB Lippincott Co, 1991, pp. 546–561.

47. Engel GL: The need for a new medical model: A challenge for biomedicine. Science *196*:129, 1977.

48. Engel GL: The clinical application of the biopsychosocial model. Am J Psychiatry *137*:535, 1980.

49. Engel GL: The biopsychosocial model and medical education. N Engl J Med *306*:802, 1981.

50. Robins LN, Helzer JE, Croughan J, Ratcliff KS: National Institute of Mental Health diagnostic interview schedule. Arch Gen Psychiatry *38*:381, 1981.

51. Spitzer RL, Williams JBW, Gibbon M, First MB: The Structured clinical interview for DSM-III-R (SCID). I: History, rationale, and description. Arch Gen Psychiatry *49*:624, 1992.

52. American Psychiatric Association: Diagnostic and Statistical Manual of Mental Disorders—Revised, Washington, DC, American Psychiatric Associations, 1987. Edition 3.

53. Walker EA et al.: Psychiatric illness and irritable bowel syndrome: A comparison with inflammatory bowel disease. Am J Psychiatry *147*:156, 1990.

54. Magni G, DiMario F, Bernasconi G, Mastropaola G: DSM-III diagnoses associated with dyspepsia of unknown cause. Am J Psychiatry *144*:1222, 1987.

55. Andrews H, Barczak P, Allan RN: Psychiatric illness in patients with inflammatory bowel disease. Gut *28*:1600, 1987.

56. Sarason IG, Johnson JH, Siegel JM: Assessing the impact of life changes: Development of the life experiences survey. J Consult Clin Psychol *46*:932, 1978.

57. Drossman DA et al.: Psychosocial factors in the irritable bowel syndrome. A multivariate study of patients and nonpatients with irritable bowel syndrome. Gastroenterology *95*:701, 1988.

58. Craig TK, Brown GW: Goal frustration and life event stress in the aetiology of painful gastrointestinal disorder. J Psychosom Res *28*:411, 1984.

59. Creed FH, Craig T, Farmer RG: Functional abdominal pain, psychiatric illness and life events. Gut *29*:235, 1988.

60. Derogatis LR: SCL-90-R: Administration, Scoring, and Procedures Manual II—For the R(evised) Version, Towson: Clinical Psychometric Research, 1983.

61. Sarason IG, Levine HM, Basham RB, Sarason BR: Assessing social support: The social support questionnaire. J Pers Soc Psych *44*:127, 1983.

62. Lazarus RS, Folkman S: Stress, Appraisal and Coping. New York, Springer Publishing Company, 1984.

63. Bergner M, Bobbitt RA, Carter WB: The sickness impact profile: Development and final revision of a health status measure. Med Care *19*:787, 1981.

64. Bech P: Quality of life in psychosomatic research. Psychopathology *20*:169, 1987.

65. Guyatt G et al.: A new measure of health status for clinical trials in inflammatory bowel disease. Gastroenterology *96*:804, 1989.

66. Drossman DA et al.: The rating form of IBD patient concerns: A new measure of health status. Psychosom Med *53*:701, 1991.

67. Love JR, Irvine EJ, Fedorak RN: Quality of life in inflammatory bowel disease. J Clin Gastroenterol *14*:15, 1992.

68. Patrick DL, Deyo RA: Generic and disease-specific measures in assessing health status and quality of life. Med Care *27*: S217, 1989.

69. Mitchell A et al.: Quality of life in patients with inflammatory bowel disease. J Clin Gastroenterol *10*:306, 1988.

70. Drossman DA et al.: Health related quality of life in inflammatory bowel disease: Functional status and patient worries and concerns. Dig Dis Sci *34*:1379, 1989.

71. Drossman DA et al.: Health status and health care use in persons with inflammatory bowel disease: A national sample. Dig Dis Sci *36*:1746, 1991.

72. Farmer RG, Easley KA, Farmer JM: Quality of life assessment by patients with inflammatory bowel disease. Cleve Clin J Med *59*:35, 1992.

73. McLeod RS et al.: Quality of life of patients with ulcerative colitis preoperatively and postoperatively. Gastroenterology *101*: 1307, 1991.

74. Kohler LW, Pemberton JH, Zinsmeister AR, Kelly KA: Quality of life after proctocolectomy. A comparison of Brooke ileostomy, Kock pouch, and ileal pouch-anal anastomosis. Gastroenterology *101*:679, 1991.

75. Drossman DA, Sandler RS, McKee DC, Lovitz AJ: Bowel patterns among subjects not seeking health care. Use of a questionnaire to identify a population with bowel dysfunction. Gastroenterology *83*:529, 1982.

76. Thompson WG, Heaton KW: Functional bowel disorders in apparently healthy people. Gastroenterology *79*:283, 1980.

77. Sandler RS, Drossman DA, Nathan HP, McKee DC: Symptom complaints and health care seeking behavior in subjects with bowel dysfunction. Gastroenterology *87*:314, 1984.

78. Whitehead WE et al.: Symptoms of psychologic distress associated with irritable bowel syndrome. Comparison of community and medical clinic samples. Gastroenterology *95*:709, 1988.

79. Smith RC et al.: Psychosocial factors are associated with health care seeking rather than diagnosis in irritable bowel syndrome. Gastroenterology *98*:293, 1990.

80. Drossman DA et al.: Sexual and physical abuse in women with functional or organic gastrointestinal disorders. Ann Intern Med *113*:828, 1990.

81. Mayer EA, Raybould HE: Role of visceral afferent mechanisms in functional bowel disorders. Gastroenterology *99*:1688, 1990.

82. Shavit Y, Martin FC: Opiates, stress and immunity: Animal studies. Ann Behav Med *9*:11, 1987.

83. Burks TF, Galligan JJ, Hirning LD, Porreca F: Brain, spinal cord and peripheral sites of action of enkephalins and other endogenous opioids on gastrointestinal motility. Gastr Clin Biol *11*:44B, 1987.

84. Baile CA, McLaughlin CL, Della Fera MA: Role of cholecystokinin and opioid peptides in control of food intake. Physiol Rev *66*: 172, 1986.

85. Shavit Y et al.: Stress, opioid peptides, the immune system, and cancer. J Immunol *135*:834s, 1985.

86. Valori RM, Kumar D, Wingate DL: Effects of different types of stress and or "prokinetic" drugs on the control of the fasting motor complex in humans. Gastroenterology *90*:1890, 1986.

87. Welgan P, Meshkinpour H, Beeler M: Effect of anger on colon motor and myoelectric activity in irritable bowel syndrome. Gastroenterology *94*:1150, 1988.

88. Svensson TH: Peripheral, autonomic regulation of locus coeruleus noradrenergic neurons in brain: Putative implications for psychiatry and psychopharmacology. Psychopharmacology *92*:1, 1987.

89. Clouse RE, Lustman PJ, McCord GS, Edmundowicz SA: Clinical correlates of abnormal sensitivity to intraesophageal balloon distention. Dig Dis Sci *36*:1040, 1991.

90. Mearin F, Cucala M, Azpiroz F, Malagelada JR: The origin of symptoms on the brain-gut axis in functional dyspepsia. Gastroenterology *101*:999, 1991.

91. Whitehead WE et al.: Tolerance for rectosigmoid distention in irritable bowel syndrome. Gastroenterology *98*:1187, 1990.

92. Bradley LA et al.: Psychosocial and psychophysical assessments of patients with unexplained chest pain. Am J Med *92*:65S, 1992.

93. Scarinci IC et al.: Pain perception and psychosocial correlates of sexual/physical abuse among patients with gastrointestinal disorders. Gastroenterology *102*:A509, 1992 (Abstract).

94. Camara EG, Danao TC: The brain and the immune system: A psychosomatic network. Psychosomatics *30*:140, 1989.

95. Sternberg EM, Chrousos GP, Wilder RL, Gold PW: The stress response and the regulation of inflammatory disease. Ann Intern Med *117*:854, 1992.

96. Kiecolt-Glaser JK, Glaser R: Psychosocial moderators of immune function. Ann Behav Med *9*:16, 1989.

97. Cohen S, Tyrrell AJ, Smith AP: Psychological stress and susceptibility to the common cold. N Engl J Med *325*:606, 1991.

98. Daruna JH, Morgan JE: Psychosocial effects on immune function: Neuroendocrine pathways. Psychosomatics *31*:4, 1990.

99. MacQueen G et al.: Pavlovian conditioning of rat mucosal mast cells to secrete rat mast cell Protease II. Science *243*:83, 1989.

100. Ader R, Cohen N: Behaviorally conditioned immunosuppression and murine systemic lupus erythematosus. Science *215*: 1534, 1982.

101. Berkman LF, Leo-Summers L, Horwitz RI: Emotional support and survival after myocardial infarction. A prospective, population-based study of the elderly. Ann Intern Med *117*:1003, 1992.

102. Reading A: Illness and disease. Med Clin North Am *61*:703, 1977.

26

Gastrointestinal Defenses Against Injury and Inflammation

IAN R. SANDERSON AND W. ALLAN WALKER

The barriers that defend the gastrointestinal tract, both physical and immunologic, have been studied increasingly during the 20th century. From ancient times until the present, the most important defense against gastrointestinal injury has been cognitive; that is, we learn not to ingest noxious agents. The importance of this fact is played out daily as pediatricians, gastroenterologists, and surgeons contend with the consequences of the accidental ingestion of poisons and caustic agents, especially among children. For the poisonous flowers and berries of earlier times we have substituted the chemical and pharmaceutical agents of our industrial age. The measures required to control this problem more effectively are beyond the scope of this review. Rather, the purpose of this chapter is to describe the resources and mechanisms whereby the gastrointestinal tract protects the body from injury and disease.

An appreciation of the topology of the intestinal tract has increased our understanding of mucosal defense. Topology is a branch of mathematics concerned with shapes. It has been developed to a very advanced stage by mathematicians in the earlier part of this century (1). However, in its simplest form it is concerned with what defines the change from the interior of an object to its exterior. When these ideas were applied to the gastrointestinal tract, it was apparent that the boundary between inside the body and its exterior was not across the mouth as had previously been supposed,

but lay in the wall of the intestine itself. This change allowed researchers to examine mucosal defense more logically. There are mechanisms that act within the lumen of the gastrointestinal tract (the extrinsic barrier) to modify the luminal contents or to reduce the movement of potential pathogens. There also is the intrinsic barrier of the gastrointestinal wall containing the physical barrier of cell membrane and tight junctions behind which lie a vast array of immune cells.

These arrangements are complex because, unlike the skin, for example, which is virtually impermeable, the small intestine is a selective barrier. The primary function of the small intestine is to absorb nutrients into the circulation (2). During the course of this activity, the intestine is exposed to a wide variety of antigens derived from foods, resident bacteria, and invading microorganisms. These need to be limited by a barrier that allows absorption of nutrient molecules. In addition, the intestine transports macromolecules that are important for growth and development (for example, epidermal growth factor (EGF) (3,4) and maternal IgG (5,6)). Thus any mechanism that acts as a barrier also must allow entry of physiologically important molecules, both large and small.

The lumen of the intestine is capable of harboring harmful microorganisms (7). To mount an immune response against these potential pathogens, the mucosal immune system must survey antigens in the lumen.

There is good evidence that immunosurveillance by the small intestine depends on the transport of antigens across the gut (8). However, such transport must occur in a controlled manner to avoid harmful immune responses. Nevertheless, there are times when the control of antigen entry breaks down, and this may lead to an excessive influx of antigens, which may ultimately cause disease (9).

MACROMOLECULAR ABSORPTION

To maintain immunosurveillance, antigens are transported across the intestine in physiologic amounts, but unrestricted (pathologic) transport may occur when the mucosal barrier is breached. This barrier consists of two main components (Fig. 26–1). Extrinsic mechanisms will limit the amount of antigen reaching the surface of the intestine; the intrinsic barrier consists of the structural and functional properties of the intestinal wall itself.

The production of immunoglobulins directed towards luminal antigen depends on immunologically intact antigen interacting with membrane bound immunoglobulins on the surface of B-cells (10,11). Mechanisms that allow passage of antigen through the intestinal epithelium in controlled amounts therefore are an essential prelude to B-cell activation.

T-cell responses, on the other hand, are initiated by the presentation of short peptides bound to major histocompatibility complexes (MHC) (12). As luminal antigen can activate mucosal T-cells (13), the intestine must process luminal antigen to peptides of the correct size which can then bind

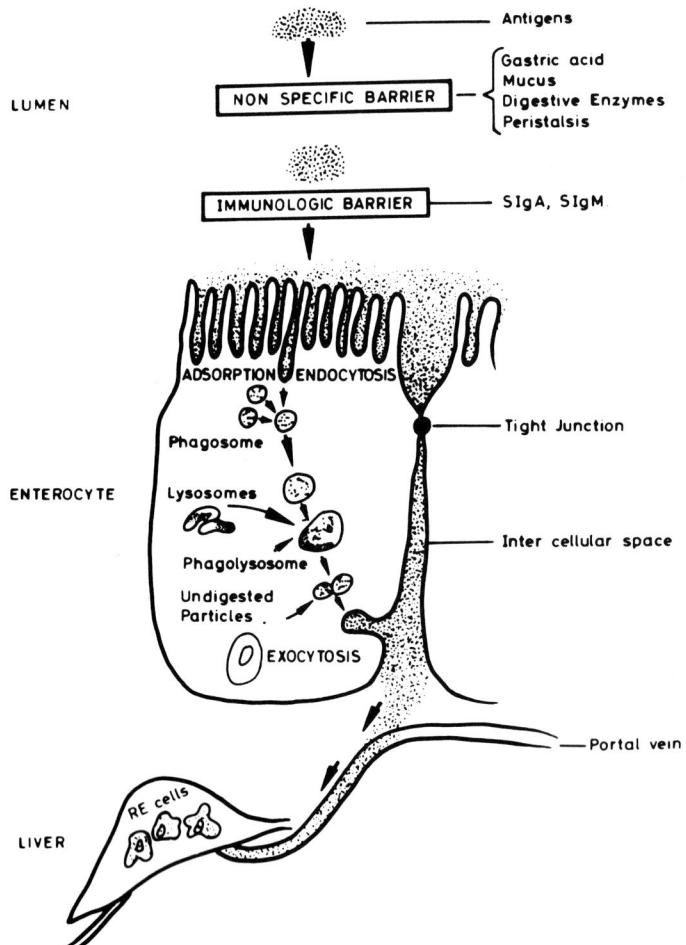

Fig. 26-1. Barriers to macromolecular absorption. Antigen entry is prevented by nonspecific and immunologic mechanism in the gastrointestinal tract as well as by the physical structure of the epithelium itself. Reproduced from Iyngkaran and Abidin: Intolerance to food proteins. *In* Pediatric Nutrition. Lifshitz F (Ed.), 1981, p. 453. Courtesy of Marcel Dekker, Inc.

Table 26–1
Physiologic Transport of Macromolecules
across the Intestinal Epithelium

---

1. Receptor-bound transport across enterocytes
2. Passage across M cells
3. Uptake, processing, and presentation in association with class II MHC molecules.

---

to MHC molecules and in turn interact with T-cell receptors. Antigens may be processed in two ways by the intestine. First, epithelial transport may generate peptide fragments; second, antigen could be processed from whole antigen that has traversed the epithelium, reaching antigen-presenting cells in the mucosal immune system. In either case, uptake of antigen by the epithelium is essential. Moreover, the pathway by which an antigen or its products reach the immune system of the gut may critically affect the type of immune reaction that ensues. Thus, an understanding of the mechanisms whereby antigen is handled is central to the study of the mucosal immune response.

Sampling of luminal antigen by the mucosa is likely to be a physiologic phenomenon, which will result in appropriate immune responses by the gut. These include the local production of secretory IgA and mechanisms that lead to oral tolerance (14). Such reactions often are beneficial. There will be times, however, when excessive antigen crosses the intestine, causing more widespread immune reactions. These reactions could result in gastrointestinal disease or systemic illness (9).

Macromolecules cross intestinal epithelial cells in two ways (Table 26–1). They can be shuttled through absorptive cells on specific receptors, in which case only those macromolecules that bind to a receptor will pass, or they can pass through specialized epithelial cells, M cells (Fig. 26-2). A further possibility is that antigenic fragments cross epithelial cells for presentation by class II MHC molecules at the basolateral surface. The definitive evidence for this mode of uptake is not yet available but, if established, this would constitute a third form of macromolecular transport.

Receptor-Bound Transport

For example, certain growth factors including epidermal growth factor, transform-

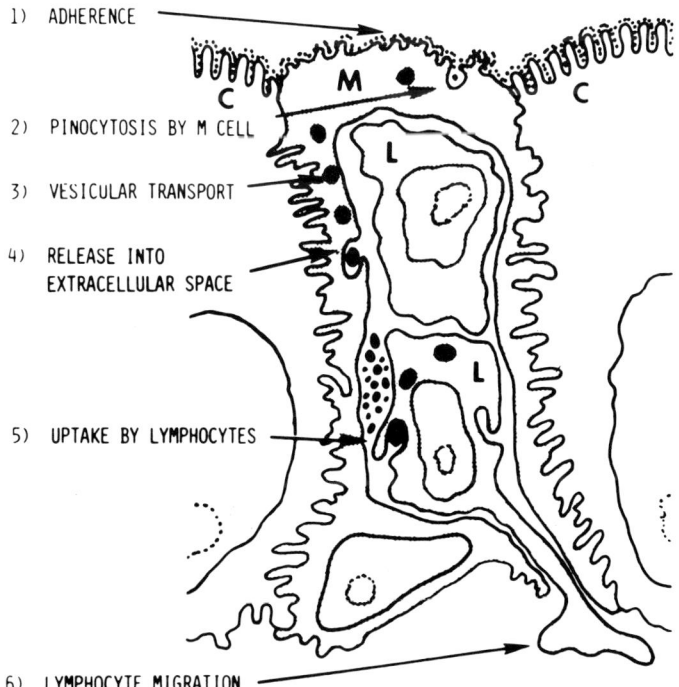

1) ADHERENCE
2) PINOCYTOSIS BY M CELL
3) VESICULAR TRANSPORT
4) RELEASE INTO EXTRACELLULAR SPACE
5) UPTAKE BY LYMPHOCYTES
6) LYMPHOCYTE MIGRATION

Fig. 26-2. M cell after adherence and endocytosis. Macromolecules need travel only a short distance from the apical surface to the basal pole where they are released close to immune cells that have migrated into the "pocket" at the basal surface of the M cells. Reproduced with permission from Owen RL: Sequential uptake of horseradish peroxidase by lymphoid follicle epithelium of Peyer's patches in the normal unobstructed mouse intestine: An ultrastructural study. Gastroenterology *72*:440, 1977.

ing growth factor-α, and nerve growth factor are transported across the intestine (15). IgG also can be transported across the intestine at times (5). The newborn makes very little immunoglobulin, and most circulating antibody is IgG derived passively from the mother. In humans IgG is transferred by the placenta during late gestation, but in many animals the transfer occurs from maternal milk through the proximal small intestine. The transfer of IgG across the gut is mediated by receptors that are similar to those present in human placenta (16). They bind to the Fc portion of the immunoglobulin molecule.

Intact proteins are transferred by mechanisms that are altogether different from those that transport nutrients such as glucose and amino acids. Nutrient molecules enter the intestinal cell cytoplasm at the apical membrane and exit through the basolateral membrane. Macromolecules, on the other hand, transverse the cell (Fig. 26–3) in membrane-bound compartments that invaginate from the apical membrane.

Cells Specialized for Macromolecular Transport (Microfold cells—M cells)

Generation of secretory immune responses by the intestinal mucosa depends on transfer of antigens across the epithelium. Any loss of the molecular structure of the antibody recognition sites, the epitopes, during transport would render them unrecognizable by B-cells. The passage of intact macromolecules across the gut is at variance with the role of the gut as a macromolecular barrier. For macromolecules to cross the gut in a controlled manner, specialized epithelial cells have evolved that overlay lymphoid follicles (17,18). These "M" cells (Fig. 26-2) have features that facilitate controlled entry of antigens and

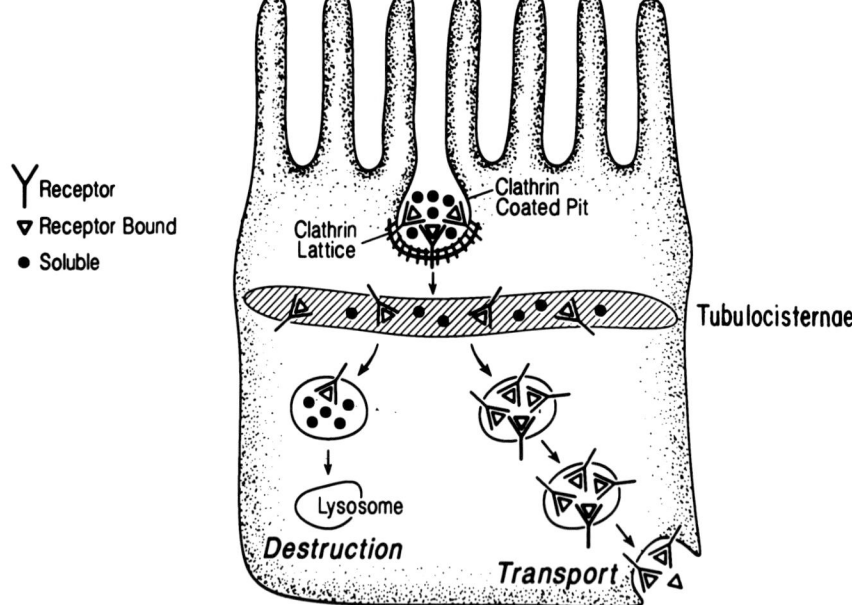

Fig. 26-3. Macromolecular endocytosis in enterocytes. Plasma membrane between microvilli invaginates to form vesicles. Clathrin, a protein that forms a membrane lattice, controls the curvature of the membrane. Macromolecules can enter the vesicle bound to surrounding membrane by its own receptor or by nonspecific attraction; they also can enter free in solution. After entry, they move to the tubulocysternae, where they are sorted and pass either to vesicles that travel towards the lysosome or to vesicles that traverse the cell to the basolateral pole. Membrane-bound molecules are more likely than those in solution to traverse the cell. Reproduced with kind permission from Sanderson IR, Walker WA: Uptake and transport of macromolecules by the intestine: Possible role in clinical disorders (an update). Gastroenterology *104*:622, 1993.

larger particles through the intestinal epithelium.

Enterocytes as Antigen Presenting Cells

Effective immune responses to antigenic proteins require T-lymphocytes. Stimulation of T-cells, in turn, depends on exogenous antigen being presented by antigen-presenting cells (APC) (12). The APC must internalize, digest, and link a small fragment of the antigen to a surface glycoprotein (the major histocompatibility complex class II or HLA-D in man) that interacts with a T-cell receptor. Numerous cells of the immune system can act as antigen-presenting cells, including B-cells, macrophages, and dendritic cells. The ability of these cells to present antigen depends on the expression of class II MHC on their surface (12). Class II MHC also are present in epithelia of the normal small intestine, particularly on villus cells, of the small intestine in both man (19) and rodents (20). In vitro studies (21–23) have demonstrated that isolated enterocytes from rodent and human small intestine can present antigens to appropriately primed T-cells. This raises the possibility that, in the intestine, class II MHC might present peptides from cellular membrane compartments to cells of the immune system that are localized below the epithelium. In support of this concept, class II MHC molecules have been detected in rat villous epithelium in association with intracellular organelles (24). Class II molecules were not observed in the microvillus brush border or in vesicles at the base of microvilli. However, organelles below the terminal web and throughout the apical cytoplasm were stained specifically. Basolateral membranes clearly manifested class II MHC molecules. These molecules, therefore, are in an ideal position for binding with polypeptides that may have been taken up and processed within the epithelial cell (Fig. 26–4). Interestingly, the expression of class II MHC in the gastrointestinal epithelium is increased in several diseases. In Crohn's disease (25–27), there is enhanced expression of enterocytes from inflamed areas (27). Increased expression of class II MHC also is evident in the small intestine in patients with autoimmune enteropathy (28) and in graft-versus-host disease (29). Certain infections increase class II MHC expression, for example in the stomach infected with Helicobacter pylori (30) and in the intestine infested with nematode parasites (31). If class II MHC molecules transport peptides derived from luminal macromolecules, these diseases result in increased presentation of

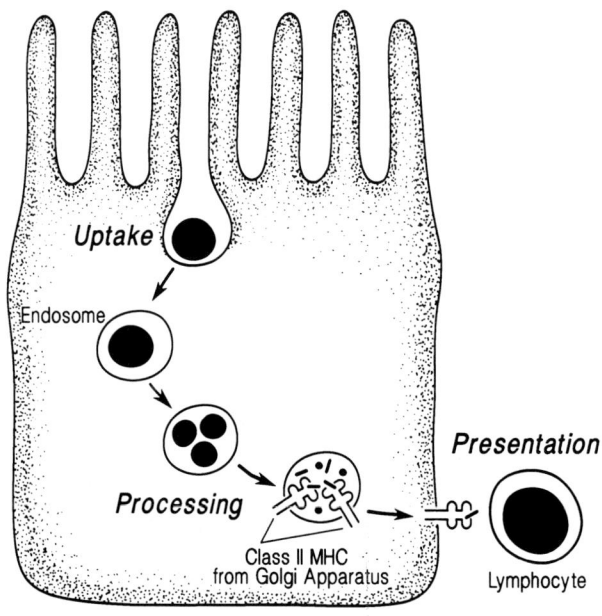

Fig. 26-4. Model of antigen presentation by enterocyte. Macromolecules can enter membrane-bound organelle of the enterocyte. Instead of binding to the surrounding membrane or being destroyed in lysosomes, antigen is processed within the endosomal component into fragments that can bind to class II MHC on the inner membrane of the components. From there, they are presented on the basolateral surface of the cell. Drawing prepared with the help of Dr. L. Mayer. Reproduced with kind permission from Sanderson IR, Walker WA: Uptake and transport of macromolecules by the intestine: Possible role in clinical disorders (an update). Gastroenterology *104*:622, 1993.

peptides to the gastrointestinal immune system. This may result in more inflammation and further presentation of luminal antigens leading to a vicious cycle. Some drugs used to treat inflammatory bowel disease reduce class II MHC expression in epithelial cells. 5-ASA, for example, reduces the class II MHC expression that occurs in cultured cells expressing class II MHC in response to interferon-γ (32).

BARRIERS PREVENTING PATHOLOGIC TRANSPORT

Physiologic passage of macromolecules is essential for the development of immune responses by the intestine, but uncontrolled penetration of antigens could initiate pathologic processes that lead to gastrointestinal diseases. For antigen transport to be controlled, nonspecific entry into the circulation must be limited. This is done in two ways: first, by restricting the amount of antigen reaching the surface of the intestine (extrinsic barrier); and second, by the physical characteristics of the intestine itself (intrinsic barrier) (see Fig. 26-1).

Many barrier mechanisms are not fully developed at birth, and there is good evidence that antigen transport in the neonatal period is less restricted than in adults. In animals, the changes in antigen absorption from newborn to adulthood is particularly evident, a phenomenon known as closure. Initially, the phenomenon was applied to the transport of immunoglobulins (33), but significant changes in absorption have been documented for antigens that do not have specific transport receptors. Radiolabeled bovine serum albumin (BSA) (34) was fed in physiologic amounts to rabbits at birth, 1 week, 2 weeks, 6 weeks, and 1 year of age and the plasma radioactivity measured. The study was designed to ensure that the radioactivity measured corresponded to protein absorption. From 1 week of age, there was a marked fall in the transport of BSA across the intestine. Moreover, a later study (35) demonstrated that the development of the mucosal barrier depended on the type of feeding during the neonatal period. Naturally fed (breast-fed) rabbits had lower plasma BSA levels than did formula-fed rabbits, suggesting that breast milk affects the

development of the mucosal barrier. A fall in antigen absorption has been demonstrated in humans also. Milk proteins penetrate more readily in infants than in adults. In one study α-lactalbumin absorption decreased with age in breast fed babies (36). In a second study, formula-fed neonates had greater levels of β-lactoglobulin than older infants (37).

Extrinsic Barrier

Proteolysis

There are many ways by which access to the epithelium can be limited (see Fig. 26-1). Proteolysis can destroy the structure of antigens and thus eliminate epitopes for immunologic recognition. Altering the proteolytic capacity of the gastrointestinal tract affects macromolecular uptake. In everted gut sacs (38) taken from rats who had previously undergone ligation of the pancreatic duct, transport of horseradish peroxidase (HRP) was greater than in sacs made from sham-operated animals. Furthermore, prior feeding of pancreatic extract decreased the uptake of HRP. The effects of digestion on macromolecular uptake have been elegantly confirmed by feeding rats aprotinin (a trypsin inhibitor) together with lysine vasopressin (39). This peptide hormone is absorbed through the intestine in sufficient quantities to have a noticeable effect on fluid retention when fed orally. When it is given together with aprotinin, however, the effects of vasopressin are more marked, implying that more has reached the surface of the intestine because of reduced proteolysis.

Neutralizing gastric acidity (which reduces the activity of gastric enzymes) also increases antigen transport. When oral feeds of sodium bicarbonate were given to rats at the same time as bovine serum albumin (BSA), increased BSA was found in the gut (38). These findings have potentially important consequences in rodents with deficiencies of pancreatic enzymes. In cystic fibrosis, for example, where pancreatic activity is severely limited, there is an increased incidence of cows' milk allergy, presumably because of increased antigen uptake. Also, gastric acidity (40) and pancreatic activity (41) may be reduced in the newborn, and this deficiency may influence the development of the mucosal barrier.

Peristalsis

The time available for absorption depends on the rapidity of passage of luminal contents down the bowel. It is a common experience in clinical gastroenterology that uptake of nutrients in patients with limited absorptive capacity (such as short bowel syndrome) is improved by reduced intestinal motility induced by agents such as loperamide (42). There is good reason to believe that the effect of damaging agents including antigens will be limited by peristaltic action. An association between motility and antigen absorption has important implications. First, motility patterns change in development (43), and this may contribute to alterations in antigen uptake with age. Second, gastrointestinal disease can affect the motility of the intestine (44) and may alter antigen absorption, although such a change may be small relative to the greater effect that an intestinal disease has on the physical barrier created by the intestine itself. Nevertheless, antibody-antigen complex formation in the mucus coat, coupled with peristalsis, causes rapid expulsion of antigens from small intestine (45).

Mucous Coat

Structure. The mucous coat lining the intestine is comprised of a solution of glycoproteins (mucin) of molecular weights ranging from one to several million daltons. Intestinal mucin molecules are composed of carbohydrate side chains (70 to 80%) bound to a protein skeleton. This protein core has a high proportion of serine, threonine and proline residues (46,47), and the carbohydrate moieties are attached to it by means of N-acetylgalactosamine. Five carbohydrate moieties (N-acetyl galactosamine, N-acetyl glucosamine, fucose, galactose and sialic acid) are arranged in side chains of 2 to 22 sugars in length.

The exact composition of the molecules of mucin can vary greatly. Distinct differences exist among animal species. Even within localized regions of the intestinal tract, mucus molecules appear to be a heterogeneous group. At least 6 different mucin species have been identified after separation on DEAE-cellulose chromatography from both rat and human (48). Each species has a distinct carbohydrate and amino acid composition. Marked changes in the composition of mucin occur with development. The mucin from the small intestine of newborn rats contains more protein than does adult rat mucin (49). The carbohydrate content also changes as the animals grow. Not only does the total carbohydrate ratio increase with age, but the types of sugar moieties change also: newborn rat mucin has less fructose and N-acetyl galactosamine than does mucin from adult rats.

Function of Mucus Coat—Viscous Coat. Numerous ways exist whereby mucus offers protection to the intestinal wall (Fig. 26–5). It provides a mucus blanket. The physical characteristics of this blanket are determined by the chemical structure of the glycoprotein molecules. The sticky quality of the mucus is an important mechanism for preventing penetration of organisms. The motility of Entamoeba histolytica trophozoites (50), for example, is significantly decreased by mucus. The increased viscosity that mucus gives to the luminal solution enhances the depth of the unstirred layer overlying the surface of the intestine. This reduces the diffusion of molecules toward the intestinal surface (51). The effect is most marked for larger molecules and limits absorption of antigens more than the smaller nutrient molecules.

Competitive Binding. The carbohydrate moieties that comprise most of the structure of mucus are analogous to the glycoprotein and glycolipid receptors that exist on the enterocyte membrane (52). They could therefore act as competitors to the binding of proteins and microorganisms at the enterocyte surface. Many infectious agents adhere to epithelial cells through cell surface appendages (fimbria, pili and flagella) (53), which have carbohydrate binding properties. Indeed, competition between salivary mucus glycoproteins and receptors on buccal epithelium has already been demonstrated for binding of pathogenic streptococci (54). Furthermore, it is possible that the invasiveness of Shigella flexneri in primates depends partly on the lack of barrier function of mucus (55). Guinea pig colonic mucus inhibits invasion of HeLa cells by Shigella; whereas monkey colonic mucus (and by implication, human mucus) does not.

A. Mucus Release

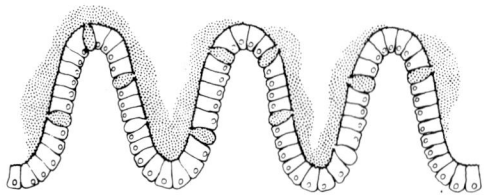

B. Physical Barrier

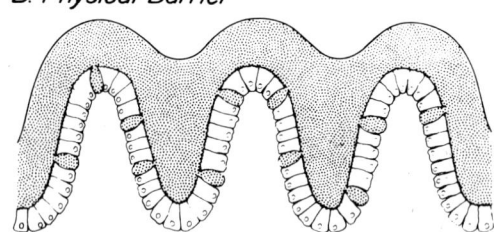

C. Inhibitory Binding Sites

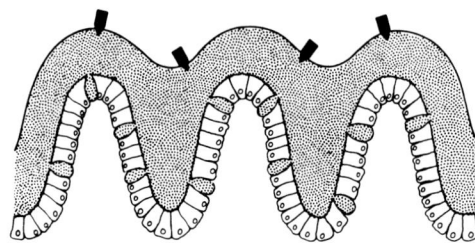

D. Link to Immune System

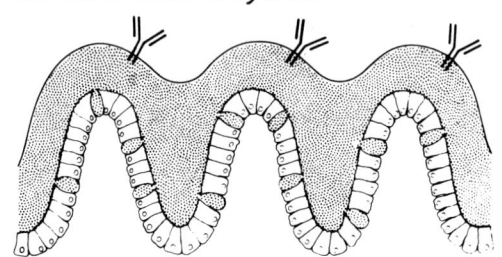

Fig. 26-5. Four proposed mechanisms for mucus protection: Rate and quantity of mucus release, viscous blanket (physical barrier), competitive binding sites, link to the intestinal immune system. Reproduced from Snyder JD, Walker WA: Structure and function of intestinal mucin: Developmental aspects. Int Arch Allergy Appl Immunol 82:351, 1981. Courtesy of S. Karger AG.

Mucin Release. Release of mucus into the gastrointestinal tract acts as a barrier by generating a stream that draws luminal contents away from epithelial cells. Both nonspecific and immunologic agents can initiate mucus release. The role of nonimmunologic agents and their relationship to endogenous agents that alter mucus secretion are not well understood (45). Cholinergic compounds (56) and mustard oil (57) induce goblet cell release, but regulatory peptides (including histamine, serotonin, and adrenergic agents) have no effect.

Immunologic Barrier

The adequacy of immune function in the gastrointestinal tract affects the attachment and penetration of bacteria and toxins. This has been elegantly shown (8) by the implantation of IgA-secreting hybridomas under the skin of infant mice, which are then inoculated with cholera. IgA appears in large amounts in the small intestine as secretory IgA. The hybridoma-secreting IgA interacts with the antigen on the surface of V. cholera, dramatically reducing the mortality.

It also is likely that IgA prevents the transfer of antigens across the gut. This hypothesis is supported by studies of patients with selective IgA deficiency. These patients have increased circulating immune complexes and precipitating antibodies to absorbed bovine milk proteins (58), peak concentrations occurring between 1 and 2 hours after milk ingestion (59).

Combined Effects of Immunologic and Non-immunologic Barriers

Both oral and parenteral immunization with specific antigens can reduce their uptake by the intestine (60,61). These observations may well represent a combined effect of immunologic and nonimmunologic components of the mucosal barrier. Proteolysis of intestinal antigens was considerably greater in immunized animals than in nonimmunized controls (38). This enhanced proteolysis is probably the result of interaction of immune complexes in the mucus coat. This augmented protective process is illustrated in Figure 26–6.

Another example of combined protection is the increased discharge of goblet cell mucus occurring in intestinal anaphylaxis.

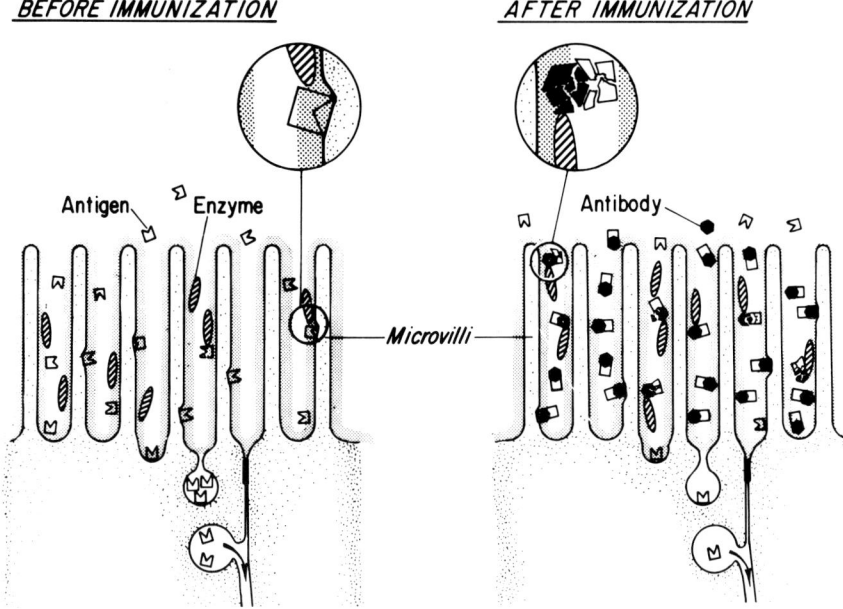

Fig. 26-6. Schematic representation of the processing of protein antigen at the surface of the gut. Before immunization, a small portion of ingested protein escapes intraluminal digestion and is taken up by the enterocyte and transported to the intercellular spaces. After immunization, antibodies present on the gut surface interact with antigen to form complexes, thereby preventing or decreasing the binding of antigen to, and subsequent pinocytosis of antigen by, intestinal epithelial cells. Antigens complexed with antibodies in the mucus coat (glycocalyx) may be degraded by pancreatic enzymes absorbed to the gut surface: consequently, there is less antigen available by intestinal epithelial cells. Reproduced with permission from Walker WA et al.: Intestinal uptake of macromolecules IV. The effect of duct ligation on the breakdown of antigen and antigen-antibody complexes on the intestinal surface. Gastroenterology *69*:1223, 1975.

Lake and colleagues (62) have shown, using radiolabeled goblet cell mucus to quantitate release, that IgE mediated-mast cell discharge of histamine results in enhanced mucus release into the intestinal tract. This may explain why parasites are eventually expelled from the intestine, together with mucus (63). Figure 26-5 illustrates possible mechanisms of immune complex-mediated goblet cell mucus release on the intestinal surface.

Intrinsic Barrier

Once antigens have negotiated the many components of the extrinsic barrier mechanism, a considerable physical barrier to further penetration remains. This barrier is formed by the surface of the enterocytes and the tight junctions that are formed between them. However, it is not impervious to the passage of antigens, as was once

thought, and its integrity is often reduced in disease of the gastrointestinal tract.

Microvillus Structure

Microvilli may constitute a significant barrier because of their size and charge. In the intestinal epithelium of children (64) are 40 microvilli, each of 100 nm diameter every 5 nm. Thus, if microvilli beat in unison, the distance between them is only 25 nm, which is the same order of magnitude as some macromolecules. The dimensions of albumin, for example, are 3×13 nm. Microvilli also are negatively charged and therefore stain easily with ruthenium red (65); therefore a charged molecule may be significantly inhibited even if its diameter is well below 25 nm.

The site of invagination of apical plasma membrane has been demonstrated as being between microvilli (66–68). Thus, it is likely that antigens must pass the microvillus "barrier" to enter the cell. This has direct relevance to disease processes; any agent that diminishes or removes microvilli or affects their formation alters the barrier function of the intestine. Microvillus structure is greatly altered by infections of cryptosporidia (69) or enteropathogenic Escherichia coli (70).

Further support for the concept of a microvillous barrier comes from morphologic studies on M cells. The function of these cells is macromolecular transport. Unlike absorptive cells, they do not have well-developed microvilli. Since every morphologic feature of these cells correlates with their function, this suggests that microvilli constitute a significant barrier.

Enterocyte Surface Membrane

At the base of the microvilli, the surface of the enterocyte consists of plasma membrane. As in other cells, this is composed of a lipid bilayer through which are situated membrane-bound proteins. This bilayer presents a considerable barrier to antigen transport because of its physical structure. In fact, it is very unlikely that antigens can cross this lipid bilayer into the enterocyte cytosol. However, invagination of apical membranes occurs regularly, allowing macromolecules to be carried into the cell within membrane-bound compartments (Fig. 26-3). Indeed, there is a large number of compartments beneath the apical surface of the enterocyte into which antigens can be transferred. Some of this activity is physiologic and has been described in an earlier section; however, bystander molecules also can be carried into the cell by this process. This was clearly demonstrated in electron micrographs, which indicated horseradish peroxidase inside membrane bound compartments (71). Stern and Walker (72) have shown that binding to the surface of the enterocyte is an important determinant as to whether macromolecules are transported across the cell. For both BSA and BLG, absorption was nonsaturable and correlated with binding to the intestinal surface. Membrane-bound macromolecular transport can be distinguished from molecules moving freely in lumen of compartments of the enterocyte (67) in newborn rat ileum.

Binding to the surface of the cell depends on the structure of the antigen and the chemical composition of the microvillus membrane. Both of these factors can vary. The structure of the antigen depends on the actual antigen itself. BSA binds less efficiently to the surface of the intestine than BLG, and consequently is transported less readily (72). In addition, structural alterations in antigen caused by proteolysis also might affect its binding by altering the physicochemical characteristics of the molecule. For example, the gliadin fraction B3 (73) binds less well to MVM protein than the pure gliadin peptide B3142.

The composition of the microvillus membrane has a significant effect on antigen binding. Plasma membrane consists of both lipids and proteins, and changes in either will affect binding to antigen. Partial digestion of microvillus membrane can alter binding to macromolecules (74). Damage to the protein in membranes is unlikely to occur in health because the intestinal surface is protected by mucus. However, if the mucus layer were affected by resident bacteria, for example, some digestion of the surface membrane might occur, leading to increased antigen binding and transport. Changes in lipid composition, on the other hand, are regularly encountered because lipid composition changes with development. Differences in membrane composition can be detected by electron spin resonance (ESR). In this technique, the movements of the lipid-soluble probe can be followed by a spectrophotometer (75). Movements of the probe in the membrane of the newborn rabbit were less confined than in adults, suggesting a more disorganized membrane structure. Indeed, chemical analysis of the membrane (76) demonstrated changes in the phospholipid headgroups with age as well as alterations in protein-lipid ratios (75). Changes in membrane fluidity noted by ESR were found to correlate with alteration in lectin binding (77). These alterations were noted to be under hormonal control because alterations in the fluidity were affected by both cortisone and thyroxine (78).

Intracellular Organelles and Enzymes

Antigens that enter enterocytes from the lumen are affected by different factors that influence transport to the basolateral membrane. This depends on the rate of endocytosis, the proportion of vesicles being divided towards the lysosome, and the speed of travel of membrane-bound compartments. The rate of breakdown of products held in membrane compartments is determined by lysosomally derived enzymes. These include proteases such as cathepsin B&D and those that catalyze carbohydrate breakdown such as acid phosphatase and mannosidase. It is the degree to which the organellar contents encounter such enzymes that determines the rate of intracellular destruction of macromolecules. This encounter can be in the lysosome or in endocytic vesicles (79). We know that such enzymes are present in intestinal epithelial cells and at levels of activity that can influence macromolecular transport. In the rat (80), cathepsin B&D activity can be found throughout the length of intestine, particularly in the mid and distal thirds. Interestingly, this activity peaks in the second week of age and then progressively falls. The ontogeny of macromolecular transport (34) in no way reflects this pattern, emphasizing that it is the importance of *interaction* between membrane-bound compartment flow and enzyme activity, that is of prime importance. This interaction is seen more clearly in the piglet, in which intestinal cathepsin B&D levels do not change with age (81), yet closure occurs in the second day of life.

Although cathepsins are capable of destroying macromolecular biologic activity, they may not completely digest the protein molecule and the final steps in digestion of peptides may be by peptidases (82) in the cytoplasm.

Junctions Between Cells

The physical barrier that prevents penetration of antigen across the intestinal epithelium consists of two main components: the epithelial cells (the transcellular route) and the spaces between cells (the paracellular route). The pathophysiology of the latter pathway has been well reviewed in recent years (83–85). The pathway consists of the tight junctions (or zonulae occludentes) and the subjunctional space.

The subjunctional space does not act as a significant barrier because molecules as large as horseradish peroxidase can diffuse freely between the serosa and this space. However, the tight junctions (TJ) offer a substantial barrier to diffusion of large molecules, although it is permeable to water and small ions (86). Claude and Goodenough (87) demonstrated a correlation between the structure of the TJ as seen in freeze fracture preparations and passive electrical permeability in a number of epithelial preparations. The preparations, when viewed under the electron microscope, show a network of characteristic anastomosing strands. The composition of these strands is unknown, but it is likely that they are proteins of high tensile strength. In tight epithelia (such as the gallbladder) there are many such strands, but in more permeable epithelia (like mammalian proximal small intestine) few are seen. These relationships have been confirmed in intestinal epithelial cell monolayers (88). During the first 10 days after passage, the junctions of TE 84 cells become increasingly tight, as estimated by transepithelial resistance. This resistance correlates with the number of strands formed between cells.

The barrier formed by tight junctions is preserved even when epithelial cells themselves are extruded at the villous tip. Younger cells beneath the extruding cell form tight junctions at the very moment when old cells are lost (89). Preservation of the TJ network is a function whose importance appears to override that of epithelial cell viability.

The tight junction is a dynamic structure whose resistance varies. Changes in paracellular absorption occur during active transport of nutrients by epithelial cells, particularly in relation to smaller molecules. Pappenheimer and colleagues (90–92) have calculated that the rate of uptake from the lumen of molecules smaller than 5500 daltons was proportional to the rate of fluid absorption, a concept known as solvent drag. The application of an alternating current across isolated intestine, with and without mucosa, gave an estimate of the impedance of the intestinal mucosa. The impedance fell with the stimulation of sodium-coupled solute transport across the enterocyte. It is therefore possible that Na-coupled solute transport triggers contraction of cytoskeletal elements of the enterocyte, which in turn pull open tight junctions. These predictions have been confirmed by electron microscopy (92). Sodium-dependent solutes such as glucose and amino acids induce expansion of intercellular spaces associated with condensation of microfilaments of the actinomycin ring associated with the TJ. Although these observations have enormous importance for the physiology of absorption of nutrients, their impact on our understanding of macromolecular transport has yet to be fully assessed. The calculated pore radius of the open TJ (5 nm) is similar to that of small macromolecules: glucose-Na transport in fact allows the passage of polypeptide 11 amino acids long (MP-1) (93), but larger immunogenic proteins may not pass through this route under physiological conditions. HRP, for example, does not pass the TJ (93), even when they have been rendered permeable to MP-1. On the other hand, insults to the intestine may open these pores sufficiently to allow the passage of antigens.

The permeability of the TJ can be examined in vitro. Monolayers of epithelial cells (T84) have effective tight junctions producing a resistance of approximately 1500 cm^2. Application of interferon-γ (94) reduces the resistance and allows easier permeation of large sugars. Interferon-γ levels are increased in the mucosal of patients with Crohn's disease. Bowel inflammation is characterized by the transepithelial passage of polymorphonuclear cells (PMN) as observed in vitro by placing chemotactic agents and PMN on different sides of the monolayer (95). The passage of neutrophils opens tight junctions, reducing the monolayer resistance and allowing transfer of large sugars.

INFLAMMATION

Inflammation, whether initiated by infection, allergens, or idiopathic immunologic derangements, is an important problem when it occurs in the gastrointestinal tract. The field of pediatric gastroenterology has largely developed from the need to combat inflammatory diseases in children: celiac disease, food-sensitive enteropathies, dysentery, Crohn's disease, and ulcerative colitis. It is reasonable, therefore, to think of inflammation as a harmful and misdirected series of events. To a large extent, this is true. Progress has been made in understanding the mechanisms of the inflammatory response with a view to combatting disease. The cellular components of the immune system and their interaction in different inflammatory conditions also has been determined. The chemical messages between cells have been described, and the process whereby the cell produce their effects are well understood. Detailed description of these elements (Fig. 26–7) is beyond the scope of this chapter, and the reader is referred to a number of excellent reviews in this area (10,11,96). There are, however, several general points which should be made.

The inflammatory response is well coordinated, even during severe disease states. Recent efforts to examine the mechanisms that control this process have been fruitful. T-cell activation, in particular, may result in inflammatory reactions that damage the gastrointestinal tract. The density of activated T cells is increased in Crohn's disease (97,98) and in autoimmune enteropathy (99). Furthermore, activation of T cells results in mucosal changes in vitro. MacDonald and colleagues (100,101) have examined the effects of T-cell activation in human intestinal lamina propria. In fetal small intestinal explants cultured in vitro addition of nontoxic lectin and anti-CD3 antibody directly activates the T cell in the lamina propria. Within 72 hours this results in villus atrophy, crypt hypertrophy, and increase in the rate of crypt cell proliferation. These effects are inhibited by cyclosporin A, and the degree of tissue damage is related to the mucosal T-cell activation. Clinical evidence also supports the primary role of T-cell activation. Patients with malignant histiocytosis of the intestine (MHI) exhibit villous atrophy and crypt hypertrophy indistinguishable from celiac disease, yet patients are refractory to gluten withdrawal for the onset of the lymphoma. It is possible that the flat mucosa in MHI is a consequence of activated malignant T cells within the lamina propria (102). In addition, James (98) has reported that the activity of Crohn's disease subsides when HIV patients exhibit helper T cells depletion in AIDS. The inference from this observation is that, as the helper

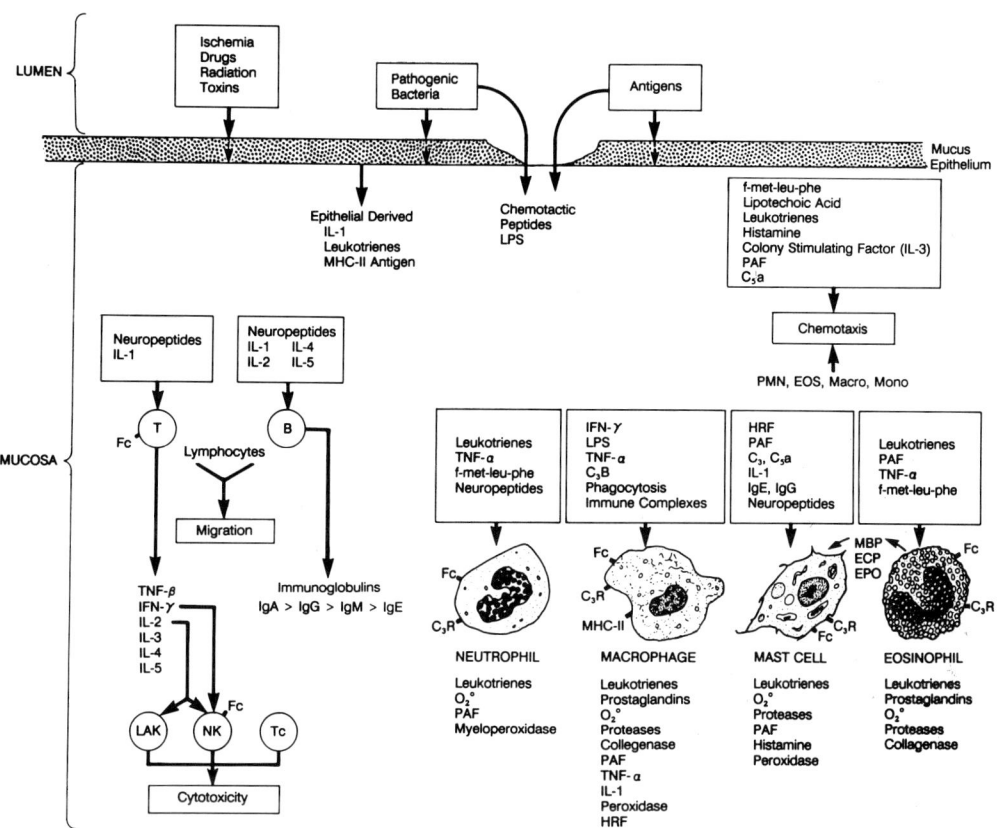

Fig. 26-7. Diagrammatic representation of the mucosa with the principal cells involved in inflammation and injury. The cell surface receptors, the most important stimulants for each cell (in boxes) and the major cellular products contributing to inflammation are shown. The colonic mucosa is protected by physical and immune mechanisms. Intestinal ischemia, radiation, toxins, and drugs all may affect the production and integrity of the mucous barrier and the underlying epithelium. Damage to these layers allows bacteria and their products, as well as foreign antigens, to enter the mucosa and initiate a complex cascade of events resulting in inflammation. Cells may be recruited to the mucosa by chemotactic agents and, together with resident cells, interact to eradicate invading organisms. The colonic epithelium itself may contribute to these processes. Whether this results in a limited acute injury or in chronic inflammation depends on poorly understood cellular regulatory mechanism. PMN = polymorphonuclear leukocytes; EOS = eosinophils; Macro = macrophages; Mono = monocytes; LAK = lymphokine-activated killer lymphocytes; NK = natural killer lymphocyte; Tc = cytotoxic T lymphocyte; TNF = tumor necrosis factor; PAF = platelet activating factor; HRF = histamine releasing factor; LPS = lipopolysaccharide (endotoxin); INF = γ-interferon gamma, O_2^0 = oxidative burst metabolites; MBP = major basis protein; ECP = eosinophil cationic protein; EPO = eosinophil peroxidase; IL = interleukin; MHC = major histocompatibility complex; f-met-leu-phe = formyl methionyl peptides; CR3 = complement C3 receptors; Fc = Fc receptor. From Martin S, Walker WA: Responses of the colon to injury: inflammation, immunity, mucus. *In* The Large Intestine: Physiology, Pathophysiology and Disease. New York, Raven Press, 1990, pp. 181–185. Reproduced with kind permission of Raven Press.

T cells disappear, the driving force behind the inflammation is removed.

Although the identification of cells controlling inflammation may provide a rationale for the treatment of T cell-mediated disease (numerous strategies are available for inactivation of T cells), the circular nature of inflammatory reactions should not be overlooked. The mucosal immune system may not be a simple hierarchy where some cells "direct operations" and others effect changes in the mucosa. Instead, it is possible that each different cell type may have the capability to respond to local conditions, perform specialized functions *and* alter the activity of other cell types in the immune response. The combination of cell types could act as a single unit where levels of activity increase or decrease in concert, without a central command. On this basis, the distinction between primary or secondary changes during the inflammatory response may be artificial.

Finally, the notion that gastrointestinal inflammation is exclusively harmful cannot be left unchallenged. In this chapter on gastrointestinal defense, it is relevant to ask whether the processes of inflammation may at times protect the host, albeit at some cost in terms of growth and general well being. Amebic dysentery is an example whereby inappropriate reduction of inflammation can result in fatal outcomes. The lesions seen in amebic dysentery may be indistinguishable from those of inflammatory bowel disease (103,104), and inadvertent treatment with corticosteroids alone is well documented (105). However, the outcome of such anti-inflammatory treatment is uniformly poor (106–108).

PERSPECTIVES FOR THE 21ST CENTURY

The progress that has taken place during this century is a prelude to discoveries that are likely to come in the next century. These will include an increased understanding of how the appropriate defense mechanisms of the gastrointestinal tract might be enhanced to prevent diseases by pathogens that presently also are associated with social disruption (such as cholera and HIV), how inappropriate inflammatory reactions to foods (as seen in celiac disease and food sensitive enteropathy) can be reduced, and how the inflammatory mechanisms of Crohn's disease and ulcerative colitis are initiated and sustained.

REFERENCES

1. Von Meumann J: Continuous Geometry. Princeton, Princeton University Press, 1960.

2. Field M, Frizell RA: Intestinal absorption and secretion. *In* Schultz SG (ed): The Gastrointestinal System. Vol. IV. Bethesda, American Physiology Society, 1991.

3. Weaver LT, Gonnella PA, Israel EJ, Walker WA: Uptake and transport of epidermal growth factor by the small intestinal epithelium of the fetal rat. Gastroenterology 98:828, 1990.

4. Carpenter G, Wahl MI: The epidermal growth factor family. *In* Sporn MB, Roberts AB (eds): Peptide Growth Factors and Their Receptors I. New York, Springer-Verlag, 1991.

5. Simister NE, Rees AR: Isolation and characterization of an Fc receptor from neonatal rat small intestine. Eur J Immunol 15:733, 1985.

6. Rodewald R, Kraehenbuhl JP: Receptor-mediated transport of IgG. J Cell Biol 99:159s, 1984.

7. Snyder JD: Bacterial infections. *In* Walker WA et al. (eds): Pediatric Gastrointestinal Disease: Pathophysiology, Diagnosis, Management. Philadelphia, B.C. Decker, Inc., 1991.

8. Winner LS: New model for analysis of mucosal immunity: Intestinal secretion of specific monoclonal immunoglobulin A from hybridoma tumors protects against Vibrio cholerae infection. Infect Immunol 59:977, 1991.

9. Sanderson IR, Walker WA: Uptake and transport of macromolecules by the intestine: Possible role in clinical disorders (An update). Gastroenterology 104:622, 1993.

10. Kagnoff MF: Immunology and the digestive system. *In* Johnson LR (ed): Physiology of the Gastrointestinal Tract. New York, Raven Press, 1987.

11. Elson CO et al.: Intestinal immunity and inflammation: Recent progress. Gastroenterology 91:746, 1986.

12. Unanue ER: Antigen presenting function of the macrophage. Ann Rev Immunol 2:395, 1984.

13. Marsh MN: Gluten, major histocompatibility complex, and the small intestine. A molecular and immunobiologic approach to the spectrum of gluten sensitivity (celiac sprue). Gastroenterology 102:330, 1992.

14. Thompson HSG, Staines NA: Could specific oral tolerance be a therapy for autoimmune disease? Immunology Today 11:396, 1991.

15. Chu SW, Walker WA: Growth factor signal transduction in human intestinal cells. Adv Exp Med Biol 310:107, 1991.

16. Sedmak DD, Davis DH, Singh U, van de Winkel JG: Expression of IgG Fc receptor

antigens in placenta and on endothelial cells in humans. An immunohistochemical study. Am J Pathol *138*:175, 1991.

17. Bockman DE, Cooper MD: Pinocytosis by epithelium associated with lymphoid follicles in the Bursa of Fabricus, appendix and Peyer's patches. An electron microscopic study. Am J Anat *136*:455, 1973.

18. Owen RL: Sequential uptake of horseradish peroxidase by lymphoid follicle epithelium of Peyer's patches in the normal unobstructed mouse intestine: An ultrastructural study. Gastroenterology *72*:440, 1977.

19. Wiman K et al.: Occurrence of la antigen on tissue of non-lymphoid origin. Nature *276*:711, 1978.

20. Kirby WN, Parr EL: The occurrence and distribution of H-2 antigens on mouse intestinal epithelial cells. J Histochem Cytochem *27*:746, 1979.

21. Bland PW, Warren LG: Antigen presentation by epithelial cells of the rat small intestine. I. Kinetics, antigen specificity and blocking by anti-la antisera. Immunology *58*:1, 1986.

22. Mayer L, Shlien R: Evidence for function of la molecules on gut epithelial cells in man. J Exp Med *166*:1471, 1987.

23. Kaiserlian D, Vidal K, Revillard J-P: Murine enterocytes can present soluble antigen to a specific class II-restricted CD4$^+$ T cells. Eur J Immunol *19*:1513, 1989.

24. Mayrhofer G, Spargo LDJ: Distribution of class II major histocompatibility antigens in enterocytes of the rat jejunum and their association with organelles of the endocytic pathway. Immunology *70*:11, 1990.

25. Selby WS, Janossy G, Maso DY, Jewell DP: Expression of HLA-DR antigens by colonic epithelium in inflammatory bowel disease. Clin Exp Immunol *53*:614, 1983.

26. Mayer L: Expression of class II molecules on intestinal epithelial cells in humans. Differences between normal and inflammatory bowel disease. Gastroenterology *100*:3, 1991.

27. Mayer L, Eisenhardt D: Lack of induction of suppressor T cells by intestinal epithelial cells from patients with inflammatory bowel disease. J Clin Invest *86*:1255, 1990.

28. Hill SM, Milla PJ: Infantile colitis (editorial). Br Med J *302*:545, 1991.

29. Mason DW, Dallman M, Barclay AN: Graft-versus-host disease induces expression of la antigen in rat epidermal cells and gut epithelium. Nature *293*:150, 1981.

30. Engstrand L et al.: Association of Campylobacter pylori with induced expression of class II transplantation antigen on gastric epithelial cells. Infect Immun *57*:827, 1989.

31. Masson SD, Perdue MH: Changes in distribution of la antigen on epithelium of the jejunum and ileum in rats infected with Nippostrongylus brasiliensis. Clin Immunol Immunopathol *57*:83, 1990.

32. Crotty B, Hoang P, Dalton HR, Jewell DP: Salicylates used in inflammatory bowel disease and colchicine impair interferon-y inducted HLA-DR expression. Gut *33*:59, 1992.

33. Brambell FW: The transmission of immunity from mother to young and the catabolism of immunoglobulins. Lancet *ii*:1087, 1986.

34. Udall JN: Development of gastrointestinal mucosal barrier. I. The effect of age on intestinal permeability to macromolecules. Pediatr Res *15*:241, 1981.

35. Udall JN: Development of gastrointestinal mucosal barrier. II. The effect of natural versus artificial feeding on intestinal permeability to macromolecules. Pediatr Res *15*:245, 1981.

36. Axelsson I et al.: Macromolecular absorption in preterm and term infants. Acta Paediatr Scand *78*:532, 1989.

37. Roberton DM, Paganelli R, Dinwiddie R, Levinsky RJ: Milk antigen absorption in the preterm and term neonate. Arch Dis Child *57*:369, 1982.

38. Walker WA, Wu M, Isselbacher JK, Bloch KJ: Intestinal uptake of macromolecules IV. The effect of duct ligation on the breakdown of antigen and antigen-antibody complexes on the intestinal surface. Gastroenterology *69*:1123, 1975.

39. Saffron M: A model for the study of oral administration of peptide hormones. Can J Biochem *57*:548, 1979.

40. Hyman PE et al.: Gastric acid secretory function in preterm infants. J Pediatr *106*:467, 1985.

41. Lebenthal E, Lee PC: Alternate pathways of digestion and absorption in early infancy. J Pediatr Gastroenterol Nutr *3*:1, 1982.

42. Remington M, Malagelada JR, Zinsmeiste A, Fleming CR: Abnormalities in gastrointestinal motor activity in patients with short bowels: Effect of a synthetic opiate. Gastroenterology *85*:629, 1983.

43. Bissett WM, Watt JB, Rivers RPA, Milla PJ: Ontogeny of fasting small intestinal motor activity in the human infant. Gut *29*:483, 1988.

44. Mayer EA, Raybould H, Koelbel C: Neuropeptides, inflammation and motility. Dig Dis Sci *33*:71S, 1988.

45. Snyder JD, Walker WA: Structure and function of intestinal mucin: Develop-

mental aspects. Int Arch Allergy Appl Immunol *82*:351, 1987.

46. Allen A: Structure and function of gastrointestinal mucus. *In* Johnson LR (ed): Physiology of the Gastrointestinal Tract. Vol. 1, New York, Raven Press, 1981.

47. Forstner J: Intestinal mucins in health and disease. Digestion *17*:234, 1978.

48. Podolsky DK: Oligosaccharide structure of isolated human colonic mucin species. J Biol Chem *260*:15510, 1985.

49. Shub MD, Pang KY, Swann DA, Walker WA: Age-related changes in chemical composition and physical properties of mucus glycoproteins from rat small intestine. Biochem J *215*:405, 1983.

50. Leitch GJ, Dickey AD, Udezuler IA, Bailey GB: Entamoeba histolytica trophozoites in the lumen and mucus blanket of rat colons studied in vivo. Infect Immun *47*:68, 1985.

51. Strocchi A, Levitt MD: A reappraisal of the magnitude and implications of the intestinal unstirred layer. Gastroenterology *101*:843, 1991.

52. Gibbons RA: Mucus of the mammalian genital tract. Br Med Bull *34*:4, 1981.

53. Freter R: Mechanisms of association of bacteria with mucosal surfaces. Ciba Found Symp *80*:36, 1981.

54. Williams RC, Gibbons RJ: Inhibition of streptococcal attachment of receptors on human buccal epithelial cells by antigenically similar salivary glycoproteins. Infect Immun *11*:711, 1975.

55. Denari G, Hale TL, Washington O: Effect of guinea pig or monkey colonic mucus on Shigella aggregation and invasion of HeLa cells by Shigella flexneri 1b and 2a. Infect Immunity *51*:975, 1986.

56. Specian RD, Neutra MR: Mechanism of rapid mucus secretion in goblet cells stimulated by acetylcholine. J Cell Biol *85*:626, 1990.

57. Neutra MR, O'Malley LJ, Specian RD: Regulation of intestinal goblet cell secretion. II. A survey of potential secretagogue. Am J Physiol *242*:G380, 1982.

58. Cunningham-Rundles C, Brandeis WE, Good RA, Day NK: Milk precipitin circulating immune complexes and IgA deficiency. Proc Natl Acad Sci USA *75*:3387, 1978.

59. Cunningham-Rundles C, Brandeis WE, Good RA, Day NK: Bovine antigens and the formation and the circulating immune complexes in selective immunoglobulin A deficiency. J Clin Invest *64*:272, 1979.

60. Walker WA, Isselbacher KJ, Bloch KJ: Intestinal uptake of macromolecules: Effect of oral immunization. Science *177*:608, 1972.

61. Walker WA, Isselbacher KJ, Bloch KJ: Intestinal uptake of macromolecules. II. Effect of parenteral immunization. J Immunol *111*:221, 1973.

62. Lake AM, Bloch KJ, Sinclair KJ, Walker WA: Anaphylactic release of intestinal goblet cell mucus. Immunology *39*:173, 1980.

63. Miller HRP, Nawa Y: Immune regulation of intestinal goblet cell differentiation. Nouv Rev fr Hemat *21*:31, 1979.

64. Phillips AD, France NE, Walker-Smith JA: The structure of the enterocyte in relation to its position on the villus in childhood: An electron microscopical study. Histopathology *3*:117, 1979.

65. Jacobs LR: Biochemical and ultrastructural characterization of the molecular topography of the rat intestinal microvillous membrane. Asymmetric distribution of hydrophilic groups and anionic binding sites. Gastroenterology *85*:46, 1983.

66. Knutton S, Limbrick AR, Robertson JD: Regular structures in membranes: Membranes in the endocytic complex of ileal epithelial cells. J Cell Biol *62*:679, 1974.

67. Gonnella PA, Neutra MR: Membrane-bound and fluid-phase macromolecules enter separate prelysosomal compartments in absorptive cells of suckling rat ileum. J Cell Biol *99*:909, 1984.

68. Shibata Y, Arima T, Arim T, Yamamoto T: Regular structures on the microvillar surface membrane of ileal epithelial cells in suckling rat intestine. J Ultrastruct Res *85*:70, 1983.

69. Phillips AD, Thomas AG, Walker-Smith JA: Cryptosporidium, chronic diarrhoea and proximal small intestinal mucosa. Gut *33*:1057, 1992.

70. Ulshen MH, Rollo JL: Pathogenesis of escherichia coli gastroenteritis in man—another mechanism. N Engl J Med *302*:99, 1980.

71. Cornell R, Walker WA, Isselbacher KJ: Small intestinal absorption of horseradish peroxidase. A cytochemical study. Lab Invest *25*:42, 1971.

72. Stern M, Walker WA: Food proteins and the gut mucosal barrier. I. Binding and uptake of cow's milk proteins by rat jejunum in vivo. Am J Physiol *246*:G556, 1984.

73. Stern M, Gellermann B: Food proteins and maturation of small intestinal microvillus membranes (MVM). I. Binding characteristics of cow's milk proteins and concanavalin A to MVM from newborn and adult rats. J Pediatr Gastroenterol Nutr *7*:115, 1988.

74. Stern M, Gellermann B, Belitz HD, Wieser

H: Food proteins and maturation of small intestinal microvillus membranes (MVM). II. Binding of gliadin hydrolysate fractions and of the gliadin peptide B3142. J Pediatr Gastroenterol Nutr *7*:122, 1988.

75. Chu SW, Walker WA: Development of the gastrointestnal mucosal barrier: VII. Changes in phospholipid head groups and fatty acid composition of intestinal microvillus membranes from newborn and adult rats. Pediatr Res *23*:439, 1988.

76. Pang KY, Bresson JL, Walker WA: Development of the gastrointestinal mucosal barrier: Evidence of structural differences in microvillus membranes from newborn and adult rabbits. Biochim Biophys Acta *727*:201, 1983.

77. Pang KY, Newman AP, Udall JN, Walker WA: Development of the gastrointestinal mucosal barrier. VI. In utero maturation of the microvillus surface by cortisone. Am J Physiol *249*:G85, 1985.

78. Israel EJ, Pang KY, Harmatz PR, Walker WA: Structural and functional maturation of rat gastrointestinal barrier with thyroxine. Am J Physiol *252*:762, 1987.

79. Dinsdale D, Healy PJ: Enzymes involved in protein transmission by the intestine of the newborn lamb. Histochem J *14*:811, 1982.

80. Davies PH, Messer M: Intestinal cathepsin B and D activities of suckling rats. Biol Neonate *45*:197, 1984.

81. Ekstrom GM, Westrom BR: Cathespin B and D activities in intestinal mucosa during postnatal development in pigs. Relation to intestinal uptake and transmission of macromolecules. Biol Neonate *59*:314, 1991.

82. Vaeth GF, Henning SJ: Postnatal development of peptidase enzymes in rat small intestine. J Pediatr Gastroenterol Nutr *1*:111, 1982.

83. Madara JL: Loosening TJs. Lessons from the intestine. J Clin Invest *83*:1089, 1989.

84. Gumbiner B: The structure, biochemistry, and assembly of epithelial TJs. Am J Physiol *253*:C749, 1987.

85. Madara JL: Maintenance of the macromolecular barrier at cell extrusion sites in intestinal epithelium: Physiological rearrangement of tight junction. J Membr Biol *116*:177, 1990.

86. Frizzell RA, Schultz SG: Ionic conductancc of extracellular shunt pathway in rabbit ileum. J Gen Physiol *59*:318, 1982.

87. Claude P, Goodenough DA: Fracture faces of zonulae accludentes from "tight" and "leaky" epithelial. J Cell Biol *58*:390, 1973.

88. Madara JL, Dharmsathaphorn K: Occluding junction structure-function relationships in a cultured epithelial monolayer. J Cell Biol *101*:2124, 1985.

89. Madara JL: Pathobiology of the intestinal epithelial barrier. Am J Pathol *137*:1273, 1990.

90. Pappenheimer JR, Reiss KZ: Contribution of solvent drag through intercellular junctions to absorption of nutrient by the small intestine of the rat. J Membr Biol *100*:123, 1987.

91. Pappenheimer JR: Physiological regulation of transepithelial impedance in the intestinal mucosal of rat and hamster. J Membr Biol *100*:137, 1987.

92. Madara JL, Pappenheimer JR: Structural basis for physiological regulation of paracellular pathways in intestinal epithelial. J Membr Biol *100*:149, 1987.

93. Atisook K, Madara JL: An oligopeptide permeates intestinal tight junctions at glucose-elicited dilatations. Implications for oligopeptide absorption. Gastroenterology *100*:719, 1991.

94. Madara JL, Stafford J: Interferon-y directly affects barrier function of cultured intestinal epithelial monolayers. J Clin Invest *83*:724, 1989.

95. Nash S, Stafford J, Madara JL: Effects of polymorphonuclear leukocyte transmigration of the barrier function of cultured intestinal epithelial monolayers. J Clin Invest *80*:1104, 1987.

96. MacDonald TT: The pathogenesis of intestinal inflammation. *In* Walker WA et al. (Eds): Pediatric Gastrointestinal Disease. Philadelphia, B. C. Decker Inc., 1990, pp. 574.

97. Choy MY, Walker-Smith JA, Williams CB, MacDonald TT: Differential expression of CD25 (interleukin-2 receptor) on lamina propria T cells and macrophages in the intestinal lesions in Crohn's disease and ulcerative colitis. Gut *31*:1365, 1990.

98. James SP: Cellular immune mechanisms in the pathogenesis of Crohn's disease. In Vivo *2*:1, 1988.

99. Sanderson IR, Phillips AD, Spencer J, Walker-Smith JA: Response of autoimmune enteropathy to cyclosporin A therapy. Gut *32*:1421, 1991.

100. MacDonald TT, Spencer J: Evidence that activated mucosal T cells play a role in the pathogenesis of enteropathy in human small intestine. J Exp Med *167*:1341, 1988.

101. Evans CM, Phillips AD, Walker-Smith JA, MacDonald TT: Activation of lamina propria T cells induces crypt epithelial proliferation and goblet cell depletion in cultured human fetal colon. Gut *33*:230, 1992.

102. Isaacson PG et al.: Malignant histiocytosis of the intestine: A T-cell lymphoma. Lancet *ii*:57, 1985.

103. Sanderson IR, Walker-Smith JA: Indigenous amoebiasis: An important differential diagnosis of chronic inflammatory bowel disease. Br Med J *289*:823, 1984.

104. Krogstad DJ et al.: Amebiasis: Epidemiologic studies in the United States, 1971–1974. Ann Intern Med *88*:89, 1978.

105. Editorial: Misdiagnosis of amoebiasis. Br Med J *ii*:452, 1975.

106. Mody VR: Corticosteroids in latent amoebiasis. Br Med J *ii*:1399, 1959.

107. Eisert J, Hannibal JE, Sanders SL: Fatal amebiasis complicating corticosteroid management of pemphigus vulgaris. N Engl J Med *261*:843, 1959.

108. Pittman FE, el-Hashimi WK, Pittman JC: Studies of human amebiasis. I. Clinical and laboratory findings in eight cases of acute amebic colitis. Gastroenterology *65*:581, 1973.

27

Immunology of the Gastrointestinal Tract: Selected Aspects

STEPHAN R. TARGAN AND LOREN KARP MURPHY

Immunology emerged as a major scientific discipline during the 20th century, and today its mechanisms are fundamental to understanding the pathogenesis of many disease processes. Although references to immunologic concepts date back to the 6th century, the current body of knowledge has evolved from the latter 19th century to the present time. With the technologic explosion of the 1980s, the pace of scientific discovery in immunology has markedly accelerated and immunity is being examined at the molecular level to determine normal and abnormal immune response. Early in this century, the findings regarding the gastrointestinal tract significantly modified assumptions concerning the mechanisms of immunity. And once again, nearing the close of the 20th century, mucosal immunology is defining new pathways of immunologic understanding. During the interim years, however, mucosal immunology yielded to systemic immunology in investigation and discovery. This chapter, reviewing the evolution of the discipline of gastrointestinal immunology, delineates several important advances in theories of mucosal immunity within the context of what was known about immunology in general. Table 27–1 depicts those topics selected and their actual or potential relevance to the pathogenesis and treatment of clinical disease.

EARLY CONCEPTS OF IMMUNITY

At the turn of the 20th century, the discipline of immunology was dominated by two opposing schools of thought. The "cellularists" focused on the phagocyte, macrophage, and polymorphonuclear cells as the means by which the body combatted infection. The "humoralists" maintained that defense against infection was within the domain of the blood, bile, etc. At the center of the debate were Elie Metchnikoff of the Pasteur Institute (France), well known for his work on the role of phagocytes and studies in bacteriology and Robert Koch of the Koch Institute (Germany), discoverer of the tubercle bacillus and cholera vibrio. The dialectic between the "cellularists" and "humoralists" gave momentum to the discipline, and although the "humoralists" prevailed at the time, much value was later found in the views of the "cellularists."

The outcome of this debate was new emphasis on the antibody as a fundamental unit in the immune process, but its relevance to human illness was less clear. For half a millennium, the role of the cellular aspect of the immune system was virtually ignored. The following discussion, organized chronologically by topic, describes the evolution of major concepts in gastrointestinal immunology, charts the discoveries, and describes the relationship of the findings to the metamorphosis of immunology as a whole.

ORAL TOLERANCE

Oral tolerance refers to the ingestion of an antigen, inducing a local mucosal response

451

Table 27–1

Discoveries in Mucosal Immunology and Their Clinical Application

Area of Mucosal Immunity	Clinical Relevance
Oral tolerance	Treatment of systemic autoimmune disease
Local immunity	Oral vaccination (i.e., polio, cholera, traveler's diarrhea)
	Understanding of immunodeficiency diseases (HIV, common variable immunodeficiency, IgA deficiency)
Lymphocyte trafficking	Treatment of inflammatory bowel disease, celiac disease, gut allergies
Cellular elements within the mucosa:	
Intraepithelial lymphocytes	Celiac disease, microscopic colitis, initiation of autoimmunity (?)
Lamina propria T cells	Pathogenesis and treatment of Crohn's disease and ulcerative colitis
Mucosal neuroimmunology	Role of stress in flaring of inflammatory bowel disease
Immunophysiology	A mechanism of diarrhea, stricture formation, and cell trafficking in inflammatory bowel disease

that inhibits a systemic response to a subsequent challenge with the same antigen. Many of the earliest recorded references to immunity were those describing the phenomenon of individuals with apparently a "natural" resistance to the bacterial causes of various plagues. Also, political rulers were known to experiment with the ingestion of poisons as a means of protection from assassination attempts. In retrospect, these primitive experiences provide an historical background for modern studies of oral tolerance.

One hundred and sixty-five years ago, Dakin became aware that the oral ingestion of antigens might prevent the systemic body response to antigen (1). He reported that native Americans ingested poison ivy leaves to prevent dermatitis on subsequent contact with the plant. The first scientific description of oral tolerance was in 1911 by H. Gideon Wells (2), a time dominated by heightened awareness of bacterial pathogens, and when scientists were concerned with methods of prevention and treatment of tuberculosis, cholera and other infectious illnesses. In Wells's classical experiments on anaphylaxis, guinea pigs were fed ovalbumin, to which they were reactive (2). With continued feeding, they became less and less sensitive to the protein until they displayed a refractory, or immune, condition in which the animals did not react to repeated subcutaneous injections of the fed protein. These

observations represent the first descriptions of the phenomenon of oral tolerance, although the existence of a mucosal immune system was not known at the time, nor was it recognized that the feeding of antigens had a profound effect on systemic responsiveness. The observations by Wells were expanded in 1946 by Merrill Chase (3), who demonstrated inhibition of a delayed-type hypersensitivity to dinitrochlorobenzene by prior feeding with the same compound. The state of refractory or absence of response to antigens following oral feeding came to be known as the Sulzberger-Chase phenomenon.

Over the next several decades, for reasons not apparent today, oral tolerance lost its scientific appeal. In the mid-1960s, interest in oral tolerance returned as part of a general upsurge of research stimulated by the discovery of IgA and its role in local immunity (see below). Much of the early work focused on testing the applicability of the oral tolerance phenomenon to different classes of antigens. By the late 1970s, immunologic studies centered on mechanisms of oral tolerance, including cellular mediation. Following the oral ingestion of ovalbumin, T-suppressor cells originating from the intestine were found to have the ability to suppress systemic antigen-specific proliferation as well as immunoglobulin production (4). In addition to this cellular mechanism, and furthering the cellular versus humoral dialectic, Andre et al. in 1975 showed that soluble factors also play a role in the induction of oral tolerance (5) by demonstrating that the intragastric administration of erythrocytes induced serum factors that inhibited systemic responses. These factors initially were thought to be related solely to an IgA complex, but IgG1 antibodies also were shown to be capable of inducing systemic tolerance.

These investigations intensified when IgE specific suppressor cells were found within the intestinal mucosa. It was hypothesized that the feeding of allergens could lead to suppression of systemic or mucosal allergic reactions, suggesting a possible therapeutic approach to the treatment of asthma and other allergic diseases. Stimulated by these studies, the applicability of the phenomenon of oral tolerance to the treatment of systemic immune disease came under investigation in the mid to late 1970s. A series of experiments in the 1980s using animal models of allergic encephalitis, uveitis, and arthritis demonstrated antigen-specific inhibition of these chronic autoimmune diseases by prior feeding with the individual antigens. Recent studies demonstrated that oral feeding could prevent not only disease occurrence, but also disease recurrence by oral feeding during times of disease remission.

Not until 1992 was it demonstrated that a soluble antigen, keyhole limpet hemocyanin, taken orally, prevented a delayed type of hypersensitivity systemic response to the antigen injected subcutaneously (Husby, personal communication). This observation suggested that systemic T cell responses could be abrogated by prior oral antigen feeding in humans; providing a rational basis for applying the process of antigen-specific oral tolerance to the treatment of well-defined autoimmune disease. The feeding of myelin basic protein to patients with chronic relapsing multiple sclerosis in an attempt to induce remission of the disease reflects the profound clinical impact of the findings on oral tolerance.

LOCAL IMMUNITY

As opposed to the description of oral tolerance, which evolved from attempts to control systemic anaphylaxis of the immune response, the concept of local immunity developed from a keen interest in generating protection from specific pathogens (immunity). Local immunity is defined as an induced immune response that is confined to a particular region of the immune system. The concept of a mucosal immune response specific to the gastrointestinal tract evolved from observations by Besredka (6), who studied oral infections caused by the ingestion of enteric bacteria. The importance of systemic antibodies in protecting against gut infections was acknowledged and suggested the possibility that local immunity might be responsible for this protection. Support for Besredka's idea of intestinal immunity was provided when Davies (7) demonstrated the presence of coproantibodies in the feces of patients suffering from bacteria-induced dysentery before the appearance of serum antibodies. The importance of these coproantibodies in the protection of guinea pigs from infection was suggested by the correlation between the appearance of coproantibodies concurrently with the development of protective immunity. There was no correlation with the appearance of serum antibodies. These findings clearly indicated the importance of local antibodies in protection against local infection.

The origin of these coproantibodies has remained controversial. In spite of the interesting observations of Walsh and Cannon in the 1930s demonstrating the local production of antibodies in the nasal cavities of animal models, twenty years later the local antibodies were assumed to represent serum antibody "spilled over" into external secretions (8). The concept that circulating antibodies may not reflect the local immune status and that antibodies, in fact, may be produced locally, emerged in the early 1960s. The "spill-over" concept finally was discarded with the demonstration of IgA as the major local mucosal immunoglobulin. Heremans described the new isotype of antibody IgA in the serum (9). Hanson and Tomasi subsequently demonstrated that this isotype formed the major immunoglobulin component of human and animal secretions, i.e., saliva, breast milk, and intestinal secretions (10,11). Crabbe, in 1965, was the investigator responsible for the first indication that IgA was the dominant isotype of the body (12).

Once the concept of local immunity was established, the IgA in external secretions was found to have a different structure than serum IgA. Serum IgA proved to be a monomer whereas mucosal IgA was a dimer. These findings led to the discovery of an additional polypeptide chain associated with secretory IgA. In immunochemical studies it was found that monomeric IgA was linked by a J-piece in the subepithelial plasma cells and transported across the epithelium by secretory component. Secretory component was originally described as glycoprotein produced by epithelial cells lying in the gastrointestinal and respiratory tracts. Secretory component-IgA complex was shown to resist proteolysis, thereby protecting IgA from destruction by luminal protease. These characteristics permitted IgA to function in the lumen to prevent bacteria from mucosal adherence and subsequent invasion. Following the observation that intravenously injected monomeric IgA could not be found in nasal secretions, it was apparent that circulating IgA did not contribute to polymeric IgA in secretions.

These findings were of enormous significance because, for the first time, many immunologists were receptive to the possibility of a separate identifiable immune system operant in gastrointestinal mucosa. The regulation of IgA production as well as the studies of the mechanisms of its transport into the secretions became the focus of many subsequent investigations. Further research identified the gut mucosa as containing the qualitatively most important B-cell system of the body (13). The overwhelming dominance of IgA signaled an important role for this immunoglobulin in maintaining host defense. Throughout the 1970s, scientists focused their studies on the role of IgA in the mucosal immune response and the unique features of the mucosal immune compartment.

RELATING FUNCTIONS TO THE PHYSICAL STRUCTURE OF THE MUCOSAL IMMUNE SYSTEM

Further Compartmentalization

The phenomenon of preferential homing of activated cells to repopulate the mucosa

is a distinctive feature of the mucosal compartment. This phenomenon defines afferent and efferent limbs of the mucosal immune system. A major advance toward defining the anatomy and the function of the afferent immune system was the discovery of the specialized epithelium that overlies lymphoid nodules, known as Peyer's patches. These patches, first described by J.C. Peyer in 1677, are defined as groups of subepithelial lymphoid follicles located throughout the small and large intestines. Studies in the early 1970s suggested that Peyer's patches were the primary organ for the generation of mucosal immune responses. The 1974 classic ultrastructural studies of Owen and Jones (14) identified "M" (microfold) cells, overlying these patches, and suggested that these cells possess the special function of transporting luminal antigens across the gut. Subsequent observations by Owen confirmed the ability of these cells to take up antigen and transport it to macrophages overlying the actual lymphoid follicle. These findings stimulated much interest in the process of antigen presentation in the mucosal immune system. Owen and colleagues were the first to describe the function of the epithelial cell, and solidified the concept of a separate afferent limb within the mucosal immune compartment.

The link between the afferent compartment and the lamina propria was suggested even before the discovery of M cells, and was first proposed after study of the mechanism of preferential lymphocyte homing to the mucosa observed in 1963 (15). These studies indicated that blast cells derived from the mesenteric lymph nodes or thoracic duct had a predilection to return to both the small intestine and large intestine. With the increased focus on the mucosal immune system in the 1970s, many studies were directed toward understanding this repopulation phenomenon. Early investigations focused on the homing of IgA blasts and later were followed by studies on T cell homing. The extent to which gut-derived lymphocytes home was redefined in 1973, when Bienenstock et al. first described the existence of bronchial as well as gut associated lymphoid tissue (16–18). This observation led to experiments demonstrating that cells from the bronchial-associated lymphoid tissue home to the gut in addition to the lung and vice versa. On the basis of such findings, Bienenstock and colleagues advanced the concept of the "common mucosal immune system," and then to the view that an immune response initiated at a specific site within the intestine could be disseminated throughout the entire mucosal immune system, including the bronchus, salivary glands, breast, urinary tract, and gut.

In the 1970s, investigators began to characterize the mechanism of preferential lymphocyte homing, including the central role of the high endothelial venules in the cell trafficking of circulating lymphocytes. Selected binding was noted on lymph node high endothelial venules. In 1979, Butcher and Weissman (19) demonstrated selected binding of lymphocytes originating from the gut to the Peyer's patch or to gut-specific high endothelial venules by means of particular ligands on circulating lymphocytes that could direct homing either to the lymph node or to the Peyer's patch. With the advent of molecular technology, many of these ligands, including the mucosal specific ligand 4 7, now have been cloned and identified, providing the opportunity to study the mechanisms not only of homing and binding to high endothelial venules of selected organs, but also of trafficking to specific tissue.

The concept of a common mucosal immune system with afferent and efferent limbs was solidified by discovery of the cell surface molecules that control the flow of trafficking cells. The cloning and sequencing of these molecules allow the development of reagents to prevent selective homing of cells to the mucosa without affecting trafficking of cells to lymph nodes and other organs of the body. These reagents represent an important method whereby mucosal inflammation can be controlled without altering the function of the general immune system, and may facilitate the specific treatment of diseases of the intestine, which are mediated by local immune responses such as inflammatory bowel disease, celiac disease, or microscopic colitis.

THE STUDY OF CELLULAR ELEMENTS WITHIN THE MUCOSA

The first suggestion that the cellular elements of the gastrointestinal mucosa were different from their counterparts in other tissues was first described in studies of mast cells. Histopathologic studies of these cells in the 1960s and 1970s led to the appreciation that mast cells existing within the mucosa were different from the mast cells of other tissues (20,21). Subsequently, it was shown that the two types of mast cells release histamine differently. Indeed, it was found that modalities used to treat allergic reactions, based on their effects on basophils, eosinophils, and tissue mast cells, were not necessarily effective in altering intestinal mast cell responses. With the advent of molecular technology, the differences between the mast cells of the mucosa and mast cells of other tissues were further defined by the demonstration of the release of different types of proteases. These observations have indicated the need to investigate the role of intestinal mast cells in gastrointestinal inflammation independently from other mast cell types.

The intriguing discoveries regarding IgA during the 1960s and early 1970s rekindled interest in the cellular constituents of the mucosal compartment as had been identified for the systemic immune system. Extrapolating from the research on IgA, Kawanishi and Strober (22) were motivated to examine cellular components of the Peyer's patches that might specifically direct intestinal B cells to produce IgA. These components, known as switch T cells, were found to be capable of switching the isotype of B-cells from IgM to IgA. This finding represented major progress in the effort to determine the selective IgA dominance over other immunoglobulins within the mucosa. Identification of the switch T cells stimulated the application of molecular techniques to investigate the presence of other isotype specific switch T cells within the system immune system. The concept of switching encouraged a series of studies on the cytokines responsible for this T cell–B cell communication. The IgA switch T cell is an example of a cell unique to the mucosal immune system and is another instance of a mucosal immunologic finding influencing research on systemic immunology.

Additional differences among mucosal T cells were appreciated in the study of the intraepithelial lymphocyte compartment. Observations in the early 1970s indicated that T lymphoblasts as well as B lymphoblasts from mesenteric lymph nodes preferentially home to the intestines. Interest focused on the epithelial compartment because the cells of the epithelium were found to be exclusively T cells. Studies in rodents initially demonstrated that intraepithelial T cells were functionally and phenotypically distinct from those of the peripheral blood and the lamina propria, defining this compartment as the "first line of defense" of the host against the environment. Intraepithelial lymphocytes resurfaces as a focus for investigation in the late 1980s with the discovery of a second class of T cells (Tγ Δ cells). Animal studies demonstrated that the small intestinal intraepithelial compartment was the major locus for these cells. This discovery encouraged many immunologists interested in Tγ Δ cells to include investigations of the unique properties of intraepithelial lymphocytes, yet another example of a unique feature of the mucosal immune system influencing research in general immunology. Studies now are under way to test the hypothesis that the intraepithelial compartment represents an extrathymic organ capable of independently shaping the T cell repertoire.

T cells of the lamina propria were found to be unique as well, and distinct from their counterparts in the peripheral blood and the intraepithelial compartment which were first performed on rodents, studies of the lamina propria T-cells were performed predominantly in humans. Experiments in the early 1980s demonstrated that lamina propria T-cells did not respond by way of the conventional antigen activation pathway. It was found that, to assess lamina propria T-cell activation, the conventional measures of proliferation were invalid, and the actual indicator of activation was cytokine expression. In contrast to peripheral blood T cells, in which the antigen specific pathway of activation was dominant, an alternate pathway of activation prevailed for the mucosal T cells. These findings demonstrated that different measurements were required to determine whether or not there was a selected mucosal T-cell response to a specific pathogen, an issue of vital importance in defining the role of any pathogen in immunologically mediated disease of the intestine. In addition, the unique mucosal T-cell profile mandates the study of alterations in this compartment in the investigation of various immunologic diseases. The development of therapeutic interventions for such diseases, perhaps a mucosally specific immune modulator, depends on recognition of the unique mucosal T-cell response, as systemically useful modalities do not necessarily effect the same changes in the mucosa. Current research indicates that such products are likely to be developed as we approach the 21st century.

IMMUNOLOGIC COMMUNICATIONS WITHIN THE INTESTINE

The prevailing thought before 1970 was that communication between the cellular and humoral immune components occurred among cells traditionally involved in the immune response; i.e., macrophages, T cells, and B cells. It had not yet been appreciated that supposedly immunologically dormant cells within the gut (e.g., fibroblasts) might also communicate with known elements of the immune response. The first evidence that cells thought to be uninvolved in immune response could participate in modulation of the immune response came from studies of the relationship between the brain and the immune system.

For decades, emotions were considered to affect the gut by inducing standard physiologic responses such as altering motility and secretion. The clinical observation that stress apparently induced flares of immune-mediated intestinal illness, suggested that affective conditions also could alter intestinal inflammation, perhaps through communication of nerves with these cell populations. Perhaps the first evidence of neuroendocrine influences on such immunologic function came from experiments performed during the early 1970s demonstrating the effects of specific lesions created in the hypothalamus and adjacent sensory structures. Such lesions could profoundly modify the amount of antibody production and alter the numbers and function of natural killer cells and T lymphocytes in the systemic immune compartment. Scientists endeavored to define mechanisms of these changes, which led to investigations of how the nervous system contacts and communicates with such cells. Felten and Bulloch subsequently demonstrated the innervation of lymphoid tissues, thereby suggesting that neurotransmitters originating in peripheral nerves could act as conduits for local and direct distribution of substances from these nerves in high concentrations to immune cells. The concept of bidirectional communication between neurons as well as the lymphoid tissue was extended in Blalock's classic studies, which suggested lymphocytes and monocytes were actually circulating endocrine organs (23). Blalock postulated that the immune system could act as a sensory efferent organ for the central nervous system surveying and discriminating between the constant influx of new molecules to which the body is exposed.

The 1972 demonstration of free axons within the intracellular spaces of the Peyer's patches was the first indication that such communication exists within the mucosa. Subsequent studies demonstrated that different types of peptidergic nerves are localized within these patches. Further evidence of neuroimmune communication within the mucosa was presented in the late 1970s and early 1980s in demonstrating that nerve cell bodies of the enteric nervous system predominantly lie within the myenteric and submucosal plexi, but processes arising within these cells actually ramify extensively throughout the wall of the intestine.

It had long been known that nerve stimulation could cause degranulation of intestinal mast cells. Proof of the close association between nerves and the immune cells of the gut was most elegantly demonstrated in the 1980s in studies which showed substance P-like nerves to be intimately associated with gut mast cells. These studies have led to the overall concept of a significant relationship among the nervous system, the mediators, and the immune system. In fact, studies have demonstrated that neurally derived peptides, such as VIP and substance P profoundly influence various aspects of mucosal immune function, including T-cell activation and production of IgA.

The discovery that neurons are capable of influencing the immune response within the mucosa and, in turn, can be influenced by immunologically active mucosal cells, launched the discipline of neuro-immuno-physiology. The first theory to arise from the concept of bidirectional communication was that the immune system could profoundly affect the functioning of epithelial cells, smooth muscle cells and fibroblasts located within the mucosa. The actual mediators involved included multiple types of inflammatory cytokines released by immune cells. Evidence has been presented that mucosal cells thought to be immunologically dormant (fibroblasts, smooth muscle cells, and epithelial cells) indeed are capable of producing factors that modulate the function of immune cells, thus closing the communication loop. The progress in mucosal immunology now has recruited not only general immunologists, but also physiologists and other scientists. The phrase "gut level communication," first used casually in the 1960s, obviously has taken on a much more complex biologic significance.

CONCLUSION

In the early 1900s, the predominant objective of medicine was the elimination of infections that decimated large populations. Use of the oral route of "immunization" to protect against bacterial invaders, represents the earliest understanding of what was to be become recognized as the mucosal immune system. Following a long dormant period through the 1930s and the 1940s, renewed interest in oral tolerance as an approach to treat anaphylaxis extended to the possible immunologic role of the mucosa. Thus, in the late 1960s, with the discovery of IgA and its predominance in the gut mucosa, the gastrointestinal immune system once again was the focus of scientific investigation. The concept of the common mucosal immune system, cellular trafficking, and the discovery of T-cells in Peyer's patches that could initiate switching of immunoglobulin isotypes provided impetus to study the role of the T-cell in system isotype conversions. The recognition of nontraditional immune interactions and evidence of the ability of the gut to mold the immune response extrathymically provides emphasis and expectation that further study of the mucosal immune system will generate many new immunologic concepts, and significantly influence the future understanding of immunology as a whole.

REFERENCES

1. Richman LK: Immunological unresponsiveness after enteric administration of protein antigens. *In* Ogra PL, Dayton D (eds): Immunology of Breast Milk. New York, Raven Press, 1979.
2. Wells HG: Studies on the chemistry of anaphylaxis (III). Experiments with isolated proteins, especially those of the hen's egg. J Infect Dis 9:147, 1911.
3. Chase MW: Inhibition of experimental drug allergy by prior feeding of the sensitizing agent. Proc Soc Exp Biol Med *61*:257, 1946.
4. Miller SD, Hanson DG: Inhibition of specific immune responses by feeding protein antigens. IV. Evidence for tolerance and specific active suppression of cell-mediated immune responses to ovalbumin. J Immunol *123*:2344, 1979.
5. Andre C, Heremans JF, Vaerman JP, Cambiaso CL: A mechanism for the induction of immunological tolerance by antigen feeding: Antigen-antibody complexes. J Exp Med *142*:1509, 1975.
6. Besredka A: De la vaccination contre les états typhoides par la voie buccale. Ann Inst Pasteur *33*:882, 1919.
7. Davies A: An investigation into the serological properties of dysentery stools. Lancet *ii*:1009, 1922.
8. Walsh TE, Cannon PR: Immunization of the respiratory tract: A comparative study of the antibody content of the respiratory and other tissues following active, passive and regional immunization. J Immunol *35*:31, 1938.
9. Heremans JF, Heremans M-TH, Schultze HE: Isolation and description of a few properties of the 2A-Globulin of human serum. Clinica Chimica Acta *4*:96, 1959.
10. Hanson LA: Comparative immunological studies of the immune globulins of human milk and of blood serum. Int Arch Allergy Appl Immunol *18*:241, 1961.
11. Tomasi TB, Zigelbaum S: The selective occurrence of g1A globulins in certain body fluids. J Clin Invest *42*:1552, 1963.
12. Crabbe PA, Carbonnara AO, Heremans JF: The normal human intestinal mucosa as major source of plasma cells containing yA-immunoglobulin. Lab Invest *14*:235, 1965.
13. Delacroix DL: The human immunoglobulin a system: Its vascular compartment. Thesis, Université Catholique de Louvain. Brussels, Brugge, European Medical Press, 1985.
14. Owen RL, Jones AL: Epithelial cell specialization within human Peyer's patches: An ultrastructural study of intestinal lymphoid follicles. Gastroenterology *66*:189, 1974.
15. Gowans JL, Knight EJ: The route of re-circulation of lymphocytes in the rat. Phil Trans Royal Soc (London) *159*:257, 1964.
16. Bienenstock J, Johnston N, Perey DYE: Bronchial lymphoid tissue. I. Morphologic characteristics. Lab Invest *28*:686, 1973.
17. Bienenstock J, Johnston N, Perey DYE: Bronchial lymphoid tissue. II. Morphologic characteristics. Lab Invest *28*:693, 1973.
18. Bienenstock J: The physiology of the local immune response and the gastrointestinal tract. Progr Immunol II *4*:197, 1974.
19. Butcher EC, Scollay RG, Weissman IL: Lymphocyte adherence to high endothelial venules: Characterization of a modified in vitro assay, and examination of the binding of syngeneic and allogeneic lymphocyte populations. J Immunol *123*:1996, 1979.
20. Enerback L: Mast cells in rat gastrointestinal mucosa. I. Effects of fixation. Acta Path Microbiol Scand *66*:289, 1966.
21. Enerback L: Mast cells in rat gastrointestinal mucosa. II. Dye-binding and metachromatic properties. Acta Pathol Microbiol Scand *66*:303, 1966.
22. Kawanishi H, Strober W: Regulatory T-cells in murine Peyer's patches directing IgA-specific isotype switching. Ann NY Acad Sci *409*:243, 1983.
23. Blalock JE, Smith EM: A complete regulatory loop between the immune and neuroendocrine systems. Fed Proc *44*:108, 1985.

28

Circulation of the Gastrointestinal Tract

EUGENE D. JACOBSON

The beginnings of current information about the splanchnic circulation constitute a rich scientific history spanning nearly two centuries.

It is not possible within the confines of a brief chapter to document the thousands of historical contributions to present views of gastrointestinal circulatory functions and malfunctions. Furthermore, the perspective of a single scholar poring through the archives is likely to be too limited by personal views and perhaps biases. In addition, work of very recent origin is difficult to assess historically because its long-term impact is yet speculative. For these reasons, my backward look has been restricted almost entirely to 20th-century original research papers published before 1986.* The reader is referred to topical reviews for more recent contributions.

The historical account is divided into three parts reflecting the largest subsets of current information dealing with components of the splanchnic circulation, namely, the gastric circulation, the mesenteric circulation, and the hepatic circulation.

THE GASTRIC CIRCULATION

Research on the gastric circulation began more than 150 years ago with Beaumont's

* I restricted citations to the first one or two in a series of germinal reports on a subject from a single laboratory. Finally, I turned to internationally respected scholars for help with my project, and they generously aided my cause. Thus, I am indebted to 10 colleagues: C. C. Chou, D. Neil Granger, Clive V. Greenway, Roberto J. Groszmann, Paul C. Johnson, Jeffrey W. Kiel, W. Wayne Lautt, Ove Lundgren, A. P. Shepherd, and John L. Wallace.

observations of a patient with a gastric fistula (1). The frontier physician noted a red suffusion of the mucosal surface when the stomach secreted its juice at mealtime. A century later, Wolf and Wolff made similar observations in a more sophisticated setting in their patient with a gastric fistula (2). These observers inferred that mucosal blood flow had increased during stimulation of gastric secretion. In neither situation could actual measurements of flow be obtained, although Wolf and Wolff quantified the changes in mucosal color (2).

The gross anatomy of the complex gastric circulation was elucidated in the last century by Mall (3). From his morphologic investigations of the human stomach, he estimated that the gastric mucosa receives about three quarters of the blood supplied to the organ. By the early part of this century, Burton-Opitz had used the strohmühr to measure blood flow to the canine stomach, which he determined to be 0.2 mL/min per gram of tissue (4).

By midcentury, careful histology of the stomach wall had been reported by Barlow et al., who also inferred arteriovenous shunts (5). Later studies employing in vivo microscopy by Guth and Rosenberg failed to verify shunts (6). Subsequent observations from Guth's laboratory demonstrated the key role of the submucosal network of arterioles in regulating gastric mucosal blood flow (7).

Probably no publication of the past 50 years had as large an impact in gastric circulatory physiology as the 1966 paper by Jacobson et al. (8). This report was to become one of the five most frequently cited papers in all of the gastrointestinal literature over the next 15 years. Its importance was based upon two features. First the paper described a quantitative method for measuring gastric mucosal blood flow in conscious or anesthetized animal subjects, and the method was apparently validated. Second, relationships between gastric secretion and mucosal blood flow were posited and confirmed. Subsequently, many laboratories worldwide adopted the aminopyrine clearance method for the investigation of gastric circulation. Although the method later was found to be flawed (9) and was replaced by other clearance techniques, this report was seminal in the history of gastric circulatory physiology. Furthermore, some of the experimental approaches and concepts emphasized by this 1966 paper have yet to be abandoned.

Other methods for measuring gastric mucosal blood flow, which supplanted the aminopyrine clearance, include the clearance of radiolabeled microspheres, the hydrogen clearance method, laser Doppler velocimetry, and in vivo microscopy. Application of microsphere distribution to the stomach and its tissues was the result of work by Delaney and Grim (10). This method has been used widely for nearly 30 years because of technical ease, low cost, and its sound scientific basis, although there are also significant limitations with its use (11,12). The H_2 clearance technique for measuring gastric mucosal blood flow was first reported by Murakami et al. (13) and has since been championed by Guth and his collaborators (9). Application of laser Doppler velocimetry to estimation of changes in gastric mucosal and muscularis blood flows was made by Kiel et al. (14). In vivo microscopy has been used for over two decades in Guth's laboratory (6) to observe microvascular activity in mucosal vessels.

Specific vasodilator responses of the gastric mucosa to prostaglandins, acetylcholine, gastrin, and histamine were quantified in conscious animals over 25 years ago (8). Previously, measurements of total gastric blood flow in anesthetized animal preparations also had demonstrated that the foregoing naturally occurring secretagogues were vasodilator agents (15,16). Main and Whittle (17) and Kauffman et al. (18) first demonstrated that inhibition of prostaglandin synthesis reduced resting gastric mucosal blood flow. Whittle et al. (19) were first to find that thromboxane A_2, prostaglandin F_2 alpha, and leukotriene C_4 were potent constrictors of gastric microvessels. Bond et al. (20) first quantified gastric blood flow increases as a consequence of feeding in conscious animals. The earliest reports about gastric pressure-flow autoregulation indicated very little vasodilation, with a falling perfusion pressure (21).

An early study that implicated the mucosal microcirculation in ulcerogenesis was Key's 1950 histopathologic analysis (22). In the next decade of this century, Davenport and L.R. Johnson (23,24) found that experimental injury of dog and rat stomach with topical acid solutions containing aspirin provoked release of local histamine, extravasation of albumin, and bleeding into the lumen. Later, Robert and his colleagues demonstrated the cytoprotective effects of prostaglandins against aspirin and ethanol (25) but failed to implicate a circulatory mechanism (26). Subsequently, Wallace et al. (27) presented strong evidence that cytoprotective agents prevented the vascular injury induced by ethanol, thereby protecting the mucosa. This laboratory also demonstrated the gastric ulcerogenicity of the potent mucosal vasoconstrictor, PAF, and suggested the key role of neutrophil adherence and activation in ulcer pathogenesis (28). Pihan et al. (29) demonstrated mucosal ischemia and microvascular stasis with different topical ulcerogens and prevented these circulatory responses with cytoprotective agents. They suggested that the microcirculatory endothelium is the first target of these gastric ulcerogens.

Menguy and Masters (30) implicated deranged oxidative metabolism in stress ulceration of the mucosa. Itoh and Guth (31) reported the involvement of oxygen-free radicals in hemorrhage-induced mucosal injury. Moody et al. (32) showed that blood flow augmentation was a major mechanism involved in cytoprotection against erosive gastritis provoked by topical noxious agents.

THE MESENTERIC CIRCULATION

Important physiologic discoveries often have had to await the emergence of reliable techniques for measuring functional parameters. Early technological applications by Burton-Opitz (33) permitted estimation of intestinal blood flow with the strohmühr. Shortly after midcentury, Grim and Lindseth (34) had utilized the distribution of microspheres to track the distribution of blood flow to the gut and to its tissue layers. Within the next few decades, dynamic and continuous measurement of mesenteric blood flow without invading the arteries became a reality with externally implanted blood flowmeters (35) and laser Doppler velocimetry (36,37).

Mealtimes pose the most recurrent physiological challenges to intestinal circulatory regulation, when central nervous and local regulatory factors must respond to ingestion, propulsion, digestion, and absorption of food. By 1910, Brodie and Vogt had demonstrated that intestinal absorption was accompanied by increased blood flow and oxygen consumption (38). Vatner et al. (39,40) noted that the cephalic phase of prandial and postprandial events increased cardiac dynamics generally and evoked an increase in visceral blood flow in conscious animals. Chou and his colleagues observed that the instillation of chyme into the upper small intestine was associated with a localized hyperemia (41,42). This laboratory also found that different alimentary constituents elicited variable vasodilator responses, with micellar lipid being the most potent stimulus (43,44). In addition, Chou and his collaborators extensively explored the role of paracrine substances (histamine, prostaglandins) in the mediation of postprandial hyperemia (45,46).

Another recurrent influence on intestinal blood flow is imposed by the mechanical movements of the bowel wall. Lawson and Chumley (47) reported that elevations of luminal pressure up to 30 mm Hg diminished blood flow briefly, whereas greater pressures evoked flow reductions which were longer lasting. Sidky and Bean (48) recorded the decrease in intestinal blood flow and venous capacitance with tonic contractions of visceral smooth muscle. Shehadeh et al. (35) demonstrated that several naturally occurring stimulants of intestinal motility also possessed inherent vasoactive properties that were the major determinants of blood flow changes. For example, acetylcholine

and angiotensin II stimulated motility equally, but the former agent increased and the latter agent decreased mesenteric blood flow. Chou and Grassmick (49) showed that rhythmic contractions of the gut wall increased muscularis blood flow, whereas tonic contractions of the wall decreased intestinal blood flow mainly by restricting mucosal and submucosal perfusion.

Autoregulatory phenomena in the mesenteric circulation have long been subjects of intense exploration, partly because of their variety, i.e., postprandial hyperemia, pressure-flow autoregulation, reactive hyperemia, autoregulatory escape, etc. For the last several decades of this century, the two competing, hypothetical explanations for mesenteric autoregulation have been the metabolic and myogenic mechanisms. The former theory posits that a changing chemical environment (pO_2, pH, released paracrine substances such as adenosine, etc.) is the critical local mechanism mandating the vasodilator response of mesenteric autoregulatory phenomena. The myogenic theory implicates microvascular resistance responses to changes in transmural pressure as the key local regulatory mechanism. Although the metabolic hypothesis dates back to the work of Barcroft nearly 100 years ago (50), the more recent research has focused on identifying the local vasodilator mediator. These investigations received a vital stimulus with a publication by H.J. Granger and Norris (51) in 1980. They clearly defined the criteria under which a putative paracrine vasoactive agent had to be judged, and they showed that adenosine met most of their criteria rather well. Reports by Walus et al. (52) and Mailman et al. (53) lent further support to adenosine and related nucleotides as dilator metabolites in mesenteric autoregulation.

The myogenic theory was proposed by P.C. Johnson (54,55) to account for intestinal pressure-flow autoregulation. His laboratory also performed some of the initial research on mesenteric capillary filtration (56). The earliest description of autoregulatory escape in the mesenteric circulation was reported by Folkow's laboratory (57,58). Intestinal reactive hyperemia (59) and veno-arterial autoregulatory dynamics (60) were explored initially by Selkurt and his colleagues. Lundgren et al. (61,62) contributed the definitive initial investigations of countercurrent exchange and multiplication in the microcirculation of the intestinal villi. The first mathematical modeling of autoregulatory escape in the mesenteric circulation was delineated more than 20 years ago by Shepherd and H.J. Granger (63). Shepherd also documented the role of capillary recruitment in maintaining tissue oxygenation as the regulatory force in the mesenteric circulation (64,65).

Microvascular physiology in the gut was first addressed by Koniges and Otto (66), who measured pressures in blood and lymphatic capillaries of the villi more than 50 years ago. The topic of capillary permeability was the subject of early studies by Mayerson et al. (67). Related ultrastructural features of mesenteric microvessels were described by Casley-Smith et al. (68). The effects of glucose absorption on intestinal microcirculatory hemodynamics and tissue pO_2 were investigated by Bohlen (69). The same laboratory also contributed an extensive early study of microvascular pressure in the gut wall (70). Mortillaro and Taylor (71) analysed the forces which influence fluid exchange across the capillaries of the gut. Folkow and his colleagues (57,58) reported initially on sympathetic neural regulation of resistance, exchange, and capacitance components of the intestinal microcirculation.

The first major circulatory disease unique to the gut was described by Wilson and Qualheim 40 years ago (72). Nonocclusive intestinal ischemia is a vasospastic disorder of considerable importance in that the disease is not rare, is difficult to diagnose, and in its severe forms usually is fatal. Cardiac glycosides appear to play a role in the pathogenesis of nonocclusive intestinal ischemia, and the vasoconstrictive, congestive effect of ouabain on splanchnic hemodynamics was first explored by Harrison et al. (73). The key role of the intestinal circulation in the pathogenesis of endotoxin shock was emphasized in the work of Fine (74) and Jacobson et al. (75), and in oligemic shock in the studies of Lillehei (76). The importance of mucosal injury to overall circulatory hemodynamics during shock was identified in studies by Lundgren, Haglund, and their collaborators (77,78). The histopathology of intestinal ischemia was reported and semi-quantified more than 20 years ago (79).

The new thrust in exploring intestinal ischemic injury and endotoxin effects on the gut began with a 1981 paper that combined the talents of a microvascular physiologist and an oxygen radical biochemist. This report from the laboratories of D.N. Granger and McCord (80) opened up a new connection between immunology and the circulation in mucosal damage. They reported that an active oxidant scavenger attenuated ischemia-induced or endotoxin-provoked capillary leakage, whereas histamine receptor antagonists were not protective. These laboratories also demonstrated attenuation of the pathological lesions provoked with protracted hypotension and ischemia by either scavenging the oxidants or blocking their synthesis (81). These two papers initiated the subsequent exciting investigations of neutrophil adhesion and migration, multiple vascular and inflammatory mediators, and the role of the endothelium in gastrointestinal mucosal ischemia/reperfusion injury.

THE HEPATIC CIRCULATION

Although the hepatic circulation is equal to the entire splanchnic arterial circulation, relatively little attention was directed to important aspects of liver hemodynamics until relatively recently. For example, the first quantitative studies of hepatic capacitance responses and fluid exchange appeared in studies by Greenway et al. less than 25 years ago (82). This work demonstrated the reservoir function of the liver. Other investigations from this laboratory showed that more than half of the blood mobilized from the entire body following hemorrhage was derived from the great splanchnic organ reservoir (83).

Burton-Opitz (84) first documented the fact that the relationship between portal venous and hepatic arterial blood flows is autoregulated within the liver. This "buffer response" permits maintenance of hepatic blood flow within limits by reciprocal changes between hepatic arterial conductance and portal vein blood flow, i.e., a fall in portal blood flow prompts hepatic arterial vasodilation. The laboratory of Lautt and his associates was responsible for identifying adenosine as the local mediator of the buffer response (85–87). The myogenic factor in hepatic pressure-flow autoregulation was first delineated by Hansen and P.C. Johnson (88). Autoregulatory escape from vasoconstrictor nerve stimulation or norepinephrine was studied with modern hemodynamic techniques initially in the liver by Greenway et al. (89). The same laboratory also investigated hepatic circulatory effects of hemorrhage in an animal model and demonstrated hepatic arterial vasodilation which maintained oxygenation of the liver (90).

The damping of portal pressure responses to increasing portal blood flow was shown by Fasth et al. (91) to depend on changes in hepatic lobar venous resistance. In this report, the authors also explored the different portal pressure responses to stimulation of mesenteric versus hepatic nerves. Rappaport (92) generated evidence to support his concept that the acinus of the liver, rather than the liver lobule, is the functional microvascular unit in the hepatic circulation.

Selkurt and P.C. Johnson (93) delved into the effects of elevating portal venous pressure on mesenteric capacitance, interstitial fluid volume, and intestinal hemodynamics. The understanding of portal hypertensive pathophysiology was advanced materially with the development of a novel animal model from Groszmann's laboratory (94). This report characterized the hyperdynamic splanchnic circulation and described portocaval shunting in the noncirrhotic liver.

The safe measurement of hepatic blood flow in human subjects became feasible at mid-century with the application of blood-borne chemical clearance by the liver. The theoretic basis of the technique rests on mathematical models (95), as well as on earlier empirical studies (96). Bradley et al. (97) used dye clearances to study effects of cirrhosis on hepatic blood flow, and Price et al. (98) used indicator dilution methods to delineate the reservoir function of the human liver during hemorrhage. The safe measurement of wedged and free hepatic venous pressures with a balloon catheter was first reported by Groszmann et al. (99). This technique quickly became a standard method for the clinical study of portal hypertension.

FURTHER READING

The reader who is inclined to study more comprehensively the information contained in this chapter is referred to several review articles and book chapters. These are listed after the historical research citations as an alphabetical bibliography.

REFERENCES

1. Beaumont W: Experiments and Observations on the Gastric Juice and the Physiology of Digestion. New York, Dover Publications Inc., 1959.
2. Wolf S, Wolff HG: Human Gastric Function. An Experimental Study of a Man and his Stomach. London, Oxford University Press, 1943.
3. Mall F: The vessels and walls of the dog's stomach. Johns Hopkins Hosp Rep *1*:1, 1896.
4. Burton-Opitz R: Über die Ströhmung des Blutes in dem Gebiete der Pfortader. III. Pflüger's Arch für ges. Physiol. *205*:245, 1910.
5. Barlow TE, Bentley FH, Walder DN: Arteries, veins, and arteriovenous anastomoses in the human stomach. Surg Gynecol Obstet *93*:657, 1951.
6. Guth PH, Rosenberg A: *In vivo* microscopy of the gastric microcirculation. Am J Dig Dis *17*:391, 1972.
7. Guth PH, Smith E: Neural control of gastric mucosal blood flow in the rat. Gastroenterology *69*:935, 1975.
8. Jacobson ED, Linford RH, Grossman MI: Gastric secretion in relation to mucosal blood flow studied by a clearance technic. J Clin Invest *45*:1, 1966.
9. Leung FW et al.: Regional gastric mucosal blood flow measurements by hydrogen gas clearance in the anesthetized rat and rabbit. Gastroenterology *87*:28, 1984.
10. Delaney JP, Grim E: Canine gastric blood flow and its distribution. Am J Physiol *207*:1195, 1964.
11. Greenway CV, Murthy VS: Effects of vasopressin and isoprenaline infusions on the distribution of blood flow in the intestine; criteria for the validity of microsphere studies. Br J Pharmacol *46*:177, 1972.
12. Shepherd AP Jr, Maxwell LD, Jacobson ED: Limitation in the use of the microsphere method for the measurement of intramural distribution of intestinal blood flow. *In* Granger DN, Bulkley GB (eds): The Measure-

ment of Splanchnic Blood Flow. Baltimore, Williams and Wilkins, 1981.

13. Murakami M, Moriga M, Miyaki T, Uchino H: Contact electrode method in hydrogen gas clearance technique: A new method for determination of regional gastric mucosal blood flow in animals and humans. Gastroenterology *82*:457, 1982.

14. Kiel JW, Riedel GL, DiResta GR, Shepherd AP: Gastric mucosal blood flow measured by laser-Doppler velocimetry. Am J Physiol *249*:G539, 1985.

15. Jacobson ED: Effects of histamine, acetylcholine and norepinephrine on gastric vascular resistance. Am J Physiol *204*:1013, 1963.

16. Jacobson ED: Hemodynamic effects of bradykinin and gastrin in the stomach. Am Heart J *68*:214, 1964.

17. Main IHM, Whittle BJR: Investigation of the vasodilator and antisecretory role of prostaglandins in the rat gastric mucosa by use of non-steroidal anti-inflammatory drugs. Br J Pharmacol *53*:217, 1975.

18. Kauffman GL Jr, Aures D, Grossman MI: Indomethacin decreases basal gastric mucosal blood flow. Gastroenterology *76*:1165, 1979.

19. Whittle BJR, Oren-Wolman N, Guth PH: Gastric vasoconstrictor actions of leukotriene C_4, prostaglandin F_2 and a thromboxane mimetic (U-46619) on the rat submucosal microcirculation *in vivo*. Am J Physiol *248*:G580, 1985.

20. Bond JH, Prentiss RA, Levitt MD: The effects of feeding on blood flow to the stomach, small bowel, and colon of the conscious dog. J Lab Clin Med *93*:594, 1979.

21. Jacobson ED, Scott JB, Frohlich ED: Hemodynamics of the stomach: I. Resistance-flow relationship in the gastric vascular bed. Am J Dig Dis *7*:779, 1962.

22. Key JA: Blood vessels of a gastric ulcer. Br Med J *2*:1464, 1950.

23. Davenport HW: Fluid produced by the gastric mucosa during damage by acetic and salicylic acids. Gastroenterology *50*:487, 1966.

24. Johnson LR: Histamine liberation by gastric mucosa of pylorus-ligated rats damaged by acetic or salicylic acids. Proc Soc Exp Biol Med *121*:384, 1966.

25. Robert A, Nezamis JE, Lancaster C, Hanchar AJ: Cytoprotection by prostaglandins in rats. Prevention of gastric necrosis produced by alcohol, HCl, NaOH, hypertonic NaCl and thermal injury. Gastroenterology *77*:433, 1979.

26. Robert A et al.: Cytoprotection by prostaglandins occurs in spite of penetration of absolute ethanol into the gastric mucosa. Gastroenterology *88*:328, 1985.

27. Wallace JL, Morris GP, Krause EJ, Greaves SE: Reduction of ethanol-induced gastric mucosal damage by cytoprotective agents: A morphological and physiological study. Can J Physiol Pharmacol *60*:1686, 1982.

28. Rosam A-C, Wallace JL, Whittle BJR: Potent ulcerogenic actions of platelet-activating factor on the stomach. Nature *319*:54, 1986.

29. Pihan G et al.: Early microcirculatory stasis in acute gastric mucosal injury in the rat and prevention by 16,16-dimethylprostaglandin E_2 or sodium thiosulfate. Gastroenterology *91*:1415, 1986.

30. Menguy R, Masters YF: Gastric mucosal energy metabolism and "stress ulceration." Ann Surg *180*:538, 1974.

31. Itoh M, Guth PH: Role of oxygen-derived free radicals in hemorrhagic shock-induced gastric lesions in the rat. Gastroenterology *88*:1162, 1985.

32. Moody FG et al.: The cytoprotective effect of mucosal blood flow in experimental erosive gastritis. Acta Physiol Scand (Special Suppl) 1977, p. 35.

33. Burton-Opitz R: Über die Strömung des Blutes in dem Gebiete der Pfortader. Pflüger's Arch ges Physiol *124*:469, 1908.

34. Grim E, Lindseth EO: Distribution of blood flow to the tissues of the small intestine of the dog. Univ Minn Med Bull *30*:138, 1958.

35. Shehadeh Z, Price WE, Jacobson ED: Effects of vasoactive agents on intestinal blood flow and motility in the dog. Am J Physiol *216*:386, 1969.

36. Shepherd AP, Riedel GL: Continuous measurement of intestinal mucosal blood flow by laser-Doppler flowmetry. Am J Physiol *242*:G668, 1982.

37. Feld AD, Fondacaro JD, Holloway GA Jr, Jacobson ED: Measurement of mucosal blood flow in the canine intestine with laser Doppler velocimetry. Life Sci *31*:1509, 1982.

38. Brodie TG, Vogt H: The gaseous metabolism of the small intestine. Part 1. The gaseous exchange during the absorption of water and dilute salt solutions. J Physol (London) *40*:135, 1910.

39. Vatner SF, Franklin D, Van Citters RL: Mesenteric vasoactivity associated with eating and digestion in the conscious dog. Am J Physiol *219*:170, 1970.

40. Vatner SF, Patrick TA, Higgins CB, Frank D: Regional circulatory adjustments to eating and digestion in conscious unrestrained primates. J Appl Physiol *36*:524, 1974.

41. Gallavan RH Jr, Chou CC, Kvietys PR, Sit SP: Regional blood flow during digestion in the conscious dog. Am J Physiol *238*:H220, 1980.

42. Chou CC, et al.: Localization of mesenteric hyperemia during digestion in dogs. Am J Physiol *230*:583, 1976.

43. Chou CC, Kvietys PR, Post J, Sit SP: Constituents of chyme responsible for postprandial intestinal hyperemia. Am J Physiol *235*:H677, 1978.

44. Kvietys PR, Gallavan RH Jr, Chou CC: Contribution of bile to postprandial intestinal hyperemia. Am J Physiol *238*:G284, 1980.

45. Chou CC, Siregar H: Role of histamine H_1- and H_2-receptors in postprandial intestinal hyperemia. Am J Physiol *243*:G248, 1982.

46. Gallavan RH Jr, Chou CC: Prostaglandin synthesis inhibition and the postprandial intestinal hyperemia. Am J Physiol *242*:G140, 1982.

47. Lawson H, Chumley J: The effect of distension on blood flow through the intestine. Am J Physiol *131*:368, 1940.

48. Sidky M, Bean JW: Influence of rhythmic and tonic contraction of intestinal muscle on blood flow and blood reservoir capacity in dog intestine. Am J Physiol *193*:386, 1958.

49. Chou CC, Grassmick B: Motility and blood flow distribution within the wall of the gastrointestinal tract. Am J Physiol *235*:H34, 1978.

50. Barcroft J: The gaseous metabolism of the submaxillary gland. Part III. The effect of chorda activity on the respiration of the gland. J Physiol (London) *27*:31, 1901–02.

51. Granger HJ, Norris CP: Role of adenosine in local control of intestinal circulation in the dog. Circ Res *46*:764, 1980.

52. Walus KM, Fondacaro JD, Jacobson ED: Effects of adenosine and its derivatives on the canine intestinal vasculature. Gastroenterology *81*:327, 1981.

53. Mailman D et al.: Relationship of cyclic nucleotide uptake and metabolism to vasodilation in the canine mesenteric artery. Am J Physiol *232*:H191, 1977.

54. Johnson PC: Autoregulation of intestinal blood flow. Am J Physiol *199*:311, 1960.

55. Johnson PC: Myogenic nature of increase in intestinal vascular resistance with venous pressure elevation. Circ Res *6*:992, 1959.

56. Johnson PC, Hanson KM: Capillary filtration in the small intestine of the dog. Circ Res *19*:766, 1966.

57. Folkow B et al.: The effect of graded vasoconstrictor fibre stimulation on the intestinal resistance and capacitance vessels. Acta Physiol Scand *61*:445, 1964.

58. Folkow B et al.: The effect of the sympathetic vasoconstrictor fibre on the distribution of capillary blood flow in the intestine. Acta Physiol Scand *61*:458, 1964.

59. Selkurt EE, Rothe CF, Richardson D: Characteristics of reactive hyperemia in the canine intestine. Circ Res *15*:532, 1964.

60. Selkurt EE, Johnson PC: Effect of acute elevation of portal venous pressure on mesenteric blood volume, interstitial fluid volume and hemodynamics. Circ Res *6*:592, 1958.

61. Lundgren O: Studies on blood flow distribution and countercurrent exchange in the small intestine. Acta Physiol Scand Suppl *303*:1, 1967.

62. Haljamae H, Jodal M, Lundgren O: Countercurrent multiplication of sodium in intestinal villi during absorption of sodium chloride. Acta Physiol Scand *89*:580, 1973.

63. Shepherd AP, Granger HJ: Autoregulatory escape in the gut: A systems analysis. Gastroenterology *65*:77, 1973.

64. Shepherd AP: Intestinal O_2 consumption and Rb extraction during arterial hypoxia. Am J Physiol *234*:E248, 1978.

65. Shepherd AP: Intestinal capillary blood flow during metabolic hyperemia. Am J Physiol *237*:E548, 1979.

66. Koniges HG, Otto M: Studies on the filtration mechanism of the intestinal lymph and on the action of acetylcholine on it and on the circulation of the intestinal villi. Quart J Exp Biol *26*:319, 1937.

67. Mayerson HS, Wolfrom CE, Shirley HH, Wasserman K: Regional difference in capillary permeability. Am J Physiol *198*:155, 1960.

68. Casley-Smith JR, O'Donoghue PJ, Crocker KWJ: Quantitative relationships between fenestrae in jejunal capillaries and tissue channels: Proof of "tunnel capillaries." Microvasc Res *9*:78, 1975.

69. Bohlen HG: Intestinal tissue PO_2 and microvascular responses during glucose exposure. Am J Physiol *238*:H164, 1980.

70. Gore RW, Bohlen HG: Microvascular pressure in rat intestinal muscle and mucosal villi. Am J Physiol *233*:H685, 1977.

71. Mortillaro NA, Taylor AE: Interaction of capillary and tissue forces in the cat small intestine. Circ Res *39*:348, 1976.

72. Wilson R, Qualheim RE: A form of acute hemorrhage enterocolitis afflicting chronically ill individuals. Gastroenterology *27*:431, 1954.

73. Harrison LA et al.: Effects of ouabain on the splanchnic circulation. J Pharm Exp Therap *169*:321, 1969.

74. Fine J: The bacterial factor in traumatic shock. N Engl J Med *260*:214, 1959.

75. Jacobson ED, Mehlman B, Kalas JP: Vasoactive mediators as the "trigger mechanism" of endotoxin shock. J Clin Invest *43*:1000, 1964.

76. Lillehei RC: The intestinal factor in irrever-

sible hemorrhagic shock. Surgery *42*:1043, 1957.

77. Haglund U et al.: The intestinal mucosal lesions in shock. II. The relationship between the mucosal lesions and the cadiovascular derangement following regional shock. Eur Surg Res 8:448, 1976.

78. Haglund U, Lundgren O: Cardiovascular effects of blood borne material released from the cat small intestine during simulated shock conditions. Acta Physiol Scand *89*: 558, 1973.

79. Chiu CJ et al.: Intestinal mucosal lesions in low flow states. Arch Surg *10*:478, 1970.

80. Granger DM, Rutili G, McCord JM: Superoxide radicals in feline intestinal ischemia. Gastroenterology *81*:22, 1981.

81. Parks DA et al.: Ischemic injury in the cat small intestine: Role of superoxide radicals. Gastroenterology *82*:9, 1982.

82. Greenway CV, Stark RD, Lautt WW: Capacitance responses and fluid exchange in the cat liver during stimulation of the hepatic nerves. Circ Res 25:277, 1969.

83. Greenway CV, Lister GE: Capacitance effects and blood reservoir function in the splanchnic vascular bed during non-hypotensive haemorrhage and blood volume expansion in anaesthetized cats. J Physiol (London) *237*:279, 1974.

84. Burton-Opitz R: The influence of the portal blood flow upon flow in the hepatic artery. Quart J Exp Physiol *4*:93, 1911.

85. Lautt WW, Legare DJ: The use of 8-phenyltheophylline as a competitive antagonist of adenosine and inhibitor of the intrinsic regulatory mechanism of the hepatic artery. Can J Physiol Pharmacol *63*:717, 1985.

86. Lautt WW, Legare DJ, D'Almeida MS: Adenosine as putative regulator of hepatic arterial flow (the buffer response). Am J Physiol *248*:H331, 1985.

87. Lautt WW, Legare DJ, Daniels TR: The comparative effect of administration of substances via the hepatic artery or portal vein on hepatic arterial resistance, liver blood volume, and hepatic extraction in cats. Hepatology *4*:927, 1984.

88. Hansen KM, Johnson PC: Local control of hepatic arterial and portal venous flow in the dog. Am J Physiol *211*:712, 1966.

89. Greenway CV, Lawson AE, Mellander S: The effects of stimulation of the hepatic nerves, infusions of noradrenaline and occlusion of the carotid arteries on liver blood flow in the anaesthetized cat. J Physiol (London) *192*:21, 1967.

90. Greenway CV, Lawson AE, Stark RD: The effect of haemorrhage on hepatic artery and portal vein flows in the anaesthetized cat. J Physiol (London) *193*:375, 1967.

91. Fasth S, Hulten L, Nordgren S: Adjustments of hepatic and small intestine blood flow on selective vasoconstrictor fibre stimulation. Acta Physiol Scand *110*:343, 1980.

92. Rappaport AM: The microcirculatory hepatic unit. Microvasc Res 6:212, 1973.

93. Selkurt EE, Johnson PC: Effect of acute elevation of portal venous pressure on mesenteric blood volume, interstitial fluid volume and hemodynamics. Circ Res 6:592, 1958.

94. Vorobioff J, Bredfeldt JE, Groszmann RJ: Hyperdynamic splanchnic circulation in a portal hypertensive rat model. A primary factor for the maintenance of chronic portal hypertension. Am J Physiol *244*:G52, 1983.

95. Bass L: Models of hepatic drug elimination. J Pharm Sci *72*:1229, 1983.

96. Caesar J et al.: The use of indocyanine green in the measurement of hepatic blood flow and as a test of hepatic function. Clin Sci *21*: 43, 1961.

97. Bradley SE, Ingelfinger FJ, Bradley GP: Hepatic circulation in cirrhosis of the liver. Circulation *5*:419, 1952.

98. Price HL et al.: Hemodynamic and metabolic effects of hemorrhage in man, with particular reference to the splanchnic circulation. Circ Res *18*:469, 1966.

99. Groszmann RJ et al.: Wedged and free hepatic venous pressure measured with a balloon catheter. Gastroenterology *76*:253, 1979.

BIBLIOGRAPHY

Granger DN, Shepherd AP: The intestinal circulation: A historical perspective. *In* Shepherd AP, Granger DN (eds): Physiology of the Intestinal Circulation. New York, Raven Press, 1984.

Greenway CV, Lautt WW: Hepatic circulation. *In* Schultz S, Woods J (eds): Handbook of Physiology, The Gastrointestinal System, Section 6, Volume 1, Chapter 41. Bethesda, The American Physiological Society, 1989.

Guth PH, Leung FW: Physiology of the gastric circulation. *In* Johnson LR (ed): Physiology of the Gastrointestinal Tract. 2nd Ed. New York, Raven Press, 1987.

Jacobson ED: The circulation of the stomach. Gastroenterology 48:85, 1965.

Jacobson ED (ed): Recent advances in the gastrointestinal circulation and related areas. Gastroenterology 52 (part 2):332, 1967.

Tepperman BL, Jacobson ED: Mesenteric circulation. *In* Johnson LR (ed): Physiology of the Gastrointestinal Tract. New York, Raven Press, 1981.

29

Observations on Gastrointestinal Neoplasia

SIDNEY J. WINAWER

THE BEGINNING OF THE MODERN ERA

Until the 19th century, cancer was considered primarily in terms of its gross pathology, and fundamental differences among various types of cancers were not recognized. In 1836, Johannes Müller, Professor of Anatomy, Physiology, and Pathology at the University of Berlin, undertook a microscopic study of his large collection of tumor specimens to ascertain whether:

"There are any important internal differences in their organization and chemical composition and, if they do exist exactly to determine their nature."

In his investigations, Müller discovered that cancer was composed of cells and demonstrated the "harmony" between pathological and embryonic tumor development (1). In 1847, Rudolf Virchow, also from Berlin, stated his then revolutionary thesis that new cells were formed by the division of the old: "omnis cellula a cellula."

The concept of proliferation of cancer cells as espoused by Virchow kindled new thought in medical research (2). This was heretical thought, not foreign to Virchow, a perennial rebel against established doctrine in medicine, politics, or public health. Since those early times, considerable progress in cell biology has been accomplished, and it is now recognized that neoplastic diseases represent the uncontrolled growth of abnormal cells with the potential to spread from the anatomic site of origin to distant areas, invading vital organs and ultimately resulting in death. Today, it also is known that many cancers can be cured if they are detected early and treated promptly; and other cancers can be controlled for long periods with a variety of therapeutic modalities.

PATHOGENESIS OF CANCER

The mechanisms involved in the regulation of cellular growth have been clarified at least partially in recent years. Various proteins involved in the complex metabolic pathways regulating the proliferation and differentiation of cells, such as those that bind to DNA and participate in regulating DNA replication, now have been identified. Many of these proteins have been isolated and their biological activity defined. Among the growth factors, the hematopoietic colony stimulating factors (CSF) are of particular interest in ameliorating the toxic effects of drugs in protecting against suppression of the bone marrow during the chemotherapy of neoplastic disease.

Gastrointestinal cancers do not develop in normal tissue but evolve after a period of hyperproliferation of normal-appearing cells that have not undergone differentiation. M. Lipkin's pioneering experiments demonstrated in animals and humans that increased cell proliferation was the first step in the flat mucosa of the gastrointestinal tract, preceding the development of a cancer (3). This abnormality in cell proliferation has been utilized in tissue biopsy studies to identify patients at increased risk of developing cancer and to initiate possible preventive measures. A prime example is the study

467

of colonic biopsies for evidence of dysplasia in the cancer-preventing colonoscopic surveillance of patients with ulcerative colitis. Obviously, the control of pre-neoplastic abnormal cell growth is critical to the prevention and the successful treatment of cancer.

The term cancer actually is a misnomer and in reality is more properly termed carcinogenesis to signify an evolving cellular reaction, as indicated by Sporn (4). The process is a dynamic rather than a static one, involving biologic and molecular changes in cells. Classical terminology, which originated more than a century ago, tends to ignore the importance of the critical dimension of time in the development of epithelial carcinogenesis.

ENVIRONMENTAL FACTORS AND CANCER REVERSIBILITY

External (environmental) factors responsible for the development and progression of neoplasia of the gastrointestinal tract have been studied extensively. This approach to the etiology of cancer apparently was first implicated by Sir Percivall Pott, who in 1775, in a study of chimney sweepers in London with scrotal cancer, observed that: "The disease in these people seems to derive its origin from a lodgment of soot in the rugae of the scrotum." This observation has been hailed as the beginning of interest in environmental causes of cancer (5). Since then, many studies have emphasized and expanded this relationship. The modern era of epidemiologic cancer research probably followed demonstration of the link between smoking and lung cancer by Lombard in his 1928 report on cancer in Massachusetts (6). The geographically related differences in cancer risk are of particular interest in relation to environmental carcinogens. For example, the risk of colorectal cancer is higher in the United States than in Japan; and equally intriguing, the risk of gastric cancer is much higher in Japan than in the United States. The factors involved are yet to be fully revealed. The changing cancer risk in subsequent generations of migrant populations, as among the Japanese migrating to Hawaii (7), further emphasizes the critical role of external environmental factors in the causation of cancer. The most recently im-

plicated environmental agent is the unique spiral organism found in the stomach, Helicobacter pylori. This organism actually was described more than a century ago, but its potential importance was not recognized until B. Marshall's pioneering studies in the 1980s. While current information is suggestive, long-term epidemiological, case control, and intervention studies will be required to clarify this important question (8). This organism can be eradicated with appropriate double antibiotic and bismuth medications, presumably eliminating this cancer risk.

Additional environmental (external) agents related to carcinogenesis include certain dietary risk factors for colorectal cancer, such as fat, noted by Reddy et al. (9); and the intestinal bacterial flora and bile acids emphasized by Hill (10). Certain "protective factors" include dietary fiber, emphasized by Burkitt (11), and calcium, reported by Garland (12). Other predisposing relationships include hepatitis B and C viruses to hepatocellular carcinoma; and of smoking, alcohol, and acid reflux to the development of the cancer-prone Barrett's esophagus. This type of information, together with endoscopic visualization and biopsy and cell proliferation markers (e.g., proliferating cell nuclear antigen expression), now permit the assessment of cancer risk within days or a few weeks, contrasting with the years of observation required in earlier times. We also appreciate that a latency period, as long as 20 years or more, may antedate the initiation of carcinogenesis and its subsequent progression. Studies of colon cancer within the framework of the National Polyp Study have demonstrated a period of approximately 10 years from normal mucosa to colon cancer, encompassing approximately 5 years from adenoma to cancer in general and 7 or 8 years from small adenoma to cancer, findings (13) in agreement with prior observations from St. Mark's Hospital, London, by Morson and colleagues (14). This time span is important from a practical viewpoint since it provides "windows of opportunity" for the earlier diagnosis and removal of precancerous lesions such as colonic adenomas and gastrointestinal lesions associated with severe dysplasia.

GENETICS

The concept of genetics in the pathogenesis of cancer can be presumptively traced back to ancient times, when physicians were intrigued by the familial clustering of breast cancer. Modern interest in the relationship between genetics and cancer is credited to Aldred S. Warthin (15). In 1895, he noticed that his seamstress was very depressed and questioned her about her grief. She told him: "All of my relatives have cancer and will die and I will die too." She died 4 years later of endometrial cancer. Her family, meticulously studied and documented by Warthin, is known as "Warthin's Family G." Such perceptive observations have generated an extensive literature linking genetics and cancer and have made possible interesting descriptions of specific inherited syndromes. The St. Mark's group clarified familial adenomatous polyposis (16), and other syndromes of an inherited nature were described by Gardner (17), Lynch (18), and Jeghers (19). More recently, studies of the inherited susceptibility to gastrointestinal cancer have focused on colorectal carcinoma. The important studies of Vogelstein, White, and Bodmer, among others, have identified several genes important in this process. It now has been demonstrated that, as the neoplastic process evolves from normal mucosa to cancer of the colon, there is an accumulation of abnormalities in genes located on chromosomes 2, 5, 13, 17, and 18 (20–23).

The first cytogenetic observation that called attention to a chromosome 5 deletion as the putative genetic area linked to familial adenomatous polyposis (FAP) was made by Herrera (22) in a patient with FAP and mental retardation. Bodmer (20) and others then focused on this area in the long arm of chromosome 5 and eventually described the APC gene. This now is being tested as a clinical genetic screening tool in FAP. Vogelstein subsequently described abnormalities in chromosome 5, 17, and 18 and later in chromosome 2, and proposed a model of colon tumorigenesis that included all of these changes in association with the adenoma-carcinoma progression (23). A series of elegant pathologic studies from St. Mark's Hospital demonstrated, in the colon especially, that carcinogenesis evolves from the hyperproliferation state through a series of progressively advancing premalignant neoplastic stages, the adenomatous polyp, and then cancer (14). This sequence has been confirmed in the large multicenter National Polyp Study reported by O'Brien, Winawer, and colleagues (24). Obviously, the surveillance of genetically susceptible high-risk individuals sharpens the focus of cancer prevention and increases the likelihood of earlier detection of premalignant conditions. Advances in the understanding of the mechanisms controlling gene expression have been facilitated by transgenic technology, a procedure involving the insertion of specific genes into fertilized mouse eggs and then identifying the expression and function of the genes in the developed organisms. Carcinogenesis thus may be considered as a dysregulation of gene function, leading first to clonal expansion and clonal heterogeneity of selected cells, proceeding to local tissue invasion, and finally to metastases.

In considering the pathogenesis of gastrointestinal neoplasia, the important area of neuroendocrine tumors also requires mention. These tumors, embryological neural crest cells, have a very different pathogenetic mechanism from the other gastrointestinal tract neoplasms. The first report of a systemic syndrome associated with such tumors was by Thorson (25) and colleagues, who characterized the carcinoid syndrome. Since then, considerable knowledge has been obtained about a wide variety of neuroendocrine tumors and their secretions and pharmacological treatment. The most significant recent advances include not only laboratory assays of secretory products, but also more effective pharmacological and chemotherapeutic agents to control these hormonally active tumors. Although such tumors are rare, they are important clinical and research challenges (26).

PREVENTION

The importance of preventive approaches in medicine has been recognized for more than a century. Thomas Huxley, in his 1876 address at Johns Hopkins University, stated (27): "The objective of medical education is to train physicians to prevent diseases and, where disease is already established, to alleviate or to cure it."

The concept of earlier identification and removal of precancerous states has received increasing emphasis in recent years with the development of new diagnostic resources, especially fiberoptic endoscopy (28). This procedure not only allows direct visualization of much of the gastrointestinal tract but also facilitates biopsy sampling for histologic, genetic, and other studies. Gastrointestinal endoscopy is discussed in detail in Chapter 30. Preventive surveillance based on the examination of asymptomatic patients at increased risk of gastric cancer has been pioneered especially in Japan, where early endoscopy and high-quality double-contrast x-ray studies have improved cancer diagnosis and earlier staging has made possible curative surgery (29). This approach also has been extended to hepatocellular carcinoma complicating cirrhosis of the liver and viral hepatitis (hepatitis C). The clearest demonstration of successful cancer prevention has been in the endoscopic and biopsy surveillance of patients with inflammatory bowel disease, adenomatous polyps of the colon and rectum, and in individuals with prior colon cancer, and/or a familial history of cancer. The ability to safely remove polyps at endoscopy has been a major advance in the prevention of colonic cancer, as initially documented by Shinya and Wolf (30) and later by the National Polyp Study. Mathematical models also have projected a significant mortality reduction (80%), resulting from colonoscopic screening of first degree relatives of probands with colorectal cancer (31). Today, approximately 10% of the population has a first-degree relative with colorectal cancer, and it now is generally accepted that a large proportion of individuals developing colorectal cancer probably have a familial susceptibility. Indeed, the studies of Burt, Skolnick, and Bishop suggest that so-called "sporadic" colorectal cancer occurs largely through inheritance of the adenomatous polyp, most likely in an autosomal-dominant partially penetrant manner. In the future, more individuals with a familial predisposition probably will be identified through genetic testing. This resource now is available only for FAP families with the APC gene (32,33).

Screening procedures for gastrointestinal malignancy, of course, have long included testing the stools for occult blood, beginning initially with the screening of patients with pernicious anemia at increased risk of gastric carcinoma, and later in patients suspected of having colorectal neoplasia. However, the value of the stool blood test was recognized generally only after David Greegor of Ohio demonstrated the earlier detection of colorectal cancers in asymptomatic individuals utilizing this procedure (34). The stool blood test again has been undergoing rigorous evaluation within the framework of clinical trials, and its efficacy based on reduction of mortality recently has been determined (35,36). It is now generally accepted that annual fecal blood testing involving six guaiac impregnated paper studies with two smears from each of three consecutive stools reduces colorectal cancer mortality. Chu et al. have demonstrated an earlier-stage neoplasm in patients coming to surgery after undergoing stool blood testing, although this change in cancer staging does not completely account for the decreasing mortality (37).

DIAGNOSIS AND STAGING

The diagnosis of gastrointestinal cancer is critical to its management and originally was made possible by Röntgen's discovery of the x-ray in 1895 (38). The development of radiology is authoritatively discussed in Chapter 31. Imaging has advanced tremendously since the early 20th century and today most of the gastrointestinal tract can be visualized far more accurately than in the past. New developments have included CT scanning, MRI, and improved double-contrast and barium enemas. The recently developed endoscopic ultrasound extends the diagnostic capacity of endoscopy in allowing the endoscopist to "see" beyond the visible inner surface of the bowel and helps determine transmural invasion, involvement of adjacent lymph nodes, and the presence of small tumors in adjacent organs, such as the pancreas not detectable by external imaging.

SURGERY

Surgery for gastrointestinal cancer was initiated by Theodor Billroth, who in 1881 removed an advanced cancer from the stomach of a patient named Theresa Heller, performing what is now known as a gastric resection with a Billroth I anastomosis. The patient lived for 4 ½ months. It is not clear whether the patient's survival was a result of her biology, Billroth's surgical skill, or the postoperative care, which included "frequent administration of enemas containing peptones, sour milk and wine." Billroth was dismayed by the high operative mortality among his next 37 resections, which were done with a Billroth II anastomosis, but he persisted and provided a systematic recording of successes and failures (39). Important clinical correlations with the stage of cancer were made possible later when Cuthbert Dukes developed the model of modern staging of cancer based on his studies of rectal cancer (40). The principles of oncologic surgery now are well established and new techniques seek to localize tumors more precisely and develop curative operations that also are aesthetically acceptable to the patient.

CHEMOTHERAPY

On a dark winter night at 7:30 pm on December 3, 1943 during World War II, the Allied air raid warning system failed and vast cargoes of fuel explosives were hit by enemy bombers in the harbor of Bari on the southern part of the Italian peninsula. One of the ships, the Liberty, contained not only tons of explosives but also 100 tons of mustard gas in airplane bombs. The poison gas produced many casualties. As a result of this disaster, a chemical agent with anticancer action was serendipitously discovered. Cornelius P. Rhoads of New York played a major role in the investigation and the promotion of nitrogen mustard as an antitumor agent. He subsequently advocated the use of these agents for the treatment of cancer. Thus was born the age of cancer chemotherapy (41).

Chemotherapy of advanced gastrointestinal cancer has been limited by the toxicity to normal cells and the resistance of cancer cells to treatment. Growth factors may be able to counteract some of this toxicity on the hematopoietic system and insight into the mechanisms of tumor resistance should provide more effective agents. The best chance for improving survival with chemotherapy in gastrointestinal cancers today is in the adjuvant setting in patients with Dukes C colon cancer and in an adjuvant setting in combination with radiation therapy in patients with Dukes B_2 and C rectal cancer. Surgical results for both cure and palliation can be enhanced thereby when combined with other treatment modalities such as chemotherapy, radiation therapy, and biological response modifiers. The concept of adjuvant chemotherapy received important support in the studies by Moertel and colleagues demonstrating improved survival in individuals after surgical removal of identifiable tumor following adjuvant chemotherapy (42). The improved survival of patients with rectal cancer also has been demonstrated with the adjuvant combination of chemotherapy and radiation (43). A further major advance in terminology was made with introduction of the TNM staging system throughout the GI tract. This system eventually will replace the various confusing modifications of the Dukes system (43).

Newer approaches to treatment are focusing on biological response modifiers, substances that stimulate or modulate the host cellular and/or humoral responses that may play a role in killing cancer cells. Examples include the interferons, interleukins, and tumor necrosis factors. The genes for many of these factors have been cloned and the application of recombinant DNA techniques has made these substances available in sufficient quantities to permit evaluation of their clinical usefulness. Another basis for treatment is related to the concept that tumor cells may retain their capability to differentiate. Differentiation of many tumor cells can be induced by a variety of structurally diverse agents, including polar compounds, hormones, vitamin derivatives, low doses of certain toxic drugs, physiologically active growth factors, and tumor promoters. Hexamethylene bisacetamide, for example, has been shown in primary tissue culture to terminally differentiate colon cancer cells, which then lose their malignant epitopes. Several polar cytodifferentiation agents are in Phase I and II experimental studies. There also is great interest in the development as therapeutic agents of monoclonal antibodies targeted to the oncogenes among the 50,000 genes in the genome that are responsible for abnormal proliferation and differentiation of cancer cells.

THE FUTURE

As we conclude the final decade of the 20th century and look ahead to the next century, exciting progress can be anticipated in the fundamental understanding of neoplasia, particularly in such areas as cellular and molecular biology, genetic vulnerability and genetic resistance, and the molecular basis of cancer therapy. While we cannot yet see the light at the end of the tunnel, the road ahead probably is no more difficult for us than it was for Pott, Virchow, Billroth, Muller, Warthin, Rhoads, and other "giants" of generations past. A major difference today, considering the remarkable scientific advances during the past half century, is the realistic expectation of the eventual control and cure of gastrointestinal neoplasia. Einstein may be correct: "The mere formulation of a problem is often far more essential than its solution which may be merely a matter of mathematical or experimental skill."

REFERENCES

1. Muller J: On the nature and structural characteristics of cancer and of those morbid growths which may be confounded with it. London, Sherwood, Gilbert and Piper, 1840. As cited in Holleb AI, Randers-Pehrson MB (eds): Classics in Oncology. New York, American Cancer Society, 1987.
2. Virchow R: Cellular pathology: As based upon physiological and pathological history. Philadelphia, JB Lippincott, 1863. As cited in Holleb AI, Randers-Pehrson MB (eds): Classics in Oncology. New York, American Cancer Society, 1987.
3. Lipkin M: Phase 1 and phase 2 proliferative lesions of colonic epithelial cells in diseases leading to colon cancer. Cancer *34*:878, 1974.
4. Sporn MB: Carcinogenesis and cancer: Different perspectives on the same disease. Cancer Research *51*:6215, 1991.
5. Potts P: Chirurgical Observations Relative to the Cataract, the Polypus of the Nose, the Cancer of the Scrotum, the Different Kinds of Ruptures and the Mortification of the Toes and Feet. London, Hawes L, Clarke W, and Collins R, 1775. As cited in Holleb AI, Randers-Pehrson MB (eds): Classics in Oncology. New York, American Cancer Society, 1987.
6. Lombard HL, Doering CR: Cancer studies in Massachusetts: 2. Habits, characteristics, and environment of individuals with and without cancer. N Engl J Med *198*:481, 1928.
7. Haenszel W, Kurihara M: Studies of Japanese migrants. I. Mortality from cancer and other diseases among Japanese in the United States. J Natl Cancer Inst *40*:43, 1968.
8. Marshall BJ, Warren JR: Unidentified curved bacilli in the stomach of patients with gastritis and peptic ulceration. Lancet *i*: 1311, 1984.
9. Reddy BS, Weisburger JH, Wynder EL: Effect of high risk and low risk diets for colon carcinogenesis of fecal microflora and steroid in man. J Nutr *105*:878, 1975.
10. Hill MJ: The effect of some factors on the fecal concentration of acid steroids, neutral steroids and mobilins. J Pathol *104*:239, 1971.
11. Burkitt DP: Some neglected leads to cancer causation. J Natl Cancer Inst *47*:913, 1971.
12. Garland C, et al.: Dietary vitamin D and calcium and risk of colorectal cancer: A 19 year prospective study in men. Lancet *i*:307, 1985.
13. Winawer SJ et al.: Randomized comparison of surveillance intervals after colonoscopic removal of newly diagnosed adenomatous polyps. N Engl J Med *328*:901, 1993.
14. Muto T, Bussey HJR, Morson BC: The evolution of cancer of the colon and rectum. Cancer *36*:2251, 1975.
15. Warthin AS: Heredity with reference to carcinoma as shown by the study of the cases examined in the pathological laboratory of the University of Michigan, 1895–1913. Arch Intern Med *12*:546, 1913. As cited in Holleb AI, Randers-Pehrson MB (eds): Classics in Oncology. New York, American Cancer Society, 1987.
16. Bussey HJR: Familial Polyposis Coli. Family Studies, Histopathology, Differential Diagnosis and Results of Treatment. Baltimore, The Johns Hopkins University Press, 1975.
17. Gardner EJ, Burt RW, Freston JW: Gastrointestinal polyposis: Syndromes and genetic mechanisms. West J Med *132*:488, 1980.
18. Lynch HT, et al.: Familial heterogeneity of colon cancer risk. Cancer *57*:2089, 1986.
19. Jeghers H, McKusick VA, Katz KH: Generalized intestinal polyposis and melanin spots of the oral mucosa, lips and digits: A syn-

drome of diagnostic significance. N Engl J Med *241*:993 and 1031, 1949.

20. Bodmer WF et al.: Localization of the gene for familial adenomatous polyposis on chromosome 5. Nature *328*:614, 1987.

21. Leppert M, Dobbs M, Scambler P: The gene for familial polyposis coli maps to the long arm of chromosome 5. Science *238*:1411, 1987.

22. Herrera L et al.: Brief clinical report. Gardner syndrome in a man with an interstitial deletion of 5q. Am J Med Genet *25*:473, 1986.

23. Vogelstein B et al.: Genetic alterations during colorectal tumor development. N Engl J Med *319*:525, 1988.

24. O'Brien MJ et al.: The National Polyp Study: Patient and polyp characteristics associated with high-grade dysplasia in colorectal adenomas. Gastroenterology *98*:371, 1990.

25. Thorson A, Bjork G, Bjorkman G, Waldenstrom J: Malignant carcinoid of the small intestine with metastases to the liver, valvular disease of the right side of the heart (pulmonary stenosis and tricuspid regurgitation without septal defects), peripheral vasomotor symptoms, bronchoconstriction and an unusual type of cyanosis; a clinical and pathological syndrome. Am Heart J *47*:795, 1954.

26. Brennan MF: Endocrine tumors of the gastrointestinal tract. In Winawer SJ (ed): Management of Gastrointestinal Diseases. (Vol 2) New York, Gower Medical Publishing, 1992, pp. 29.1–29.30.

27. Huxley T: American Addresses. New York, Appleton, 1877, pp. 99–127 and 110–112.

28. Hirschowitz BI, et al.: Demonstration of a new gastroscopy—the fiberscope. Gastroenterology *35*:50, 1958.

29. Murakami T: Studies on the histogenesis of early gastric cancer. Acta Pathol Jpn *2*:10, 1952.

30. Shinya H, Wolff WI: Removal of colonic polyps by fiberoptic colonoscopy. N Engl J Med *288*:329, 1973.

31. Eddy DM et al.: Screening for colorectal cancer in a high-risk population: Results of a mathematical model. Gastroenterology *92*: 682, 1987.

32. Cairns J: A survey of cancer sites by kinship in the Utah Mormon population. In Cairns J, Lyon JL, Skolnick M (eds): (Banbury Report #4). Cancer Incidence in Defined Populations. New York, Cold Spring Harbor Laboratory, 1980, pp. 299–318.

33. Cannon-Albright LA et al.: Common inheritance of susceptibility to colonic adenomatous polyps and associated colorectal cancers. N Engl J Med *319*:533, 1988.

34. Greegor DH: Diagnosis of large bowel cancer in the asymptomatic patient. JAMA *201*: 943, 1967.

35. Mandel JS et al.: Reducing mortality from colorectal cancer by screening for fecal occult blood. N Engl J Med *328*:1365, 1993.

36. Winawer SJ, Flehinger BJ, Schottenfeld D, Miller DG: Screening for colorectal cancer with fecal occult blood testing and sigmoidoscopy. JNCI *85*:(16): 1311, 1993.

37. Chu KC, Kramer BS, Smart CR: Analysis of the role of cancer prevention and control measures in reducing cancer mortality. JNCI *83*:(22):1636, 1991.

38. Rontgen WK: Uber eine neve Art von Strahlen. Sitzungsberichte der Wurzburger physik medic. Gesellschaft, 1895. Translated by Arthur Stanton for Nature, 1896. Reprinted from Science *NS3*:227, 1896. As cited in Holleb AI, Randers-Pehrson MB (eds): Classics in Oncology. New York, American Cancer Society, 1987.

39. Billroth T: Letter, Wiener medizinische Wochenschrift *31*:161, 1881. Translated by Dr. C Wertheimer and published in Hurwitz A, Degenshein GA (eds): Milestones in Modern Surgery. Courtesy of Hoeber-Harper, New York. As cited in Holleb AI, Randers-Pehrson MB (eds): Classics in Oncology. New York, American Cancer Society, 1987.

40. Dukes CE: The surgical pathology of rectal cancer. Permission from Journal of Clinical Pathology *2*:95, 1949. As cited in Holleb AI, Randers-Pehrson MB (eds): Classics in Oncology. New York, American Cancer Society, 1987.

41. Rhoads CP: The sword and the ploughshare. Permission from Journal of the Mount Sinai Hospital (now the Mount Sinai Journal of Medicine) *13*:299, 1947. As cited in Holleb AI, Randers-Pehrson MB (eds): Classics in Oncology. New York, American Cancer Society, 1987.

42. Moertel CG et al.: Levamisole and fluorouracil for adjuvant therapy of resected colon carcinoma. N Engl J Med *322*(6):352, 1990.

43. Winawer SJ, Enker WE, Levin B: Colorectal cancer. *In* Winawer SJ (ed): Management of Gastrointestinal Diseases. New York, Gower Medical Publishing, 1992, pp. 27.1–27.40.

30

Gastrointestinal Endoscopy

WILLIAM S. HAUBRICH

The remarkable evolutionary advance of gastrointestinal endoscopy over the past century is a testament to human ingenuity. It is also a prime example of achievement made possible by continuing cooperation between clinicians and experts in the various technical and bio-engineering fields. Although much of the modern impetus to endoscopy and its practical application originated in America, largely in the 20th century, the story begins in Europe (Fig. 30–1).

THE CONCEPT OF ENDOSCOPY

Endoscopy was conceived as, and remains, a means of visualizing the interior of accessible viscera for the purpose of diagnosis and facilitating appropriate therapy.

In this regard, it is instructive to note that the term "endoscopy" was contrived by combining the Greek prefix endo- (within) and the verb skopein (to view or observe). The lexical sum is an apt designation for the procedure of peering into the recesses of the living body. The Greek skopein means not merely to look at something but rather to view with a purpose, to observe with intent, to monitor.

The bodily orifices most amenable to inspection are, of course, the mouth, the nares, and the ears, and these were surely explored, insofar as possible, by primitive man. The esophagus, the trachea and bronchi, the urethra, the vagina, and the anus also were promising portals, but the problems in probing them were basically two: the design of a proper instrument that could

convey the desired image and provision of adequate illumination of dark recesses. Materials with which to construct any form of tube or catheter were limited, as was the means of fashioning them. In the early 19th century, various metallic alloys were available, but machines to manufacture small, thin tubes of high tensile strength were relatively crude. Rubber, as a plastic material, was known, but the process of vulcanization, whereby rubber is rendered strong and elastic, was not discovered until 1839. Plastics as we know them were nonexistent. Moreover, once an orifice was penetrated, how was visualization to be achieved? The only available sources of illumination were sunlight, direct or reflected, or the glow of a burning candle or the wick of an oil or gas lamp, none of which was readily adaptable or sufficiently intense. What was needed was an incandescent light. This was provided in 1879 by Thomas Alva Edison. A footnote to the history of endoscopy concerns the celebrated William Osler, who attended the 1879 meeting of the American Association for the Advancement of Science. He encountered Edison, who had just demonstrated his newly created incandescent bulb. Osler recalled their conversation, wherein Edison advanced his belief that now "it would be possible to illumine the interior of the body by passing a small electric burner into the stomach" (1).

The earliest recorded attempt at endoscopy beyond a bodily orifice was in the first decade of the 19th century by Phillip Bozzini (2), who devised a tin tube illuminated by a wax candle fitted with a mirror, which

Chronological Development GI Endoscopy

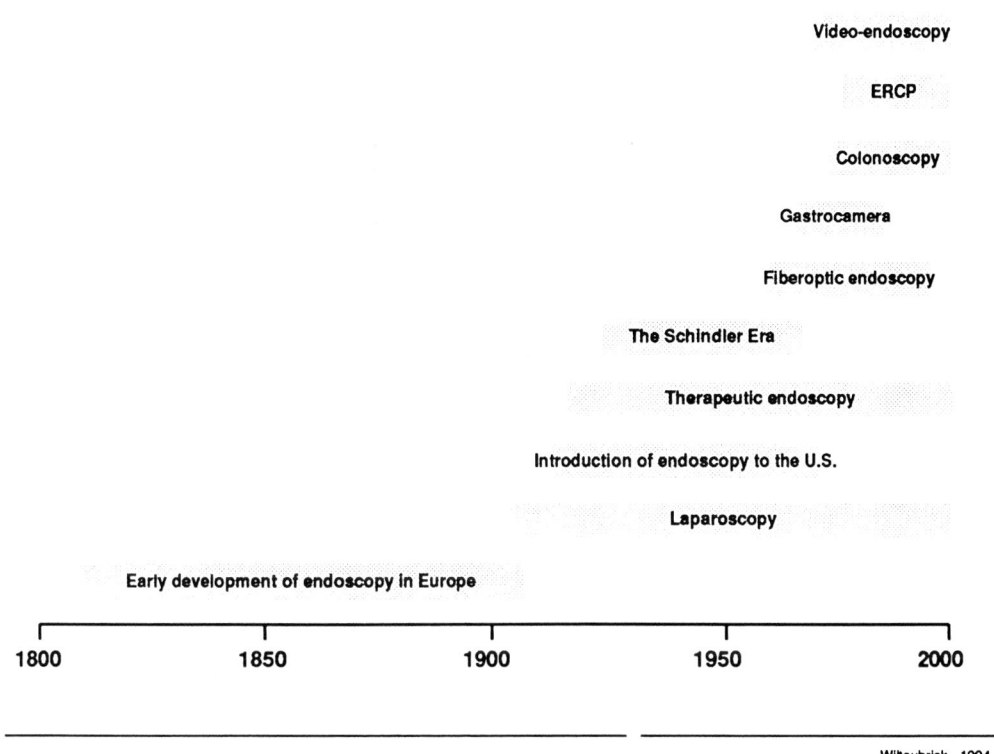

Fig. 30–1. Time chart depicting the advent of major advances in the evolution of gastrointestinal endoscopy.

he called a *Lichtleiter* (light conductor). He tried to peer into the urethra and urinary bladder. On hearing of this, the medical faculty at Vienna dismissed the device as "a magic lantern in the human body."

Much of the subsequent development of the endoscope, as applied to visualization of the urethra and urinary bladder and before the advent of gastroscopy, took place in France. In 1826, Pierre-Salomen Segalas introduced a "urethro-cystic speculum" (the term speculum implies use of a mirror), the first endoscope of any practical use in diagnosis (3). Not surprisingly, faulty illumination hampered the use of Segalas' primitive endoscope. Jean-Pierre Bonnafont in the late 1830s offered modifications that partially solved this problem, and his designs were incorporated in the endoscope devised by Antonin-Jean Desmoreaux in the 1850s (4,5). An excellent, more detailed

and illustrated account of these early devices is provided in Edmonson's monograph (6).

THE FIRST ATTEMPTS
AT GASTROSCOPY

Adolf Kussmaul, a German physician whose 80 years spanned most of the 19th century, is known to most students for his description of air hunger as a symptom of diabetic acidosis. Kussmaul also is credited with fashioning and using in 1868 what might be regarded as the first gastroscope (7). Oddly, in numerous publications related to the gastrointestinal tract, Kussmaul hardly mentioned his efforts to devise a gastroscope, the account having been given by others (8).

Kussmaul's instrument was a straight,

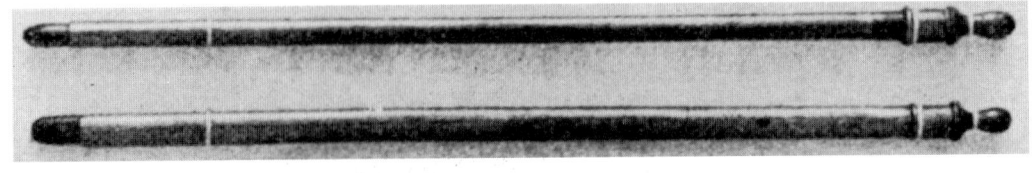

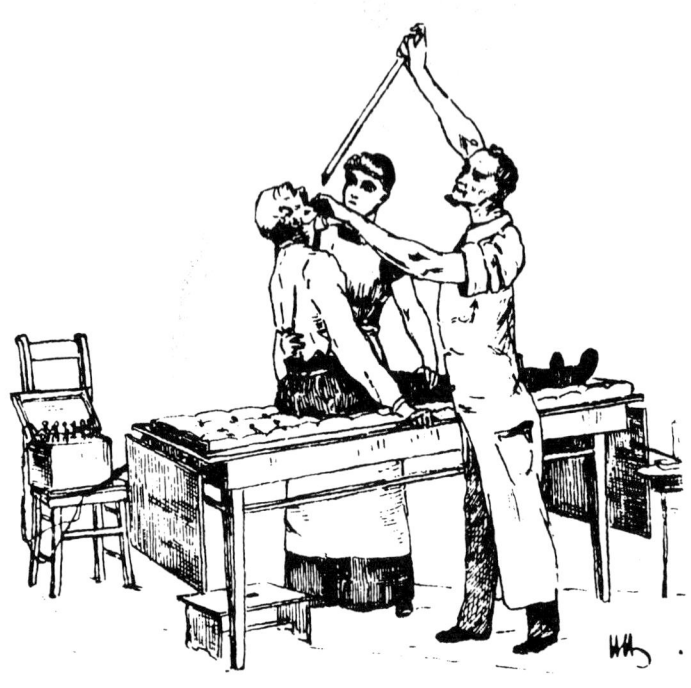

Fig. 30–2. *A,* Kussmaul's straight rigid gastroscope and obturator (1868). *B,* The brusque manner in which this crude instrument was inserted. Courtesy of Dr. James Edmondson, Historical Division, Cleveland Medical Library Association.

rigid metal tube intended to be passed over a previously inserted flexible obturator (Fig. 30–2). The light source was a Desmoreaux lamp that burned a mixture of alcohol and turpentine, illumination being concentrated by a reflector and lens. Kussmaul is said to have recruited his first subjects from the ranks of sword swallowers, commonly found at country fairs, whose unscathed performance required an ability to align the mouth, esophagus, and proximal stomach. Apparently, Kussmaul succeeded in getting his tube swallowed, but illumination was so feeble that no useful image was obtained. In the 1880s, Joseph Leiter, a Viennese instrument maker, impressed by Kussmaul's demonstration, collaborated with Johann von Mikulicz-Radecki, a surgeon widely known for a variety of innovative operations, in the design of an improved gastroscope (Fig. 30–3) (9). Originally, illumination was supplied by an exposed, electrically activated, glowing platinum wire, but this was soon replaced by a minia-

ture incandescent globe devised by Max Nitze and called, by an incongruous coupling of French and German, a "Mignon Lampchen."

A Cleveland surgeon, F. C. Herrick, in 1911 proposed intraoperative gastroscopy by inserting a modified cystoscope through a small incision in the exposed stomach wall. The aim was to locate possible sources of bleeding from the gastric mucosa (10). Meanwhile, early accounts of peroral esophagogastroscopy were coming from Chevalier Jackson (11) of Philadelphia and from Janeway and Greene (12) of New York.

The compulsion of early investigators to seek a means, however crude, of detecting diseases affecting the interior of the esophagus and stomach can be understood by recalling that their efforts preceded by decades the advent of gastrointestinal fluoroscopy and radiography. Not until 1895 did Wilhelm Röntgen discover the remarkable property of x-rays to penetrate soft tissues.

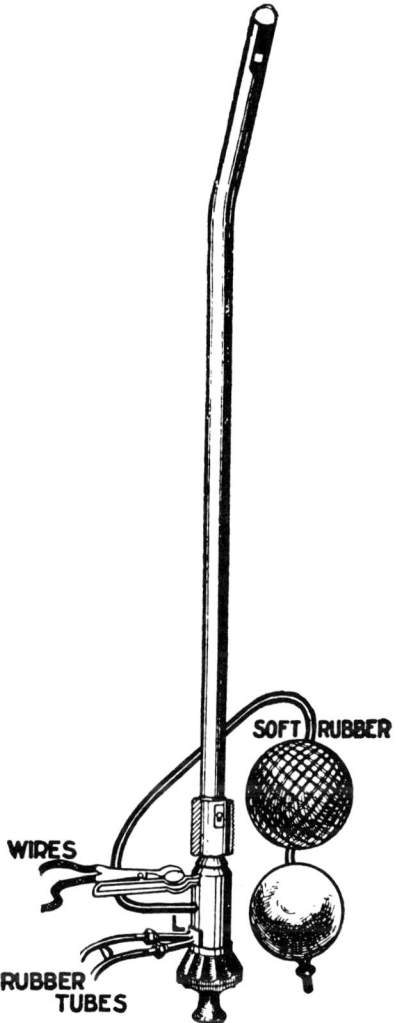

Fig. 30–3. The Mikulicz-Leiter gastroscope (1881). The tube, while rigid, was slightly angulated at its distal end to accommodate the configuration of the esophagogastric junction.

At the juncture of the 19th and 20th centuries, the most notable advances in endoscopy were by German workers. The reason was the technical supremacy in optics and instrument fabrication by German artisans. However, these skills were soon imported and mastered by American craftsmen. Among the foremost of these was Reinhold Wappler of New York, who later organized the firm of American Cystoscope Makers, Incorporated, now better known by its initials ACMI.

THE 20TH CENTURY CATALYST

Rudolf Schindler was born in Berlin in 1888, the son of a prosperous banker and an artistically gifted mother who encouraged his early interest in classical music, poetry, and natural history. Young Schindler's decision to study medicine derived from his respect and admiration for his maternal uncle, Richard Simon, a Berlin ophthalmologist (13,14). His medical degree from the University of Berlin in hand, Schindler undertook a rural practice that was soon interrupted by World War I. Schindler enrolled for service as a medical officer, a position from which he observed, at first hand, the prevalence of digestive ills in both the military and civilian populations. He became convinced that much digestive disability could be attributed to morbid changes in the gastric mucosa undetectable by conventional methods of examination. He concluded that a proper diagnosis, and hence effective therapy, would emerge only by direct observation of the internal milieu of the living stomach—in short, by gastroscopy.

After the war, Schindler attended patients at the Munich-Schwabing Hospital where, in 1920, he gained access to a rigid Elsner gastroscope. With this instrument, and later with an improved model modified according to his own specifications, Schindler performed hundreds of gastroscopic examinations, each procedure meticulously documented. Often gastroscopy was sequentially repeated in the same subject to observe the natural progress of mucosal lesions. Nor did Schindler neglect to study the normal stomach. He is said to have examined on a number of occasions the stomach of his accommodating housekeeper. This early work, conducted in a scholarly manner, culminated in the 1923 publication of Schindler's monumental *Lehrbuch und Atlas der Gastroskopie* (15).

Intragastric photography, although attempted (16) then, was inadequate as a means of documenting endoscopic observations. Therefore, gastroscopic images were vividly reproduced as colored drawings or paintings, usually rendered by professional artists who were allowed glimpses through the endoscope, their sketches later embellished with advice by the examining doctor. Artistically inclined clinicians would sometimes illustrate their own cases. Both Schindler's 1923 classic and the atlas compiled in 1937 by Kurt Gutzeit and Heinrich Teitge (17) can still be perused for their accurate depiction of stomach lesions now seldom seen (18). Among the most adept artists was Gladys McHugh, who illustrated the American editions of Schindler's *Gastroscopy* for the University of Chicago Press (19).

Meanwhile, Schindler was far from satisfied with the utility and safety of the rigid gastroscope. He devoted himself to the design of a partially flexible instrument that could be inserted with less discomfort and risk to the patient and that would provide clearer, more extensive images. Gordon and Kirsner (14) relate the story as told by Schindler's daughter, Ursula Gibson, that in 1928, following a family dinner, her father was inspired to create an instrument using certain optical principles described in 1911 by Michael Hoffmann (20). The optical principle employed lenses of short focal length, positioned sequentially within a flexible wire frame, thereby transmitting an image "around a corner." Schindler deftly sketched his design on the convenient tablecloth, which was then folded, packaged, and forwarded to George Wolf, a leading instrument maker in Berlin with whom Schindler had been acquainted. After months of anxious waiting, Schindler received from Wolf a prototype instrument constructed exactly according to Schindler's impromptu sketch. Thus began a fruitful, if sometimes, turbulent, collaboration of Schindler, the imaginative clinician, and Wolf, the consummate artisan. At first, Wolf proposed an optical gastroscope that would be flexible throughout its length, but Schindler, based on his personal clinical experience, insisted on combining a rigid proximal half with a flexible distal half to ensure a more easily handled instrument that conveyed a brighter, sharper image. Within a few years evolved the famous Schindler-Wolf semiflexible gastroscope, first produced in 1932 (Fig. 30–4) (21).

Schindler's achievement of an acceptably safe, workable gastroscope was widely acclaimed, and clinicians flocked to Munich to observe and learn of the use of the new instrument. Among these were Francois Moutier of France (who published his own *Traité de Gastroscopie et de Pathologie de L'estomac* (22), Norbert Henning of Leipzig and Kurt Gutzeig of Breslau. Visitors from America included Samuel Weiss, a New York gastroenterologist, and Edward Benedict, a Boston ear-nose-and-throat surgeon. At that time in certain prominent US medical centers, peroral endoscopy was considered solely in the province of a specialty then known as bronchoesophagology.

In the early 1930s, Rudolf Schindler, whose grandfather was nominally Jewish, was subjected to increasing persecution by the anti-Semitic Nazi regime. He was befriended by two American colleagues, Dr. Marie Ortmayer and Dr. Walter Lincoln Palmer of Chicago, both of whom had visited Schindler's clinic in the 1920s. Knowing of his plight, they arranged for Schindler to come to the University of Chicago as a visiting professor. Despite his incarceration in the concentration camp at Dachau, Schindler was rescued, largely by the incessant efforts of his wife Gabrielle. In 1934, the Schindler family arrived in Chicago, the father clutching the long wooden box that bore his "magic lantern" (19).

Schindler's publications, now in English, proliferated. Walter Palmer, together with others of the University of Chicago faculty, provided unstinting assistance to Schindler in arranging publication of his textbook *Gastroscopy* in 1937. This, with subsequently revised editions (23) appearing in 1950 and 1966, was the gospel of gastroscopy for a generation of clinicians. Schindler subtitled his book *The Endoscopic Study of Gastric Pathology*. By this, Schindler made clear his belief in the endoscopic method, not as an end in itself, but rather as an approach to an overall understanding of digestive diseases and to the care of patients. Schindler always thought of himself first as a physician and only secondarily as an endoscopist.

In Chicago, Schindler allied himself with William J. Cameron, head of Cameron Surgical Company, which became the world's foremost supplier of illuminated diagnostic instruments. With the supply of German-made equipment cut off during World War II, the Cameron Omni-angle gastroscope, modeled closely after the original Wolf-Schindler design, became the standard instrument throughout the US. On Cameron's

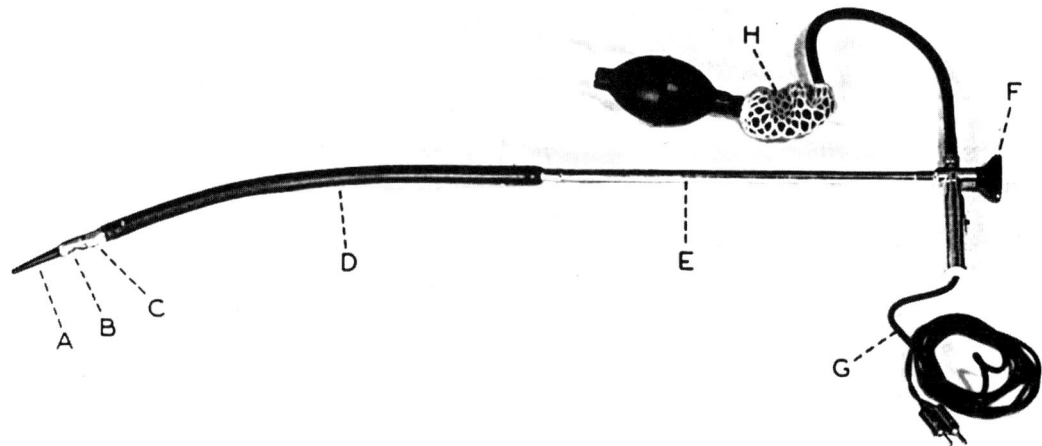

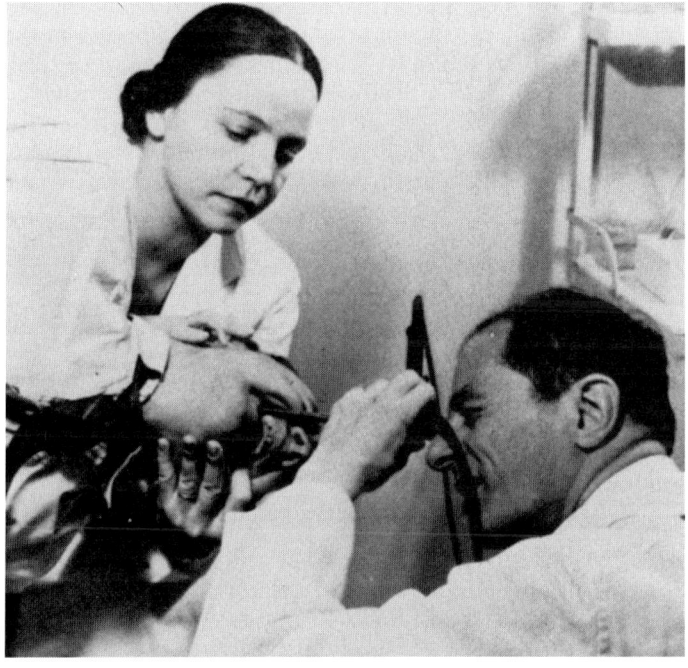

Fig. 30–4. *A,* The Wolf-Schindler semiflexible lens-and-prism gastroscope (1932). This was the prototype of instruments generally used in Europe and the U.S. through the 1950s. *B,* Rudolf Schindler, right, performing gastroscopy at the University of Chicago, assisted by his wife Gabrielle, left.

staff in Chicago was a talented instrument maker, Louis Streifeneder, with whom Scindler developed a close rapport. Streifeneder later formed his own firm, the Eder Instrument Company, which continues a tradition of meticulous workmanship, now mainly directed to the production of laparoscopes.

By 1943, the climate in Chicago had become clouded by what Schindler perceived as a lack of support for his view of gastritis as a central cause of digestive disturbance. Moving to Los Angeles, he taught at the College of Medical Evangelists (now Loma Linda University) and also served as consultant to the Long Beach Veterans Administration Hospital in association with Dr. Stephen Stempien and Dr. Angelo Dagradi. At age 70, Schindler learned Portuguese and accepted appointment to the faculty of the University of Minas Gerais at Belo Horizonte, Brazil. His wife's ill health necessitated a return to the US in 1960.

A proper account of Rudolf Schindler's career would be incomplete without mention of his wife Gabrielle (née Winkler), to whom he was wed in 1922. Not only had Frau Schindler played a major role in freeing her husband from the threat of the Nazi regime in Germany, but she had become his trusted clinical aide. The use of both the rigid and the semiflexible gastroscope required a capable assistant who could hold and manipulate the patient's head in the course of the procedure. Moreover, the assistant was charged with closely monitoring the patient's reaction to the examination and continuously soothing the patient's apprehension and discomfort. Although untrained as a nurse, Gabrielle readily acquired the necessary skill to an indispensable degree (see Fig. 30-3). It is said that, on the rare occasions when Gabrielle was unavailable to assist him, Schindler declined to perform gastroscopy.

In 1962, the American Society for Gastrointestinal Endoscopy bestowed its first Rudolf Schindler Award, its highest honor. The recipient, fittingly, was the man for whom the award was named. That occasion was Schindler's last attendance at an annual meeting of the group he had originally founded as the American Gastroscopic Club in 1941 (24). Schindler's beloved wife Gabrielle died in 1964. The following year, Schindler returned to Munich, Germany, where much of his early work had been accomplished. There he married Marie Koch, a friend of long standing, and occupied his last years by preparing an atlas based on his lifetime performance of 10,300 gastroscopic examinations. In addition, he found time to enjoy his music and his collection of sea shells. He died of cardiac complications in Munich in 1968 (25).

DOCUMENTING GASTROSCOPY

A major impediment to acceptance of the findings of early gastroscopy was that views of the internal milieu of the stomach, including such lesions as might be seen, were limited to the visual cognizance of the examiner, or to such fleeting glimpses as might be permitted an observer peering over the examiner's shoulder.

The widely adopted Wolf-Schindler gastroscope and its successors bore no channel through which a biopsy forceps could be inserted. In retrospect, one would think this could have been managed by adapting the channel through which air was insufflated. Unfortunately, Schindler seemed convinced that an accurate appraisal of the status of the gastric mucosa could be derived from its endoscopic appearance alone. The Boston surgeon Edward Benedict, perhaps because he was more accustomed to the need for histologic verification, devised what he called an operating gastroscope, which incorporated a biopsy forceps (26). However, this cumbersome and unwieldy instrument never gained widespread acceptance.

The first challenge to subjective endoscopic interpretation was the introduction of the gastric mucosal biopsy tube by Ian Wood and his Australian coworkers in the late 1940s (27). Such biopsy required a separate procedure, but at least this provided the pathologist with a section of tissue for microscopic examination. Not surprisingly, the gastroscopic diagnosis and the actual histologic findings did not always agree.

The advent of photography, earlier in the 19th century, offered a means of recording and preserving the endoscopic image. As previously mentioned, primitive attempts at gastroscopic photography had been described (16), but insufficient illumination and the insensitivity of then-available film emulsions discouraged further efforts to adapt photography to endoscopy. Later, these impediments were largely overcome (28,29).

An alternative development was the construction of a miniature camera, small enough to be swallowed by the patient and attached to a tube through which the camera could be activated and then retrieved. Originally conceived in the West (30), the idea was ideally suited to implementation by the technologically skillful Japanese. Thus a workable gastrocamera was developed by Tatsuno Uji (31) of the University of Tokyo in collaboration with his engineering colleagues at the Olympus Optical Company.

Dr. John Morrissey has related the story (32,33) of how Dr. Yoshio Hara introduced gastrocamera photography at the University of Wisconsin in 1962. Hara had come to the Madison campus with the primary intent of studying new advances in cancer chemotherapy. Perhaps not incidentally, he brought along a set of vivid, full-color photographs of lesions as they appeared in the living stomach, as well as the tiny camera that had captured them. Morrissey, given the opportunity to view Hara's pictures, was quick to recognize the utility of the device and became adept in its use. Shortly thereafter, scores of clinicians flocked to Madison from across the land, eager to learn the new technique.

No more vivid photographs of the interior of the intact stomach have ever been obtained, as evidenced by perusal of the color plates in Morrissey's 1965 article (34). However, the early gastrocamera had a major drawback: the operator could not see the result of his work until the film had been developed. Pictures (32 exposures on a tiny roll of 5 mm film) were taken according to a rote sequence (the shutter was opened, the flash activated, and the film advanced as the camera was aimed at each of four circumferential quadrants, at eight prescribed levels from the pylorus to the cardia). If all went well (which was not always the case), the result was a fairly complete photographic survey of the stomach's interior. A gastroscope was still needed to provide a visual image and guidance.

In 1963, the problem was solved by simply incorporating the tiny camera in a standard gastroscope. By this time, however the acuity of the fiberoptic gastroscope and its light source had been improved to such an extent that most endoscopists found it easier to attach an external 35 mm camera to the eyepiece of the gastroscope and thereby record the image conveyed by the fiberglass bundle. The pictures thus obtained were not as sharp, but they were adequate. Ease of use prevailed. The gastrocamera, marvelous as it was, soon became obsolete.

THE ADOPTION OF FIBEROPTIC TECHNOLOGY

The era of fiberoptic gastrointestinal endoscopy might be said to have begun in Ann Arbor, Michigan, when Basil Hirschowitz, then a fellow in gastroenterology from South Africa by way of England, noted in the January 1954 issue of *Nature* two articles on the optical properties of fine glass fibers. One of them in particular, by Hopkins and Kapany (35) of the Imperial College of Science and Technology in London, fired his imagination of how an endoscopic image might be transmitted by a coherent bundle of fully flexible glass fibers from the alimentary lumen of a patient to the eye of an examiner. The ensuing events have been described in fascinating accounts by Hirschowitz (36,37) and Hopkins (38).

That light would follow the curved path of a stream of water pouring from a tank was first demonstrated by John Tyndall, a British physicist, in 1870. The idea of using flexible glass fibers to propagate light was proposed in patent applications by J. L. Baird of England in 1927 and by C. W. Hansell of the US in 1930. Schindler credited Heinrich Lamm (39) with being the first to recommend the adaptation of fiberoptics to gastroscopy. Unfortunately, Schindler gave no further thought to the matter because he was then preoccupied with developing his own optical design.

The principle of transmission of light by a fine glass fiber is easy to comprehend; implementation of that principle in endoscopy is difficult. Light-carrying glass fibers can be bundled in two ways. A randomly collected bundle can be readily assembled and serves to transmit light effectively from one end to the other; in the case of endoscopy, this is from a source of illumination to the interior of a body cavity. But endoscopy further requires that a readable image be conveyed in the opposite direction, i.e., from the body cavity to the eye of the examiner. Thus the need is for a second type of bundle, a coherent bundle, wherein many thousands of hair-thin glass fibers must be meticulously assembled in such a manner that their array is precisely the same at one end as at the other. This is only part of the problem. Any appreciable leakage of light from one fiber to its neighbor defeats the purpose of a coherent bundle. This principal impediment to devising a workable endoscope was overcome by Lawrence Curtiss, then an undergraduate physics student at the University of Michigan. Curtiss conceived of a process whereby an individual fiber of optical glass could be clad in a thin layer of glass of lower refractive index, the latter serving as an insulating coat. Hirschowitz, with whom Curtiss collaborated (40), credits this as the single most important innovation in the advent of fiberoptic endoscopy.

I can remember visiting the physics laboratory of the University of Michigan to witness a demonstration of the prototype coherent fiberoptic bundle. The hose-like device had been mounted on a stand and festooned to show its remarkable flexibility. The objective was aimed at a well-illuminated postage stamp that had been affixed to the wall. The stamp happened to be of the 5-cent denomination that bore the likeness of Abraham Lincoln. One by one, the visitors stepped up to peer into the eyepiece where we could make out a rather grainy image of Lincoln's familiar face. Although, the fiberoptic image, at that early stage of development, was not as vivid as the image projected by the then standard optical gastroscope, we recognized that we were witnessing a remarkable achievement.

Three years of endeavor had elapsed since Hirschowitz's initial inspiration, and in February 1957 a prototype fiberscope, adapted for gastroscopy, was finally constructed at Ann Arbor (Fig. 30–5). Hirschowitz himself undertook to be the first to swallow the fully flexible instrument

that resembled an oversized Ewald tube. Unscathed by the experience, within a few days he performed at the University of Michigan Hospital the first fiberoptic gastroscopy, his patient being a young woman with a duodenal ulcer. Later that spring, Hirschowitz demonstrated his new instrument at the annual session of the American Gastroenterological Association in Colorado Springs (41).

It was not until the 1960s that meticulous technicians, working both in Japan and the US, succeeded in refining commercial construction of the first clinically useful fiberoptic gastrointestinal endoscopes. Notably improved were illumination, optical clarity, wieldability, and control of the distal tip. Channels were provided for air insufflation and biopsy under direct visual guidance. The Japanese were especially intent on this endeavor, largely because of the prevalence of gastric cancer in their population.

The first of the new instruments to gain widespread use in the US was the fully flexible fiberoptic esophagoscope with a working length of 75 cm. This had the enormous advantage of an end-viewing objective

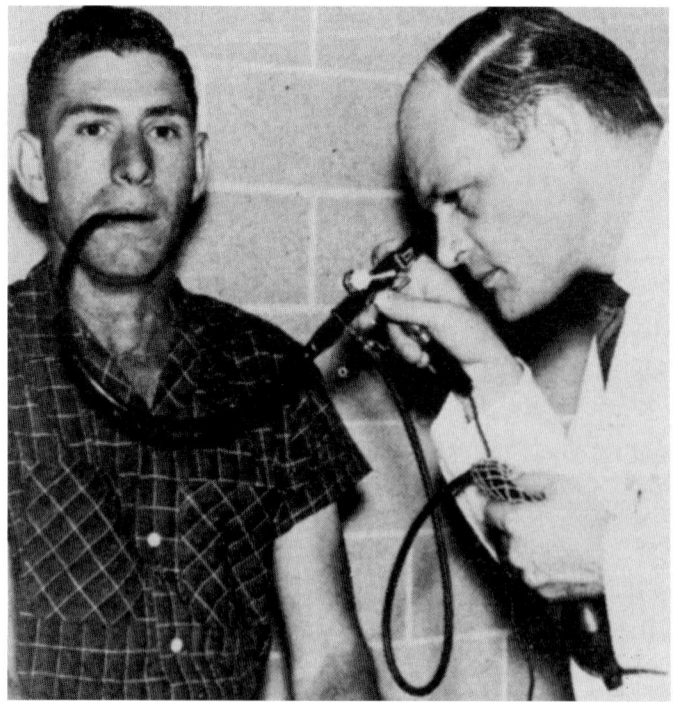

Fig. 30–5. Basil Hirschowitz examining a patient by means of a prototype of the fully flexible fiberoptic gastroscope developed at the University of Michigan (1961). Courtesy of Dr. Basil Hirschowitz.

rather than the traditional side-viewing objective, a carryover from the Schindler design, with which Hirschowitz's early fiberscope was equipped. To clinicians previously obliged to attempt endoscopy of the esophagus by means of a straight, rigid, unyielding, steel tube, the flexible fiberoptic esophagoscope was a marvel. Soon thereafter, the improved coherent fiberoptic bundle was extended to a working length of 110 cm, thus providing an easily insertable instrument with which the esophagus, stomach, and duodenum could be thoroughly examined at the same sitting. Bringing the duodenum within the range of endoscopy was a signal advance.

In the 1970s, improvements in endoscope design, one after another, were introduced so rapidly that one could hardly purchase a new instrument and become acquainted with its use before it was rendered obsolete by a new model. The ungainly device that had its inauspicious beginning in the corner of the physics laboratory in Ann Arbor was transformed into a diagnostic instrument that most gastroenterologists found invaluable. In the hands of a host of clinicians, for a full generation, fiberoptic endoscopy notably advanced the diagnosis and management of a widely ranging variety of gastrointestinal diseases.

The success of the fiberoptic endoscope introduced through the mouth naturally led to its adaptation for insertion at the lower end of the alimentary tract. Simple specula designed for examination of the anus and rectum had been in wide use since the late 1800s. Essentially, these were no more than hollow tubes of varying diameter and length, beveled at the end intended for insertion and fitted with an obturator and a handle. Illumination of the shorter anoscopes was external, by flashlight or reflection from a headmirror; longer proctoscopes carried a small incandescent bulb placed at either the proximal or distal end. For practical purposes, the maximum length of a straight, hollow, rigid proctosigmoidoscope was 25 cm. Thought was given to adapting for examination of the colon an instrument similar in design to the Wolf-Schindler gastroscope, but the tortuosity of the sigmoid segment was far beyond the bending capacity of a lens-and-prism construction. Even the early fiberscope could not be properly advanced

in a retrograde manner through the sigmoid colon although a few venturesome examiners tacitly tried this with the fiberoptic esophagoscope from time to time.

Development of a workable fiberoptic colonoscope also began at the hospital of the University of Michigan. According to Bergein F. Overholt (42,43), who pioneered adaptation of the fiberoptic principle to endoscopy of the large intestine, the work was stimulated in 1961 by an unusually disagreeable proctosigmoidoscopy suffered by the person of Dr. J. Howard Gowan in the course of a routine but somewhat trying physical evaluation at the hospital. Coincidentally, Overholt, then serving his internship, was being interviewed by Gowan in connection with an application for a U.S. Public Health Service fellowship. Overholt expressed due commiseration, then followed up with a remark on the prospect that a fully flexible instrument might provide a more comfortable sigmoidoscopy procedure. This, apparently, ensured Gowan's support.

Meanwhile, others had been tempted to set aside esthetics and insert the fiberoptic gastroscope in the anus (44). At the same time, all manner of contrivance had been suggested to pull back through the colon a flexible fiberscope hooked onto the end of a swallowed string that had been allowed to traverse the alimentary canal. None proved practicable. Just as the anatomy of the proximal alimentary tract had posed a problem for Kussmaul and the earliest would-be gastroscopists, so did the serpentine anatomy of the lower bowel present a problem to would-be colonoscopists.

Overholt, with the support of his mentor, Dr. H. Marvin Pollard (45), strove to overcome this difficulty. From a silicone-rubber cast, Overholt made a lifelike model of the human distal colon, which enabled him to make the necessary adjustments in torque and control of a fiberoptic endoscope suited to retrograde insertion by way of the rectum. The result was a prototype instrument first clinically used in 1963. Further refinement was required, and it was not until the 1967 meeting of the American Society for Gastrointestinal Endoscopy that Overholt described, to a somewhat skeptical audience, his experience in examining the first 40 patients (46). By coincidence this event took place at the same locale, the Broadmoor Hotel in Colorado Springs, where a decade earlier Hirschowitz, also representing the University of Michigan, had first described fiberoptic gastroscopy. Meanwhile, Japanese workers had been busily engaged in creating their version of a colonoscope and advancing its clinical application (47,48).

Colonoscopy gained rapid acceptance by clinicians who had been recently introduced to the marvel of fiberoptic gastroscopy, although most operators soon found that successful colonoscopy was much more tedious and demanding than examination of the upper gastrointestinal tract. Christopher Williams (49) in England and Hiromi Shinya (50) and Jerome Waye (51) of New York were among the early proponents and most proficient teachers of the new art of fiberoptic colonoscopy. Thus, the effort initiated by Burgein Overholt, refined and promoted by colleagues around the globe, resulted in placing an additional major segment of the alimentary tract within the purview of gastrointestinal endoscopists.

ENDOSCOPY IS UNITED TO TELEVISION

Fiberoptics, which dominated the field for barely 25 years, now has been superseded, for most gastroenterologic applications, by the burgeoning technology of videoendoscopy, whereby vivid images are transmitted electronically from within the patient to a television screen.

In the 1950s, availability of television cameras and monitors naturally suggested their application to endoscopy, especially valuable in objective documentation. Black-and-white televised images of bronchoscopy were reported in 1957 (52). J. Alfred Rider and Basil Hirschowitz collaborated in a demonstration of televised images of upper gastrointestinal endoscopy at the 1963 meeting of the American Society for Gastrointestinal Endoscopy in San Francisco. Television cameras that could be attached to the eyepiece of a standard fiberoptic gastroscope were employed (53), but the cameras were unwieldy and heavy (even the lightest weighed about 7 pounds) and had to be suspended from the ceiling of the examining room.

What was needed was to incorporate within the tip of the endoscope itself an electronic device capable of registering and transmitting signals that could be translated into a visible, vivid image. This became feasible with the development of the charge-coupled device (CCD), which could function, in effect, as a miniature television camera, small enough to be accommodated within the end of a slender, flexible tube. A necessary adjunct was a computer capable of transforming the electronic signals thus generated into a recognizable image.

The first video-endoscope was introduced by Welch Allyn, Inc., a long-established maker of illuminated diagnostic instruments. Among the early reports of clinical experience with prototype videoendoscopes were those of Sivak and Fleischer (54) in the US, and by Classen and Phillip (55) and Demling and Hagel (56) in Europe. The many advantages of supplanting the coherent fiberoptic bundle with a CCD coupled with a computer were foreseen in 1988 by Silverstein (57) and have now been realized by gastrointestinal endoscopists worldwide. Videoendoscopy has emerged as the current standard.

EXPLORING THE PANCREATIC AND BILIARY DUCTS

Imaging the intact biliary and pancreatic ducts had long defied clinicians. The story of attempts to visualize the biliary tree begins in 1924 when the surgeons Evarts Graham and Warren Cole succeeded in showing that intravenously administered iodinated phenolphthalein was selectively excreted in bile, a property that prompted development of contrast media whereby the configuration of the intact biliary tree could be recorded radiographically. The method soon led to oral cholecystography, the mainstay of diagnosis of gallbladder disease for over half the 20th century. However, even with the use of improved media, the radiographic image of the biliary duct was often incomplete and indistinct, and the pancreatic duct could not be visualized even dimly. Doubilet et al. in 1955 (58) described intraoperative pancreatography, but what was needed was a means of recording a clear image of the pancreatic duct without surgical intervention. In 1965, Rabinov and Simon (59) reported transduodenal cannulation of the ampulla of Vater by means of a swallowed catheter manipulated under fluoroscopic guidance. However, their painstaking procedure succeeded in only one of eight patients.

A solution was to guide a cannula into the ampulla under endoscopic control. This was first accomplished by William S. McCune, a surgeon, and his associates (60) at George Washington University in 1968. They were principally interested in demonstrating the pancreatic duct. Having achieved his aim, McCune declined to pursue the technique. Again, it remained for the Japanese to perfect the technique, now extended to include the biliary tree, as subsequently described by Oi and his coworkers (61) and by Kasugai et al. (62). The procedure was thus termed "endoscopic retrograde cholangiopancreatography," a cumbersome name quickly shortened to ERCP. Foremost among proponents of ERCP in the US were Jack Vennes and his colleagues (63,64) at the Minneapolis Veterans Administration Hospital.

In some cases, a radiographic delineation of the ducts was not enough, and means were sought to actually view by endoscopy the lumina and their contents directly. The first attempt was in 1923 by Bakes (65), a German surgeon better known for devising the graduated probes commonly used at operation to dilate the ampulla of Vater and the ducts beyond. A right-angled telescope specifically designed for insertion in the common bile duct was reported by McIver (66) in 1941. Improved instruments were later described by Wildegans (67) and by Berc (68). An attempt was made to adapt fiberoptic technology to choledochoscopy (69), but surgeons found that the rigid optical instruments conveyed a brighter, sharper image (70). This is one of the few instances in the development of endoscopy wherein the fixed lens system prevailed over the flexible fiberoptic bundle. A more recent innovation, however, has been adaptation of a video-urethroscope for the purpose of both diagnostic and therapeutic choledochoscopy under laparoscopic guidance (71).

With the demonstrated feasibility of endoscopically guided cannulation of the ampulla of Vater with a catheter for the purpose of contrast radiography, it was inevitable that substitution of the small-caliber endoscope would be proposed. This remarkable technical feat was reported in 1978 by Nakajima et al. (72). These workers modified a duodenoscope (the "mother 'scope") by enlarging to 2.8 mm the bore of its catheter channel, through which they passed a 2.3 mm fiberoptic endoscope (the "baby 'scope") that, in turn, could be guided under direct vision into either the common bile duct or the pancreatic duct. Because the exceedingly slender caliber of the probing endoscope could accommodate only 3000 fibers and the view was through a fluid medium, the image lacked the clarity provided by other endoscopic techniques. Peroral cholangiopancreatography did not gain wide use. Nevertheless, its accomplishment must be regarded as a technical tour de force.

LAPAROSCOPY

The percutaneous endoscopic approach to the peritoneal cavity and its visceral contents has gained recent widespread attention, particularly in its therapeutic applications; however, the idea of endoscopic penetration of the abdominal wall is not new. The history of the concept is somewhat confusing because of the various names that have been applied to the procedure: peritoneoscopy, organoscopy, and coeliscopy, all with the same frame of reference. "Laparoscopy," a term contrived from a combination of the Greek *lapara,* "the soft parts of the body between the lower rib margins and the hips," and *skopein,* "to observe," has the advantage of historical precedence and, largely because of its adoption by gynecologists and surgeons, has now achieved almost universal currency.

In 1902, Georg Kelling (73) reported, at the 73rd meeting in Hamburg of a group known as German Natural Scientists and Physicians, his observations of the abdominal viscera of a dog by means of a Nitze cystoscope. In the same year, Dimitri Ott (74), a Russian gynecologist, deliberately introduced a speculum into the pelvic cavity of a female patient through an incision in the posterior vaginal fornix, a procedure he called "ventroscopy." Working independently in Sweden, H. D. Jacobaeus (75,76) reported his percutaneous endoscopic examination of the abdominal and thoracic cavities and in 1912 proposed the term "laparoscopy." Thereafter, Kelling and Jacobaeus long disputed priority of discovery. In what may have been one of the earliest efforts at cost containment, Kelling (77) in 1923 wrote that he used "coelioscopy" as a means of sparing his patients the expense of surgical laparotomy.

Use of the procedure in the US was first reported in 1911 by Bertram Bernheim (78), a surgeon at the Johns Hopkins Hospital in Baltimore. He had inserted a proctoscope with a half-inch bore through the abdominal wall of a jaundiced patient to confirm the presence of a Courvoisier gallbladder. Benjamin Orndoff (79) of Chicago used a similar device for the procedure called "peritoneoscopy." Meanwhile, the procedure became widely applied in Europe, where Korbsch (80) published his *Lehrbuch und Atlas der Laparo- und Thorakoskopie* in 1927. Heinz Kalk, a renowned German proponent of laparoscopy, culminated a series of publications with his own textbook and atlas, prepared in collaboration with Egmont Wildhirt in 1961 (81), which emphasized the additional advantage of endoscopically guided liver biopsy.

John Ruddock (82) of Los Angeles was almost a lone champion of the procedure in the US during the 1930s. Ruddock used a slightly modified cystoscope in hundreds of cases and proposed what was then an astonishing number of therapeutic applications, including sterilization of female patients and herniorrhaphy. Such proposals were, at that time, deemed unduly radical, and, ironically, had the effect of retarding rather than promoting further use of endoscopic exploration of the peritoneal and pelvic cavities. As it turned out, Ruddock was a half-century ahead of his time.

After World War II, with resumed importation of refined German instruments and the arrival of immigrant physicians trained in their use, laparoscopy won renewed adherents, especially among gynecologists. Prominent among endoscopically oriented gynecologists was Peter Steptoe of England, who found laparoscopy essential in his

development of the technique that ushered in the "test-tube baby boom" (83).

Recent years had seen an astonishing adaptation of the laparoscopic approach to numerous intra-abdominal manipulations, notably those directed to management of calculous biliary tract disease. Pioneered in France (84,85), laparoscopic cholecystectomy has come, in many centers, to supersede largely the traditional open operation. Endoscopic appendectomy was first reported by Semm in 1983 (86), but only more recently has this procedure been adopted by surgeons having gained confidence in their skill at laparoscopic manipulation.

THERAPEUTIC ENDOSCOPY

Until recently, endoscopists could describe and record what they saw but were relatively powerless to intervene therapeutically (87). Early in the 20th century, those who styled themselves bronchoesophagologists were adept in extracting foreign objects deliberately or inadvertently choked down by unwitting children and misguided adults. In years past, the walls of the Chevalier Jackson Clinic on the 10th floor of the Graduate Hospital in Philadelphia were adorned by an astonishing display of trophies of incredible variety, extracted from various recesses. Endoscopists no longer so decorate their workplaces (the array of foreign bodies extracted by Jackson and his associates is now part of the Mutter Museum collection at the College of Physicians of Philadelphia), but the ingenious application of a variety of techniques employing gastrointestinal endoscopy became widely promulgated (88).

The treatment procedure currently and most widely used by gastrointestinal endoscopists, and probably of benefit to the greatest number of patients, is colonoscopic polypectomy (89). In Miami at the 1971 session of the American Gastroenterological Association, Shinya and Wolff (50) astonished the audience by showing motion pictures depicting their innovative technique of snaring, then cauterizing and severing the stalk of a pedunculated colon polyp, a procedure now regarded as commonplace.

Control of active bleeding from lesions within the range of endoscopy by electrocoagulation, heater probe, or laser, was accomplished as a result of intensive investigation during the decade following 1970. Endoscopically guided percutaneous gastrostomy was first performed in 1979, using a jury-rigged applicance (90). Remarkably, improvisation has often led to a notable advance in gastrointestinal endoscopy. Enteric and ductal strictures are now amenable to dilation under endoscopic guidance. Obstructing neoplasms can be at least partially obliterated under direct vision by endoscopically aimed laser beams or electrodessicators. Even more dramatic is endoscopic intervention in calculous disease in the biliary and pancreatic ducts.

In some instances, as application of the endoscopic method has evolved, what may seem relatively new is not. An example is endoscopic sclerotherapy of esophageal varices, a procedure first reported by Clarence Crafoord and Paul Freckner (91) in Europe in 1939 and, a few years later, in the US by Herman Moersch (92) and by Cecil Patterson and Milford Rouse (93). Being aware of what has gone before can clarify one's perspective.

Repeated emphasis has been given to the benefit of collaborative effort by clinicians and artisans in the advance of endoscopic technology. Today, similar cooperation between gastroenterologic internists is leading to even more innovative approaches to the management of digestive diseases (94).

EPILOGUE

Several recurring themes stand out in this account of the origins and evolution of knowledge of gastrointestinal endoscopy.

First, almost without exception, advances in endoscopy have come about by close collaboration of clinicians and technicians. Neither could have succeeded without the other. One need only recall the paired names of Mikulicz and Leiter, of Schindler and Wolf, of Palmer or McCune and Streifeneder. Further advance has evolved from a merging of basically unrelated technologies. An example is the development of endoscopic ultrasonography (95–98).

Second, clinicians who have notably advanced endoscopy have done so in the broader context of advancing medical practice overall. A notable case in point is Rudolf Schindler.

Third, innovative instrumentation has often been prompted by technical advances made far afield of the recognized domain of gastrointestinal endoscopy or even beyond the broad purview of medicine. Instructive examples are the adaptation of fiberoptics and, later, the charge-coupled device to endoscopy.

Fourth, progress of instrumentation and its clinical application does not always proceed in a smoothly linear or logical fashion but rather by an irregular, and sometimes unpredictable, sequence of initial surprise, often followed by skepticism, then evaluation, and finally acceptance or rejection, depending on careful study and experience.

The history of endoscopy is an account of accomplishment facilitated by the cooperative interaction between science and technology and serves to point the way to still more marvelous advances yet to come.

REFERENCES

1. Cushing H: The Life of Sir William Osler. Vol. I, p 174. Oxford, The Clarendon Press, 1925.
2. Bozzini PH: Lichtleiter, eine Erfindung zur Anshauung innere Teile und Krankheiten. J Prakt Heilk *24*:207, 1806.
3. Segal A: Pierre-Salomen Segalas l'Etcheparé, précurseur de l'endoscopie moderne. Bull Acad Nat Méd *162*:709, 1978.
4. Segal A: Le medecin principal de première classe Jean-Pierre Bonnafont (1805–1891); sa place préponderante dans l'histoire de l'endoscopie au XIXe siècle. Histoire des Médicales *17*(1):63, 1983.
5. Millemand P, Gilbrin E: Antonin-Jean Desmoreaux (1815–1894), le créateur de l'endoscopie. Bull Acad Nat Méd *160*:95, 1976.
6. Edmondson JM: History of the instruments for gastrointestinal endoscopy. Gastrointest Endosc (supplement) *37*:S27, 1991.
7. Kluge F, Seidler E: Briefe von Adolf Kussmaul und seinen Mitarbeitern. Medizin historisches J *21*:288, 1986.
8. Killian G: Zur Geschichte der Oesophago- und Gastroskopie. Dtsch Z Chir *58*:499, 1901.
9. Mikulicz J: Über Gastroskopie und Oesophagoskopie. Wien Med Presse *52*:1629, 1881.

10. Herrick FC: Profuse recurrent gastric hemorrhage, with report of cases and description of an instrument for viewing the gastric interior at operation. Cleveland Med J *10*:969, 1911.

11. Jackson C: Tracheobronchoscopy, Esophagoscopy, and Gastroscopy. St Louis, Laryngoscope Company, 1907.

12. Janeway HH, Green N: Esophagoscopy and gastroscopy. Surg Gynecol Obstet *13*:245, 1911.

13. Davis AB: Rudolf Schindler's role in the development of gastroscopy. Bull Hist Med *46*: 150, 1972.

14. Gordon ME, Kirsner JB: Rudolf Schindler, pioneer gastroscopist; glimpses of the man and his work. Gastroenterology *77*:354, 1979.

15. Schindler R: Lehrbuch und Atlas der Gastroskopie. Munich, IF Lehmann, 1923.

16. Lange GM, Meltzing D: Die Photographis des Magenintern. München med Wochenschr *45*:1585, 1898.

17. Gutzeit K, Teitge H: Die Gastroskopie; Lehrbuch und Atlas. Berlin, Urban & Schwartzenberg, 1937.

18. Palmer ED: Gutzeit and Teitge revisited. Gastrointest Endosc *23*:244, 1977.

19. Kirsner JB: American gastroscopy; yesterday and today. Gastrointest Endosc *37*:643, 1991.

20. Hoffmann M: Optische Instrumente mit beweglicher Achse und ihre Verwendlung für die Gastroskopie. München med Wochenschr *58*:2446, 1911.

21. Schindler R: Ein vollig ungefahrliches flexibles Gastroskop. München med Wochenschr *79*:1268, 1932.

22. Moutier F: Traite de gastroscopie et de pathologie endoscopique de l'estomac. Paris, Masson, 1935.

23. Schindler R: Gastroscopy: The Endoscopic Study of Gastric Pathology. Chicago, University of Chicago Press, 1937; revised 1950; 2nd ed. New York, Hafner Publishing Company, 1966.

24. Gerstner P: The American Society of Gastrointestinal Endoscopy; a history. Gastrointest Endosc *37*:suppl 1–26, 1991.

25. Dagradi AE, Stempien SJ: In memorium: Rudolf Schindler. Gastrointest Endosc *15*: 121, 1968.

26. Benedict EB: An operating gastroscope. Gastroenterology *11*:281, 1948.

27. Wood IJ et al.: Gastric biopsy. Lancet *1*:18, 1949.

28. Nelson RS: Routine gastroscopic photography. Gastroenterology 1956 *30*:661, 1956.

29. Segal HL, Watson JS Jr: Color photography through the flexible gastroscope. Gastroenterology *35*:50, 1958.

30. Editorial (unsigned): Photography of the stomach wall. Lancet *1*:371, 1931.

31. Uji T: The gastrocamera. Tokyo Med J *61*: 135, 1952.

32. Morrissey JF: Gastrointestinal endoscopy; 20 years of progress. Gastrointest Endosc *29*:53, 1983.

33. Morrissey JF: The use of the gastrocamera for the diagnosis of gastric ulcer. Gastroenterology *48*:711, 1965.

34. Perna G, Honda T, Morrissey JF: Gastrocamera photography. Arch Intern Med *116*: 434, 1965.

35. Hopkins HH, Kapany NS: A flexible fiberscope, using static scanning. Nature (London) *173*:39, 1954.

36. Hirschowitz BI: A personal hsitory of the fiberscope. Gastroenterology *76*:864, 1979. (See also Powell DW, Levinson DJ: Presentation of the Julius Friedenwald Medal to Basil I Hirschowitz. Gastroenterology *103*: 1720, 1992.)

37. Hirschowitz BI: Videotaped interview and demonstration. On file in the archives of the American Society for Gastrointestinal Endoscopy, Historical Division, Cleveland Medical Library Association, 1989.

38. Hopkins HH: The 1991 Lister Oration, delivered at the Royal College of Surgeons, London. Audiotape on file in the A/S/G/E Archives, Cleveland Health Sciences Museum.

39. Lamm H: Beigesamte optische Gerate. Zeitschrift Instrumentenk *50*:57, 1930.

40. Curtiss LE, Hirschowitz BI, Peters CW: A long fiberscope for internal medical examinations. J Am Optical Soc *46*:1030, 1956.

41. Hirschowitz BI et al.: Demonstration of a new gastroscope, the "fiberscope." Gastroenterology *35*:50, 1958.

42. Overholt BF: The history of colonoscopy. *In* Hunt RH, Waye JD (eds.): Colonoscopy: Clinical Practice and Colour Atlas. London, Chapman Hall Ltd, 1981.

43. Overholt BF: Videotape and demonstration. On file in the archives of the American Society for Gastrointestinal Endoscopy, Historical Division, Cleveland Medical Library Association, 1991.

44. Lemire S, Cocco AE: Visualization of the left colon with the fiberoptic gastroduodenoscope. Gastrointest Endosc *13*:29, 1966.

45. Pollard HM: Presentation of 1975 Schindler Award to B.F. Overholt. Gastrointest Endosc *22*:62, 1975.

46. Overholt BF: Clinical experience with the fibersigmoidoscope. Gastrointest Endosc *15*:27, 1968.

47. Oshiba S, Watanabe A: Endoscopy of the colon. Gastroenterol Endosc (Tokyo) *7*:440, 1965.

48. Niwa H: Endoscopy of the colon. Gastroenterol Endosc (Tokyo) 7:402, 1965.

49. Williams CB, Muto T: Examination of the whole colon with the fiberoptic colonoscope. Br Med J 3:278, 1972.

50. Wolff WI, Shinya H: Colonofiberoscopy. JAMA 217:1509, 1971.

51. Waye JD: Colonoscopy. Surg Clin North Am 52:1013, 1972.

52. Soulas A: Bronchoscopy and television. Dis Chest 31:580, 1957.

53. Rider JA, Puletti EJ, Rider RD, Columbine PN: Color television gastroscopy; A critical analysis. Gastrointest Endosc 18:66, 1971.

54. Sivak MJ Jr, Fleischer DE: Colonoscopy with a video-endoscope; A preliminary experience. Gastrointest Endosc 30:1, 1984.

55. Classen M, Phillip J: Electronic endoscopy of the upper gastrointestinal tract; Initial experience with a new type of endoscope that has no fiberoptic bundle for imaging. Endoscopy 16:16, 1984.

56. Demling L, Hegel HJ: Video-endoscopy; Fundamentals and problems. Endoscopy 17:167, 1985.

57. Silverstein FE: The future of video-endoscopy. Gastrointest Endosc 34:361, 1988.

58. Doubilet H, Poppel MH, Mulholland JH: Pancreatography: Technics, principles, and observations. Radiology 64:325, 1955.

59. Ravinov KR, Simon M: Peroral cannulation of the ampulla of Vater for direct cholangiography and pancreatography; Preliminary report of a new method. Radiology 85:693, 1965.

60. McCune WS, Shorb PE, Moscovitz H: Endoscopic cannulation of the ampulla of Vater; a preliminary report. Ann Surg 167:752, 1968.

61. Oi I: Fiberduodenoscopy and endocopic pancreatocholangiography. Gastrointest Endosc 17:59, 1970.

62. Kasugai T et al.: Endoscopic pancreatocholangiography. I. The normal endoscopic pancreatocholangiogram. Gastroenterology 63:217, 1972.

63. Vennes JA, Silvis SE: Endoscopic visualization of the bile and pancreatic ducts. Gastrointest Endosc 18:147, 1972.

64. Silvis SE: Presentation of 1978 Schindler Award to Jack Vennes. Gastrointest Endosc 24:263, 1978.

65. Bakes J: Die Choledochopapilloskopie nebst Bemerkungen über Hepaticusdrainage und Dilatation de Papill. Archiv Klin Chir 126:473, 1923.

66. McIver MA: An instrument for visualizing the interior of the common duct at operation. Surgery 9:112, 1941.

67. Wildegans H: Die operative Gallengangen-doskopie. Munich, Urban & Schwartzenberg, 1960.

68. Berci G: Choledochoscopy; the exploration of the extrahepatic biliary system under visual control; preliminary report. Med J Aust 2:862, 1961.

69. Shore JM, Lippman HN: Operative endoscopy of the biliary tract. Ann Surg 156:951, 1962.

70. Shore JM, Berci G: The clinical importance of cholangiography. Endoscopy 2:117, 1970.

71. Sackier J, Berci G, Paz-Partlow M: Transcystic laparoscopic choledocholithotomy. Amer Surg 57:323, 1991.

72. Nakajima M et al.: Direct endoscopic visualization of the bile and pancreatic duct systems by peroral cholangiopancreatoscopy (PCPS). Gastrointest Endosc 24:141, 1978.

73. Kelling G: Über Oesophagoskopie, Gastroskopie, und Kölioskopie. Münch med Wochenschr 49:21, 1902.

74. Ott DO: Die Beleuchtung der Bauchhöhle Ventroskopie als Methode bei vaginaler Köliotomie. Centralbl Gynäkol 31:817, 1902.

75. Jacobaeus HC: Über Laparo- und Thorakoskopie bei Untersuchung seroser Hohlungen anzuwenden. Münch med Wochenschr 58:2090, 1910.

76. Jacobaeus HC: Über Laparo- und Thorakoscopie. Beitr klin Erforsch Tuberk 25:183, 1912.

77. Kelling G: Kölioskopie und Gastroskopie. Arch Klin Chir 136:226, 1923.

78. Bernheim BM: Organoscopy; Cytoscopy of the abdominal cavity. Ann Surg 53:764, 1911.

79. Orndorff BH: The peritoneoscope in diagnosis of diseases of the abdomen. J Radiology 1:305, 1920.

80. Korbsch R: Lehrbuch und Atlas der Laparo- und Thorakoskopie. Munich, IF Lehmann V, 1927.

81. Kalk H, Wildhirt E: Lehrbuch und Atlas der Laparoskopie und Leberpunktion. Stuttgart, Georg Thieme, 1962.

82. Ruddock JC: Peritoneoscopy. Surg Gynec Obstet 65:629, 1937.

83. Steptoe PC: Laparoscopy in Gynecology. Edinburgh, E & S Livingstone Ltd, 1967.

84. Dubois F, Berthelots G, Levard H: Cholecystectomy par coelioscopie. Presse Méd 18:980, 1989.

85. Perissat J, Belliard R, Collet DC, Bikandou C: Cholecystectomy par laparoscopie. J Chir (Paris) 123:347, 1990.

86. Semm K: Endoscopic appendectomy. Endoscopy 15:159, 1983.

87. Soergel KH, Hogan WJ: Therapeutic endoscopy. Hosp Practice 18:81, 1983.

88. Vizcarrondo FJ, Brady PG, Nord HJ: For-

eign bodies of the upper gastrointestinal tract. Gastroint Endosc 29:208, 1983.

89. Winawer SJ et al.: Reduction in colorectal cancer incidence following colonoscopic polypectomy; Report of the national polyp study. Gastroenterology 100:A410, 1991.

90. Gauderer MWL, Ponsky JL, Izant RJ: Gastrostomy without laparotomy; A percutaneous endoscopic technique. J Pediatr Surg 15:872, 1980.

91. Crafoord C, Frenckner P: Nonsurgical treatment of varicose veins in the esophagus. Acta Otolaryngol 27:422, 1939.

92. Moersch HJ: Further studies on the treatment of esophageal varices by injection of a sclerosing solution. Ann Otol Rhinol Laryngol 50:1233, 1941.

93. Patterson CO, Rouse MO: Injection treatment of esophageal varices. JAMA 130:384, 1946.

94. Cotton PB: Therapeutic gastrointestinal endoscopy; problems in proving efficacy. (Editorial) N Engl J Med 326:1626, 1992.

95. Tio TL, Tytgat GN: Endoscopic ultrasonography in normal and pathologic upper gastrointestinal wall structure; comparison of studies in vivo and in vitro with histology. Scand J Gastroent (Suppl) 123:27, 1986.

96. Cotton PB, Shorvon PJ, Lees WR: Endoscopic ultrasonography; A new look from within. Br Med J 290:1373, 1985.

97. Sivak MV Jr: Is there an ultrasonographic endoscope in your future? Gastrointest Endosc 34:64, 1988.

98. Supplement (46 pp) to Volume 36, Number 2 (March/April), Gastrointest Endosc 1990.

31

Gastrointestinal Radiology

M. MAZEN ANBARI AND IGOR LAUFER

The development of gastrointestinal radiology is a fundamental part of the history of gastroenterology. Before the discovery of x-rays and their application to the GI tract, gastroenterology relied entirely on clinical science and symptoms for diagnosis. Short of surgery, there was no direct way to achieve access to most of the GI tract. The discovery of the x-ray and, in particular, the development of contrast media for opacification of the bowel opened new vistas for the investigation of normal and abnormal states in the GI tract and for direct rather than indirect diagnosis.

The field had its beginnings soon after the discovery of x-rays in 1895, and has since progressed rapidly, leading to unprecedented developments in gastrointestinal physiology and pathology. This chapter considers some of the most important contributions to the field. A contribution may take the form of a fundamental idea or the solution to a problem, a practical application of a theoretical insight, or the standardization and popularization of a known application. In addition, the role of technology in radiology is perhaps unique in all the medical specialties, and the history of gastrointestinal radiology necessarily includes the history of imaging techniques. Table 31–1 lists selected landmark developments in the history of GI radiology.

THE HOLLOW VISCERA

Early Days

As soon as news of the discovery of x-rays was widely disseminated, attempts at medical application were undertaken. The instinct of the very early pioneers was simply to expose different parts of the human body and observe the resulting images. Thus the earliest clinical applications of the new rays centered on the bones in the limbs, and on the detection of foreign bodies, since natural differences in opacity resulted in meaningful images (1–4). Exposing the abdomen to x-rays produced nothing useful because of the poor penetration of the beam. The first gastrointestinal applications, therefore, went no further than the occasional visualization of an air-filled stomach or the detection of foreign bodies in the gastrointestinal tract (5–6). Surgically removed gallstones were visualized about 3 months after Roentgen's discovery. The true beginning of gastrointestinal radiology required a simple but fundamental idea: artificial contrast.

The Upper Gastrointestinal Tract

Given that metals are opaque to x-rays, the first idea of an artificial contrast method was to image the stomach with a metallic wire. Carl Wegele suggested that a thin metal wire could be passed through a gastric tube to outline the stomach (7). Radiographic images illustrating this technique subsequently were published (8). A variation on this theme was the use of a bag swallowed whole, then filled with lead acetate through a tube until the bag outlined the stomach entirely (9). Another change was the use of gelatin capsules, containing opaque material, which were swallowed and observed fluoroscopically.

Table 31–1
Selected Milestones in the Development of Gastrointestinal Radiology*

1895	W. C. Roentgen discovers x-rays
1896	Foreign body is detected in the esophagus
1896	Gastrointestinal study, on a guinea pig, is reported by Becher
1897	Rumpel reports bismuth study of the stomach
1898	Cannon reports radiologic observations on peristalsis
1900	American radiographs of gallstones in vivo
1904	Rieder meal method
1904	Single-contrast examination of colon is reported by Schule
1910	Barium is popularized by Bachem and Gunther
1911	Lewis Gregory Cole reports first use of duodenal tube
1914	George and Gerber describe the radiologic appearance of duodenal ulcer
1914	Coolidge tube
1917	Carman and Miller publish first comprehensive gastrointestinal radiology book
1921	Carman's meniscus sign
1921	Direct gallbladder puncture
1923	Double-contrast study of the colon
1924	Cholecystography is developed by Graham and Cole
1929	Thorium is discovered
1929	Enteroclysis
1932	Crohn's disease is described
1937	Hampton reports double-contrast study of stomach
1937	Percutaneous transhepatic cholangiography
1945	The beginnings of nuclear magnetic resonance spectroscopy
1947	Thorium-related neoplasm
1951	Iopanoic acid (telepaque) is introduced
1953	Seldinger introduces percutaneous catheterization technique
1950s	Early gastric cancer detection studies in Japan
1960s	Welin's double contrast technique for study of the colon is reported
1962	Retained gallstones are extracted through the T-tube
1963	Holmes and Howry report on ultrasound abdominal scanning
1963	Cormack publishes mathematical basis of computed tomography
1971	Damadian uses NMR to distinguish normal from malignant tissue
1971	Society of Gastrointestinal Radiologists is founded
1973	Retained gallstones are extracted by remote-controlled catheter
1973	Hounsfield publishes description of first computed tomographic apparatus
1973	Lauterbur reports magnetic resonance images of various rat tissues
1974	Skinny needle for invasive diagnostic procedures
1975	Appearance of gastric erosions on double contrast examination
1975	Technetium-labeled dimethylaminodiacetic acid is introduced for gallbladder imaging
1975	Earliest computed tomographic images of liver and pancreas
1976	A new journal, Gastrointestinal Radiology, is published
1977	First in-vivo magnetic resonance human images
1978	Herlinger introduces a methylcellulose enteroclysis technique
1981	First magnetic resonance images of liver and pancreas
1992	Human immunodeficiency virus-related ulcers of esophagus are described

* Reproduced with permission from Anbari M, Laufer I: Development of gastrointestinal radiology. *In* RM Gore, MS Levine, I Laufer (eds): Textbook of Gastrointestinal Radiology. Philadelphia, WB Saunders Co, 1993.

These cumbersome and dangerous examinations were to be replaced by examinations with a liquid contrast medium. Ironically, one possible substance that would fulfill that role was already in existence and in common use: bismuth. In the latter part of the 19th century, bismuth was known as a medication for ulcer. It was usually given in very large doses. This made incidental observations on x-ray radiographs likely; indeed, such prominent early radiologists as Charles Lester Leonard and George E.

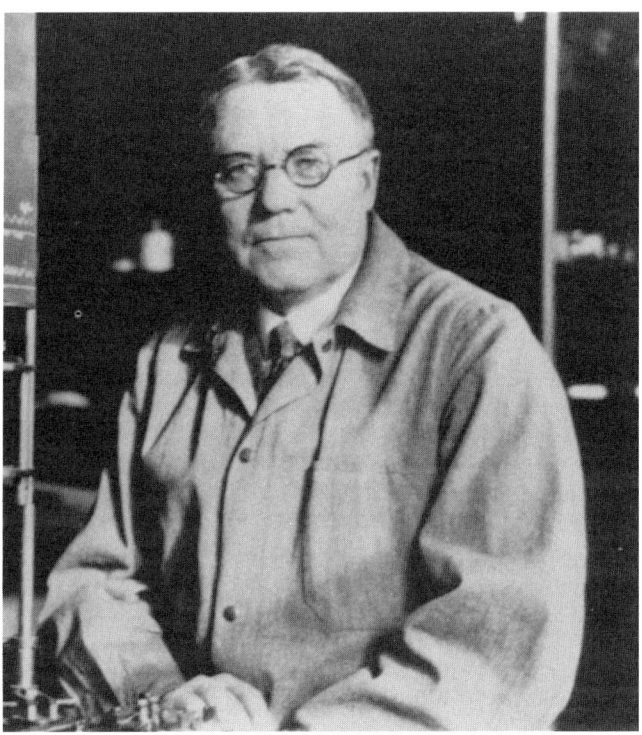

Fig. 31–1. Walter B. Cannon (1871–1945). Eisenberg R. L.: Radiology: An illustrated history. St. Louis, Mosby-Yearbook, 1992, p. 259, and Francis A. Countway Library of Medicine, Boston, MA.

Pfahler made such observations, but they did not appreciate the diagnostic potential of what they saw (9). It was Rumpel of Germany who published the first report describing the purposeful use of bismuth subnitrate in the imaging of the stomach (10). Two months later, the first American observations were made by Walter B. Cannon, then a Harvard medical student (Fig. 31–1).

The use of bismuth made it possible to make useful diagnostic observations, but there was a need for a standard procedure. Hermann Rieder of Germany filled that need by describing a specific method of using large amounts of bismuth, either with food or water or as a thick paste (11). His method became known to all as the "Rieder method" and his meal as the "Rieder meal." Standardization facilitated the widespread use of bismuth in Europe and then in America. Reports of bismuth toxicity followed and there was a need for a safer contrast agent. Again, as with bismuth, the answer was already in existence. Walter Cannon had used barium as early as 1896 in his studies, and had reported on its advantages in 1904 (12). The widespread use of barium awaited a standard-setting article,

which was provided in 1910 by Bachem and Gunther (13).

The Lower Gastrointestinal Tract

Although attempts to image the colon lagged a few years behind upper gastrointestinal imaging, they followed a similar path. Naturally existing air in the colon did not provide adequate contrast for most purposes, and an artificial contrast was needed. In 1901, Francis Henry Williams suggested in his book, *The Roentgen Rays in Medicine and Surgery,* two ways that this could be achieved (14). One was air that "may be pumped into the large bowel, and the outline of the sigmoid flexure and the descending colon may be easily followed." The other was bismuth. Williams mentioned the idea that the large intestine "may be injected with fluid containing an opaque substance like subnitrate of bismuth, and its outline and position studied." On the whole, however, he disapproved of the idea, fearing that the "heavy" opaque liquid might threaten the integrity of the bowel.

Such fears were not universal. Schule of Germany performed the first single contrast enema in 1904 (15). As a contrast medium, he used a mixture of bismuth and oil. In 1910, a standard-setting article was written by Georg Fedor Haenisch (16). He did not change the basic idea of giving a contrast medium in enema form, but he introduced improvements that brought the procedure closer to current standards. Unlike Schule, he used a horizontal table equipped with facilities for fluoroscopy so that he could follow the progress of the contrast in the bowel. He emphasized the prior cleansing of the colon with cathartics and enemas. He also pointed out the importance of a post-evacuation examination.

Direct versus Indirect Diagnosis

The introduction of contrast media and the popularization of radiographic imaging made it possible for physicians to see what they had previously been able to visualize only at surgery or autopsy. At that time, there were two methods of imaging, fluoroscopy and radiography. With fluoroscopy, one or more physicians would obtain a real-time view of the GI tract and observe its form and function (indirect method) (Fig. 31–2). With radiography, multiple images were made serially of the GI tract to be developed and studied later (direct method). There was a conflict among physicians revolving around the respective merits of these two techniques. For example, Russell D. Carman, author of a major early work on gastrointestinal radiology (17), preferred fluoroscopy and the use of "symptom-complexes" to reach diagnoses. In contrast, Lewis Gregory Cole (18), a leader in radiologic-pathologic correlation (which he called "retrospectoscopy") opted for the use of a vast number of plates. Interestingly, the descendants of these two schools can still be identified today. The "Mayo School" (19) places heavy emphasis on fluoroscopic observation while the "Double Contrast School" relies on high quality radiographs (20). The two schools may be reaching a common ground with the development of high resolution fluoroscopy and digital spot filming (21).

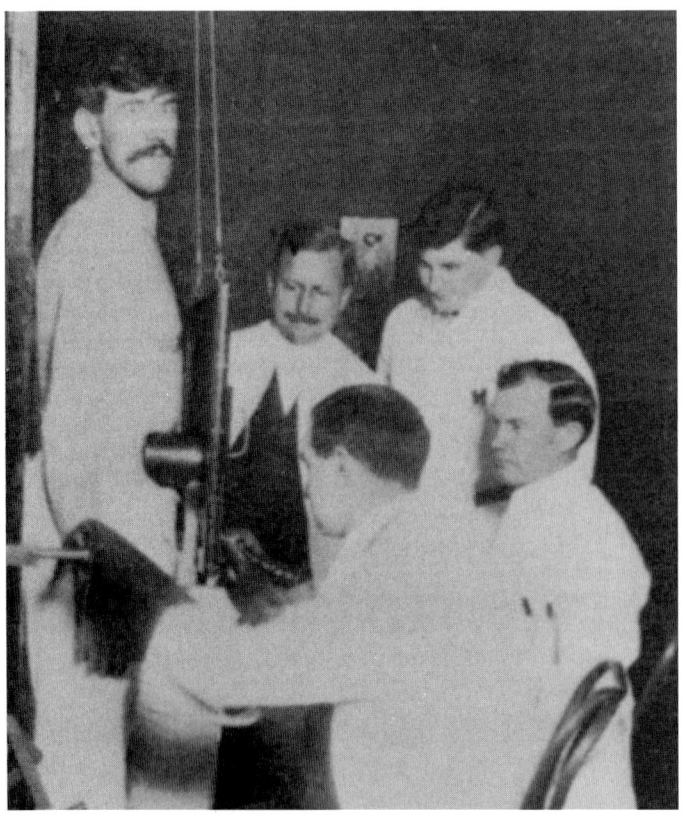

Fig. 31–2. Fluoroscopy as a group activity. A group of physicians performing direct fluoroscopy in 1915 (from Lippman, CW: Cylinder with Bucky effect. Am J Roentgenol *3*:452, 1915)

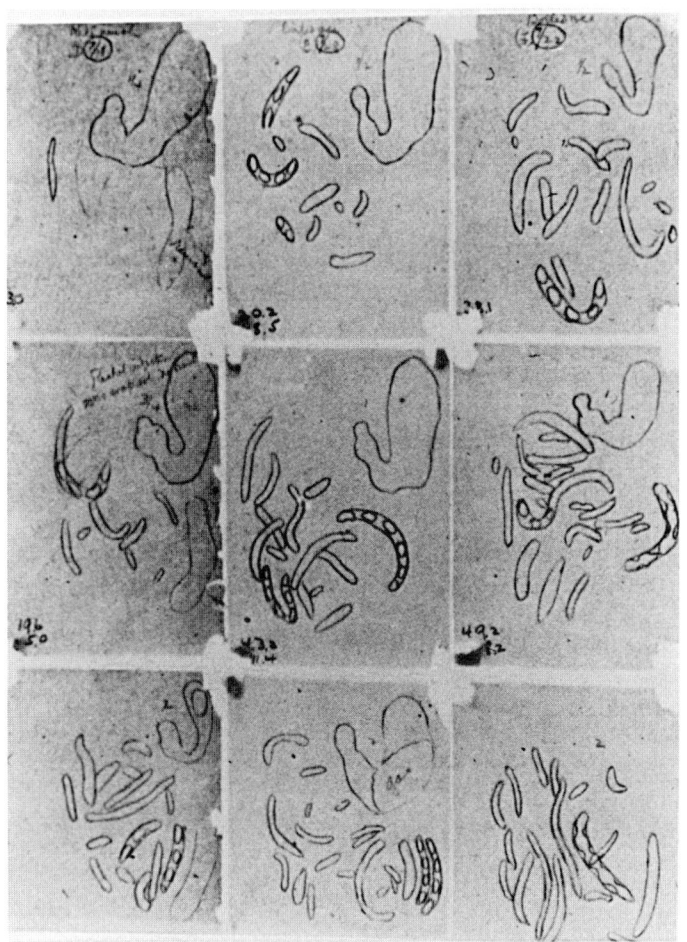

Fig. 31–3. Radiologic Observation by Walter B. Cannon. This is a photograph of Cannon's toilet paper tracings made during gastrointestinal motility studies. Reproduced with permission from Barger AC: New technology for a new century: Walter B. Cannon and the invisible rays. Am J Roentgenol *136*:187, 1981, and Francis A. Countway Library of Medicine, Boston, MA.)

Radiology and Physiology

The early use of radiology was directed not only at diagnosis of disease, but also at the elucidation of normal physiology (22). This is best exemplified by Walter B. Cannon, who was a pioneer in both radiology and physiology. Cannon first published reports on the movement of food in the esophagus by peristalsis. He then reported on gastric peristalsis and the function of the pylorus (Fig. 31–3) (23). He made one of his most important observations while studying gastric contractions in a cat. He noticed that, when the cat struggled to get loose, gastric peristalsis stopped and the pylorus relaxed. When the cat relaxed, the contractions gradually resumed. Cannon's observation led to his distinction between functional and mechanical disorders of the gastrointestinal tract and subsequently became the im-

petus for additional research of vital importance on the autonomic nervous system.

Another example of physiologic radiology is provided by A. E. Barclay of England, a radiologist who became interested in the physiology of swallowing. He combined radiology with pressure measurements to demonstrate the role of negative esophageal pressure in swallowing. He later worked with physiologists to demonstrate vascular shunts in the gastric mucosa (24). Examples like these are abundant and represent the precedent for the current frequent cooperation among radiologists, gastroenterologists, and surgeons in research.

Radiologic Pathology

Once useful imaging techniques were well known, the next step was the orderly description of the normal and pathologic appearance of the gastrointestinal tract. For example, in 1910, Martin Haudek described the "niche" of gastric ulcer, the barium-filled protrusion from the wall of the stomach (25). George and Gerber characterized the radiologic appearance of duodenal ulcer in 1914 (26). Eisler and Lenk in 1921 discussed gastric mucosal fold patterns and provided an early description of "single streaks which run diagonally, often almost transversely across the stomach and converge toward a point on the lesser curvature. In the region of this point they appear to be blunt-ended, broken off and pushed more closely together" (27). This is the earliest description of what we now know as the radiating folds of a benign gastric ulcer. Richard Rendich stressed the appearance of the gastric rugal folds in his attempt to distinguish between atrophic and hypertrophic gastritis (28). Russell Carman of the Mayo Clinic published extensive reports on the diagnosis of gastric carcinoma. In 1921, he described the meniscus sign that bears his name, which indicates an ulcerating gastric cancer (29). Ironically, Carman ended up diagnosing gastric cancer on his own radiographs in October 1925, and died of the disease 8 months later (1,9).

Much also was learned about colonic disease during that period. By the time Russell Carman and Albert Miller published the first and second editions of their comprehensive gastrointestinal radiology textbook in 1917 and 1920, topics such as carcinoma, tuberculosis, diverticulosis, megacolon, and polyps were included (17).

The Principle of the Negative Diagnosis

This is perhaps the single most important contribution of gastrointestinal radiology to gastroenterology. Physicians of that time knew that patients usually had the lesion, be it ulcer or cancer, that the radiologist predicted. But what if the radiologist saw nothing of note on fluoroscopy or on the radiographs? It was for Lewis Gregory Cole to show that this usually meant that indeed there was no lesion. He worked with a surgeon, George E. Brewer, to prove that point. Brewer operated on a small series of patients whose clinical symptoms suggested to him the existence of an operable lesion

and whose radiographs were negative. Not one of them had a cancer or an ulcer (9).

This was one of the earliest demonstrations of the specificity of the new diagnostic tool. The benefit was the avoidance of exploratory laparotomy, with its associated morbidity and mortality. This basic principle would continue to be paramount in radiology and would even increase in importance in later decades.

Double Contrast Studies

Even though single contrast studies achieved a high degree of accuracy and usefulness by the 1920s, there still was much room for improvement. The concept of double contrast slowly emerged. Interestingly, the original idea of distending the stomach with gas to facilitate diagnosis dates back to 1901. It was in that year that Francis Henry Williams alluded in his book to the idea of ingesting "Seidlitz powder" to produce gas in the stomach (14). Guido Holzknecht of Vienna used a combination of bismuth and gas in 1906 (9). In 1913, Charles Lester Leonard of the University of Pennsylvania had this insight: "if a method of coating the mucosa uniformly with an opaque salt can be combined with [gas distention of the stomach], the lesser lesions of the mucosa might be revealed" (30).

The first application of these concepts came from Germany in 1923. Double contrast was first used in the colon, when Fischer combined the contrast medium enema with insufflation of air (31). This technique soon made its way to the United States, and was improved upon by Weber and Kirklin at the Mayo Clinic during the 1930s (9). They concentrated their efforts on developing criteria for identifying malignancy in the colon. Much attention also was directed to the characterization and description of the radiologic appearance of colitis. In 1932, Crohn, Ginzburg, and Oppenheimer reported the radiologic appearance and clinical characteristics of an inflammatory process in the terminal ileum without a recognizable causative organism (32). This entity, then called terminal ileitis, eventually was found to occur throughout the gastrointestinal tract, and became known as regional enteritis or Crohn's disease.

The standardized application of double

contrast to the upper GI tract started with a report by Hampton in 1937 showing examples of duodenal ulcers and a prepyloric carcinoma (33). Hampton is, of course, famous for both his "line" in benign gastric ulcer and his "hump" indicating pulmonary embolism. For his GI studies, Hampton used swallowed air and a barium suspension. Other important contributions elaborated on this theme in the following years. For example, Wasch and Epstein showed the special value of double contrast radiography in demonstrating tumors of the cardia (34). In 1958, Schatzki and Gary demonstrated the importance of en-face views of the stomach for the diagnosis of ulcers (35).

The 1950s saw the beginning of developments in double contrast radiology that constitute the precursor of current day-to-day gastrointestinal radiology practice. Two giant figures of that time are Shirakabe of Japan and Welin of Sweden. Professor Hikoo Shirakabe led a group of Japanese gastroenterologists in efforts to develop an accurate double-contrast technique for the examination of the stomach (36). Their initial interest was the diagnosis of gastric ulcers, but they soon directed their attention to the early diagnosis of, and screening for, gastric cancer, which is particularly prevalent in Japan. Their techniques became standard and the result was a marked improvement in outcome for patients with early gastric cancer, for whom the 5-year survival rate was 90% or better (37). Initially, these results generated little interest in the West because of the much lower incidence of gastric cancer, but eventually, these techniques were adopted for a variety of diagnoses (38,39). Important modifications of the Japanese techniques were published in the late 1960s and early 1970s (40). New barium suspensions were developed and were specifically designed to produce high-quality radiographs of the stomach (41). Soon thereafter, double contrast examination techniques were used by Laufer (42,43) and Poplack (44,45) to diagnose entities more prevalent in the West, such as gastric erosions, linear ulcers, and ulcer scars—lesions that were rarely diagnosed with older techniques.

Concurrent with these developments were intensive efforts to demonstrate small polypoid lesions of the colon. Major progress in this area was accomplished by Welin in Malmo, Sweden, where over 70,000 double contrast examinations had been performed by 1967 (46). Welin's 1963 report on the rates and patterns of growth of colonic and rectal tumors followed by double contrast imaging (47) continues to be heavily cited in the literature (48). The Welin technique slowly achieved increasing popularity in the United States, largely through the efforts of Roscoe Miller, who made the examination more practicable through the development of new apparatus, barium suspensions, and accessories.

Small Bowel Imaging in the Modern Era

Early studies of the small bowel were follow-through studies that evolved logically from single-contrast studies of the stomach. Overlap of loops of bowel and the low resolution of early radiographic images limited the usefulness of follow-through studies. An assessment of gastrointestinal radiology published in 1956 stated that "roentgenologic examination of the small bowel is still a difficult procedure; the diagnostic yield is low and the accuracy is less than elsewhere in the gastrointestinal tract" (49). Dr. Richard Marshak sparked great interest in radiology of the small bowel and raised the standard of practice (50).

Small bowel imaging presented unique instrumentation and contrast medium problems. In 1911, Lewis Gregory Cole used a tube to obstruct the distal duodenum by balloon inflation, the purpose of which was to ensure complete filling of the duodenum with the bismuth-buttermilk mixture he was using (51). Cole suggested that a modification of the tube may permit direct introduction of the contrast material into the duodenum. Building on earlier efforts, Gilberto S. Pesquera in New York recommended in 1929 the use of a duodenal tube for continuous and controlled filling of the small intestine (52). The term barium enteroclysis was coined 10 years later by Gershon-Cohen and Shay of Philadelphia (53). The next major improvement in this procedure was the introduction of new types of tubes, including the use of a guide wire, to make intubations more manageable and easier (54–56).

The next hurdle was the choice of appropriate contrast solutions, and hydroxymethyl cellulose was found to be better than water because it did not mix readily with barium (57). The use of large volumes of barium combined with a 0.5% solution of methylcellulose in water was first introduced by Herlinger in 1978 (58). Since then, this method has been used for the characterization of various small bowel diseases, and its superiority to follow-through studies has been shown (59).

Current Status of Contrast Imaging

Although its origins go back to almost a century ago, contrast examination of the gastrointestinal tract retains its vitality and continues to provide descriptions of new entities and improve our understanding of pathologic processes. For example, the last decade has seen reports of drug-induced esophagitis (60) and carpet lesions of the colon and rectum (61). The gastrointestinal manifestations of AIDS presented new diagnostic challenges, and the response of gastrointestinal radiology has been swift. Descriptions of herpes esophagitis (62), candida esophagitis (63), CMV esophagitis (64), and esophagitis caused by the AIDS virus itself (65), as well as gastrointestinal Kaposi's sarcoma (66), quickly appeared.

Despite the continuing importance and value of contrast studies of the GI tract, their dominant role in GI diagnosis is diminishing, partly because radiologists' interest is being diverted to the evolving high-technology techniques such as CT and MRI; in addition, the aggressive use of gastrointestinal endoscopy is diminishing the number of radiographic studies. The combination of these factors poses a significant threat to the survival of contrast radiology. It remains to be seen whether the advantages of these studies, including their diagnostic value, safety, and reasonable cost, will be sufficient to ensure their survival.

CONTRAST EXAMINATIONS OF THE GALLBLADDER AND BILIARY TRACT

The early studies of the gallbladder were limited to plain films, and did no more than visualize opaque gallstones. Radiologists realized that only a minority of gallstones were radio-opaque, and that they needed a better way to visualize the gallbladder. The solution, of course, was contrast, but the difficult question was the nature of the contrast and the route of administration which would enable the contrast to reach the gallbladder.

The cholecystography pioneers were Evarts Graham and Warren H. Cole. They started with two important facts in mind. First, halogens are opaque to x-rays; second, phenolphthalein derivatives are excreted almost entirely through the gallbladder. They injected dogs with an iodine or bromine derivative of phenolphthalein. More than 200 futile attempts had been made before a gallbladder was finally visualized (67). The reason for this success turned out to be that the animal caretaker had forgotten to feed that particular dog that morning (9).

Human applications soon followed, but the increasing use of intravenous cholecystography, like the increasing use of bismuth subnitrate in the stomach, was hampered by occasional toxic reactions to the intravenous contrast agent. Rather than change the contrast (as with bismuth to barium), research focused on changing the route of administration, armed with new knowledge about enterohepatic circulation. In early 1925, two groups working independently reported successful oral cholecystography images (68,69). In 1951, Hoppe and Archer described iopanoic acid (Telepaque) (70), which was both a safer compound and one that produced increased gallbladder opacification. This became the standard for gallbladder examination until it was supplanted by ultrasound.

THE MODERN ERA

Gastrointestinal radiology has benefited from a number of new inventions and ideas since the 1940s. Examples include the universal radiographic-fluoroscopic table, automated film processing, improvements in x-ray generators, image intensification, and television display of fluoroscopic images. But the hallmark of the modern era of radiology is the introduction of new and powerful modalities of imaging: nuclear medicine, ultrasound, angiography, CT, and MRI. These were not developed for gastrointestinal use specifically; indeed, their beginnings do not rest with imaging or with medicine at all. Their application to gastrointestinal radiology led to the current possibilities for imaging the liver, spleen, and pancreas, replaced contrast imaging of the gallbladder almost entirely, and complemented the imaging of the gastrointestinal tube itself.

Ultrasound

Diagnostic ultrasound had its inception in areas far removed from medicine. The first use of ultrasound was for the purpose of detecting submarines in World War I. This was subsequently refined into the sound navigation and ranging system (SONAR). Next came the use of ultrasound to detect flaws in metals. The medical application occurred in the 1950s. Howry (70) in Denver and Wild (71) in Minneapolis were two important figures who led the way and published some of the earliest clinical applications of ultrasound. These applications borrowed heavily from their background in SONAR: the images could be obtained only when the subject was immersed in water. Obviously, it would not be possible to move sick patients into water tanks for imaging; thus a fundamental modification of the technique was needed. Ian Donald, in Glasgow, began his research on ultrasound by examining surgically removed gynecologic neoplasms; he applied the probe directly to the tumors. By 1957, he was able to report on the development of a two-dimensional contact scanner (72). This made the new technology practical and easy to use, and clinical applications proliferated.

Nuclear Medicine

This modality is built on the basic concepts of subatomic particles and radioactivity. These were discovered by physicists, and conjure up such names as Becquerel, Bohr, Rutherford, Hahn, Fermi, and Einstein (73). The first uses for radioactive traces were for basic science research in physiology and biochemistry. In 1923, Hevsey became the first to use radioactive isotopes in a biologic system, in this case, plants (74). He received the Nobel prize 20 years later for his work. Radioactive iodine was used in the 1930s and 1940s to study

thyroid metabolism (75). Around 1950, the first mapping of tracer distribution in vivo was accomplished independently by Cassen at UCLA and by Mayneord and Newberry in England (76). The orderly subsequent development of nuclear medicine benefited from the discovery or synthesis of many radioactive isotopes and constitutes a key example of the value of interdisciplinary cooperation and communication.

Angiography

The idea of opacifying vessels to obtain diagnostic information dates back to 1896, when a contrast mixture composed of lime, cinnabar, and petroleum was injected into the brachial artery of a cadaver (77). The search for contrast media safe for human injection centered on the halogens, which were known to be opaque to x-rays.

The first angiograms were obtained by direct injection of contrast into peripheral vessels through a needle placed by a surgical cutdown. Reaching such vessels as the aorta or portal vein proved problematic. Thus, angiographers relied on direct injection at laparotomy, used a translumbar approach, or waited for the peripherally injected contrast to reach the desired area in retrograde fashion (78,79).

After initial efforts by Farinas and by Peirce to use femoral artery catheterization to reach the aorta (80,81), Sven Ivar Seldinger of Sweden introduced his percutaneous catheter technique in 1953 (82). It involved the introduction of a catheter over a guide wire, and soon became internationally known. Seldinger's 1953 report describing the technique became the most frequently cited radiologic paper of all time (83). Recent advances in angiography have included the advent of digital substraction angiography and low-osmolality contrast media.

Computed Tomography

Excellent and detailed reviews of the development of CT (84,85) and MRI (84–86) have been published. The mathematical basis of computed tomography was in fact developed as early as 1917 by Radon, an Austrian mathematician, who was working with equations that described gravitational forces (84). The principles he established were used in the 1950s and 1960s to solve such imaging problems as solar astronomy and electron microscopy. In 1955, Allen MacLeod Cormack, a South African physicist, started working part-time in the radiation therapy department of a Capetown hospital. He noted the problem of tissue inhomogeneity, which created difficulty in radiation therapy planning. His 1963 paper (87) developing a mathematical approach to this problem generated virtually no response, and his ideas were not acknowledged until several years later. Unaware of Cormack's work, Godfrey Hounsfield, an engineer with Electronic Musical Instruments (EMI) in Britain, suggested in 1968 that an image might be constructed by computer from multiple x-ray images taken from multiple angles. He presented his early clinical results in April 1972 to the annual congress of the British Institute of Radiology. Hounsfield's report (88) in the British Journal of Radiology in 1973 describing the CT system became the second most frequently cited radiology paper of all time (48). The news soon reached the United States, and preliminary reports of clinical applications followed. Hounsfield and Cormack shared a Nobel Prize in 1979.

Magnetic Resonance Imaging

The development of MRI trailed that of CT by a few years. In 1945, Felix Bloch and Edward Purcell independently measured the magnetic moment of the proton to an accuracy of 1 per million. They received the Nobel prize in Physics in 1952 for their discovery, which led to the development of nuclear magnetic resonance spectroscopy (84–86). Early use centered on chemical and biochemical applications, but NMR research on biologic systems soon followed. Two investigators, Thomas Shaw and Erik Odeblad, led the way, with the latter producing articles on the NMR properties of a variety of human tissues, fluids, and secretions. In 1971, Raymond Damadian reported that NMR could distinguish malignant tumors from normal tissue (89). Then, in 1973, Paul Lauterbur published a seminal paper in Nature on the NMR spectra of different rat tissues (90). The first human in vivo image was published in 1977 (91).

GALLBLADDER IMAGING IN THE MODERN ERA

The expanding technology whose development was summarized earlier was applied to gallbladder imaging starting in the 1960s.

Isotopes and Ultrasound

The "major breakthrough" in radionuclide imaging of the gallbladder was the successful labeling of a molecule of iminodiacetic acid (IDA) with radioactive technetium. In 1975, Harvey and coworkers showed that technetium-labeled dimethyliminodiacetic acid (99m Tc-HIDA) could be used to visualize the liver, bile ducts, and gallbladder with serial gamma camera images (92). Subsequently, several other IDA molecules were produced to provide better visualization, including such compounds as technetium-labeled DISIDA, permitting visualization even in the presence of significant jaundice (93). Persistent nonvisualization of the gallbladder in a fasting individual with normal hepatic uptake and excretion is considered reliable evidence of acute cholecystitis.

Like nuclear medicine techniques, ultrasound had been developing gradually for some time, before it was finally applied to gallbladder imaging. Application of A-mode ultrasound to the abdomen was first reported in the mid-1960s. A landmark article in 1963 by Joseph Holmes and Douglass Howry, both ultrasound pioneers, reported on their experience with B-mode scanning of intraabdominal structures (94). Progress was quickly made, and gallbladder-specific applications were described in the early 1970s (95–97). Ultrasound now has virtually replaced oral cholecystography.

Interventional Radiology

The major advances of recent years related to the gallbladder are various interventional techniques, both diagnostic and therapeutic. These advances have in fact been in the making for decades. In 1921, Burckhardt and Mueller inserted a needle into the gallbladder cavity by direct transhepatic puncture. Their purpose was to inject contrast to visualize gallstones, but even at that time, the authors wondered whether it would one day be possible "by injection of a narcotic agent into the gallbladder to abort temporarily an acute attack of gallstone colic . . . to influence cholecystitis by direct injections into the gallbladder . . . by the injection of certain fluids into the gallbladder to dissolve gallstones or to reduce their size'' (98).

A few years later, the first postoperative cholangiogram was performed in 1925 by Cotte of Lyon, France, and the first intraoperative cholangiogram was performed by Mirrizzi and Losada of Argentina (9). Nonsurgical percutaneous transhepatic cholangiography (PTC) originated in Indochina in 1937 (99). The first American report of this procedure, as well as a percutaneous method for drainage of an obstructed biliary tract, appeared in 1952 (100). PTC did not become standard procedure, however, because of two common side effects, internal bleeding and bile peritonitis. The 1974 introduction of a flexible, skinny needle for use in transhepatic puncture changed that dramatically (101).

A central insight in the area of interventional radiology of the gallbladder was that the techniques used to *diagnose* an entity, such as a retained gallstone following surgery, might be useful, when properly modified, to *treat* that entity. The first step, percutaneous drainage of the obstructed biliary tree, was followed by percutaneous stone extraction. Important early contributions were made by Mondet in Argentina and Mazzariello and Mahorner in the United States. Although started by surgeons, the technique was streamlined into a standard procedure by Burhenne, who applied it not only for stone extraction but also for dilation of benign biliary strictures (102).

LIVER, SPLEEN, AND PANCREAS IMAGING IN THE MODERN ERA

Early attempts at visualizing the liver, spleen, and pancreas were, on the whole, unsatisfactory. In 1929, it was accidentally discovered that the spleen could be opacified with thorium, and that tumors, cysts, and abscesses could be demonstrated (9). In 1947, however, this came to an end when the first report of a human neoplasm attributable to thorium was published (103). Thus, useful imaging of these organs be-

came possible and widespread only after the application of modalities that developed independently, such as ultrasound, angiography, CT, and MRI, and these have become the mainstay of solid organ imaging.

Liver and Spleen

Before the advent of ultrasound and CT, three angiographic techniques played an important part in the study of the liver and spleen. In the mid-1940s, direct injection of the portal vein at laparotomy was introduced, but the diagnostic value of the images obtained was limited. Splenoportography was introduced in the 1950s. It involved the injection of contrast material directly into the spleen, with filling of the splenic and portal veins (104). As might be expected, the procedure was fraught with complications. The third technique was arterial portography, which was based on the observation that the portal system could be visualized after aortography. The images obtained in this manner became useful only after the introduction of selective catheterization of the celiac, superior mesenteric, and splenic arteries (105,106).

The application of CT imaging to the abdomen initially presented a technical problem. Bodily movements made thoracic and abdominal imaging difficult because scanning time was then measured in minutes. The industry responded promptly to medical needs with rapid technical advances to decrease the scanning time and greatly improve resolution. Applications to abdominal imaging quickly proliferated (107–110). The application of MRI to liver imaging was also dependent on technologic progress in improving resolution and decreasing imaging time. Clinical reports on the use of MRI in diagnosis started appearing frequently in the 1980s, and abdominal applications are gradually becoming standardized and widely used (111).

Pancreas

For the first 70 years of radiologic history, the pancreas was an invisible organ whose skeleton was only rarely outlined by pathologic calcification. Diseases of the pancreas could be diagnosed radiologically only by secondary abnormalities in the bile ducts or in the hollow organs such as the stomach, duodenum, or colon surrounding the pancreas (112).

Radiology of the pancreas came of age only in the past two decades or so, when invasive and cross-sectional techniques such as ultrasound, CT, and MRI were applied. Ultrasound was the first cross-sectional technique used to image the pancreas (113). Improvement in resolution and image quality made it possible to visualize the pancreatic ducts. Early reports on pancreatic CT were published in the mid 1970s (114,115).

Pancreatic imaging benefited greatly from the introduction of the skinny needle for PTC. This needle eventually was used for aspiration biopsy and direct opacification of the pancreatic duct under sonographic guidance (116). Superselective vessel catheterization and angiography resulted in significant improvement in the diagnosis of pancreatic neoplasms (117). Currently, a combination of these techniques permits the precise diagnosis of pancreatitis and of a variety of pancreatic neoplasms.

RECENT CHALLENGES

Gastrointestinal radiology has been facing a dual challenge in recent years. First, the advent and rapid progress of endoscopy made it necessary for radiologists to prove that contrast gastrointestinal radiology affords excellent accuracy, sensitivity, specificity, and cost-effectiveness.

The second challenge is to technology in general, and touches not only gastrointestinal radiology but also all subspecialties of medicine. Sometimes the challenge is philosophic, portraying our reliance on the new technologies as an undue obsession (118). More frequently, the challenge is based on health care costs. CT and MRI in particular have come to symbolize to government regulators and to the lay public the supposed "inappropriate" and "unnecessary" use of expensive technology. No other medical technology or procedure, except perhaps electronic fetal monitoring, has been mentioned so frequently by health experts when discussing increased health care costs. The proper response has been our cost-effectiveness studies which demonstrated the invaluable role of CT in diagnosis, in avoiding

unnecessary surgery, guiding therapy, and predicting prognosis (85). MRI is now in a position occupied by CT a decade or so ago, and efficacy and cost-effectiveness studies are ongoing and promising.

CONCLUSION

The history of gastrointestinal radiology has repeating themes. A fundamental idea is introduced as a solution to a problem. The idea is developed and is given concrete and practical applications. These applications are then tested and retested, and then, if successful, standardized. Recently, scientifically standardized applications have had to prove themselves in terms of cost-effectiveness and efficacy. As gastrointestinal radiology enters its second century, new applications such as endoscopic ultrasound and endoluminal MRI will be increasingly useful. New modalities such as PET and others still unimaginable will probably find gastrointestinal applications. Also in the next few years, gastrointestinal radiology, like other subspecialties of radiology, will adopt some form of computer storage and digital imaging systems that will significantly alter the day-to-day practice of the specialty.

REFERENCES

1. Brecher R, Brecher E: The Rays: A History of Radiology in The United States and Canada. Baltimore, Williams & Wilkins, 1969.
2. Goodman P, History. *In* Margulis AR, Burhenne HJ (eds): Alimentary Tract Roentgenology. 4th ed. St. Louis, CV Mosby, 1989.
3. Kirsner JB: The Development of American Gastroenterology. New York, Raven Press, 1990.
4. Bordley J, Harvey AM: Two Centuries of American Medicine, 1776–1976. Philadelphia, WB Saunders, 1976.
5. Morton WJ, Hammer EW: The X-ray. New York, American Technical Book, 1896.
6. White JW: A foreign body in the esophagus detected and located by Rontgen rays. Univ Med Magazine 8:710, 1896.
7. Wegele C: A proposal for the use of Roentgen procedures in medicine. Dtsch Med Wschr *22*:287, 1896.

8. Lindemann E: Demonstration of Roentgen pictures of the normal and distended stomach. Dtsch Med Wschr *23*:266, 1897. *In* Bruwer A: Classic Descriptions in Diagnostic Roentgenology. Springfield, IL, Charles C Thomas, 1964.

9. Eisenberg RL: Radiology: An Illustrated History. St. Louis, Mosby/Yearbook, 1992.

10. Rumpel T: Visualization of esophagus of patient with dysphagia with bismuth. Munchen Med Wschr *44*:420, 1897.

11. Rieder H: Radiologic examination of the stomach and intestines in the living man. Munchen Med Wschr *51*:1548, 1904.

12. Cannon WB: The passage of different foodstuffs from the stomach and through the small intestine. Am J Physiol *12*:387, 1904.

13. Bachem C, Gunther H: Barium sulfate as a shadow-forming contrast agent in roentgenologic examinations. Zeitschr fur Rontgenkunde *12*:369, 1910.

14. Williams FH: The Roentgen Rays in Medicine and Surgery. New York, Macmillan, 1901.

15. Schule A: Intubation and radiography of the large intestine. Arch Verdaungskr *10*: 111, 1904.

16. Haenisch GF: Roentgenologic examination in narrowing of the large intestine: The early roentgenologic diagnosis of carcinoma of the large intestine. Munchen Med Wschr *45*:2331, 1911.

17. Carman RD, Miller A: The Roentgen Diagnosis of Diseases of the Alimentary Tract. 1st Ed. Philadelphia, WB Saunders Co., 1917.

18. Cole LG: A preliminary report on the diagnostic and therapeutic application of the Coolidge tube. AJR *1*:125, 1914.

19. Teefey SA: Carlson HC: The fluoroscopic barium enema in colonic polyp detection. AJR *141*:1269, 1983.

20. Laufer I, Levine MS: Double Contrast Gastrointestinal Radiology. 2nd Ed. Philadelphia, WB Saunders Co, 1992.

21. Feczko PJ, Ackerman LV, Kastan DJ, Halpert RD: Digital radiography of the gastrointestinal tract. Gastrointest Radiol *13*: 191, 1988.

22. Brooks FP: The radiologic exploration of the gastrointestinal tract: An interdisciplinary enterprise. Radiographics *6*:160, 1986.

23. Cannon WB: The movements of the stomach studied by means of the Roentgen rays. Am J Physiol *1*:359, 1898.

24. Barclay AE: The practical importance of mechanics in digestion. AJR *40*:325, 1938.

25. Rigler LG, Weiner M: History of radiology of the gastrointestinal tube. *In* Margulis AR, Burhenne HJ (eds): Alimentary Tract Roentgenology. 3rd Ed. St. Louis, CV Mosby, 1983.

26. George AW, Gerber I: The direct method of diagnosis of duodenal ulcer by means of the Roentgen ray. AJR *1*:277, 1914.

27. Eisler F, Lenk R: The importance of the pattern of stomach folds in the diagnosis of gastric ulcer. Deutsch Med Wschr *1*:1459, 1921.

28. Rendich RA: The roentgenographic study of the mucosa in normal and pathological states. AJR *10*:526, 1923.

30. Leonard CL: The radiography of the stomach and intestines. AJR *1*:1, 1913.

31. Fischer AW: A new roentgenologic method for examination of the large intestine: A combination of the contrast material enema and insufflation of air. Klin Wschr *2*:1595, 1923.

32. Crohn B, Ginzburg L, Oppenheimer GD: Regional ileitis. JAMA *99*:1323, 1932.

33. Hampton AO: A safe method for the Roentgen demonstration of bleeding duodenal ulcers. AJR *38*:565, 1937.

34. Wasch MG, Epstein BS: The Roentgen visualization of tumors of cardia. AJR *51*:564, 1944.

35. Schatzki R, Gary JE: Face-on demonstration of ulcers in the upper stomach in a dependent position. AJR *79*:722, 1958.

36. Shirakabe H: Double Contrast Studies of the Stomach. Stuttgart, Georg-Thieme Verlag, 1972.

37. Yamada E et al.: Surgical results of early gastric cancer. Int Surg *59*:7, 1974.

38. Obata WG: A double contrast technique for examination of the stomach using barium sulfate with simethicone. AJR *115*:275, 1972.

39. Gelfand DW: The Japanese-style double contrast examination of the stomach. Gastrointest Radiol *1*:7, 1976.

40. Scott-Harden WG: Radiological investigation of peptic ulcer. Br J Hosp Med *10*:149, 1973.

41. Gelfand DW: High-density, low-viscosity barium for fine mucosal detail on double-contrast upper gastrointestinal examinations. AJR *130*:831, 1978.

42. Laufer I, Hamilton J, Mullens JE: Demonstration of superficial gastric erosions by double contrast radiology. Gastroenterology *68*:387, 1975.

43. Laufer I: Assessment of the accuracy of double contrast gastroduodenal radiology. Gastroenterology *71*:874, 1976.

44. Poplack W et al.: Demonstration of erosive gastritis by the double contrast technique. Radiology *117*:519, 1975.

45. Poplack W et al.: Linear and rod-shaped peptic ulcers. Radiology *122*:317, 1977.

46. Welin S: Results of the Malmo technique of colon examination. JAMA *199*:369, 1967.

47. Welin S et al.: The rates and patterns of growth of 375 tumors of the large intestine and rectum observed serially by double contrast enema study (Malmo technique). AJR *90*:673, 1963.

48. Chew FS: The 50 most frequently cited papers in the past fifty years. AJR *150*:227, 1988.

49. Stevenson CA: The development of gastrointestinal roentgenology. AJR *75*:230, 1956.

50. Marshak RH: Radiology of the Small Intestine. Philadelphia, WB Saunders Co., 1976.

51. Cole LG: Artificial dilatation of the duodenum for radiographic examination. Am Quart Roentgenol *3*:204, 1911.

52. Pesquera GS: A method for the direct visualization of lesions in the small intestine. AJR *22*:254, 1929.

53. Gershon-Cohen J, Shay H: Barium enteroclysis. AJR *42*:456, 1939.

54. Scott-Harden WG: Examination of the small bowel. *In* McLaren JW (ed): Modern Trends in Diagnostic Radiology. 3rd Series. London, Butterworth, 1960.

55. Bilbao MK et al.: Hypotonic duodenography. Radiology *89*:438, 1967.

56. Gianturco C: Rapid fluoroscopic duodenal intubation. Radiology *88*:1165, 1967.

57. Trickey SE, Halls J, Hobson CJ: A further development of the small bowel enema. Proc Roy Soc Med *56*:1070, 1963.

58. Herlinger H: A modified technique for the double contrast small bowel enema. Gastrointest Radiol *3*:201, 1978.

59. Herlinger H, Maglinte DT: Clinical Radiology of the Small Intestine. Philadelphia, WB Saunders, 1989.

60. Creteur V et al.: Drug-induced esophagitis detected by double-contrast radiography. Radiology *147*:365, 1983.

61. Rubesin SE et al.: Carpet lesions of the colon. Radiographics *5*:537, 1985.

62. Levine MS et al.: Herpes esophagitis: Sensitivity of double contrast esophagography. AJR *151*:57, 1988.

63. Levine MS, Macones AJ, Laufer I: *Candida* esophagitis: Accuracy of radiologic diagnosis. Radiology *154*:581, 1985.

64. Balthazar EJ, et al.: Cytomegalovirus esophagitis in AIDS: Radiographic features in 16 patients. AJR *149*:919, 1987.

65. Levine MS et al.: Giant HIV-related ulcers in the esophagus. Radiology *180*:323, 1991.

66. Wall SD, Friedman SL, Margulis AR: Gastrointestinal Kaposi's sarcoma in AIDS: Radiographic manifestations. J Clin Gastroenterol *6*:165, 1984.

67. Graham EA, Cole WH: Roentgenologic examination of the gallbladder: New method utilizing intravenous injection of tetrabromphenolphthalein. JAMA *82*:613, 1924.

68. Whitaker LR, Milliken G, Vogt EC: The oral administration of sodium tetraiodophenolphthalein for cholecystography. Surg Gynecol Obstet *40*:847, 1925.

69. Menees TO, Robinson HC: Oral administration of tetraiodophenolphthalein: Preliminary report. AJR *13*:368, 1925.

70. Hoppe JO, Archer S: Triiodoalkanoic acid derivatives as cholecystographic media. Fed Proc *10*:975, 1951.

71. Wild JJ: The use of ultrasonic pulses for the measurement of biologic tissue and the detection of tissue density changes. Surgery *27*:183, 1950.

72. Donald I, MacVicar J, Brown TG: Investigation of abdominal masses by pulsed ultrasound. Lancet *i*:1188, 1958.

73. Grigg ERN: The beginnings of nuclear medicine. *In* Gottschalk A, Hoffer PB, Potchen EJ: Diagnostic Nuclear Medicine. Baltimore, Williams & Wilkins, 1988.

74. Hevsey G: The absorption and translocation of lead by plants, a contribution to the application of the method of radioactive indicators in the investigation of changes of substance in plants. Biochem J *17*:439, 1923.

75. Lindeman JF, Quinn JL: The history of nuclear medicine instrumentation and clinical procedures. *In* Gottschalk A, Hoffer PB, Potchen EJ, (eds): Diagnostic Nuclear Medicine. Baltimore, Williams & Wilkins, 1988.

76. Mayneord WV, Newberry SP: An automatic method of studying the distribution of activity in a source of ionizing radiation. Nature *168*:762, 1951.

77. Haschek E, Lindenthal OT: A contribution to the practical use of photography according to Roentgen. Wien Klin Wschr *9*:63, 1896.

78. Whipple AO: The problem of portal hypertension in relation to the hepatosplenopathies. Ann Surg *122*:449, 1945.

79. Castellanos A, Pereiras R: Countercurrent aortography. Rev Cuba Cardiol *2*:187, 1939.

80. Farinas PL: A new technique for the arteriographic examination of the abdominal aorta and its branches. AJR *46*:641, 1941.

81. Peirce EC: Percutaneous femoral artery catheterization in man with special reference to aortography. Surg Gyncol Obstet *93*:56, 1951.

82. Seldinger SI: Catheter replacement of the needle in percutaneous arteriography: A new technique. Acta Radiol *39*:368, 1953.

83. Siegelman SS: The cat's meow: The most frequently cited papers in Radiology 1955–1986. Radiology *168*:414, 1988.

84. Hendee WR: Cross sectional medical imaging: A history. Radiographics 9:1155, 1989.

85. Evens RG: The history, economics and politics of CT and MRI. *In* Lee JKT, Sagel SS, Stanley RJ (eds): Computed Body Tomography with MRI Correlation. 2nd Ed. New York, Raven Press, 1989.

86. Mourino MR: From Thales to Lauterbur, or from the lodestone to MR imaging: Magnetism and medicine. Radiology *180*:593, 1991.

87. Cormack AM: Representation of a function by its line integrals, with some radiological application. J Appl Physiol *35*:2722, 1964.

88. Hounsfield GN: Computerized transverse axial scanning (tomography). I. Description of system. Br J Radiol 46:1016, 1973.

89. Damadian R: Tumor detection by nuclear magnetic resonance. Science *171*:1151, 1971.

90. Lauterbur PC: Image formation by induced local interactions: Examples employing nuclear magnetic resonance. Nature *242*:190, 1973.

91. Damadian R, Goldsmith M, Minkoff L: NMR in cancer, FONAR image of the live human body. Physiol Chem Phys 9:97, 1977.

92. Harvey J, Loberg M, Cooper M: 99m Tc-HIDA: A new radiopharmaceutical for hepatobiliary imaging. J Nucl Med *16*:533, 1975.

93. Feld R, Kurtz AB, Zeman RK: Imaging the gallbladder: A historical perspective. AJR *156*:737, 1991.

94. Holmes JH, Howry DH: Ultrasonic diagnosis of abdominal disease. Am J Digest Dis 8:12, 1963.

95. Doust BD, Malakad NF: Ultrasonic B-mode examination of the gallbladder. Radiology *110*:643, 1974.

96. Hublitz VF, Kahn PC, Sell LA: Cholecystosonography: An approach to the non-visualized bladder. Radiology *103*:645, 1972.

97. Leopold GR, Sokoloff J: Ultrasonic scanning in the diagnosis of biliary tract diseases. Surg Clin North Am *53*:1043, 1973.

98. Burckhardt H, Mueller W: Experiments on puncture of the gallbladder and its visualization with roentgen rays. Deutsch Ztschr Chirurgie *162*:168, 1921.

99. Huard P, Do-Xuan-Hop: Transhepatic puncture of the bile ducts. Bull Soc Med-Chir Indochine *15*:1090, 1937.

100. Carter R, Saypol GM: Transabdominal cholangiography. JAMA *148*:253, 1952.

101. Okuda K et al.: Non-surgical percutaneous transhepatic cholangiography: Diagnostic significance in medical problems of the liver. Am J Digest Dis *19*:21, 1974.

102. Burhenne HJ: The history of interventional radiology of the biliary tract. Radiol Clin North Am *28*:1139, 1990.

103. MacMahon HE, Murphy AS, Bates MI: Endothelial cell sarcoma of the liver following thorotrast injections. Am J Pathol *23*: 585, 1947.

104. Abeatici S, Campi L: On the possibilities of hepatic angiography-visualization of the portal system (experimental studies). Acta Radiol *36*:383, 1951.

105. Boijsen E, Eckman CA, Olin T: Coeliac and superior mesenteric angiography in portal hypertension. Acta Chir Scand *126*: 315, 1963.

106. Pollard JJ, Nebesar RA: Catheterization of the splenic artery for portal venography. N Engl J Med *271*:234, 1964.

107. Levitt RG, Sagel SS, Stanley RJ, Jost RG: Accuracy of computed tomography of the liver and biliary tract. Radiology *124*:123, 1977.

108. Haaga JR et al.: CT detection and aspiration of abdominal abscesses. AJR *128*:465, 1977.

109. Stephens DH, Sheedy PF, Hattery RR, MacCarty RL: Computed tomography of the liver. AJR *128*:579, 1977.

110. Alfidi RJ et al.: Computed tomography of the thorax and abdomen. Radiology *117*: 257, 1975.

111. Lee JKT, Sagel SS, Stanley RJ (eds): Computed Body Tomography with MRI Correlation. 2nd Ed. New York, Raven Press, 1989.

112. Ferruci JT et al.: The radiographic features of the normal hypotonic duodenogram. Radiology *96*:401, 1970.

113. Freeny PC: Radiology of the pancreas: Two decades of progress in imaging and intervention. AJR *150*:975, 1988.

114. Haaga JR et al.: Computed tomography of the pancreas. Radiology *120*:589, 1976.

115. Stanley RJ, Sagel SS, Levitt RG: Computed tomographic evaluation of the pancreas. Radiology *124*:715, 1977.

116. Ohto M et al.: Ultrasonically guided percutaneous contrast medium injection and aspiration biopsy: A real time puncture transducer. Radiology *136*:171, 1980.

117. Rosch J, Holman DC: Superselective arteriography of the pancreas. *In* Anacker H (ed): Efficiency and Limits of Radiologic Examination of the Pancreas. Acton, MA, Publishing Sciences, 1975, pp. 159–167.

118. Ell SR: Radiology and history. Invest Radiol *23*:956, 1988.

Index

Note: Page numbers in *italics* indicate figures; page numbers followed by t indicate tables.